FUNDAMENTAL AND CLINICAL CARDIOLOGY

Editor-in-Chief

Samuel Z. Goldhaber, M.D.

*Harvard Medical School
and Brigham and Women's Hospital
Boston, Massachusetts*

Associate Editor, Europe

Henri Bounameaux, M.D.

*University Hospital of Geneva
Geneva, Switzerland*

1. *Drug Treatment of Hyperlipidemia*, edited by Basil M. Rifkind
2. *Cardiotonic Drugs: A Clinical Review. Second Edition, Revised and Expanded*, edited by Carl V. Leier
3. *Complications of Coronary Angioplasty*, edited by Alexander J. R. Black, H. Vernon Anderson, and Stephen G. Ellis
4. *Unstable Angina*, edited by John D. Rutherford
5. *Beta-Blockers and Cardiac Arrhythmias*, edited by Prakash C. Deedwania
6. *Exercise and the Heart in Health and Disease*, edited by Roy J. Shephard and Henry S. Miller, Jr.
7. *Cardiopulmonary Physiology in Critical Care*, edited by Steven M. Scharf
8. *Atherosclerotic Cardiovascular Disease, Hemostasis, and Endothelial Function*, edited by Robert Boyer Francis, Jr.
9. *Coronary Heart Disease Prevention*, edited by Frank G. Yanowitz
10. *Thrombolysis and Adjunctive Therapy for Acute Myocardial Infarction*, edited by Eric R. Bates
11. *Stunned Myocardium: Properties, Mechanisms, and Clinical Manifestations*, edited by Robert A. Kloner and Karin Przyklenk

Additional Volumes in Preparation

Prevention of Venous Thromboembolism, edited by Samuel Z. Goldhaber

Heart Failure: Basic Science and Clinical Aspects, edited by Judith K. Gwathmey, Gordon M. Briggs, and Paul Allen

Thrombolysis and Adjunctive Therapy for Acute Myocardial Infarction

Thrombolysis and Adjunctive Therapy for Acute Myocardial Infarction

Edited by

Eric R. Bates
University of Michigan Medical Center
Ann Arbor, Michigan

Marcel Dekker, Inc.   New York • Basel • Hong Kong

Library of Congress Cataloging-in-Publication Data

Thrombolysis and adjunctive therapy for acute myocardial infarction /
    edited by Eric R. Bates.
        p.   cm. -- (Functional and clinical cardiology ; v. 10)
    Includes bibliographical references and index.
    ISBN 0-8247-8664-5
        1. Myocardial infarction--Chemotherapy.   2. Myocardial infarction-
-Adjuvant treatment.   3. Thrombolytic therapy.   I. Bates, Eric R.
II. Series.
        [DNLM: 1. Myocardial Infarction--drug therapy.   2. Thrombolytic
Therapy.   W1 FU538TD v. 10 / WG 300 T495]
    RC685.I6T486   1992
    616.1'237061--dc20
    DNLM/DLC
    for Library of Congress   92-49831
                                                                                CIP

This book is printed on acid-free paper.

Marcel Dekker, Inc.
270 Madison Avenue, New York, New York 10016

Current printing (last digit):
10 9 8 7 6 5 4 3 2 1

PRINTED IN THE UNITED STATES OF AMERICA

Series Introduction

Marcel Dekker, Inc., has focused on the development of various series of beautifully produced books in different branches of medicine. These series have facilitated the integration of rapidly advancing information for both the clinical specialist and the researcher.

My goal as editor of the Fundamental and Clinical Cardiology series is to assemble the talents of world-renowned authorities to discuss virtually every area of cardiovascular medicine. In the current monograph, *Thrombolysis and Adjunctive Therapy for Acute Myocardial Infarction*, Dr. Bates has edited a much needed and timely book. Future contributions to this series will include books on molecular biology, interventional cardiology, and clinical management of such problems as coronary artery disease and ventricular arrhythmias.

Samuel Z. Goldhaber

Preface

Thrombolytic and aspirin therapy for patients with acute myocardial infarction has produced the first major reduction in hospital mortality since electrical defibrillation and coronary care unit monitoring became part of clinical practice three decades ago. Whereas aspirin is simple to administer, inexpensive, and almost free of complications, thrombolytic therapy has been surrounded by debate and controversy. Additionally, in this era of randomized clinical trials in acute myocardial infarction, several other traditional treatment options are rigorously being tested. Furthermore, new pharmacological and mechanical interventions hold promise for reducing hospital mortality rates below the current 8-10%. Therefore, the purpose of this book is to update the clinician on the most recent data regarding the multiple present and future treatment possibilities for patients with acute myocardial infarction.

The salutary results in patients treated with thrombolytic therapy have, in the last few years, sparked intense investigative effort to again be directed toward acute myocardial infarction. The first four chapters of this book summarize the effects of thrombolytic therapy on the major endpoints of treatment, which include infarct artery patency, left ventricular function, mortality, and complications. Nitrates, beta-adrenergic blockers, and calcium channel blockers have been the mainstays of treatment for angina pectoris; results in acute myocardial infarction are summarized in Chapters 5 through 7. The recognition that infarct artery reocclusion can be as devastating as the initial acute coronary thrombosis has focused attention on antiplatelet and anticoagulant therapy. Aspirin, new antiplatelet agents, heparin, new antithrombin agents, warfarin, and combination thrombolytic therapy are the topics of Chapters 8 through 13. Angiotensin-converting enzyme inhibitors have proven beneficial in patients with congestive heart failure, and their potential use in acute myocardial infarction is summarized in Chapter 14. Preliminary investigations with free radical scavengers are detailed in Chapter 15. Chapters 16 and 17 summarize the treatment options for left ventricular dysfunction and electrical complications, respectively. Mechanical interventions are useful adjuncts in tertiary care centers and their potential roles in acute myocardial infarction are reviewed in Chapters 18 through 20. Finally, the economic ramifications of treating acute myocardial infarction are described in Chapter 21, and a summary of proven interventions is provided in Chapter 22.

It is our hope that this book will help integrate the life-saving lessons learned from clinical trials into standard clinical practice. The effort put forth by the many contributors and the editorial staff of Marcel Dekker, Inc., is gratefully acknowledged.

Eric R. Bates

Contents

Contributors

Eric R. Bates, M.D. Associate Professor, Division of Cardiology, Department of Internal Medicine, University of Michigan Medical Center, Ann Arbor, Michigan

Robert M. Califf, M.D. Associate Professor, Division of Cardiology, Department of Medicine, Duke University Medical Center, Durham, North Carolina

Stephen G. Ellis, M.D. Director, Cardiac Catheterization Laboratory, Department of Cardiology, The Cleveland Clinic Foundation, Cleveland, Ohio

Ari Ezratty, M.D. Clinical Cardiology, Department of Medicine, Brigham and Women's Hospital, Boston, Massachusetts

Valentin Fuster, M.D., Ph.D. Mallinckrodt Professor of Medicine, Harvard Medical School, and Chief, Cardiac Unit, Massachusetts General Hospital, Boston, Massachusetts

Samuel Z. Goldhaber, M.D. Associate Professor of Medicine, Harvard Medical School, and Staff Cardiologist, Brigham and Women's Hospital, Boston, Massachusetts

Cindy Grines, M.D. Medical Director, Cardiac Catheterization Laboratory, Department of Cardiology, William Beaumont Hospital, Royal Oak, Michigan

Gabriel B. Habib, M.D., F.A.C.C. Director, Coronary Care Unit, VA Medical Center, and Assistant Professor of Medicine, Baylor College of Medicine, Houston, Texas

Charles H. Hennekens, M.D. Professor, Department of Medicine and Preventive Medicine, Harvard Medical School, Brigham and Women's Hospital, Boston, Massachusetts

L. David Hillis, M.D. The Jan and Henri Bromberg Professor of Medicine, Department of Internal Medicine, University of Texas Southwestern Medical Center, Dallas, Texas

John H. Ip, M.D. Instructor, Division of Cardiology, Department of Medicine, Mount Sinai Medical Center, New York, New York

Douglas Israel, M.D. Clinical Instructor, Division of Cardiology, Department of Medicine, Mount Sinai Medical Center, New York, New York

James J. Jollis, M.D. Fellow, Division of Cardiology, Duke University Medical Center, Durham, North Carolina

Bodh I. Jugdutt, M.B.Ch.B., M.Sc., F.A.C.C., F.R.C.P.C. Professor of Medicine and Director, Adult Echocardiography, Division of Cardiology, Department of Medicine, University of Alberta, Edmonton, Alberta, Canada

Steven J. Kalbfleisch, M.D. Fellow in Cardiovascular Electrophysiology, Division of Cardiology, University of Michigan Medical Center, Ann Arbor, Michigan

Dean J. Kereiakes, M.D., F.A.C.C. Director, Division of Cardiovascular Intervention, The Christ Hospital Cardiovascular Research Center, Cincinnati, Ohio

A. Michael Lincoff, M.D. Interventional Cardiology Fellow, Department of Cardiology, The Cleveland Clinic Foundation, Cleveland, Ohio

Joseph Loscalzo, M.D., Ph.D. Associate Professor of Medicine, Harvard Medical School, and Director, Center for Research in Thrombolysis, Brigham and Women's Hospital, and Chief, Cardiology Section, Brockton/West Roxbury VA Medical Center, Boston, Massachusetts

Daniel B. Mark, M.D., M.P.H. Assistant Professor of Medicine and Director of Economic and Quality of Life Studies, Division of Cardiology, Department of Medicine, Duke University Medical Center, Durham, North Carolina

Fred Morady, M.D., F.A.C.C. Professor of Internal Medicine and Director, Clinical Electrophysiology Laboratory, Division of Cardiology, University of Michigan Medical Center, Ann Arbor, Michigan

John M. Nicklas, M.D. Associate Professor of Internal Medicine, and Director, Coronary Care Unit, University of Michigan Medical Center, Ann Arbor, Michigan

William O'Neill, M.D., F.A.C.C. Director of Cardiology, Department of Medicine, William Beaumont Hospital, Royal Oak, Michigan

Bertram Pitt, M.D., F.A.C.C. Professor of Internal Medicine and Associate Chairman for Industrial and Academic Programs, Division of Cardiology, Department of Internal Medicine, University of Michigan Medical Center, Ann Arbor, Michigan

Jeffrey J. Popma, M.D. Director, Angiographic Core Laboratory, Washington Cardiology Center, Washington, D.C.

Robert Roberts, M.D., F.A.C.C.   Professor of Medicine and Cell Biology, Baylor College of Medicine, and Chief, Division of Cardiology, Methodist Hospital, Houston, Texas

Allan M. Ross, M.D., F.A.C.P., F.A.C.C.   Professor of Medicine and Director, Division of Cardiology, George Washington University, Washington, D.C.

David C. Sane, M.D.   Assistant Professor, Division of Cardiology, Department of Medicine, Duke University Medical Center, Durham, North Carolina

Koon K. Teo, M.B.B.Ch., Ph.D.   Assistant Professor, Division of Cardiology, Department of Medicine, University of Alberta Hospital, Edmonton, Alberta, Canada

Eric Topol, M.D.   Chairman, Department of Cardiology, and Director, Center for Thrombosis and Arterial Biology, The Cleveland Clinic Foundation, Cleveland, Ohio

Steven W. Werns, M.D.   Assistant Professor of Internal Medicine, Division of Cardiology, University of Michigan Medical Center, Ann Arbor, Michigan

Thrombolysis and Adjunctive Therapy for Acute Myocardial Infarction

I

---

*THROMBOLYTIC THERAPY FOR
ACUTE MYOCARDIAL
INFARCTION:
CLINICAL ENDPOINTS*

1

Infarct Artery Patency

Eric R. Bates
University of Michigan Medical Center, Ann Arbor, Michigan

CORONARY THROMBOSIS

Herrick (1) suggested in 1912 that postmortem coronary thrombi were related to the clinical events that precipitated myocardial necrosis. More than six decades later, DeWood et al. (2) demonstrated angiographically that as many as 85% of patients had thrombotic coronary artery occlusion during the early hours of acute transmural myocardial infarction. Although thrombolytic therapy had been given to patients as early as 1958 (3), early trials were inconclusive owing to small sample sizes, late initiation of therapy, and inadequate doses of streptokinase. The modern era of thrombolytic therapy began 15 years ago with the angiographic demonstration that acute reperfusion of a coronary artery occluded by thrombus could be accomplished with thrombolytic therapy (4,5).

Acute myocardial infarction is usually precipitated by plaque fissuring or rupture (6,7). Plaques most likely to rupture have a soft core of lipid, are eccentric, and produce only mild to moderate angiographic luminal stenosis (8,9). Thinning of the fibrous cap tissue associated with macrophage infiltration precedes plaque rupture, which is presumably initiated by hemodynamic or mechanical factors (8,9). Exposure of collagen and other vascular wall constituents activates platelets and the coagulation cascade system. As explained by Davies (8,10), thrombus predominantly composed of platelets forms initially within the plaque, altering

3

plaque configuration and reducing luminal blood flow. Intimal flaps and platelet activation may increase arterial tone, further reducing flow. Subsequently, thrombus projects into the lumen and can embolize distally or become occlusive and propagate distally or sometimes proximally. The intraluminal thrombus is composed mostly of red blood cells entrapped in a fibrin network, a structure very susceptible to natural or therapeutic fibrinolysis. In the early stages of thrombus formation and after successful thrombolysis, repeated transitions between mural and occlusive thrombosis can occur. Unsuccessful lysis appears to be associated with more complex plaque tears where intraplaque thrombus may be externally compressing the lumen or where an intimal flap is raised (10). Reocclusion after thrombolysis appears to be stimulated by increased shear rates from luminal encroachment by the residual thrombus and plaque and by exposure of thrombin bound to fibrin in the thrombus (11,12). These conditions result in platelet and clotting reactivation.

INFARCT ARTERY PATENCY

Early Patency

The driving theory behind thrombolytic therapy in acute myocardial infarction is that early restoration of infarct artery patency can salvage ischemic muscle, preserve left ventricular function, and decrease mortality. Reimer et al. (13) demonstrated in a dog model that myocardial necrosis after coronary artery occlusion spread from the endocardial surface to the epicardial surface over a period of hours. Early reperfusion before transmural necrosis developed preserved an epicardial rim of viable muscle. Little preservation of muscle occurred after 3 hr of ischemia, a finding corroborated clinically in the Netherlands Interuniversity Trial (14), where enzyme release, a measure of infarct size, was equal in treated and control patients when symptoms were present for over 3 hr. The best recovery of left ventricular function occurs when therapy is initiated within 1 hr of symptom onset (15). Concordantly, both the Gruppo Italiano per lo Studio della Streptochinasi nell'Infarto Miocardico (GISSI-1) (16) trial and the Second International Study of Infarct Survival (ISIS-2) trial (17) demonstrated the greatest reduction in mortality in the first hour of symptoms, with declining benefit as time to treatment increased. Thus, great emphasis has been placed on educating patients with persistent ischemic chest pain to report as soon as possible to a medical facility for evaluation, and prehospital administration of thrombolytic therapy is being tested. Likewise, the 90-min angiogram after initiation of therapy has become the standard by which to measure patency status and compare the relative efficacy of thrombolytic agents.

Late Patency

The surprising survival benefit from achieving infarct artery patency several hours after symptom onset, in a time frame beyond which myocardial salvage could be expected, was first demonstrated in the Western Washington Intracoronary Streptokinase Trial (18). Although no improvement in infarct size or ejection fraction was demonstrated in patients treated with streptokinase (19), mortality at 1 year in patients with complete reperfusion, partial reperfusion, and no reperfusion during the acute cardiac catherization was 2.5%, 23.1%, and 14.6%, respectively. Similarly, restoring patency after approximately 5 hr of ischemia conveyed a prolonged survival benefit to patients enrolled in the first Thrombolysis in Myocardial Infarction (TIMI-1) trial (20). Mortality benefit with treatment initiated 6–12 hr and maybe up to 24 hr after onset of symptoms has been suggested by the ISIS-2 trial (17), the Estudio Multicentrico Estreptoquinasa Republica de America del Sur (EMERAS) trial (21), and a meta-analysis of older intravenous thrombolytic trials (22). Importantly, patency rates in patients treated with rt-PA with 6–24 hr of chest pain were 64% versus 23% in controls at 36 hr after symptom onset in the sixth Thrombolysis and Angioplasty in Myocardial Infarction (TAMI-6) trial (23). Similar data for the other thrombolytic agents are not available.

Spontaneous Patency

The intrinsic fibrinolytic system restores infarct artery patency in a small percentage of patients early after arterial thrombosis and eventually achieves patency rates approaching those resulting from thrombolytic therapy. In the landmark study by DeWood and colleagues (2), patency rates after 0–4 hr, 4–6 hr, 6–12 hr, and 12–24 hr were 12.7%, 14.7%, 31.6%, and 35.1%, respectively. A 67% patency rate was seen in a small number of patients studied by Rentrop and co-workers (24) 10–14 days after acute myocardial infarction. Cigarroa and co-workers (25) retrospectively reviewed the coronary angiograms of patients with one-vessel disease studied a mean of almost 1 month after myocardial infarction. Over a 4-year follow-up period, patients with infarct artery patency had a significantly lower incidence of unstable angina, congestive heart failure, or death. The same group (26) found lower left ventricular volumes, higher ejection fractions, and lower mortality in patients with multivessel disease and spontaneous reperfusion of the infarct artery following first myocardial infarction.

CLINICAL REPERFUSION TRIALS

Differences in Study Design

Determining the relative ability of thrombolytic agents to reperfuse infarct arteries has been an obvious endpoint for comparison since thrombotic arterial occlusion is the predominant etiology for acute myocardial infarction. Numerous reviews have tabulated results from several studies to determine the most successful lytic agent. However, several differences in study design need to be kept in mind when interpreting these efforts.

First, reperfusion is a broad term that can be used to mean recanalization or patency. Recanalization rates are determined by first documenting the presence of an occluded artery by angiography and then determining opening rates after administration of a lytic agent. In contrast, patency rates are determined only from posttreatment angiograms. Patency rates are higher than recanalization rates because they include a small percentage (10–20%) of patients with open arteries that never occluded or spontaneously reperfused.

Second, differences can exist in the scoring systems used to determine the degree of blood flow in the infarct artery. The most frequently used methodology was developed by the TIMI Study Group (27) (Table 1). Most studies using this classification define patency as grade 2 plus grade 3 flow.

Third, it is clear that clinical markers of reperfusion, including relief of chest pain, normalization of ST-segment elevation, or bursts of accelerated idioventricular rhythm, do not accurately reflect reperfusion (28,29). Determining the time of peak creatine kinase (CK) release has been used as a surrogate for angiography in some studies (30). Early reperfusion has been associated with peak CK levels occurring within 15 hr of chest pain onset, whereas peak CK levels occur later in persistently occluded arteries (31). Newer techniques involving CK-MB isoenzyme release (32) or continuous 12-lead ST-segment monitoring (33,34) may allow more rapid and accurate noninvasive determination of infarct artery patency. For the present, however, angiographic documentation remains the standard by which to evaluate reperfusion.

Fourth, doses of thrombolytic agents and infusion times have varied widely. Higher doses or more rapid infusion times have improved patency rates in some studies and longer infusions may have reduced reocclusion rates in other studies. Patency rates with alteplase, in particular, appear to be influenced by infusion times. With conventional dosing of 100 mg over 3 hr, only 70 mg has been infused when the 90-min angiogram is recorded versus 100 mg in the front-loaded regimens. In contrast, angiographic studies with anistreplase, streptokinase, urokinase, or saruplase have been performed after completion of the drug infusion.

Fifth, time to treatment and time to angiography are important. Organization of the thrombus begins to occur after the first few hours, decreasing acute reperfusion rates in patients who present later for treatment. Patency rates are also time dependent. Sixty- or ninety-minute patency rates are "snapshots" in time, arbitrarily chosen because of the logistics involved in transporting the patient into the catherization laboratory for evaluation. Later evaluations will result in higher reperfusion rates because of continued thrombolysis or spontaneous reperfusion.

Table 1   Definitions of Perfusion in the TIMI Trial

Grade 0 (no perfusion):   There is no antegrade flow beyond the point of occlusion.

Grade 1 (penetration without perfusion):   The contrast material passes beyond the area of obstruction but "hangs up" and fails to opacify the entire coronary bed distal to the obstruction for the duration of the cineangiographic filming sequence.

Grade 2 (partial perfusion):   The contrast material passes across the obstruction and opacifies the coronary bed distal to the obstruction. However, the rate of entry of contrast material into the vessel distal to the obstruction or its rate of clearance from the distal bed (or both) are perceptibly slower than its entry into or clearance from comparable areas not perfused by the previously occluded vessel—e.g., the opposite coronary artery or the coronary bed proximal to the obstruction.

Grade 3 (complete perfusion):   Antegrade flow into the bed distal to the obstruction occurs as promptly as antegrade flow into the bed proximal to the obstruction, and clearance of contrast material from the involved bed is as rapid as clearance from an uninvolved bed in the same vessel or the opposite artery.

Source: Ref. 27.

Because reperfusion is a dynamic process, early measurements reflect velocity of opening whereas later measurements are more reflective of final patency rates. A fair comparison of agents should be done at the same time.

Sixth, some studies have used the flow status on the first angiographic injection as the endpoint, whereas others have used the final injection. Since the hydrostatic force of injecting contrast into the artery can result in reperfusion in 5–10% of patients, reperfusion rates will be slightly higher if the final angiographic evaluation is used as the reference point.

Finally, studies reporting results with fewer than 50 patients should not be given equal weight to studies reporting on 100–200 patients. Similarly, patients have occasionally been counted twice when results from both a preliminary abstract and the final manuscript have been included separately.

The following review of patency rates associated with currently available thrombolytic agents has been organized with these considerations in mind. Studies employing noninvasive detection techniques have been excluded, as have angiographic recanalization studies. Standard dosing regimens have been analyzed, and time to angiography is emphasized. Although symptom duration could not easily be controlled, mean symptom duration was consistently 2.5–4 hr.

Early Angiographic Patency Results

Streptokinase

Streptokinase is a bacterial-derived protein that binds indirectly to circulating plasminogen to activate fibrinolysis. It is antigenic and occasionally produces

8   **Bates**

Table 2   Streptokinase—Patency Data

Study	Dose (IU)	Angio (hr)	Patency (%, n)
Cribier (36)	1.5×10^6	1.0	52 (11/21)
PRIMI (37)	1.5×10^6	1.0	48 (82/171)
Schwartz (38)	1.5×10^6	1.5	45 (25/55)
ECSG-1 (39)	1.5×10^6	1.5	55 (34/62)
Lopez-Sendon (40)	1.5×10^6	1.5	60 (15/25)
Stack (41)	1.5×10^6	1.5	44 (95/216)
PRIMI (37)	1.5×10^6	1.5	64 (124/174)
Charbonnier (42)	1.5×10^6	1.5	51 (27/53)
Hogg (43)	1.5×10^6	1.5	53 (31/58)
Mean	1.5×10^6	1.5	53 (351/663)
Brochier (44)	1.5×10^6	1.7	56 (24/43)
Anderson (45)	1.5×10^6	2.3	73 (129/176)
Six (46)	1.5×10^6	2.8	60 (32/53)
Vogt (47)	1.5×10^6	3.0	72 (21/31)

drug rash, fever, serum sickness, and anaphylactic reactions. Hypotension can occur via activation of kinins and the complement system. The half-life is relatively long (20 min) and marked fibrinogenolysis is produced. The dose of 1.5 million units infused over 1 hr was empirically recommended by Schroder and colleagues (35). There is no evidence that this dose is superior to lower doses such as 500,000 units (35). The current charge to the hospital pharmacy for streptokinase is approximately $300.

Reperfusion velocity is slower with streptokinase than with other agents (Table 2). Patency at 60 min is just under 50% (36,37) and at 90 min is just over 50% (37–43). However, from 2 to 3 hr after treatment, patency rates reach 70% (44–47), the rate achieved with alteplase, anistreplase, duteplase, or saruplase at 90 min. These data suggest that equivalent patency to tissue plasminogen activator is not reached at 3 hr, as suggested in a recent review by Sherry and Marder (48), but occurs sometime later as patency rates with rt-PA also improve after 90 min due to continued thrombolysis (49).

Alteplase

Alteplase is a recombinant, predominantly single-chain form of tissue plasminogen activator (t-PA). A serine protease enzyme, it directly activated the fibrin-plasminogen complex, producing both local and systemic fibrinolysis. No antigenic activity has been reported and hypotension is not directly induced. The half-life of alteplase is only a few minutes, and it produces relatively mild fibrinogenolysis. The conventional dose of 100 mg over 3 hr (6-mg bolus, 54 mg/1 hr, 20

Table 3   Alteplase—Patency Data

Study	Dose	Angio (hr)	Patency (%, n)	
RAAMI (51)	100 mg/3 hr	1.0	62	(81/130)
GAUS (52)	70 mg/90 min	1.5	69	(84/121)
TAMI-4 (53)	100 mg/3 hr	1.5	60	(19/25)
RAAMI (51)	100 mg/3 hr	1.5	75	(107/143)
TAMI-5 (54)	100 mg/3 hr	1.5	71	(67/95)
CRAFT (55)	100 mg/3 hr	1.5	63	(126/199)
Mean	70 mg/90 min	1.5	68	(399/583)

mg/1 hr, 20 mg/1 hr) was chosen because of equal thrombolytic 90-min efficacy and a lower incidence of intracerebral hemorrhage compared with the 150-mg dose (50). The cost of alteplase is approximately $2300.

With the conventional dose of 100 mg over 3 hr, patency rates at 60 min are approximately 10 percentage points higher than with streptokinase, and the difference is 15 percentage points at 90 min (51–55) (Table 3). However, only 70 mg of the 100-mg dose has been infused at the time of the 90-min angiogram. Unlike streptokinase, alteplase appears to be associated with a dose-response curve. This point is illustrated in Table 4, where results from studies using weight-adjusted dosing schedules have been analyzed according to the dose infused at the time of the 90-min angiogram. Patency rates increased from 67% to 84% as the dose increased from 0.75 mg/kg to 1.4 mg/kg (39,49,56–59). Similarly, infusing the total dose of 100 mg within 90 min instead of 3 hr, known as accelerated or front-loaded dosing, improves patency rates to approximately 85%, according to results from the studies summarized in Table 5 (51,60,61). The dose schedule used in these studies (15-mg bolus, 50 mg over 30 min, 35 mg over 60 min) appears to result in 90-min patency rates approximately 30 percentage points higher than

Table 4   Weight-Adjusted Alteplase

Study	90-min dose	Patency (%, n)	
ECSG 1 + 2 (39,56)	0.75 mg/kg	67	(81/121)
Topol (49)	0.875 mg/kg	69	(49/71)
Smalling (57)	0.875 mg/kg	70	(61/87)
Johns (58)	1.0 mg/kg	76	(52/68)
Topol (59)	1.16 mg/kg	79	(104/131)
Smalling (57)	1.4 mg/kg	84	(68/81)

Table 5   Front-Loaded Alteplase (100 mg/90 min)

Study	60-min patency (%, *n*)		90-min patency (%, *n*)	
Neuhaus (60)	74	(54/73)	91	(67/74)
RAAMI (51)	76	(93/123)	82	(113/138)
TAPS (61)	74	(146/198)	85	(168/198)
Mean	74	(293/394)	85	(348/410)

seen with intravenous streptokinase. In other terms, the 60-min patency rate of approximately 75% is higher than patency rates 2–3 hr after streptokinase therapy (Table 2) and equivalent patency rates are certainly not achieved until after 3 hr. Other accelerated dosing schemes have been somewhat less successful (62), but all have achieved patency rates and reocclusion rates at least equal to those seen with the conventional 3-hr infusion, and bleeding complications have not been increased.

Bolus dosing has also been attempted. Tebbe and colleagues (63) injected 50 mg of alteplase into 20 patients; 15 patients had patent infarct arteries at 60 min. However, Tranchesi and co-workers (64) achieved a patency rate of only 48% in 28 patients with the same dose. They also noted a 32% patency rate (9/29) at 60 min after a 60-mg bolus and a 72% patency rate (18/25) after a 70-mg bolus. Purvis et al. (65) administered two bolus doses 30 min apart. Patency rates after 20 mg and 50 mg, 50 mg and 20 mg, and 50 mg and 50 mg were 75% (9/12), 92% (11/12), and 92% (11/12), respectively. Two other groups gave a 20-mg bolus followed 30 min later by 80 mg in a 2-hr infusion; patency rates were 94% in one study, but only 73% in the other (62,66). Thus, the potential value of "ultrathrombolysis" requires further evaluation (67).

Alteplase has also been used in combination with streptokinase, urokinase, and saruplase (Chapter 13). The patency rate with alteplase/streptokinase was 79% in 198 patients (68–70) and was 78% in 481 patients with alteplase/urokinase (54,62,71,72). The alteplase/saruplase studies have been dose-finding studies involving small doses of each drug (73–75).

Duteplase

Duteplase is a predominantly two-chain form of t-PA. Duteplase differs from alteplase in the substitution of a methionine for a valine amino acid at position 245. Although there are subtle biochemical differences between the two agents, comparative trials have not been performed to evaluate clinical differences. Duteplase was withdrawn from further development after a patent infringement legal suit was lost to the manufacturer of alteplase.

Table 6   Duteplase—Patency Data (76)

Study	Dose	Angio (hr)	Patency (%, n)
ESPRIT	0.4 MU/kg/1 hr; 0.2 MU/kg/3 hr	1.5	71 (117/251)
P52:02	0.4 MU/kg/1 hr; 0.2 MU/kg/3 hr	1.5	67 (155/230)
P52:10	0.4 MU/kg/1 hr; 0.2 MU/kg/3 hr	1.5	69 (330/478)
Mean		1.5	69 (622/959)

Source: Ref. 76.

Duteplase was the form of t-PA used in the ISIS-2 trial. A dose of 0.6 MU/kg was given over 4 hr with 0.4 MU/kg given in the first hour (including a 10% bolus) and 0.2 MU/kg given over the subsequent 3 hr. Thus, as with the conventional alteplase dose of 100 mg over 3 hr used in the GISSI-2 trial, 2/3 of the dose was administered by 90 min. Three unpublished angiographic studies (76) involving this dose of duteplase (Table 6) showed equal patency compared with the alteplase studies (Table 3). Kalbfleisch (77) recently infused the 0.6 MU/kg dose over 1 hr, achieving a 76% patency rate at 90 min in 87 patients.

Anistreplase

Anisoylated plasminogen streptokinase activator complex (APSAC), or anistreplase, is a stoichiometric combination of streptokinase and human lysplasminogen. An anisoyl group reversibly bound to the catalytic center of the plasminogen

Table 7   Anistreplase—Patency Data

Study	Dose	Angio (hr)	Patency (%, n)
Kasper (78)	30 U	1.0	64 (32/50)
TAPS (61)	30 U	1.0	60 (123/204)
Kasper (78)	30 U	1.25	84 (42/50)
Been (79)	30 U	1.5	100 (16/16)
Lopez-Sendon (40)	30 U	1.5	86 (19/22)
Charbonnier (42)	30 U	1.5	70 (38/54)
Visser (80)	30 U	1.5	75 (107/142)
Hogg (43)	30 U	1.5	55 (32/58)
TAPS (61)	30 U	1.5	70 (142/202)
Mean	30 U	1.5	72 (354/494)
Anderson (45)	30 U	2.3	72 (132/183)
Vogt (47)	30 U	2.6	76 (23/30)

moiety slowly undergoes deacylation prior to plasminogen activation, permitting rapid injection of the drug because of the slow onset of activity. The plasma half-life of 90 min is long relative to streptokinase, but the risk of antigenic complications and hypotension is similar. The conventional dose is 30 units infused over 2–5 min, and the cost is approximately $1700.

Patency rates at 60 min are over 60% (61,78) and at 90 min are over 70% (40, 42,43,61,78–80) (Table 7), supporting a higher patency velocity than seen with streptokinase. However, patency rates do not appear to improve further between 90 min and 2–3 hr after injection. Compared with the conventional alteplase dose, early patency rates are equivalent, although patency at 2–3 hr may be somewhat lower. In the Tissue Plasminogen Activator-APSAC Patency Study (TAPS) (61), patency at 90 min was 70%, compared with 85% for the front-loaded alteplase dose given over 90 min. The major advantage of anistreplase is its ease of administration, which may be of particular benefit for out-of-hospital thrombolytic therapy.

Urokinase

Urokinase is a nonantigenic direct plasminogen activator that has been used more for intracoronary than intravenous administration. Three million units costs approximately $2200. It can be given as a bolus, like anistreplase, or infused over 60–90 min. Mathey et al. (81) injected a bolus of 2 million units and documented a 60% patency rate at 60 min in 50 patients (Table 8). Four other trials have noted similar patency rates at 90 min with infusion protocols (52,54,55,82). Mortality trials have not been performed, and intravenous urokinase is not formally approved by the Food and Drug Administration for use in acute myocardial infarction.

Saruplase

Saruplase (pro-urokinase) is the single chain proenzyme of urokinase. Like alteplase, it is produced by recombinant DNA technology, lacks antigenicity, has a

Table 8   Urokinase—Patency Data

Study	Dose	Angio	Patency (%, n)
GAUS (52)	1.5×10^6 unit bolus/1.5×10^6 units @ 90 min	1.5	66 (77/117)
Wall (82)	3×10^6 units/60 min	1.5	58 (57/98)
TAMI-5	1.5×10^6 unit bolus/1.5×10^6 units @ 90 min	1.5	62 (59/95)
CRAFT (55)	1.5×10^6 unit bolus/1.5×10^6 units @ 90 min	1.5	53 (105/198)
Mean		1.5	59 (298/508)

Table 9   Saruplase—Patency Data

Study	Dose	Angio (hr)	Patency (%)
PRIMI (37)	80 mg/60 min	1.0	72 (122/170)
		1.5	71 (131/184)
Vermeer (83)	80 mg/60 min	1.5	72 (>500)

short half-life, and is relatively fibrin selective. A dose of 80 mg is administered over 60 min, with 20 mg given as a bolus. In the PRIMI trial (37), 90-min patency was 71% versus 64% for streptokinase (Table 9). A preliminary report (83) of a larger experience showed a 72% patency rate at 90 min for over 500 patients (Table 9).

Later Angiographic Patency Results

Somewhere between 3 and 24 hr after initiation of thrombolytic therapy, equivalent patency rates are probably achieved regardless of the thrombolytic agent employed (37,40,43,52,61,84–85) (Table 10). Patency is seen in 85–90% of infarct

Table 10   Patency Data—24–36 hr

Drug	Study	Dose	Angio (hr)	Patency (%, n)
Alteplase	TEAM-3 (84)	100 mg	24	84 (114/135)
	TIMI-2 (89)	100 mg	33	85 (1040/1229)
	Mean			85 (1154/1364)
Anistreplase	Lopez-Sendon (40)	30 U	24	91 (20/22)
	Hogg (43)	30 U	24	81 (47/58)
	TEAM-3 (84)	30 U	24	90 (123/137)
	TAPS (61)	30 U	24–36	93 (183/196)
	Mean			90 (373/413)
Saruplase	PRIMI (37)	80 mg/60 min	24–36	85 (150/177)
Streptokinase	Lopez-Sendon (40)	1.5×10^6 IU	24	75 (18/24)
	PRIMI (37)	1.5×10^6 IU	24–36	88 (160/181)
	Hogg (43)	1.5×10^6 IU	24	88 (49/56)
	Mean			87 (227/261)
Urokinase	GAUS (52)	3×10^6 IU	24	73 (77/105)

Table 11   Patency Data—Late

Drug	Study	Dose	Angio	Patency (%, n)
Alteplase	PAIMS (86)	100 mg	4 days	81 (63/78)
	ECSG-6 (87)	100 mg	3–5 days	79 (515/652)
	Machecourt (88)	100 mg	3–7 days	75 (68/84)
	NHF (89)	100 mg	5–7 days	70 (43/61)
	White (90)	100 mg	3 wk	76 (103/135)
Anistreplase	Bassand (91)	30 U	4 days	77 (82/112)
	Machecourt (88)	30 U	3–7 days	73 (61/84)
	TAPS (61)	30 U	14 days	90 (158/176)
Streptokinase	PAIMS (86)	1.5×10^6 IU	4 days	74 (55/74)
	WWIVSK (92)	1.5×10^6 IU	10 days	69 (132/191)
	White (93)	1.5×10^6 IU	3 wk	75 (80/107)
	White (90)	1.5×10^6 IU	3 wk	75 (101/135)
Urokinase	GAUS (52)	3×10^6 IU	>10 days	71 (59/83)

arteries, approximating patency rates achieved with direct coronary angioplasty. In the following days and weeks, reocclusion occurs in a few arteries, reducing sustained patency rates to approximately 75% (Table 11) (52,61,86–93).

REOCCLUSION

Reocclusion of the infarct artery negates the potential benefits associated with early reperfusion. Whereas successful reperfusion in patients clinically selected for thrombolytic therapy in the United States is associated with a hospital mortality of approximately 5% (94), patients with reocclusion after successful thrombolysis have a hospital mortality of 10–15% (94,95). The pathophysiological basis for reocclusion is probably the same as for initial thrombotic occlusion and involves a severe residual stenosis with disruption of its intimal surface, increased shear forces, and exposed thrombin on the surface of the residual thrombus promoting platelet activation and aggregation. The impact of vasomotor tone and the no-reflow phenomenon on this process are not defined but may contribute.

It has become clear through following patients with the continuous 12-lead ST-segment monitor that reperfusion is a dynamic process in the early hours after thrombolytic therapy (34). Thrombus dissolution and reformation can occur several times before the final patency status is determined. Higher fibrinogen levels may contribute to rethrombosis; lower fibrinogen levels and the resulting increase in the products of fibrinogen degradation that exert a potent antiplatelet effort may favor continued patency (96). In support of this concept is the suggestion that patients treated with t-PA have a higher incidence of recurrent temporary thrombosis, as measured by the continuous 12-lead ST-segment monitor, compared with streptokinase (34). If further cellular damage is caused by recurrent occlusion, this finding could explain why no difference in left ventricular function or mortality has been shown to date in clinical trials despite differences in reperfusion velocity between the thrombolytic agents. It also supports the suggestion that 24-hr patency is more reflective of final patency status and clinical benefit than is 90-min patency.

Early clinical studies with small numbers of patients suggested that the degree of residual stenosis predicted reocclusion (97,98). Thus, the efficacy of performing coronary angioplasty to reduce the residual stenosis was tested in three trials (99-101). All failed to show a benefit in reducing reocclusion rates or improving left ventricular function, and rates for blood transfusion, emergency bypass graft surgery and mortality were increased. Moreover, when large numbers of patients were studied with acute and 7-day coronary arteriograms available to analyze, none of 27 variables including residual stenosis was found to predict reocclusion (102).

Results from the TAMI trial suggest that half of clinically significant reocclusions occur within the first 24 hr; additionally half of all reocclusions are silent (94). Aspirin was shown to decrease reinfarction rates from 2% to 1% in the ISIS-2 trial (17). Intravenous heparin, compared with placebo, has been shown to yield higher later patency rates with rt-PA (87,103,104); the risk-to-benefit ratio of intravenous heparin compared with subcutaneous heparin has not been clarified. Because reocclusion continues to occur despite aspirin and heparin treatment, newer antiplatelet and antithrombin agents are being tested (Chapters 9 and 11).

Determining relative reocclusion rates for the different thrombolytic agents has been more difficult than documenting relative patency rates. First, much fewer data exist and many studies have evaluated only a few dozen patients. Second, differential initial patency rates may bias subsequent determinations of reocclusion rates by selecting arteries with different thrombotic potential. It is unclear why arteries that open early with front-loaded alteplase remain occluded early after streptokinase. Third, there has been no consistent time frame after thrombolytic therapy to compare reocclusion rates as there has been with patency rates and the 90-min angiogram. Comparing 24-hr reocclusion rates with 7-day reocclusion rates is irrelevant because of the different risk. Fourth, fewer studies have obtained paired angiograms in greater than 80% of the patients treated within a study; obtaining the second angiogram has often been influenced by clinical factors rather than incorporated into the protocol prospectively. Finally, some studies have used ECG or enzymatic evidence for infarct extension or reinfarction as a surrogate for reocclusion, rather than defining rates more precisely with arteriography.

Despite the clinical consensus that alteplase and duteplase have higher reocclusion rates than streptokinase or anistreplase, the patency results summarized in Tables 10 and 11 do not clearly support that conclusion. However, the TAMI-5 study (54) and the German Activator Urokinase Study (GAUS) (52) did show lower reocclusion rates for urokinase, a nonselective agent, compared with alteplase. Unfortunately, there are no other large comparative trials to analyze. In the TAMI data bank, the 7-day reocclusion rate with alteplase is 14%. The lowest reocclusion rates, under 5%, appear to be associated with the combination of alteplase and either streptokinase (68–70) or urokinase (54,62,71,72), an observation that requires further investigation (Chapter 13).

THE OPEN ARTERY HYPOTHESIS

Available data suggest that arterial patency independently improves survival. Explanations for the beneficial effects associated with infarct artery patency have been summarized recently by several authors (105–107). Besides limiting infarct size and preserving left ventricular ejection fraction, other potential salutary effects include improving left ventricular remodeling, decreasing left ventricular mural thrombus formation, improving electrical stability, and improving collateral blood flow. These additional benefits have attracted attention because the mortality benefits with lytic therapy have been greater than can be explained by the relatively small improvements in regional and global left ventricular function (Chapter 2).

Left Ventricular Remodeling

Transmural myocardial infarction is followed by remodeling of the left ventricle. Thinning and dilatation of the infarct zone caused by slippage of myocytes and stretching of myofibrils produces infarct expansion (108). This can lead to volume and pressure elevations, which increase ventricular wall stress and potentially expand infarct and noninfarct regional zones. The process can be progressive, leading to later complications as left ventricular cavity size correlates with subsequent congestive heart failure, ventricular arrhythmias, and mortality (109).

Successful reperfusion may modify this process in several ways. First, preservation of an epicardial rim of viable myocardium may prevent cell slippage and infarct expansion. Second, intramyocardial hemorrhage, myocellular edema, and restoration of vascular volume increase tissue turgor, which may decrease infarct expansion (110). Third, the healing process appears to be facilitated. Inflammatory cells have early access to the infarct area, less fibrosis occurs, and scar thickness is increased (111). Animal studies have demonstrated that reperfusion limits infarct expansion even when infarct size is not reduced (112), and clinical studies have demonstrated lower ventricular volumes in patients receiving thrombolytic therapy compared with controls (109,113).

Electrical Stability

Arterial patency favorably influences the electrical stability of the heart. Kersschot and colleagues (114) performed programmed electrical stimulation on 36 patients after myocardial infarction. Patients treated with streptokinase had fewer sustained ventricular arrhythmias (10/21 versus 15/15; $p < 0.001$). Sager et al. (115) studied 20 patients with transmural anterior myocardial infarction complicated by left ventricular aneurysm. Ventricular tachycardia was induced in 7/8 patients who did not receive thrombolytic therapy versus 1/12 in the thrombolytic group ($p = 0.0008$). In the following year, four of the eight patients in the control group died suddenly or were resuscitated from ventricular tachycardia, compared with no arrhythmic events in the patients treated with thrombolytic therapy.

Low-amplitude potentials that prolong the QRS complex can be recorded on a signal averaged ECG. They are associated with increased risk of ventricular tachycardia or sudden death. Gang and colleagues (116) noted that late potentials were significantly lower in patients treated with t-PA versus controls (2/44 versus 14/62; $p = 0.01$). Only 4/67 patients with patent arteries had late potentials, compared with 9/28 patients having occluded arteries ($p = 0.01$).

Infarcted tissue in patients with patent arteries appears to be more homogeneous (117). Reduced left ventricular aneurysm formation may reduce the substrate for electrical instability. Likewise, preventing abnormal volume loading could decrease variations in refractoriness that facilitate reentry arrhythmias (118). Finally, preventing transmural infarction may spare sympathetic fibers in the epicardium, decreasing vulnerability to develop ventricular fibrillation (119).

Collateral Circulation

In addition to restoring antegrade flow to the infarct zone, a patent artery can be a source of collateral circulation in patients with multivessel disease. This may reduce ischemia in the secondary zone or reduce subsequent infarct size should another artery develop thrombotic occlusion. Also, collateral circulation may offer the thoracic surgeon another site for a bypass graft should coronary artery bypass graft surgery be required.

Limitations

As attractive as it seems, the open-artery hypothesis may not explain the survival benefit seen with thrombolytic therapy. The low mortality rates reported in many trials are partly due to the exclusion of high-risk patients, such as those with age greater than 75 years, cardiogenic shock, previous bypass graft surgery, late presentation, or confounding medical conditions (120,121). Mean ejection fraction consistently approximates 50%, and patients with single-vessel disease predominate: only a minority of patients with three-vessel disease develop ST-segment elevation with coronary occlusion (122). Additionally, effective anti-ischemic medications including beta blockers, risk stratification strategies, coronary angiography and electrophysiological testing, and coronary revascularization have changed the natural history of myocardial infarction. Five-year follow-up in the Netherlands Interuniversity trial (123) did not find arterial patency predictive of outcome: rather, left ventricular function and significant multivessel disease were again the important determinants.

CONCLUSION

In summary, 90-min angiographic patency with alteplase or duteplase is approximately 15 percentage points higher compared with streptokinase, as initially reported in the first European Cooperative Study Group (ECSG) trial (56), not 25 points higher as is often quoted. However, infusing the total dose within 90 min increases the difference to almost 30 percentage points. Early patency rates with urokinase are somewhat better than with streptokinase, whereas anistreplase and saruplase yield slightly higher patency rates relative to 3-hr t-PA infusions. The highest 90-min patency rates have been seen with front-loaded alteplase infusions lasting 90 min and with the combination of alteplase and urokinase or streptokinase. Somewhere between 3 hr and 24 hr, equivalent patency rates are achieved with all the thrombolytic agents despite dosing variations. Although thrombolysis is a dynamic process and reocclusion occurs frequently during the first day of treatment, continuing fibrin dissolution appears to override the tendency toward rethrombosis, as patency rates increase with time. However, reocclusion over the next several days may reduce patency rates at hospital discharge by about 10 points compared with 24- to 36-hr patency rates.

The impact of early patency on patient survival relative to sustained late patency remains to be defined. The potential early patency advantage for t-PA suggested by experimental and small clinical studies has not been confirmed by large comparative mortality trials (124,125), perhaps because of a higher incidence of intermittent patency. The results of the Global Utilization of Streptokinase and t-PA for Occluded Coronary Arteries (GUSTO) trial will hopefully resolve this important issue. In this mortality trial, four treatment strategies will be tested. Front-loaded, weight-adjusted alteplase with intravenous heparin should produce the highest possible early patency rates, and the combination of alteplase, streptokinase, and intravenous heparin should produce high sustained patency rates. If either of these strategies is more successful than streptokinase with intravenous or subcutaneous heparin, the higher expense of alteplase may be clinically justified (Chapter 21) and other strategies aimed toward more rapid and/or more sustained infarct artery patency will need to be investigated to see whether further improvements in clinical outcome can be achieved (Chapter 3). If there are no mortality differences in GUSTO, then there is no clinical benefit associated with 90-min patency rates, and streptokinase will be the thrombolytic agent of choice for the treatment of acute myocardial infarction.

REFERENCES

1. Herrick JB. Clinical features of sudden obstruction of the coronary arteries. JAMA 1912; 59:2015-20.
2. DeWood MA, Spores J, Notske R, et al. Prevalence of total coronary occlusion during the early hours of transmural myocardial infarction. N Engl J Med 1980; 303: 897-902.
3. Fletcher AP, Alkjaersig N, Smyrniotis FE, Sherry S. Treatment of patients suffering from early myocardial infarction with massive and prolonged streptokinase therapy. Trans Assoc Am Physicians 1958; 71:287-96.
4. Chazov EI, Mateeva LS, Mazaev AV, Sargin KE, Sadovskaia GV. Intracoronary administration of fibrinolysis in acute myocardial infarction. Ter Arkh 1976; 48:8-19.
5. Rentrop KT, Blanke H, Karsch KR, Kreuzer H. Initial experience with transluminal recanalization of the recently occluded infarct-related coronary artery in acute myocardial infarction: comparison with conventionally treated patients. Clin Cardiol 1979; 2:92-105.
6. Falk E. Plaque rupture with severe pre-existing stenosis precipitating coronary thrombosis. Characteristics of coronary atherosclerotic plaques underlying fatal occlusive thrombi. Br Heart J 1983; 50:127-34.
7. Davies MJ, Thomas AC. Plaque fissuring—the cause of acute myocardial infarction, sudden ischemic death, and crescendo angina. Br Heart J 1985; 53:363-73.
8. Davies MJ. A macro and micro view of coronary vascular insult in ischemic heart disease. Circulation 1990; 82(Suppl II):II-38-II-46.
9. Fuster V, Stein B, Ambrose JA, Badimon L, Badimon JJ, Chesebro JH. Atherosclerotic plaque rupture and thrombosis. Evolving concepts. Circulation 1990; 82(Suppl II): II-47-II-59.
10. Davies MJ. Successful and unsuccessful coronary thrombolysis. Br Heart J 1989; 61: 381-4.
11. Badimon L, Badimon JJ. Mechanisms of arterial thrombosis in nonparallel streamlines: Platelet thrombi grow on the apex of stenotic severely injured vessel walls. Experimental study in the pig model. J Clin Invest 1989; 84:1134-44.
12. Francis CW, Markham RE Jr, Barlow GH, Florack TM, Dobrzynski DM, Marder VJ. Thrombin activity of fibrin thrombi and soluble plasmic derivatives. J Lab Clin Med 1983; 102:220-30.
13. Reimer KA, Lowe JE, Rasmussen MM, Jennings RB. The wave front phenomenon of ischemic cell death: 1. Myocardial infarct size vs. duration of coronary occlusion in dogs. Circulation 1977; 56:786-94.
14. Simoons ML, Serruys PW, van den Brand M, et al. Early thrombolysis in acute myo-

cardial infarction: limitation of infarct size and improved survival. J Am Coll Cardiol 1986; 7:717-28.

15. Koren G, Weiss AT, Hasin Y, et al. Prevention of myocardial damage in acute myocardial ischemia by early treatment with intravenous streptokinase. N Engl J Med 1985; 313:1384-9.

16. Gruppo Italiano per lo Studio della Streptochinasi nell 'Infarto Miocardico (GISSI). Effectiveness of intravenous thrombolytic treatment in acute myocardial infarction. Lancet 1986; 1:397-401.

17. ISIS-2 (Second International Study of Infarct Survival) Collaborative Group. Randomized trial of intravenous streptokinase, oral aspirin, both or neither among 17,187 cases of suspected acute myocardial infarction: ISIS-2. Lancet 1988; 2: 349-60.

18. Kennedy JW, Ritchie JL, Davis KB, Stadius ML, Maynard C, Fritz JK. The Western Washington randomized trial of intracoronary streptokinase in acute myocardial infarction. A 12-month follow-up report. N Engl J Med 1985; 312:1073-8.

19. Ritchie JL, Davis KB, Williams DL, Caldwell J, Kennedy JW. Global and regional left ventricular function and tomographic radionuclide perfusion: the Western Washington Intracoronary Streptokinase in Myocardial Infarction Trial. Circulation 1984; 70:867-75.

20. Dalen JE, Gore JM, Braunwald E, et al. Six- and 12-month follow-up of the phase I Thrombolysis in Myocardial Infarction (TIMI) trial. Am J Cardiol 1988; 62:179-85.

21. Paolasso E. EMERAS trial: results and discussion. Presented at the American College of Cardiology 40th Annual Scientific Session, Atlanta, GA, March 5, 1991.

22. Yusuf S, Collins R, Peto R, et al. Intravenous and intracoronary fibrinolytic therapy in acute myocardial infarction: overview of results on mortality, reinfarction and side effects from 33 randomized controlled trials. Eur Heart J 1985; 6:556-85.

23. Topol EJ, Ellis SG, Wall TC, et al. Does late reperfusion therapy for myocardial infarction improve left ventricular function? Preliminary results of the TAMI-6 randomized, controlled trial. J Am Coll Cardiol 1991; 17:45A (abstract).

24. Rentrop KP, Feit F, Blanke H, et al. Effects of intracoronary streptokinase and intracoronary nitroglycerin infusion on coronary angiographic patterns and mortality in patients with acute myocardial infarction. N Engl J Med 1984; 311:1457-63.

25. Cigarroa RG, Lange RA, Hillis LD. Prognosis after acute myocardial infarction in patients with and without residual antegrade coronary blood flow. Am J Cardiol 1989; 64:155-60.

26. Lange RA, Cigarroa RG, Hillis LD. Influence of residual antegrade coronary blood flow on survival after myocardial infarction in patients with multivessel coronary artery disease. Cor Artery Dis 1990; 1:56-63.

27. The TIMI Study Group. The Thrombolysis in Myocardial Infarction (TIMI) trial: phase I findings. N Engl J Med 1985; 312:923-26.

28. Kircher BE, Topol EJ, O'Neill WW, Pitt B. Prediction of acute myocardial infarct coronary artery recanalization after intravenous thrombolytic therapy. Am J Cardiol 1987; 59:513-5.

29. Califf RM, O'Neill WW, Stack RS, et al. Failure of simple clinical measurements to

predict perfusion status after intravenous thrombolysis. Ann Intern Med 1988; 108:658-62.

30. The I.S.A.M. Study Group. A prospective trial of intravenous streptokinase in acute myocardial infarction (I.S.A.M.). Mortality, morbidity and infarct size at 21 days. N Engl J Med 1986; 314:1465-71.

31. Blanke H, von Hardenberg D, Cohen M. Patterns of creatine kinase release during acute myocardial infarction after nonsurgical reperfusion: comparison with conventional treatment and correlation with infarct size. J Am Coll Cardiol 1984; 3:675-80.

32. Ohman EM, Christenson RH, Sigmon KN, Flanagan CH, Frid DJ, Califf RM. Noninvasive detection of reperfusion after thrombolysis using rapid CK-MB analysis. Circulation 1990; 82(Suppl III):III-281 (abstract).

33. Krucoff MW, Wagner NB, Pope JE, et al. The portable programmable microprocessor-driven real-time 12-lead electrocardiographic monitor: preliminary report of a new device for the noninvasive detection of successful reperfusion or silent coronary reocclusion. Am J Cardiol 1990; 65:143-8.

34. Kwon K, Freedman SB, Wilcox I, et al. The unstable ST segment early after thrombolysis for acute infarction and its usefulness as a marker of recurrent coronary occlusion. Am J Cardiol 1991; 67:109-15.

35. Schroder R, Biamino G, Leitner E-R, et al. Intravenous short-term infusion of streptokinase in acute myocardial infarction. Circulation 1983; 67:536-48.

36. Cribier A, Berland J, Saoudi N, et al. Intracoronary streptokinase, heparin or intravenous streptokinase in acute infarction: Preliminary results of a prospective randomized trial with angiographic evaluation in 44 patients. Haemostasis 1986; 16(Suppl 3):122-9.

37. PRIMI Trial Study Group: Randomized double-blind trial of recombinant prourokinase against streptokinase in acute myocardial infarction. Lancet 1989; 1:863-8.

38. Schwartz F, Hofmann M, Schuler G, et al. Thrombolysis in acute myocardial infarction: effect of intravenous followed by intracoronary streptokinase application on estimates of infarct size. Am J Cardiol 1984; 53:1505-10.

39. Verstraete M, Bory M, Collen D, et al. Randomized trial of intravenous recombinant tissue-type plasminogen activator versus intravenous streptokinase in acute myocardial infarction. Lancet 1985; 1:842-7.

40. Lopez-Sendon J, Seabra-Gomez R, Macaya JC, et al. Intravenous anisoylated plasminogen streptokinase activator kinase in myocardial infarction: A randomized multicenter study. Circulation 1988; 78(Suppl II):II-277 (abstract).

41. Stack RS, O'Connor CM, Mark DB, et al. Coronary perfusion during acute myocardial infarction with a combined therapy of coronary angioplasty and high dose intravenous streptokinase. Circulation 1988; 77:151-61.

42. Charbonnier B, Cribier A, Monassier JP, et al. European multicentre randomized study of APSAC (anisoylated plasminogen streptokinase activator complex) versus streptokinase in myocardial infarction. Arch Mal Coeur 1989; 82:1565-71.

43. Hogg KJ, Gemmill JD, Burns JM, et al. Angiographic patency study of anistreplase versus streptokinase in acute myocardial infarction. Lancet 1990; 335:254-8.

44. Brochier ML, Quillet L, Kulbertus H, et al. Intravenous APSAC versus intravenous streptokinase in evolving myocardial infarction. Drugs 1987; 33(Suppl 3):140-45.

45. Anderson J, Sorenson SG, Moreno FL, et al. Multicenter patency trial of intravenous anistreplase compared with streptokinase in acute myocardial infarction. Circulation 1991; 83:126-40.
46. Six AJ, Louwerenburg HW, Braams R, et al. A double-blind randomized multicenter dose-ranging trial of intravenous streptokinase in acute myocardial infarction. Am J Cardiol 1990; 65:119-23.
47. Vogt P, Schaller MD, Monnier P, et al. Systemic thrombolysis in acute myocardial infarction: Bolus injection of APSAC versus infusion of streptokinase. Eur Heart J 1988; 9(Suppl 1):213 (abstract).
48. Sherry S, Marder VJ. Streptokinase and recombinant tissue plasminogen activator (rt-PA) are equally effective in treating acute myocardial infarction. Ann Intern Med 1991; 114:417-23.
49. Topol EJ, Morris DC, Smalling RW, et al. A multicenter, randomized, placebo-controlled trial of a new form of intravenous recombinant tissue-type plasminogen activator (Activase) in acute myocardial infarction. J Am Coll Cardiol 1987; 9:1205-13.
50. Braunwald E, Knatterud GL, Passamani E, Robertson TL, Solomon R. Update from the Thrombolysis in Myocardial Infarction Trial. J Am Coll Cardiol 1987; 10:970.
51. Carney R, Brandt T, Daley P, et al. Increased efficacy of rt-PA by more rapid administration: The RAAMI Trial. Circulation 1990; 82(Suppl III):III-538 (abstract).
52. Neuhaus KL, Tebbe U, Gottwick M, et al. Intravenous recombinant tissue plasminogen activator (rt-PA) and urokinase in acute myocardial infarction; results of the German Activator Urokinase Study (GAUS). J Am Coll Cardiol 1988; 12:581-7.
53. Topol EJ, Ellis SG, Califf RM, et al. Combined tissue-type plasminogen activator and prostacyclin therapy for acute myocardial infarction. J Am Coll Cardiol 1989; 14:877-84.
54. Califf RM, Topol EJ, Stack RS, et al. An evaluation of combination thrombolytic therapy and timing of cardiac catherization in acute myocardial infarctions: the TAMI-5 randomized trial. Circulation 1991; 83:1543-56.
55. Whitlow PL, Bashore TM for the Craft Study Group. Catherization/Rescue Angioplasty Following Thrombolysis (CRAFT) study: Acute myocardial infarction treated with recombinant tissue plasminogen activator versus urokinase. J Am Coll Cardiol 1991; 17:276A (abstract).
56. Verstraete M, Bliefield W, Brower RW, et al. Double-blind randomized trial of intravenous tissue-type plasminogen activator versus placebo in acute myocardial infarction. Lancet 1985; 2:965-9.
57. Smalling RW, Schumacher R, Morris D, et al. Improved infarct-related arterial patency after high dose, weight-adjusted, rapid infusion of tissue-type plasminogen activator in myocardial infarction: results of a multicenter randomized trial of two dosage regimens. J Am Coll Cardiol 1990; 15:915-21.
58. Johns JA, Gold HK, Leinbach RC, et al. Prevention of coronary artery reocclusion and reduction in late coronary artery stenosis after thrombolytic therapy in patients with acute myocardial infarction. Circulation 1988; 78:546-56.
59. Topol EJ, George BS, Kereiakes DJ, et al. A randomized controlled trial of intravenous tissue plasminogen activator and early intravenous heparin in acute myocardial infarction. Circulation 1989; 79:281-6.

60. Neuhaus KL, Feuerer W, Jeep-Tebbe S, Niederer W, Vogt A, Tebbe U. Improved thrombolysis with recombinant tissue-type plasminogen activator in acute myocardial infarction. J Am Coll Cardiol 1989; 14:1566-9.

61. von Essen R, Vogt A, Roth M, Reib M, Tebbe U, Neuhaus KL. Early patency of infarct-related vessel after accelerated infusion of 100 mg rt-PA as compared to 30 mg APSAC: results of the TAPS study. Eur Heart J 1991; 12:30 (abstract).

62. Wall TC, Topol EJ, George BS, Elis SG, Samaha J, Kereiakes DJ, Worley SJ, Sigmon K, Califf RM. The TAMI-7 trial of accelerated plasminogen activator dose regimens for coronary thrombolysis. Circulation 1990; 82(Suppl III):III-538 (abstract).

63. Tebbe U, Tanswell P, Seifried E, Feuerer W, Scholz K-H, Herrmann KS. Single-bolus injection of recombinant tissue-type plasminogen activator in acute myocardial infarction. Am J Cardiol 1989; 64:448-53.

64. Tranchesi B, Verstraete M, Vanhove P, et al. Intravenous bolus administration of recombinant tissue plasminogen activator to patients with acute myocardial infarction. Cor Artery Disease 1990; 1:83-8.

65. Purvis JA, Trouton TG, Dolzell GW, et al. Pre-hospital double bolus alteplase in acute myocardial infarction. Circulation 1990; 82(Suppl III):III-538 (abstract).

66. McKendall GR, Attubato M, Drew TM, et al. Improved infarct artery patency using a modified regimen of t-PA: results of the pre-hospital administration of t-PA (PATS) pilot trial. J Am Coll Cardiol 1990; 15:3A (abstract).

67. Topol EJ. Ultrathrombolysis. J Am Coll Cardiol 1990; 15:922-4.

68. Grines CL, Nissen SE, Booth DC, et al. A prospective, randomized trial comparing combination half dose t-PA with streptokinase to full dose tPA in acute myocardial infarction; preliminary report. J Am Coll Cardiol 1990; 15:4A (abstract).

69. Grines CL, Nissen SE, Booth DC, et al. A new thrombolytic regimen for acute myocardial infarction using combination half dose tissue-type plasminogen activator with full dose streptokinase: a pilot study. J Am Coll Cardiol 1989; 14:573-80.

70. Bonnet JL, Bory M, D'Houdain F, et al. Association of tissue plasminogen activator and streptokinase in acute myocardial infarction: preliminary data. Circulation 1989; 80(Suppl II):II-343 (abstract).

71. Topol EJ, Califf RM, George BS, et al. Coronary arterial thrombolysis with combined infusion of recombinant tissue-type plasminogen activator and urokinase in patients with acute myocardial infarction. Circulation 1988; 77:1100-7.

72. The Urokinase and Alteplase in Myocardial Infarction Collaborative Group. Combination of urokinase and alteplase in the treatment of myocardial infarction. Cor Artery Dis 1991; 2:225-35.

73. Collen D, van de Werf F. Coronary thrombolysis with low dose synergistic combinations of recombinant tissue-type plasminogen activator and recombinant single-chain urokinase-type plasminogen activator (rscu-PA) in man. Am J Cardiol 1987; 60:431-4.

74. Tranchesi B, Bellotti G, Chamone DF, Verstraete M. Effect of combined administration of saruplase and single-chain alteplase on coronary recanalization in acute myocardial infarction. Am J Cardiol 1989; 164:229-32.

75. Bode C, Nordt T, Baumann H, et al. Combination therapy with prourokinase and

tissue plasminogen activator in acute myocardial infarction is both effective and highly specific. Circulation 1989; 80(Suppl II):II-344 (abstract).

76. ISIS-3 Update. Scientific background to the ISIS-3 comparisons. Evidence from other studies. Brookline, MA:ISIS Coordinating Center, February 1991, p. 3.

77. Kalbfleisch JM. Simplified short-term administration of rt-PA in patients with acute myocardial infarction. Circulation 1990; 82(Suppl III):III-539 (abstract).

78. Kasper W, Meinertz T, Wollschlager H, et al. Coronary thrombolysis during acute myocardial infarction by intravenous BRL 26921, a new anisoylated plasminogen-streptokinase activator complex. Am J Cardiol 1986; 58:418-21.

79. Been M, de Bono DP, Muir AL, Boulton FE, Hillis WS, Hornung R. Coronary thrombolysis with intravenous anisoylated plasminogen-streptokinase activator complex BRL 26921. Br Heart J 1985; 53:253-9.

80. Visser RF. Angiographic assessment of patency and reocclusion: preliminary results of the Dutch APSAC Reocclusion Multicenter Study (ARMS). Clin Cardiol 1990; 13:45-7.

81. Mathey DG, Schofer J, Sheehan FH, Becher H, Tilsner V, Dodge HT. Intravenous urokinase in acute myocardial infarction. Am J Cardiol 1985; 55:878-82.

82. Wall TC, Phillips HR III, Stack RS, et al. Results of high dose intravenous urokinase for acute myocardial infarction. Am J Cardiol 1990; 65:124-31.

83. Vermeer F, Massberg I, Meyer J, et al. Saruplase, a new fibrin specific thrombolytic agent; efficacy and safety in the first 1000 patients. J Am Coll Cardiol 1991; 17:152A (abstract).

84. Anderson JL, Sorenson SG, Karagounis L, et al. A double-blind, randomized comparison of anistreplase and alteplase in acute myocardial infarction: coronary patency results from the TEAM-3 Study. J Am Coll Cardiol 1991; 17:152A (abstract).

85. The TIMI Study Group. Comparison of invasive and conservative strategies after treatment with intravenous tissue plasminogen activator in acute myocardial infarction: results of the Thrombolysis in Myocardial Infarction (TIMI) phase II trial. N Engl J Med 1989; 320:618-27.

86. Magnani B. Plasminogen Activator Italian Multicenter Study (PAIMS): comparison of intravenous recombinant single-chain human tissue-type plasminogen activator (rt-PA) with intravenous streptokinase in acute myocardial infarction. J Am Coll Cardiol 1989; 13:19-26.

87. de Bono DP, Simoons ML, Tijssen J, et al. Early intravenous heparin enhances coronary patency after alteplase thrombolysis: results of a randomized double blind European Cooperative Study Group trial. Br Heart J (in press).

88. Machecourt J, Cassagnes J, Bassand JP, et al. Results of a randomized trial comparing APSAC and rt-PA for the preservation of left ventricular function after acute myocardial infarction. J Am Coll Cardiol 1990; 15:64A (abstract).

89. National Heart Foundation of Australia Coronary Thrombolysis Group. Coronary thrombolysis and myocardial salvage by tissue plasminogen activator given up to 4 hours after onset of myocardial infarction. Lancet 1988; 1:203-7.

90. White HD, Rivers JT, Maslowski AH, et al. Effect of intravenous streptokinase as

compared with that of tissue plasminogen activator on left ventricular function after first myocardial infarction. N Engl J Med 1989; 320:817-21.

91. Bassand JP, Machecourt J, Cassagnes J, et al. Multicenter trial of intravenous anisoylated plasminogen streptokinase activator complex (APSAC) in acute myocardial infarction; Effects on infarct size and left ventricular function. J Am Coll Cardiol 1989; 13:988-97.

92. Kennedy JW, Martin GV, Davis KB, et al. The Western Washington intravenous streptokinase in acute myocardial infarction randomized trial. Circulation 1988; 77: 345-52.

93. White HD, Norris RM, Brown MA, et al. Effect of intravenous streptokinase on left ventricular function and early survival after acute myocardial infarction. N Engl J Med 1987; 317:850-5.

94. Ohman EM, Califf RM, Topol EJ, et al. Consequences of reocclusion after successful reperfusion therapy in acute myocardial infarction. Circulation 1990; 82:781-91.

95. Ellis SG, Debowey D, Bates ER, Topol EJ. Treatment of recurrent ischemia after thrombolysis and successful reperfusion for acute myocardial infarction: effect on in-hospital mortality and left ventricular function. J Am Coll Cardiol 1991; 17: 752-7.

96. Stump DC, Califf RM, Topol EJ, et al. Pharmacokinetics of thrombolysis with recombinant tissue-type plasminogen activator: correlation with characteristics of and clinical outcomes in patients with acute myocardial infarction. Circulation 1989; 80: 1222-30.

97. Harrison DG, Ferguson DW, Collins SM, et al. Rethrombosis after reperfusion with streptokinase: Importance of geometry of residual lesions. Circulation 1984; 69: 991-9.

98. Gash AK, Spann JF, Sherry S, et al. Factors influencing reocclusion after coronary thrombolysis for acute myocardial infarction. Am J Cardiol 1986; 57:175-7.

99. Topol EJ, Califf RM, George BS, et al. A randomized trial of immediate versus delayed elective angioplasty after intravenous tissue plasminogen activator in acute myocardial infarction. N Engl J Med 1987; 317:581-8.

100. Simoons ML, Arnold AER, Betriu A, et al. Thrombolysis with tissue plasminogen activator in acute myocardial infarction; no additional benefit from immediate percutaneous coronary angioplasty. Lancet 1988; 1:197-203.

101. The TIMI Research Group. Immediate vs delayed catheterization and angioplasty following thrombolytic therapy for acute myocardial infarction: TIMI II A results. JAMA 1988; 260:2849-58.

102. Ellis SG, Topol EJ, George BS, et al. Recurrent ischemia without warning: analysis of risk factors for in-hospital ischemic events following successful thrombolysis with intravenous tissue plasminogen activator. Circulation 1989; 80:1159-65.

103. Hsia J, Hamilton WP, Kleiman N, Roberts R, Chaitman BR, Ross AM. A comparison between heparin and low-dose aspirin as adjunctive therapy with tissue plasminogen activator for acute myocardial infarction. N Engl J Med 1990; 323:1433-7.

104. Bleich SD, Nichols TC, Schumacher RR, Cooke DH, Tate DA, Teichman SL. Effect of heparin on coronary arterial patency after thrombolysis with tissue plasminogen activator in acute myocardial infarction. Am J. Cardiol 1990; 66:1412-7.

105. Braunwald E. Myocardial reperfusion, limitation of infarct size, and improved survival: should the paradigm be expanded? Circulation 1989; 79:441-4.
106. Califf R, Topol E, Gersh BJ. From myocardial salvage to patient salvage in acute myocardial infarction: the role of reperfusion therapy. J Am Coll Cardiol 1989; 14: 1382-8.
107. Fortin DF, Califf RM. Long-term survival from acute myocardial infarction: salutary effect of an open coronary vessel. Am J Med 1990; 88:9N-15N.
108. Weisman HF, Healy B. Myocardial infarct expansion, infarct extension, and reinfarction: pathophysiologic concepts. Prog Cardiovasc Dis 1987; 30:73-110.
109. White HD, Norris RM, Brown MA, Brandt P, Whitlock R, Wild C. Left ventricular end-systolic volume as the major determinant of survival after recovery from myocardial infarction. Circulation 1987; 76:44-51.
110. Vogel WM, Apstein CG, Briggs LL, et al. Acute alterations in left ventricular diastolic chamber stiffness: role of the "erectile" effect of coronary arterial pressure and flow in normal and damaged hearts. Circ Res 1982; 51:465-78.
111. Hale SL, Kloner RA. Left ventricular topographic alterations in the completely healed rat infarct caused by early and late coronary artery reperfusion. Am Heart J 1988; 116:1508-13.
112. Hochman JS, Choo H. Limitation of myocardial infarct expansion of reperfusion independent of myocardial salvage. Circulation 1987; 75:299-306.
113. Serruys PW, Simoons ML, Suryapranata H, et al. Preservation of global and regional ventricular function after early thrombolysis in acute myocardial infarction. J. Am Coll Cardiol 1986; 7:729-42.
114. Kersschot IE, Brugada P, Ramental M, et al. Effects of early reperfusion in acute myocardial infarction on arrhythmias induced by programmed stimulation: a prospective, randomized study. J Am Coll Cardiol 1986; 7:1234-42.
115. Sager PT, Perlmutter PA, Rosenfeld LE, McPherson CA, Wackers FJTH, Batsford ZWP. Electrophysiologic effects of thrombolytic therapy in patient with a transmural anterior myocardial infarction complicated by left ventricular aneurysm formation. J Am Coll Cadriol 1988; 12:19-24.
116. Gang ES, Lew AS, Hong M, et al. Decreased incidence in ventricular late potentials after successful thrombolytic therapy for acute myocardial infarction. N Engl J Med 1989; 321:712-6.
117. VanderWall EE, VanDijkman PRN, DeRoos A, et al. Diagnostic significance of gadolinium DTPA (diethylenetriamine penta-acetic acid) enhanced magnetic resonance imaging and thrombolytic treatment for acute myocardial infarction; Its potential in assessing reperfusion. Br Heart J 1990; 63:12-17.
118. Calkins H, Maughan WL, Weisman HF, et al. Effect of acute volume load on refractoriness and arrhythmia development in isolated, chronically infarcted dog hearts. Circulation 1989; 79:687-97.
119. Inoue H, Zipes DP. Results of sympathetic denervation in the canine heart: supersensitivity that may be arrhythmogenic. Circulation 1987; 75:877-87.
120. Pfeffer MA, Braunwald E, Cuddy TE, et al. Selection bias in the use of thrombolytic therapy in acute myocardial infarction. Circulation 1989; 80(Suppl II):II-522 (abstract).

121. Cragg DR, Bonema JD, Jaiyesimi IA, et al. Ineligibility for intravenous thrombolytic therapy predicts high mortality after acute myocardial infarction. Circulation 1989; 80(Suppl II):II-522 (abstract).

122. Topol EJ, Holmes DR, Rogers WJ. Coronary angioplasty for acute myocardial infarction: a critical appraisal. Ann Intern Med 1991; 114:877-85.

123. Simoons ML, Vos J, Tijssen JGP, Vermeer F, Verheught F, Krauss AK. Long-term benefit of early thrombolytic therapy in patients with acute MI: 5-year follow-up of trial conduction by the Interuniversity Cardiology Institute of the Netherlands. J Am Coll Cardiol 1989; 14:1609-15.

124. The International Study Group. In-hospital mortality and clinical course of 20,891 patients with suspected acute myocardial infarction randomized between alteplase and streptokinase with or without heparin. Lancet 1990; 336:71-5.

125. Sleight P. ISIS-3 Trial: results of SK versus APSAC versus t-PA. Presented at the American College of Cardiology 40th Annual Scientific Session, Atlanta, GA, March 5, 1991.

2

Left Ventricular Function After Acute Myocardial Infarction: Ventriculographic and Clinical Endpoints

Jeffrey J. Popma
Washington Cardiology Center, Washington, D.C.

L. David Hillis
University of Texas Southwestern Medical Center, Dallas, Texas

INTRODUCTION

The timely administration of thrombolytic therapy for acute myocardial infarction has reduced the in-hospital mortality for patients under age 70 years to 4-6% (1-5). A reduction in mortality of 15-20% also has been achieved after thrombolytic administration in the elderly and in patients presenting 6-24 hr after symptom onset (6). Despite these salutary effects on mortality, current thrombolytic strategies remain limited by persistent occlusion of the infarct-related artery in some patients (7), reocclusion despite initially successful thrombolysis in others (8), and an often clinically devastating intracranial hemorrhage in an occasional recipient (1-5). Moreover, certain patients, particularly women, those with prior myocardial infarction, or those with symptoms of congestive heart failure, remain at especially high risk for significant in-hospital morbidity and mortality (2,4,9).

To address these shortcomings, ongoing thrombolytic trials have been designed to define the optimal balance between the aggressive pursuit of infarct-related artery patency, with its potential to improve survival, and the risk of major bleeding events (10). With thrombolytic agents administered in virtually all study limbs, most patients in these trials are not at particularly high risk for mortality after myocardial infarction, thus necessitating the enrollment of 15,000 patients to demonstrate a 20% difference in survival (2,11).

29

Based on the prethrombolytic correlation of left ventricular ejection fraction and mortality after myocardial infarction (12,13), some authors have suggested that left ventricular function, measured as a continuous variable, be used as a surrogate endpoint for mortality in comparative thrombolytic trials, reducing the number of patients required to demonstrate significant differences amongthrombolytic strategies to less than 400 (11). Placebo-controlled thrombolytic trials have shown improvement in both left ventricular ejection fraction and regional wall motion in most (14–16), but not all (17,18), series. However, since the correlation between left ventricular ejection fraction and survival is imperfect (19), some authors have recommended that left ventricular ejection fraction be abandoned as a surrogate mortality endpoint in comparative thrombolytic trials (20).

The purposes of this review are: (a) to summarize the current indices for evaluating left ventricular function after acute myocardial infarction and to discuss factors relating to the timing and ultimate recovery of function, (b) to discuss the limitations of standard indices of left ventricular function as primary endpoints for thrombolytic trials, (c) to provide alternative clinical indices of left ventricular function that may yield relevant information to the clinician in evaluating alternative thrombolytic strategies, and (d) to examine the effects of single-agent, combination, and adjunctive thrombolytic strategies on these indices of left ventricular function after acute myocardial infarction.

INDICES OF LEFT VENTRICULAR FUNCTION

In the late 1970s, Reimer et al. (21) showed that experimental canine coronary occlusion caused progressive myocardial necrosis from endocardium to epicardium, with the extent of necrosis dependent on the duration of occlusion. With the subsequent angiographic demonstration by DeWood et al. (22) that a totally occlusive coronary thrombus was present in nearly 90% of patients with evolving Q-wave infarction, it was assumed that myocardial "salvage" was possible in patients with myocardial infarction, provided that coronary perfusion could be quickly reestablished with a thrombolytic agent. The paradigm in the early 1980s of pharmacological reperfusion of the infarct-related artery, reduction of myocardial infarct size and left ventricular dysfunction, and improvement in survival, potentially obtainable with thrombolytic therapy, represented an exciting therapeutic advance for patients with acute myocardial infarction (23).

To establish the clinical efficacy of thrombolytic therapy in patients with acute myocardial infarction, early studies using intracoronary streptokinase relied on the documentation of coronary reperfusion as a principal endpoint (24–26). The patients in these early series were often treated relatively late after symptom onset; although infarct-related artery reperfusion occurred in 70–80%, the evidence that myocardial "salvage" occurred was not convincing (17). Subsequent large-scale, placebo-controlled trials in patients treated early after symptom onset were required to establish the interactive relationship among infarct-related artery patency, myocardial "salvage," and survival after thrombolytic therapy for acute myocardial infarction. To evaluate one of these endpoints, myocardial "salvage," several indices of left ventricular function were used (Table 1).

Left Ventricular Ejection Fraction

Left ventricular ejection fraction, the most commonly used index of left ventricular function, is easily calculated from end-diastolic and end-systolic ventricular contours using single or biplane area length (27,28), volumetric (29), or radionuclide (17) methods. Quantitation of ejection using these techniques provides a useful continuous measure of global ventricular function and, therefore, a potential index of myocardial "salvage" in patients after myocardial infarction. In the prethrombolytic era, global left ventricular ejection fraction was an important predictor of survival after infarction (12,13,30); as a result, it was advocated as a surrogate endpoint for mortality in clinical thrombolytic trials (11).

The use of left ventricular ejection fraction as the sole index of myocardial "salvage" after thrombolytic therapy may have important limitations (20). In trials using left ventricular ejection fraction as the primary endpoint, contrast ventriculograms may not be obtainable in all patients (Table 2); imputed values for missing variables due to death have been used in some (31), but not all (32), trials. Furthermore, incomplete ventriculographic follow-up is often a reality, due to patient or physician refusal, medical contraindications, or early ischemic complications (20). As a result, the most seriously ill patients may be excluded from analysis (20). In those who undergo ventriculography, technical exclusions such as inadequate ventricular opacification with contrast, premature contractions, or patient movement may preclude analysis in as many as 20–30% of studies. In the patients with technically adequate studies, noninfarct-zone hyperkinesis may result in a near-normal global left ventricular ejection fraction, despite marked infarct-related regional wall motion asynergy (33–35). With recovery of infarct-related regional wall motion over days to weeks, noninfarct-related hyperkinesis lessens and little or no net change in global ejection fraction may be noted over time. Estimation of myocardial "salvage" using single-plane ventriculo-graphic methods may also be problematic (36), particularly in patients with circumflex occlusions (37).

These factors may account for the imperfect relationship among left ventricular ejection fraction, myocardial infarct size (38), and survival (19,20,39) in clinical thrombolytic trials. Furthermore, as noted by van de Werf (19), patients treated soon after the onset of symptoms of acute myocardial infarction have the greatest reduction in mortality. At least some of the patients who survive because of successful thrombolytic administration will have depressed left ventricular function, negating the improvement in global left ventricular function seen in oth-

Table 1   Indices of Left Ventricular Function After Myocardial Infarction

Index	Advantages	Disadvantages	Comments
LVEF	Widely applied Easily standard-ized	Poor correlation with survival Missing values in 20-30% Little change over time ? Correlation with symptoms	Beneficial effects demonstrated in placebo-con-trolled trials, but not in compara-tive and adjunc-tive trials
Regional wall motion	Correlated with survival Sensitive index of myocardial salvage	Requires computer-assisted analysis Missing values in 20-30% ? Correlation with symptoms	Centerline methods used in TAMI and TIMI trials
Left ventricu-lar volumes	Sensitive index of remodeling	Requires computer-assisted analysis Missing values in 20-30% Calibration often difficult Little correlation with symptoms	Absolute differ-ences in volumes have been small (Table 6)
"Extensive" LV dysfunc-tion	Useful in reduc-ing enrollment numbers for significance Incorporates clini-cal, EKG, and ECHO criteria	Correlation with survival not demonstrated	Validated in trial of > 15,000 patients
Composite clinical endpoint	Allows ranking of all adverse outcomes	Difficult to interpret clinical meaning	May be useful in comparative thrombolytic trials when LVEF is similar

LVEF = left ventricular ejection fraction; TIMI = Thrombolysis In Myocardial Infarction Trial; TAMI = Thrombolysis and Angioplasty in Myocardial Infarction Trial; LV = left ventricular.

Table 2   Factors Accounting for Incomplete
Ventriculographic Analysis

Patients enrolled	127
Ventriculography at 7-10 days	119
Technically adequate	97
Technically inadequate	22
PVCs	17
Inadequate filling	3
Patient movement	2
No follow-up ventriculography	8
Death	3
Early CABG	3
Patient refusal	2

PVCs = premature ventricular contractions; CABG =
coronary bypass surgery.
Source: Derived from the University of Michigan
Core Laboratory analysis of ventriculograms obtained from 127 consecutive patients enrolled in an
adjunctive thrombolytic trial.

ers when mean ejection fractions for treatment groups are compared (19). For
these reasons, clinical trials using left ventricular ejection fraction as the sole index of myocardial preservation may underestimate the overall efficacy of the
agent under evaluation (40).

Infarct-Related Regional Wall Motion

The quantitation of infarct-related regional wall motion may provide a useful index of myocardial "salvage" after myocardial infarction. Characterization of infarct-related regional wall motion using two-dimensional echocardiography has
the advantage of allowing repetitive studies in the postinfarction period, although
precise quantitation is sometimes difficult. Alternatively, contrast or radionuclide
ventriculography, while somewhat limited in the ability to be performed serially,
may permit a more standardized assessment of regional wall motion. At least three
methods of quantitating regional wall motion using contrast ventriculograms have
been described (Fig. 1) (41-43). With the "centerline" method used in the Thrombolysis in Myocardial Infarction (TIMI) and Thrombolysis and Angioplasty in
Myocardial Infarction (TAMI) trials, the left ventricular contour is divided into
100 chords constructed perpendicular to a centerline drawn midway between the
end-diastolic and end-systolic contours (Fig. 2). Based on the mean regional wall
motion obtained from a normal reference population, infarct-related regional wall

motion, expressed in units of standard deviation/chord, provides a useful index of myocardial injury and recovery in patients with acute myocardial infarction. Quantitation of infarct-related regional wall motion may provide a more sensitive index of the recovery of left ventricular function than global ejection fraction in patients after myocardial infarction (33–35).

Noninfarct-Related Regional Wall Motion

In the peri-infarction period, noninfarct-related hyperkinesia may result from increased catecholamines, elevated left ventricular end-diastolic pressure, and/or intraventricular unloading of the noninfarct zone. A more favorable prognosis has been demonstrated in patients with noninfarct-related hyperkinesis after acute myocardial infarction compared to those with normal or depressed noninfarct-related regional wall motion (44). In a series of 332 patients treated with intravenous t-PA reported by Grines et al. (44), in-hospital mortality was closely related to function of the noninfarct zone and to the number of diseased vessels, as assessed 90 min after thrombolytic administration. Notably, in 266 patients with paired 90-min and 7-day ventriculograms, little change was noted in noninfarct-zone wall motion from the acute to convalescent period. Noninfarct-related hyperkinesis in the acute phase tended to recede by the time of convalescent evaluation, whereas depressed noninfarct-zone wall motion tended to improve during the follow-up period (44). The implications of these changes are not known.

Left Ventricular End-Diastolic and End-Systolic Volumes

In the absence of thrombolytic therapy, left ventricular dilatation, defined as a ≥20% increase in end-diastolic volume, occurs in up to one-third of patients within 6 months of myocardial infarction (45). Resulting from infarct expansion, slippage of myofibrils, and lengthening of the necrotic myocytes, left ventricular dilatation is most pronounced in patients with anterior infarction (45,46) and in those with extensive infarct-related regional wall motion abnormalities (47,48). Cavity dilatation may begin within hours of infarction (46) and progressively increase during the subsequent weeks to months (45,46,48,49). Importantly, the magnitude of cavity dilatation may have prognostic significance, since left ventricular end-systolic volume is a more important predictor of 5-year survival than left ventricular ejection fraction, particularly when the ejection fraction is <50% (30).

Left ventricular cavity dilatation after myocardial infarction may be ameliorated by early spontaneous or pharmacologically induced coronary reperfusion or by altering left ventricular stress and/or loading conditions. Left ventricular volumes, measured 1 month after myocardial infarction, were unchanged in patients

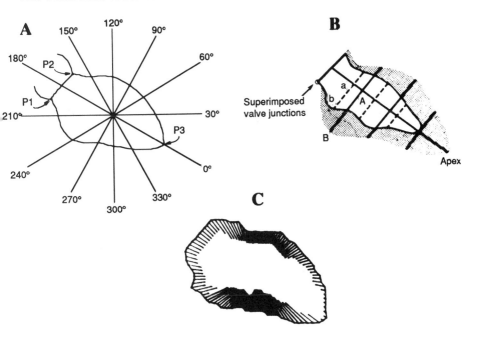

Figure 1   Three methods of analysis of regional wall motion using contrast ventriculography. Using the polar coordinate reference or "center-of-gravity" method, reported by Cole et al. (43), the center of the left ventricular silhouette is determined from the margins of the aortic annulus and the apex (A). End-diastolic and end-systolic contours are superimposed, and the radial shortening/second is determined for the particular region of interest. Using the second method, described by Sniderman et al. (42), the valve junctions are superimposed from the end-diastolic and end-systolic contours (B). Regional wall motion is expressed as the fractional change from hemilength AB (end-diastole) to hemilength ab (end-systole) for the particular region of interest. Using the third technique, the centerline method of Sheehan et al. (41) (C), 100 perpendicular lines are drawn between the end-diastolic and end-systolic contours. Regional wall motion, expressed as the SD/chord, is determined by comparison of the regional wall motion in patients with regional wall motion in a reference population.

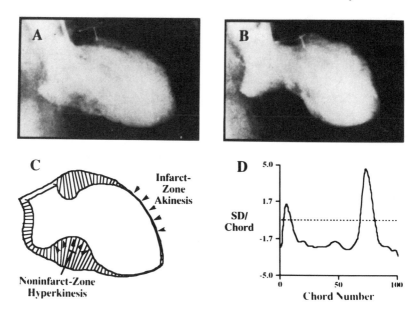

Figure 2   Centerline method of regional wall motion analysis. After acute myocardial infarction, the end-diastolic (A) and end-systolic contour (B) are digitized. End-diastolic and end-systolic images are then superimposed using a computer-assisted method, and 100 chords are constructed perpendicular to the ventricular contours (C), demonstrating anterior infarct-related akinesis and non-infarct-related hyperkinesis. In this patient with single vessel left anterior descending artery disease, chords 10–66 are used to express anterior infarct-related regional wall motion, and chords 67–80 are used to express inferior non-infarct-related regional wall motion (D).

with early reperfusion but increased significantly in those without spontaneous reperfusion (50). In 332 patients randomized to intracoronary streptokinase or conservative treatment, end-diastolic and end-systolic ventricular volumes were significantly lower 7–10 days after infarction in patients treated with streptokinase (34,51). Moreover, left ventricular volumes were significantly higher in patients with infarct-related coronary occlusion, despite attempts at pharmacological and mechanical reperfusion, than in those with sustained reperfusion (34).

A late determination of left ventricular volumes after myocardial infarction may demonstrate favorable improvements in left ventricular remodeling not apparent from the evaluation of global or regional wall motion alone. In the Thrombolysis and Angioplasty in Myocardial Infarction (TAMI-6) trial reported by Topol et al. (52), patients presenting 6–24 hr after symptom onset were randomly assigned to t-PA 100 mg over 2 hr or placebo. Although no differences were detected between groups in ejection fraction or regional wall motion at 6-month follow-up ventriculography, the t-PA-treated patients manifested no increase in cavity size, whereas the placebo-treated group had a significant increase in median end-diastolic volume (52). Thus, thrombolytic administration 6-24 hr after symptom onset may exert a beneficial effect on left ventricular remodeling, independent of its effects on regional and global left ventricular function.

Clinical Indices of Left Ventricular Function

Clinical indices of left ventricular dysfunction may serve as valuable endpoints in comparative thrombolytic trials. Several studies have examined the effect of thrombolytic therapy in reducing mortality in patients presenting with clinical manifestations of left ventricular dysfunction and in preventing the development of symptoms of congestive heart failure after myocardial infarction. In the Gruppo Italiano per lo studio della streptochinasi nell'infarto miocardico (GISSI-1) trial (1), Killip classification was used to stratify patients according to the severity of left ventricular dysfunction soon after symptom onset. In all four Killip subgroups, mortality was similar in patients treated with streptokinase or placebo, and it was nearly identical to prethrombolytic historical control data (9). In patients with Killip IV symptoms, mortality was 77% and 72% for streptokinase- and placebo-treated patients, respectively, suggesting that thrombolytic administration may have little effect in altering prognosis in patients with severely compromised left ventricular function.

Other studies have examined the effect of thrombolytic therapy in preventing symptoms of congestive heart failure during the in-hospital period. Although one placebo-controlled trial suggested that t-PA reduced the incidence of cardiogenic shock (3.8% for t-PA compared to 5.1% for placebo; $p < 0.05$) (4), most have suggested only a modest, if any, reduction in the incidence of in-hospital congestive heart failure (1,5,14,18).

To incorporate clinical criteria for congestive heart failure and objective evidence of left ventricular dysfunction, the Gruppo Italiano per lo studio della sopravvivenza nell'infarto miocardico (GISSI-2) trial (53) used a combined clinical, electrocardiographic, and echocardiographic endpoint to evaluate left ventricular function. "Extensive left ventricular damage" was defined as the presence of clinical heart failure (any two of bibasilar rales, third heart sound, dyspnea, or radiographic evidence of pulmonary congestion) or, in the absence of clinical manifestations of heart failure, evidence of extensive myocardial necrosis, as assessed by two-dimensional echocardiography and electrocardiography. Using these criteria, extensive left ventricular dysfunction developed in 14% of patients after myocardial infarction but was not affected by the thrombolytic agent administered (53). Despite the objectivity of this combined endpoint, some have sug-

Table 3   Ranking of Adverse Clinical
Endpoints

Death
Intracranial hemorrhage
Nonhemorrhagic stroke
Ejection fraction < 0.30
Reinfarction
Heart failure
Pulmonary edema
Cardiac arrest
Emergency bypass surgery
Ischemia (without reinfarction)
Reocclusion
Emergency coronary angioplasty
Ejection fraction < 0.45
Ischemia without ST-segment changes
Nonemergency CABG
Transfusion requirement

Ranking in order of decreasing clinical importance.
Source: Modified from Califf et al. (20), with
permission.

gested that the heterogeneous methods used to define left ventricular dysfunction
may limit its clinical applicability (20).

Accounting for the relative severity of each potential adverse outcome in patients after myocardial infarction, a composite endpoint, including both left ventricular ejection fraction and symptoms of congestive heart failure, may be
valuable (20). Ranking these endpoints according to their relative clinical importance would allow a statistical comparison of differing treatment strategies using a
variety of analytical methods (20). At the 1989 American Heart Association
Meeting, 407 cardiologists ranked 16 adverse clinical outcomes after myocardial
infarction by their order of clinical importance (Table 3) (20). Based on this ranking, prevention of severe left ventricular dysfunction and symptoms of congestive
heart failure were of more clinical significance than the prevention of emergency
bypass surgery, recurrent ischemia (without infarction), and reocclusion. Notably, preservation of left ventricular ejection fraction >0.45 was of lesser importance. Several trials are currently examining the value of the use of such a
composite clinical endpoint (54).

From the preceding discussion, it is apparent that several indices of left ventricular function are available to assess the efficacy of thrombolytic strategies af-

ter myocardial infarction. Left ventricular ejection fraction, the most widely used endpoint of ventricular function, is easily determined but may underestimate the degree of myocardial salvage, principally due to noninfarct zone hyperkinesis. Infarct-related and noninfarct-related regional wall motion are more sensitive indices of ventricular recovery and may have prognostic importance. Quantitation of left ventricular volumes early and late after thrombolytic therapy may provide supplemental information about left ventricular remodeling after infarction. From a clinical perspective, prevention of severe left ventricular dysfunction and symptoms of congestive heart failure may be evaluated separately or as a composite clinical endpoint. By obtaining a comprehensive assessment of left ventricular function, comparison of the relative advantages of alternative thrombolytic regimens may be possible.

TIMING OF RECOVERY OF LEFT VENTRICULAR FUNCTION

In experimental models of coronary reperfusion, brief periods of ischemia may result in marked delays in the recovery of regional left ventricular function (55). For example, in the canine model, 4–7 days may be required for regional wall motion recovery after a 60-min occlusion and 4 weeks may be required when the occlusion lasts more than 3 hr (56). This delayed recovery of left ventricular function, termed myocardial "stunning" (57,58), has been attributed to alterations in oxidative metabolism, calcium flux, and accumulation of leukocytes within the ischemic myocardium (40,57,58).

Although documentation of delayed recovery of regional myocardial function after coronary occlusion has been reproducible in the experimental model, the timing of recovery of wall motion abnormalities after thrombolytic therapy in patients with acute myocardial infarction is less well characterized. Despite angiographically documented reperfusion, little improvement in regional or global left ventricular performance is noted when ventriculography is performed 90 min after the initiation of therapy (59,60). Further, the measurement of ventricular function within 24 hr of thrombolytic administration may provide variable results (61).

After 24 hr, progressive improvement in regional wall motion occurs in some patients, with the magnitude of improvement offering insight into prognosis (62,63). In an echocardiographic series of 23 patients with successful pharmacological and/or mechanical reperfusion, regional wall motion progressively improved at day 1 and day 3 but was without further improvement by day 7 (62). Moreover, in a series of 165 patients receiving thrombolytic therapy, improvement in left ventricular ejection fraction, assessed 90 min and 3 days following thrombolytic administration, correlated with an improved prognosis (63).

Others have suggested that the full recovery of left ventricular function in pa-

tients may be more delayed (64). In 264 patients receiving intracoronary streptokinase, global ejection fraction was 54 ± 12% acutely and 52 ± 12% 3 days later
(p = NS), but it increased significantly to 57 ± 12% during the subsequent 6
months. The lack of improvement at 3 days was attributed to an early loss of noninfarct zone hyperkinesis despite improved, but persistently abnormal, infarct-
zone wall motion; the significant improvement in left ventricular ejection fraction
between 3 days and 6 months was felt due to further improvement in infarct-related hypokinesia (64). Delayed recovery of ventricular function has also been
noted in patients undergoing "rescue" coronary angioplasty (65). However, based
on serial study of 433 patients reported by Harrison et al. (66), no improvement in
global left ventricular ejection fraction or regional wall motion was noted between
10 days and 6 months after myocardial infarction. Lack of improvement of left
ventricular ejection fraction from 7 days to 6 weeks has also been noted by others
(67).

These results suggest that the optimal timing of the analysis of left ventricular
function is 7–10 days after thrombolytic therapy. Studies that evaluate left ventricular function earlier than 3 days may be limited by persistently delayed infarct-
zone hypokinesis, which may eventually resolve. Late improvements in left
ventricular ejection fraction or regional wall motion have not been demonstrated,
although ventricular remodeling may best be assessed 6 months following thrombolytic administration.

FACTORS INFLUENCING RECOVERY OF LEFT
VENTRICULAR FUNCTION

Despite the early administration of thrombolytic agents, complete recovery of left
ventricular function does not occur in many patients (33,68). In a serial echocardiographic study of patients following thrombolytic therapy for acute myocardial
infarction, left ventricular function was evaluated acutely and at 1, 2, 3, and 10
days. Surprisingly, the administration of intravenous streptokinase within 4 hr of
symptom onset resulted in an improvement of regional wall motion by 10 days in
only 33% of patients (68). To determine which patients will recover ventricular
function after thrombolytic administration, a variety of clinical and angiographic
factors have been examined.

Infarct-Related Artery Patency

Recent studies have demonstrated the prognostic importance of a patent infarct-
related artery after acute myocardial infarction (69,70). Similarly, infarct-related
artery patency, both acutely and at the time of follow-up arteriography, is the most
consistent predictor of recovery of left ventricular function after thrombolytic
therapy (71–76). The critical importance of coronary recanalization on the recov-

ery of left ventricular function was demonstrated in early, nonrandomized series of patients receiving intracoronary streptokinase after acute myocardial infarction. In these series, infarct-artery recanalization was associated with improved global and regional left ventricular function, whereas unsuccessful recanalization was associated with no improvement or worsened left ventricular function (72,73). Patients who fail to reperfuse the infarct-related artery 90 min after intravenous t-PA have lower left ventricular ejection fractions and worse regional wall motion than those with reperfusion (72). Despite successful "rescue" coronary angioplasty, ejection fraction may remain depressed in many of these patients (7), although late improvements in left ventricular ejection fraction have been noted in some (65). Furthermore, patients with in-hospital reocclusion following successful reperfusion had lesser improvements in global and regional left ventricular function at 7–10 days than those with sustained reperfusion (8). Importantly, the beneficial effects on left ventricular function of a patent infarct-related artery may not be limited to improvements in left ventricular ejection fraction; rather, they may include preservation of left ventricular cavity size, provision of collaterals to other diseased arteries (20), and/or a diminution in electrical instability, with a reduced incidence of ventricular tachyarrhythmias and sudden death (69).

Baseline Left Ventricular Function

Prior reports suggested that patients with the most pronounced left ventricular dysfunction at the time of acute arteriography have the greatest improvement in left ventricular function during the convalescent period (73,77,78). For example, infarct-related akinesia and dyskinesis at the time of intracoronary streptokinase administration are related to a delayed improvement of regional wall motion (78). In 137 patients undergoing pharmacological, mechanical, or combined reperfusion therapy in whom paired left ventriculograms were performed within 24 hr of infarction and before hospital discharge, the most important predictor of recovery of left ventricular function was depressed baseline left ventricular function (73). Similarly, in 433 consecutive patients treated with intravenous t-PA and/or urokinase, global and regional left ventricular function were analyzed at baseline and 7–10 days after infarction; only baseline left ventricular function and persistent reperfusion correlated with improvements in left ventricular function during the convalescent phase (77).

Time to Treatment

Concordant with results in the experimental model, several clinical studies have suggested that very early administration of a thrombolytic agent causes maximal recovery of left ventricular function, particularly when the thrombolytic agent is given within 2 hr of symptom onset (34,79–81). Although other reports have failed to demonstrate a relationship between time to treatment and recovery of left ventricular function (60,73,77,82), few patients in these studies actually received thrombolytic agents within 2 hr of symptom onset.

Other Factors

Coronary collaterals are infrequently found in patients with acute myocardial infarction, but their presence in the infarct territory appears to confer a protective effect on the recovery of left ventricular function after thrombolytic therapy (82–85). In addition, improved left ventricular function has been demonstrated in other subgroups, such as those with minimal residual atherosclerosis after thrombolysis (86) or those undergoing immediate surgical or percutaneous revascularization (87,88).

The importance of the residual stenosis in the infarct-related artery on the recovery of left ventricular function after thrombolysis is unsettled. Sheehan et al. (78) demonstrated that a residual diameter stenosis > 0.4 mm was associated with greater improvement in left ventricular function after intracoronary streptokinase infusion. However, in a larger, randomized trial of t-PA, urokinase, and combination t-PA and urokinase, no relationship could be demonstrated between residual coronary dimensions 90 min or 7 days after thrombolytic therapy and recovery of global or regional left ventricular function (89).

Finally, the location of infarction appears to be of little importance in determining the degree of recovery of left ventricular function after thrombolytic administration (60,78,90,91). In a subset analysis of 266 patients undergoing ventriculography 90 min and 7 days after t-PA, improvements in regional wall motion were independent of the location of the infarct-related artery (90).

LEFT VENTRICULAR FUNCTION AFTER SINGLE-AGENT, COMBINATION, AND ADJUNCTIVE THROMBOLYTIC STRATEGIES

A variety of single-agent, combination, and adjunctive thrombolytic strategies have been tested in clinical trials of patients with acute myocardial infarction. Collectively, a beneficial effect on left ventricular function has been documented, although the magnitude of the benefit is less than might be expected from the concomitantly demonstrated reductions in mortality.

Intracoronary Streptokinase

Five randomized, placebo-controlled trials of intracoronary streptokinase in acute myocardial infarction have been performed, each varying with respect to sample size, symptom duration, and the timing of ventriculography (Table 4). Notably, in trials wherein intracoronary streptokinase was administered within 4 hr of symptom onset, left ventricular function was significantly improved 1–8 weeks follow-

Table 4   Effects of Intracoronary Streptokinase on Left Ventricular Function After Acute Myocardial Infarction

Trial	No. Pts Treated	No. Pts Analyzed	Symptom Duration (Hours)	Time of Ventricular Analysis	Treatment Benefit Compared with Placebo	p Value
Anderson et al [92]	50	45	< 4 Hours	< 24 Hours	1.0	NS
				10 Days	8.0	<0.05
Serruys et al [34]	533	332	< 4 Hours	2-8 Weeks	6.0	0.0001
Khaja et al [59]	40	40	< 6 Hours	48 Hours	9.0	NS
				12 Days	8.0	NS
				5 Months	7.0	NS
Kennedy et al [70]	250	NR	< 12 Hours	14 Days	1.0	NS
Ritchie et al [17]	232	207	< 12 Hours	60 Days	0.0	NS

-10   -5   0   5   10   15
Improvement in Ejection Fraction Points

No. Pts indicates number of patients; NR = not reported; NS = not significant. Brackets demonstrate 95% confidence intervals.

ing streptokinase (34,92). Significant improvements in regional wall motion were also noted in these studies. In the report by Khaja et al. (59), limited by a small sample size, no differences in the improvement in left ventricular function in streptokinase-treated and placebo-treated patients were noted, although left ventricular ejection fraction was consistently higher in the streptokinase-treated patients at 48 hr, 12 days, and 5 months after infarction. Importantly, when streptokinase administration was delayed to within 12 hr of symptom onset, no significant differences in the treatment and placebo groups were found (70,82,93).

Thus, when administered early after symptom onset, intracoronary streptokinase improves global and regional ventricular function in patients with acute myocardial infarction. While survival benefits have been noted in patients treated both early and late after symptom onset, no differences in ventricular function have been noted in patients treated up to 12 hr after symptom onset (17,70).

Intravenous Streptokinase

Several small, randomized trials of intravenous streptokinase and placebo in patients with acute myocardial infarction have noted a variable benefit of streptokinase on left ventricular function (94-97). Because of small sample sizes (<70 patients), these improvements have been of marginal statistical significance.

Each of the three large-scale, multicenter trials of intravenous streptokinase and placebo in patients with acute myocardial infarction suggested that myocardial "salvage" results from thrombolytic administration (Table 5). In the series by White et al. (15), 219 patients presenting within 4 hr of symptom onset were randomly assigned to streptokinase 1.5 mU over 1 hr or placebo. In the subset of patients with first infarction, left ventricular ejection fraction was significantly improved by streptokinase in comparison to the placebo-treated patients, a benefit shown in patients with both anterior and inferior infarctions. In 848 patients with symptom duration < 3 hr, left ventricular ejection fraction was significantly higher in the streptokinase-treated patients than in the placebo-treated patients (16). Similar, but less significant, results were found in the Western Washington Intravenous Streptokinase Trial (98). In each of these series, salutary effects on regional wall motion and/or left ventricular end-systolic volumes were demonstrated in thrombolytic-treated patients (Table 6) (15,16,98).

Intravenous t-PA

Six large-scale randomized trials of intravenous t-PA and placebo have been performed in patients with acute myocardial infarction (14,99-103). Markedly concordant in their study designs, these trials randomized patients with symptoms of 2.5 to 5-hr duration and evaluated ventricular function 3-8 weeks afterward. Compared with placebo-treated patients, improvements of 2-7 ejection fraction points were noted in patients treated with intravenous t-PA (Table 5), particularly in those with anterior infarctions. In addition to the beneficial effect of thrombolytic therapy on left ventricular ejection fraction, improvements in infarct-related regional wall motion were noted in the t-PA-treated patients. In a randomized trial of 355 patients receiving t-PA and 366 receiving placebo, left ventricular end-diastolic and end-systolic volumes were significantly lower in the t-PA-treated patients (101).

Intravenous Anistreplase

Pilot trials (<100 patients) of anistreplase have demonstrated beneficial effects of this agent on early coronary reperfusion in patients with acute myocardial infarction. Because of small sample sizes in these trials, the effect of anistreplase on left ventricular function was somewhat variable (104-106).

Two large, multicenter trials of intravenous anistreplase in patients with acute myocardial infarction have been performed, each demonstrating somewhat disparate effects on left ventricular function (Table 5) (18,107,108). In 231 patients presenting within 5 hr of symptom onset, treatment with anistreplace, 30 U over 5 min, was compared to treatment with intravenous heparin alone. Left ventricular

Table 5   Effect of Intravenous Streptokinase, t-PA, and Anistreplase on Left Ventricular Function after Acute Myocardial Infarction

Trial	No. Pts Enrolled	No. Pts Analyzed	Symptom Duration (Hours)	Time of Ventricular Analysis (Weeks)	Treatment Benefit Compared with Placebo	p Value
Intravenous Streptokinase						
White et al [15]	219	155	< 4	3		<0.005
ISAM [16]	1741	848	< 6	3-4		<0.005
Ritchie et al [98]	368	205	< 6	8		0.08
Intravenous tPA						
VHAT [103]	352	295	≤ 2.5	4		<0.05
Guerci et al [99]	138	117	< 4	1		<0.02
NHF [14]	144	103	< 4	1		0.04
O'Rourke et al [100]	145	126	< 2.5	3		0.006
Van de Werf et al [101]	721	577	< 5	3		<0.05
Armstrong et al [102]	115	105	< 3.75	3-4		0.017
Intravenous Anistreplase						
Bassand et al [107]	231	209	< 5	1		0.002
Meinertz et al [18]	313	256	< 4	2-3		
Anterior						NS
Inferior						NS

Improvement in Ejection Fraction Points (-10, -5, 0, 5, 10, 15)

ISAM = Intravenous Streptokinase in Acute Myocardial Infarction Study Group; No. Pts indicates number of patients; NHF = National Heart Foundation of Australia Coronary Thrombolysis Group; NS = not significant; tPA = tissue plasminogen activator; VHAT = The Thrombolysis Early in Acute Heart Attack Trial Study Group. Brackets demonstrate 95% confidence intervals.

ejection fraction, measured 7 days afterward, was significantly higher in those treated with anistreplase, and this beneficial influence on left ventricular ejection fraction was noted in patients with both anterior and inferior infarctions (107). Conversely, in 313 patients presenting within 4 hr of acute infarction, no differences in global or regional left ventricular function were found in patients treated with anistreplase or heparin (18). Notably, however, mortality was significantly higher in the heparin-treated patients (12.6% compared with 5.6% in the anistreplase-treated patients). The inability to perform ventriculographic analysis in those patients expiring within the first 2-3 weeks may account for the lack of benefit of anistreplase on left ventricular function in the latter trial.

Table 6   Effect of Thrombolytic Therapy on Left Ventricular Volumes After Acute Myocardial Infarction

Trial	No. Pts	Thrombo-lytic	Symptom Duration (Hours)	Time of Ventricular Analysis (Weeks)	End-Systolic Volume	End-Diastolic Volume
Serruys[34*]	332	Placebo / IC SK	< 4	2-8	53 ‡ / 41	95 ‡ / 84
White[15]	155	Placebo / IV SK	< 4	3	73 ‡ / 55	
Van de Werf[101]	577	Placebo / tPA	< 5	3	66 / 60	124 / 118
Sheehan[71*]	145	IV SK / tPA	< 7	1	39 / 39	76 / 78
Topol[52]	132	Placebo / tPA	6-24	26	83 / 81	165 279 / 158 268

```
            0   50  100 150 200     0   50  100 150 200
                      cc                      cc
```

IC SK = intracoronary streptokinase; IV SK = intravenous streptokinase; No. Pts indicates number of patients *reported in volume index (cc/m^2); ‡ = $p < 0.01$. Brackets demonstrate 95% confidence intervals.

Combination Thrombolytic Therapy

In 146 patients receiving intravenous t-PA and a varying dose of intravenous urokinase reported by Topol et al. (109), improvement in left ventricular ejection fraction from 90 min to 7 days was significantly greater in those given combination thrombolytic therapy than in historical controls treated with t-PA alone (Δ + 5% versus Δ - 1%; $p = 0.008$). In this series, the improvement in ejection fraction may have occurred because of a reduced incidence of reocclusion in those receiving combination therapy, particularly in patients undergoing "rescue" angioplasty. Based on these preliminary findings, a randomized trial of 575 patients assigned to thrombolytic treatment with t-PA, urokinase, or combination t-PA and urokinase was performed (110). Importantly, despite significant reductions in reocclusion in the combination-treated patients, no differences in global left ventricular ejection fraction or regional wall motion early or late following thrombolysis were noted in the three treatment groups (Table 7) (110).

Table 7   Effect of Combination Thrombolytic Therapy and Adjunctive Therapy on Left Ventricular Function After Acute Myocardial Infarction

Trial	No. Pts Treated	No. Pts Analyzed	Symptom Duration (Hours)	Time of Ventricular Analysis (Weeks)	Treatment Benefit Compared with tPA Alone	p Value
Combination Thrombolytics						
tPA + Urokinase [110]	385	NR	< 6	1		NS
tPA + Streptokinase [111]	216	148	< 6	1		0.07
Thrombolytic Adjuncts						
Prostacyclin [114]	50	41	< 6	1		NS
Heparin [118]	134	NR	< 6	1		NS
Metoprolol [3]*	1390	NR	< 4	1		NS
Captopril [126]	38	33	< 6	1		NS
Nifedipine [128]	149	149	< 6	1		NS
Superoxide Dismutase [129]	114	71	< 6	1		NS

-10   -5   0   5   10   15
Improvement in Ejection Fraction Points

No. Pts indicates number of patients; NR = not reported; NS = not significant. *assumes SD = 14%. Brackets demonstrate 95% confidence intervals.

Other combination thrombolytic regimens have been used (111). In patients randomized to t-PA or to combination t-PA and streptokinase reported by Grines et al. (111), a beneficial effect on recovery of left ventricular function was noted in combination-treated patients. Ninety-minute infarct-related artery patency was significantly greater in those randomized to combination therapy (79% versus 64%; $p < 0.05$), and left ventricular ejection fraction, measured 7 days after infarction, tended to be higher in those given combination therapy than those receiving t-PA alone. Regional wall motion, measured using the centerline method, was significantly improved with combination therapy (107). These beneficial effects were attributed to a lowered incidence of reocclusion, a lower serum viscosity, or reduced afterload in the combination-treated patients.

In the series of both Califf et al. (110) and Grines et al. (111), left ventricular ejection fraction was well preserved in the patients receiving t-PA monotherapy. For this reason, it is unlikely that the standard index of ventricular function, left ventricular ejection fraction, will be sufficient to detect differences between these comparative combination treatment strategies, and other, more clinically relevant, indices may be needed.

Thrombolytic Adjuncts

The use of adjunctive pharmacological strategies, designed for concomitant use with thrombolytic agents, may result in more timely thrombolysis, thereby limiting the extent of endothelial and myocyte injury after myocardial infarction (112). Although several adjuncts have been tested in pilot and randomized trials, few have demonstrated a substantial improvement in left ventricular function over that obtained using thrombolytic therapy alone (Table 7).

Prostacyclin

Prostaglandin I2, or prostacyclin, is a potent inhibitor of platelet aggregation. It has been administered alone and as an adjunct to t-PA in patients with myocardial infarction (113,114). In 54 patients, Armstrong et al. (113) noted no difference in global or regional left ventricular function in patients randomized to prostacyclin or standard therapy for acute myocardial infarction. In a nonrandomized pilot study of 50 patients receiving t-PA and Iloprost or t-PA alone, adjunctive Iloprost did not improve 7-day regional or global left ventricular ejection fraction, and the combination was associated with a decrease in ejection fraction from initial to follow-up studies (114). This paradoxical, and potentially deleterious, effect of Iloprost was subsequently explained by the results of animal studies that demonstrated that Iloprost increased hepatic blood flow, leading to increased hepatic clearance of t-PA (115).

Heparin

Although the importance of adjunctive heparin in maintaining coronary patency 7–24 hr after t-PA administration has recently been demonstrated (116,117), few studies have examined the effect of heparin on preserving left ventricular function by preventing reocclusion after myocardial reperfusion. In 134 patients receiving t-PA and randomized to immediate intravenous heparin or to delayed elective heparin, no difference in early or late ventricular function was noted (109). Notably, a larger, randomized study of delayed subcutaneous heparin in patients with acute myocardial infarction failed to demonstrate a survival benefit in patients treated with t-PA or streptokinase (2).

β-Adrenergic Receptor Blockade

Prior to the thrombolytic era, the early administration of β-adrenergic blocking agents was shown to limit myocardial infarct size and improve survival in patients with acute myocardial infarction (119–121). Intravenous β-adrenergic blockade may exert important effects on infarct-related and noninfarct-related regional wall motion. In 33 patients with documented reperfusion after thrombolytic therapy, ventriculography performed before and after administration of 15 mg of intravenous metoprolol demonstrated no change in global left ventricular ejection fraction, but metoprolol significantly reduced non-infarct-zone motion, improved infarct-zone motion, and resulted in a smaller circumferential extent of hypokinesis (122). These changes occurred independently of myocardial salvage (122,123).

The adjunctive value of early intravenous β-adrenergic blocking agents in preventing recurrent ischemia and reinfarction was subsequently demonstrated in a study of 1390 patients treated with t-PA within 4 hr of symptom onset (3). In this trial, patients eligible for β-adrenergic receptor blockade were randomly assigned to immediate intravenous metoprolol followed by oral metoprolol or to delayed metoprolol begun on day 6. Patients assigned to immediate metoprolol had fewer nonfatal reinfarctions and recurrent ischemic events than those given delayed metoprolol. However, there was no significant difference in left ventricular ejection fraction at hospital discharge or after 6 weeks (Table 6), and exercise left ventricular ejection fraction was similar in the two groups (3).

Captopril

Left ventricular cavity dilatation commonly occurs after myocardial infarction, particularly in patients with anterior infarction and those with persistent coronary occlusion (124,125). Pharmacological intervention following myocardial infarction may prevent left ventricular dilatation by reducing afterload and promoting favorable left ventricular remodeling. In 59 patients with a first anterior myocardial infarction, captopril, begun 1–4 weeks following infarction, lessened the magnitude of ventricular cavity dilatation, as assessed by left-ventricular end-diastolic volume 1 year after infarction (125). These results were supported by data from an additional 60 patients randomized to treatment with captopril or furosemide 1 week after infarction. In those treated with captopril, significant reductions in left ventricular end-systolic volume were noted, whereas the ventricular volumes increased significantly in those given furosemide (124). These data suggest that angiotensin-converting enzyme inhibition can reduce the degree of left ventricular dilatation after myocardial infarction.

In a trial of 38 patients receiving t-PA within 3 hr of symptom onset, patients were randomly assigned to intravenous captopril, 10 mg, followed by oral captopril, or placebo (126). Although there were no differences in acute or 7-day global or regional wall motion between the two groups, the 7-day end-diastolic volume was significantly higher in the placebo group, suggesting that captopril given at the time of thrombolytic therapy may also be useful in preventing left-ventricular dilatation after myocardial infarction (126).

Calcium Antagonists

In patients with non-Q-wave myocardial infarction, diltiazem was shown to reduce the incidence of cardiac events rates in patients without left ventricular dysfunction, even though it exerted no demonstrable effect on global left ventricular ejection fraction (127). In 149 patients receiving intracoronary or intravenous thrombolytic therapy for acute myocardial infarction, patients were randomly assigned to intracoronary followed by oral nifedipine or placebo. No differences in global left ventricular ejection fraction or left ventricular end-diastolic or end-systolic volumes were noted in the two groups (128).

Superoxide Dismutase

In experimental models, superoxide dismutase has been shown to limit reperfusion injury after transient coronary occlusion. In a randomized pilot trial of 114 patients undergoing "rescue" coronary angioplasty after failed thrombolysis, a subgroup at particular risk for reperfusion injury, Werns et al. (129) reported no improvement in acute or 7-day global and regional wall motion in patients treated with superoxide dismutase. Whether other free radical scavengers, such as perfluorocarbons, have value in preventing reperfusion injury in patients with acute myocardial infarction is currently under study.

COMPARATIVE THROMBOLYTIC TRIALS

t-PA and Intravenous Streptokinase

Several randomized trials have been performed to compare the effects of t-PA and streptokinase on the recovery of left ventricular function in patients with acute myocardial infarction (Table 8). In phase I of the Thrombolysis in Myocardial Infarction Trial (TIMI), 290 patients were randomized with 7 hr of symptom onset to intravenous streptokinase or t-PA. Global and regional left ventricular function and left-ventricular volumes, measured from contrast ventriculograms at the time of hospital discharge, were similar in the two groups (71). In a comparative thrombolytic trial by White et al. (32), 270 patients with first myocardial infarction and symptom onset < 3 hr in duration were randomly assigned to t-PA or streptokinase. In the absence of recurrent ischemia, cardiac catheterization was deferred for 3 weeks after thrombolytic administration. Left ventricular ejection fraction, infarct-related regional wall motion score, and left ventricular end-systolic volume, as assessed by contrast ventriculography, were similar in the two groups (32,130). In a smaller trial of 86 patients randomly assigned to 100 mg t-PA or 1.5 mU of streptokinase within 3 hr of symptom onset, left ventricular function, as assessed by contrast ventriculography 4 days after therapy, was similar in both groups, although t-PA–treated patients were noted to have late improvements in global left ventricular function, as assessed by echocardiography (131).

Intravenous t-PA and Urokinase

Two large trials have compared the effects of t-PA and urokinase on left ventricular function in patients with acute myocardial infarction. In a German randomized

Table 8   Comparative Effects of Thrombolytic Agents on Left Ventricular Function After Acute Myocardial Infarction

Trial	No. Pts Treated	No. Pts Analyzed	Symptom Duration (Hours)	Time of Ventricular Analysis (Days)	Treatment Benefit Compared with tPA	p Value
tPA vs Streptokinase						
Sheehan *et al* [71]	290	145	< 7	7	-1	NS
White *et al* [32]	270	240	< 3	21	0	NS
Magnani [131]	171	85	< 3	4	-2	NS
				10	-5	<0.05
tPA vs Urokinase						
Neuhaus *et al* [132]	246	169	< 6	10-28	-1	NS
Califf *et al* [110]	381	NR	< 6	10	0	NS

Improvement in Ejection Fraction Points: -10   -5   0   5   10   15

No. Pts indicates number of patients; NR = not reported; NS = not significant. Brackets demonstrate 95% confidence intervals.

trial, 246 patients presenting within 6 hr of symptom onset were randomized to therapy with t-PA or urokinase. No differences in baseline or follow-up left ventricular ejection fraction were noted in the two groups (132). In a somewhat larger, randomized trial of monotherapy with t-PA or urokinase and combination t-PA and urokinase reported by Califf et al. (110), left ventricular ejection fraction and regional wall motion, measured acutely and 7 days later, were similar to each of the treatment groups.

RECOMMENDATIONS FOR CLINICAL THROMBOLYTIC TRIALS

From the preceding discussion, it is evident that compared with placebo, the early administration of thrombolytic therapy improves left ventricular ejection fraction, regional wall motion, and left ventricular remodeling in patients with acute myocardial infarction. However, in comparative and adjunctive thrombolytic trials that incorporate thrombolytic agents into virtually all study limbs, a disheartening homogeneity of ventricular function using standard endpoints has been observed. Because of the limitations of any single index of left ventricular function, future comparative thrombolytic trials should incorporate a variety of ventriculographic and clinical indices as endpoints for analysis.

The limitations of the use of left ventricular ejection fraction as the sole endpoint for ventricular function have been noted. Nevertheless, because of its simplicity and widespread applicability, left ventricular ejection fraction obtained 7–10 days following thrombolytic therapy remains a clinically useful ventriculographic endpoint. Treatment strategies resulting in major improvements in ventricular function would be detected by improvements in global ventricular function. Furthermore, quantitation of infarct-zone regional wall motion, while less clinically applicable, may provide a more sensitive index of left ventricular "salvage" and should be recommended as a ventriculographic endpoint in comparative thrombolytic trials. When the treatment strategy may potentially enhance late left ventricular remodeling, left ventricular volumes, determined 6 months following thrombolytic therapy, may be useful.

Increasingly, composite clinical endpoints will be used to evaluate the benefit of alternative thrombolytic strategies. Objective ventriculographic indices of left ventricular dysfunction may be related to other adverse outcomes, such as increased risk of major bleeding events, and allow a more accurate assessment of risk-benefit ratio associated with novel thrombolytic approaches. Weighted-sum or ordinal rank statistical analysis of a combined clinical outcome in this fashion may allow timely, cost-effective, and accurate information about alternative thrombolytic strategies in patients with acute myocardial infarction without recruitment of the prohibitively large numbers of patients required to demonstrate significant improvements in mortality. Once the clinical value of an alternative thrombolytic strategy has been demonstrated using this composite clinical endpoint, large trials focusing on major clinical endpoints may then be performed.

REFERENCES

1. Gruppo Italiano per lo studio della streptochinasi nell'infarto miocardico (GISSI). Long-term effects of intravenous thrombolysis in acute myocardial infarction: final report of the GISSI study. Lancet 1987; 2:871–4.
2. The International Study Group. In-hospital mortality and clinical course of 20,891 patients with suspected acute myocardial infarction randomised between alteplase and streptokinase with or without heparin. Lancet 1990; 336:71–5.
3. The TIMI Study Group. Comparison of invasive and conservative strategies after treatment with intravenous tissue plasminogen activator in acute myocardial infarction. Results of the Thrombolysis in Myocardial Infarction (TIMI) Phase II Trial. N Engl J Med 1989; 320:618–27.
4. Wilcox RG, von der Lippe G, Olsson CG, Jensen G, Skene AM, Hampton JR. Trial of tissue plasminogen activator for mortality reduction in acute myocardial infarction. Anglo-Scandinavian Study of Early Thrombolysis (ASSET). Lancet 1988; 2:525–30.
5. AIMS Trial Study Group. Long-term effects of intravenous anistreplase in acute myocardial infarction: final report of the AIMS study. Lancet 1990; 335:427–31.

6. ISIS-2 (Second International Study of Infarct Survival) Collaborative Group. Randomised trial of intravenous streptokinase, oral aspirin, both, or neither among 17,187 cases of suspected acute myocardial infarction: ISIS-2. Lancet 1988; 2: 349-60.

7. Califf RM, Topol EJ, George BS, et al. Characteristics and outcome of patients in whom reperfusion with intravenous tissue-type plasminogen activator fails: results of the Thrombolysis and Angioplasty in Myocardial Infarction (TAMI) I trial. Circulation 1988; 77:1090-9.

8. Ohman EM, Califf RM, Topol EJ, et al. Consequences of reocclusion after successful reperfusion therapy in acute myocardial infarction. Circulation 1990; 82:781-91.

9. Bater ER, Topol EJ. Limitations of thrombolytic therapy for acute myocardial infarction complicated by congestive heart failure and cardiogenic shock. J Am Coll Cardiol 1991 (in press).

10. Topol EJ. Ultrathrombolysis. J Am Coll Cardiol 1990; 15:922-4.

11. Norris RM, White HD. Therapeutic trials in coronary thrombosis should measure left ventricular function as primary end-point of treatment. Lancet 1988; 1:104-6.

12. Mukharji J, Rude RE, Poole K, et al. Risk factors for sudden death after myocardial infarction: two-year follow-up. Am J Cardiol 1984; 54:31-6.

13. The Multicenter Postinfarction Research Group. Risk stratification and survival after myocardial infarction. N Engl J Med 1983; 309:331-6.

14. National Heart Foundation of Australia Coronary Thrombolysis Group. Coronary thrombolysis and myocardial salvage by tissue plasminogen activator given up to 4 hours after onset of myocardial infarction. Lancet 1988; 1:203-7.

15. White HD, Norris RM, Brown MA, et al. Effect of intravenous streptokinase on left ventricular function and early survival after acute myocardial infarction. N Engl J Med 1987; 317:850-5.

16. The I.S.A.M. Study Group. A prospective trial of intravenous streptokinase in acute myocardial infarction (I.S.A.M.). Mortality, morbidity, and infarct size at 21 days. N Engl J Med 1986; 314:1465-71.

17. Ritchie JL, Davis KB, Williams DL, Caldwell J, Kennedy JW. Global and regional left ventricular function and tomographic radionuclide perfusion: the Western Washington Intracoronary Streptokinase in Myocardial Infarction Trial. Circulation 1984; 70:867-75.

18. Meinhertz T, Kasper W, Schumacher M, Just H. The German multicenter trial of anisoylated plasminogen streptokinase activator complex versus heparin for acute myocardial infarction. Am J Cardiol 1988; 62:347-51.

19. van de Werf F. Discrepancies between the effects of coronary reperfusion on survival and left ventricular function. Lancet 1989; 2:1367-9.

20. Califf RM, Harrelson-Woodlief L, Topol EJ. Left ventricular ejection fraction may not be useful as an endpoint of thrombolytic therapy comparative trials. Circulation 1990; 82:1847-53.

21. Reimer KA, Lowe JE, Rasmussen MM, Jennings RB. The "wavefront phenomenon" of myocardial ischemic cell death. I. Myocardial infarct-size vs. duration of coronary occlusion in dogs. Circulation 1977; 56:786-94.

22. DeWood MA, Spores J, Notske R, Mouser LT, Burroughs R, Golden MS, Lang HT. Prevalence of total coronary occlusion during the early hours of transmural myocardial infarction. N Engl J Med 1980; 303:897-902.

23. Braunwald E. Myocardial reperfusion, limitation of infarct size, reduction of left ventricular dysfunction, and improved survival. Should the paradigm be expanded? Circulation 1989; 79:441-4.

24. Rentrop P, Blanke H, Karsch KR, et al. Acute myocardial infarction: Intracoronary application of nitroglycerin and streptokinase. Clin Cardiol 1979; 2:354-63.

25. Ganz W, Buchbinder N, Marcus H, et al. Intracoronary thrombolysis in evolving myocardial infarction. Am Heart J 1981; 101:4-13.

26. Leiboff RH, Katz RJ, Wasserman AG, et al. A randomized, angiographically controlled trial of intracoronary streptokinase in acute myocardial infarction. Am J Cardiol 1984; 53:404-7.

27. Kennedy JW, Trenholme SE, Kasser IS. Left ventricular volume and mass from single-plane cineangiocardiogram. A comparison of anteroposterior and right anterior oblique methods. Am Heart J 1970; 80:343-52.

28. Wynne J, Green LH, Mann T, Levin D, Grossman W. Estimation of left ventricular volumes in man from biplane cineangiograms filmed in oblique projections. Am J Cardiol 1978; 41:726-32.

29. Chapman CB, Baker O, Reynolds J, Bonte FJ. Use of biplane cineflourography for measurement of ventricular volume. Circulation 1958; 18:1105-17.

30. White HD, Norris RM, Brown MA, Brandt PWT, Whitlock RML, Wild CJ. Left ventricular end-systolic volume as the major determinant of survival after recovery from myocardial infarction. Circulation 1987; 76:44-51.

31. The TIMI Research Group. Immediate vs. delayed catheterization and angioplasty following thrombolytic therapy for acute myocardial infarction. TIMI IIA results. JAMA 1988; 260:2849-58.

32. White HD, Rivers JT, Maslowski AH, et al. Effect of intravenous streptokinase as compared with that of tissue plasminogen activator on left ventricular function after first myocardial infarction. N Engl J Med 1989; 320:817-21.

33. Sheehan FH, Mathey DG, Schofer J, Krebber HJ, Dodge HT. Effect of interventions in salvaging left ventricular function in acute myocardial infarction: a study of intracoronary streptokinase. Am J Cardiol 1983; 52:431-8.

34. Serruys PW, Simoons ML, Suryapranata H, et al. Preservation of global and regional left ventricular function after early thrombolysis in acute myocardial infarction. J Am Coll Cardiol 1986; 7:729-42.

35. Stack RS, Phillips HR, Grierson DS, et al. Functional improvement of jeopardized myocardium following intracoronary streptokinase infusion in acute myocardial infarction. J Clin Invest 1983; 72:84-95.

36. Holmes DR Jr., Bove AA, Nishimura RA, et al. Comparision of monoplane and biplane assessment of regional wall motion after thrombolytic therapy for acute myocardial infarction. Am J Cardiol 1987; 59:793-7.

37. Sheehan FH. Left ventricular dysfunction in acute myocardial infarction due to isolated left circumflex coronary artery stenosis. Am J Cardiol 1989; 64:440-7.

38. Mortelmans L, Vanhaecke J, Lasaffre E, et al. Evaluation of the effect of throm-

bolytic treatment on infarct size and left ventricular function by enzymatic, scintigraphic, and angiographic methods. Am Heart J 1990; 119:1231-7.

39. Work JW, Ferguson JG, Diamond GA. Limitations of a conventional logistic regression model based on left ventricular ejection fraction in predicting coronary events after myocardial infarction. Am J Cardiol 1989; 64:702-7.

40. Sheehan FH. Determinants of improved left ventricular function after thrombolytic therapy in acute myocardial infarction. J Am Coll Cardiol 1987; 9:937-44.

41. Sheehan FH, Bolson EL, Dodge HT, Mathey DG, Schofer J, Woo HW. Advantages and applications of the centerline method for characterizing regional ventricular function. Circulation 1986; 74:293-305.

42. Sniderman AD, Marpole D, Fallen EL. Regional contractile patterns in the normal and ischemic ventricle in man. Am J. Cardiol 1973; 31:484-9.

43. Cole JS, Holland PA, Glaeser DH. A semiautomated technique for the rapid evaluation of left ventricular regional wall motion. Cath Cardiovasc Diagn 1976; 2: 185-97.

44. Grines CL, Topol EJ, Califf RM, et al. Prognostic implications and predictors of enhanced regional wall motion of the noninfarct zone after thrombolysis and angioplasty therapy of acute myocardial infarction. Circulation 1989; 80:245-53.

45. Jeremy RW, Allman KC, Bautovitch G, Harris PJ. Patterns of left ventricular dilatation during the six months after myocardial infarction. J Am Coll Cardiol 1989; 13: 304-10.

46. Seals AA, Pratt CM, Mahmarian JJ, et al. Relation of left ventricular dilation during acute myocardial infarction to systolic performance, diastolic dysfunction, infarct size and location. Am J Cardiol 1988; 61:224-9.

47. Lamas GA, Pfeffer MA. Increased left ventricular volume following myocardial infarction in man. Am Heart J 1986; 111:30-5.

48. McKay RG, Pfeffer MA, Pasternak RC, et al. Left ventricular remodeling after myocardial infarction: a corollary to infarct expansion. Circulation 1986; 74:693-702.

49. Warren SE, Royal HD, Markis JE, Grossman W, McKay RG. Time course of left ventricular dilation after myocardial infarction: influence of infarct-related artery and success of coronary thrombolysis. J Am Coll Cardiol 1988; 11:12-9.

50. Shen WF, Cui LQ, Gong LS, Lesbre JP. Beneficial effect of residual flow to the infarct region on left ventricular volume changes after acute myocardial infarction. Am Heart J 1990; 119:525-9.

51. van der Laarse A, Kerkhof PLM, Vermeer F, et al. Relation between infarct size and left ventricular performance assessed in patients with first acute myocardial infarction randomized to intracoronary thrombolytic therapy or to conventional treatment. Am J Cardiol 1988; 61:1-7.

52. Topol EJ, Califf RM, Vandormael M, et al. A randomized trial of late reperfusion therapy for acute myocardial infarction. N Engl J Med (submitted).

53. Gruppo Italiano per lo studio della sopravvivenza nell'infarto miocardico. GISSI-2: a factorial randomised trial of alteplase versus streptokinase and heparin versus no heparin among 12,490 patients with acute myocardial infarction. Lancet 1990; 336:65-71.

54. Boissel JP. Registry of multicenter clinical trials. Tenth report—1988. Thromb Haemost 1989; 62:1126-42.

55. Heyndrickx GR, Millard RW, McRitchie RJ, Maroko PR, Vatner SF. Regional myocardial functional and electrophysiological alterations after brief coronary artery occlusion in conscious dogs. J Clin Invest 1975; 56:978-85.

56. Lavallee M, Cox D, Patrick TA, Vatner SF. Salvage of myocardial function by coronary artery reperfusion 1, 2, and 3 hours after occlusion in conscious dogs. Circ Res 1983; 53:235-47.

57. Braunwald E, Kloner RA. The stunned myocardium: prolonged, postischemic ventricular dysfunction. Circulation 1982; 66:1146-9.

58. Kloner RA, Przyklenk K, Patel B. Altered myocardial states. The stunned and hibernating myocardium. Am J Med 1989; 86:14A-22A.

59. Khaja F, Walton JA, Brymer JF, et al. Intracoronary fibrinolytic therapy in acute myocardial infarction. Report of a prospective randomized trial. N Engl J Med 1983; 308:1305-11.

60. Reduto LA, Smalling RW, Freund GC, Gould KL. Intracoronary infusion of streptokinase in patients with acute myocardial infarction: effects of reperfusion on left ventricular performance. Am J Cardiol 1981; 48:403-9.

61. Wackers FJ, Berger HJ, Weinberg MA, Zaret BL. Spontaneous changes in left ventricular function over the first 24 hours of acute transmural myocardial infarction: implications for evaluating early therapeutic interventions. Circulation 1982; 66: 748-54.

62. Bourdillon PDV, Broderick TM, Williams ES, et al. Early recovery of regional left ventricular function after reperfusion in acute myocardial infarction assessed by serial two-dimensional echocardiography. Am J Cardiol 1989; 63:641-6.

63. Sheehan FH, Doerr R, Schmidt WG, et al. Early recovery of left ventricular function after thrombolytic therapy for acute myocardial infarction: an important determinant of survival. J Am Coll Cardiol 1988; 12:289-300.

64. Schmidt WG, Sheehan FH, von Essen R, Uebis R, Effert S. Evolution of left ventricular function after intracoronary thrombolysis for acute myocardial infarction. Am J Cardiol 1989; 63:497-502.

65. Grines CL, O'Neill WW, Anselmo EG, Juni JE, Topol EJ. Comparison of left ventricular function and contractile reserve after successful recanalization by thrombolysis versus rescue percutaneous transluminal coronary angioplasty for acute myocardial infarction. Am J Cardiol 1988; 62:352-57.

66. Harrison JK, Skelton TN, Davidson CJ, et al. Regional and global left ventricular function evaluated acutely, at 7 days, and at 6 months following thrombolytic therapy. Circulation 1989; 80(Suppl II):II-313 (abstract).

67. Henzlova MJ, Bourge RC, Tauxe L, Rogers WJ. Is preservation of left ventricular function after thrombolytic therapy sustained? Circulation 1989; 80(Suppl II):II-312 (abstract).

68. Touchstone DA, Beller GA, Nygaard TW, Tedesco C, Kaul S. Effects of successful intravenous reperfusion therapy on regional myocardial function and geometry in humans: a tomographic assessment using two-dimensional echocardiography. J Am Coll Cardiol 1989; 13:1506-13.

69. Cigarroa RG, Lange RA, Hillis LD. Prognosis after acute myocardial infarction in patients with and without residual anterograde coronary blood flow. Am J Cardiol 1989; 64:155-60.

70. Kennedy JW, Ritchie JL, Davis KB, Fritz JK. Western Washington Randomized Trial of Intracoronary Streptokinase in acute myocardial infarction. N Engl J Med 1983; 309:1477-82.

71. Sheehan FH, Braunwald E, Canner P, et al. The effect of intravenous thrombolytic therapy on left ventricular function: a report on tissue-type plasminogen activator and streptokinase from the Thrombolysis in Myocardial Infarction (TIMI Phase I) Trial. Circulation 1987; 75:817-29.

72. De Feyter PJ, van Eenige MJ, van der Wall EE, et al. Effects of spontaneous and streptokinase-induced recanalization on left ventricular function after myocardial infarction. Circulation 1983; 67:1039-44.

73. Marzoll U, Kleiman NS, Dunn JK, et al. Factors determining improvement in left ventricular function after reperfusion therapy for acute myocardial infarction: primacy of baseline ejection fraction. J Am Coll Cardiol 1991; 17:613-20.

74. Smalling RW, Fuentes F, Matthews MW, et al. Sustained improvement in left ventricular function and mortality by intracoronary streptokinase administration during evolving myocardial infarction. Circulation 1983; 68:131-8.

75. Bates ER, Topol EJ, Kline EM, et al. Early reperfusion therapy improves left ventricular function after acute inferior myocardial infarction associated with right coronary artery disease. Am Heart J 1987; 114:261-7.

76. Jang I-K, Vanhaecke J, De Geest H, Verstraete M, Collen D, van der Werf F. Coronary thrombolysis with recombinant tissue-type plasminogen activator: patency rate and regional wall motion after 3 months. J Am Coll Cardiol 1986; 8:1455-60.

77. Califf RM, Parsons WJ, Tcheng JE, et al. Baseline function, not time to treatment, is most closely associated with LV function improvement during the first week after thrombolytic therapy. Circulation 1988; 78(Suppl II):II-213 (abstract).

78. Sheehan FH, Mathey DG, Schofer J, Dodge HT, Bolson EL. Factors that determine recovery of left ventricular function after thrombolysis in patients with acute myocardial infarction. Circulation 1985; 71:1121-8.

79. Schroder R, Biamino G, Leitner ERV, et al. Intravenous short-term infusion of streptokinase in acute myocardial infarction. Circulation 1983; 67:536-48.

80. Schwartz F, Schuler G, Katus H, et al. Intracoronary thrombolysis in acute myocardial infarction: duration of ischemia as a major determinant of late results after recanalization. Am J Cardiol 1982; 50:933-7.

81. Mathey DG, Sheehan FH, Schofer J, Dodge HT. Time of onset of symptoms to thrombolytic therapy: a major determinant of myocardial salvage in patients with acute transmural infarction. J Am Coll Cardiol 1985; 6:518-25.

82. Rogers WJ, Hood WP, Mantle JA, et al. Return of left ventricular function after reperfusion in patients with myocardial infarction: importance of subtotal stenosis or collaterals. J Am Coll Cardiol 1984; 69:338-49.

83. Williams DO, Amsterdam EA, Miller RR, Mason DT. Functional significance of coronary collateral vessels in patients with acute myocardial infarction: relation to pump performance, cardiogenic shock and survival. Am J Cardiol 1976; 37:345-51.

84. Saito Y, Yasuno M, Ishida M, et al. Importance of coronary collaterals for restoration of left ventricular function after intracoronary thrombolysis. Am J Cardiol 1988; 55:1259-63.

85. Rentrop KP, Feit F, Sherman W, et al. Late thrombolytic therapy preserves left ventricular function in patients with collateralized total coronary occlusion: primary end point findings of the Second Mount Sinai-New York University Trial. J Am Coll Cardiol 1989; 14:58-64.

86. Kereiakes DJ, Topol EJ, George BS, et al. Myocardial infarction with minimal coronary atherosclerosis in the era of thrombolytic reperfusion. J Am Coll Cardiol 1991; 17:304-12.

87. Kereiakes DJ, Topol EJ, George BS, et al. Emergency coronary artery bypass surgery preserves global and regional left ventricular function after intravenous tissue plasminogen activator therapy for acute myocardial infarction. J Am Coll Cardiol 1988; 11:899-907.

88. Topol EJ, Weiss JL, Brinker JA, et al. Regional wall motion improvement after coronary thrombolysis with recombinant tissue plasminogen activator: importance of coronary angioplasty. J Am Coll Cardiol 1985; 6:426-33.

89. Popma JJ, Califf RM, Ellis SG, et al. Mechanism of benefit of combination thrombolytic therapy for acute myocardial infarction: a quantitative angiographic and hematologic study. J Am Coll Cardiol 1991 (in press).

90. Bates ER, Califf RM, Stack RS, et al. Thrombolysis and Angioplasty in Myocardial Infarction (TAMI-1) Trial: influence of infarct location on arterial patency, left ventricular function, and mortality. J Am Coll Cardiol 1989; 13:12-8.

91. Simoons ML, Serruys PW, van den Brand M, et al. Early thrombolysis in acute myocardial infarction: limitation of infarct size and improved survival. J Am Coll Cardiol 1986; 7:717-28.

92. Anderson JL, Marshall HW, Bray BE, et al. A randomized trial of intracoronary streptokinase in the treatment of acute myocardial infarction. N Engl J Med 1983; 308:1312-8.

93. Rentrop KP, Feit F, Blanke H, et al. Effects of intracoronary streptokinase and intracoronary nitroglycerin infusion on coronary angiographic patterns and mortality in patients with acute myocardial infarction. N Engl J Med 1984; 311:1457-63.

94. Wisenberg G, Finnie KJ, Jablonsky G, Kostuk WJ, Marshall T. Nuclear magnetic resonance and radionuclide angiographic assessment of acute myocardial infarction in a randomized trial of intravenous streptokinase. Am J Cardiol 1988; 62:1011-6.

95. Olson HG, Butman SM, Piters KM, et al. A randomized controlled trial of intravenous streptokinase in evolving myocardial infarction. Am Heart J 1986; 111:1021-9.

96. Schreiber TL, Miller DH, Silvasi DA, Moses JW, Borer JS. Randomized double-blind trial of intravenous streptokinase for acute myocardial infarction. Am J Cardiol 1986; 58:47-52.

97. Durand P, Asseman P, Pruvost P, Bertrand ME, La Blanche JM, Thery C. Effectiveness of intravenous streptokinase on infarct-size and left ventricular function in acute myocardial infarction. Prospective and randomized study. Clin Cardiol 1987; 10:383-92.

98. Ritchie JL, Cerqueira M, Maynard C, Davis K, Kennedy JW. Ventricular function

and infarct size: the Western Washington intravenous streptokinase in myocardial infarction trial. J Am Coll Cardiol 1988; 11:689-97.

99. Guerci AD, Gerstenblith G, Brinker JA, et al. A randomized trial of intravenous plasminogen activator for acute myocardial infarction with subsequent randomization to elective coronary angioplasty. N Engl J Med 1987; 317:1613-8.

100. O'Rourke M, Baron D, Keogh A, et al. Limitation of myocardial infarction by early infusion of recombinant tissue-type plasminogen activator. Circulation 1988; 77: 1311-5.

101. Van de Werf F, Arnola AER. Intravenous tissue plasminogen activator and size of infarct, left ventricular function, and survival in acute myocardial infarction. Br Med J 1986; 297:1374-9.

102. Armstrong PW, Baigrie RS, Daly PA, et al. Tissue plasminogen activator: Toronto (TPAT) placebo-controlled randomized trial in acute myocardial infarction. J Am Coll Cardiol 1989; 13:1469-76.

103. The Thrombolysis Early in Acute Heart Attack Trial Study Group. Very early thrombolytic therapy in suspected acute myocardial infarction. Am J Cardiol 1990; 65: 401-7.

104. Been M, de Bono DP, Muir AL, Boulton FE, Hillis WS, Harnung R. Coronary thrombolysis with intravenous anisoylated plasminogen-activator complex BRL 26921. Br Heart J 1985; 53:253-9.

105. Taeymans Y, Meterne P. Assessment of left ventricular function in a randomised study of intravenous anisoylated plasminogen streptokinase activator complex versus heparin in acute myocardial infarction. Preliminary results of the European Multicenter Study. Drugs 1987; 33:216-20.

106. Buchalter MB, Bourke JP, Jennings K, et al. The effect of thrombolytic therapy with anisoylated plasminogen streptokinase activator complex on the indicators of myocardial salvage. Drugs 1987; 33:209-15.

107. Bassand JP, Machecourt J, Cassegnes J, et al. Multicenter trial of intravenous anisoylated plasminogen streptokinase activator complex (APSAC) in acute myocardial infarction: Effect on infarct size and left ventricular function. J Am Coll Cardiol 1989; 13:988-97.

108. Maublant JC, Peycelon P, Cardot JC, Verdenet J, Fagret D, Comet M. Value of myocardial defect size by thallium-201 SPECT: results of a multicenter trial comparing heparin and a new fibrinolytic agent. J Nucl Med 1988; 29:1486-91.

109. Topol EJ, Califf RM, George BS, et al. Coronary arterial thrombolysis with combined infusion of recombinant tissue-type plasminogen activator and urokinase in patients with acute myocardial infarction. Circulation 1988; 77:1100-7.

110. Califf RM, Topol EJ, Stack RS, et al. An evaluation of combination thrombolytic therapy and timing of cardiac catheterization in acute myocardial infarction: the TAMI 5 randomized trial. Circulation 1991; 83:1543-56.

111. Grines CL, Nissen SE, Booth DC, et al. A prospective, randomized trial comparing combination half dose tissue plasminogen activator with streptokinase to full dose tissue tissue plasminogen activator. Circulation (in press).

112. Popma JJ, Topol EJ. Adjuncts to thrombolysis for myocardial reperfusion. Ann Intern Med 1991; 115:34-44.

113. Armstrong PW, Langevin LM, Watts DG. Randomized trial of prostacyclin infusion in acute myocardial infarction. Am J Cardiol 1988; 61:455-7.

114. Topol EJ, Ellis SG, Califf RM, et al. Combined tissue-type plasminogen activator and prostacyclin therapy for acute myocardial infarction. J Am Coll Cardiol 1989; 14:877-84.

115. Kerins DM, FitzGerald GA, Fitzgerald DJ. The influence of platelet inhibitors on the efficacy and disposition of tissue plasminogen activator (T-PA). Clin Res 1989; 37:4A (abstract).

116. Hsai J, Hamilton WP, Kleiman N, Roberts R, Chaitman BR, Ross AM. A comparison between heparin and low-dose aspirin as adjunctive therapy with tissue plasminogen activator for acute myocardial infarction. N Engl J Med 1990; 323:1433-7.

117. Bleich SD, Nichols TC, Schumacher RR, Cooke DH, Tate DA, Teichman SL. Effect of heparin on coronary arterial patency after thrombolysis with tissue plasminogen activator in acute myocardial infarction. Am J Cardiol 1990; 66:1412-7.

118. Topol EJ, George BS, Kereiakes DJ, et al. A randomized controlled trial of intravenous tissue plasminogen activator and early intravenous heparin in acute myocardial infarction. Circulation 1989; 79:281-6.

119. ISIS-1 (First International Study of Infarct Survival) Collaborative Group. Randomised trial of intravenous atenolol among 16,027 cases of suspected acute myocardial infarction: ISIS-1. Lancet 1986; 1:57-66.

120. Hjalmarson A, Herlitz J, Holmberg S, et al. The Goteborg metoprolol trial. Effects on mortality and morbidity in acute myocardial infarction. Circulation 1983; 67: I-26-I-32.

121. The International Collaborative Study Group. Reduction of infarct size with the early use of timolol in acute myocardial infarction. N Engl J Med 1984; 310:9-15.

122. Grines CL, Booth DC, Nissen SE, Gurley JC, Bennett KA, DeMaria AN. Acute effects of parenteral beta-blockade on regional ventricular function of infarct and noninfarct zones after reperfusion therapy in humans. J Am Coll Cardiol 1991; 17: 1382-7.

123. Steingart RM, Matthews R, Gambino A, Kantrowitz N, Katz S. Effects of intravenous metoprolol on global and regional left ventricular function after coronary arterial reperfusion in acute myocardial infarction. Am J Cardiol 1989; 63:767-71.

124. Sharpe N, Murphy J, Smith H, Hannan S. Treatment of patients with symptomless left ventricular dysfunction after myocardial infarction. Lancet 1988; 1:255-60.

125. Pfeffer MA, Lamas GA, Vaughan DE, Parisi AF, Braunwald E. Effect of captopril on progressive ventricular dilatation after anterior myocardial infarction. N Engl J Med 1988; 319:80-6.

126. Nabel EG, Topol EJ, Galeana A, et al. A randomized, placebo-controlled, trial of combined early intravenous captopril and recombinant tissue-type plasminogen activator therapy in acute myocardial infarction. J Am Coll Cardiol 1991; 17:467-73.

127. The Multicenter Diltiazem Postinfarction Trial Research Group. The effect of diltiazem on mortality and reinfarction after myocardial infarction. N Engl J Med 1988; 319:385-92.

128. Erbel R, Pop T, Meinertz T, et al. Combination of calcium channel blocker and thrombolytic therapy in acute myocardial infarction. Am Heart J 1988; 115:529-38.

129. Werns SW, Brinker J, Gruber J, et al. A randomized, double-blind trial of recombinant human superoxide dismutase (SOD) in patients undergoing PTCA for acute MI. Circulation 1989; 80(Suppl II):II-113 (abstract).
130. Cross DB, Ashton NG, Norris RM, White HD. Comparison of the effects of streptokinase and tissue plasminogen activator on regional wall motion after first myocardial infarction: analysis by the centerline method with correction for area at risk. J Am Coll Cardiol 1991; 17:1039-46.
131. Magnani B. Plasminogen Activator Italian Multicenter Study (PAIMS): comparison of intravenous recombinant single-chain human tissue-type plasminogen activator (rt-PA) with intravenous streptokinase in acute myocardial infarction. J Am Coll Cardiol 1989; 13:19-26.
132. Neuhaus KL, Tebbe U, Gotturick M, et al. IV recombinant rt-PA and urokinase in acute myocardial infarction: results of the German Activator Urokinase Study (GAUS). J Am Coll Cardiol 1988; 12:581-7.

3

Thrombolytic Mortality Trials

Eric R. Bates
University of Michigan Medical Center, Ann Arbor, Michigan

Eric Topol
The Cleveland Clinic Foundation, Cleveland, Ohio

INTRODUCTION

The major endpoints by which to judge thrombolytic drug efficacy have been infarct artery patency, left ventricular function, and mortality. Although reestablishing infarct artery patency remains the primary goal, it is unclear whether acute patency, late patency, or sustained patency without reocclusion predicts the best clinical outcome (Chapter 1). Likewise, whereas left ventricular function is the major determining factor in prognosis, there are limitations in measuring this endpoint, and the small changes documented in previous studies do not completely explain the salutary results associated with thrombolytic therapy (Chapter 2). Mortality is the most definitive, easiest to measure endpoint. In this chapter, we will review the results from the five controlled mortality trials, summarize results for several clinically important subgroups, and discuss comparative mortality trial results.

CONTROLLED THROMBOLYTIC MORTALITY TRIALS

There have been five controlled trials of thrombolytic therapy where at least 1000 patients were enrolled (1-5). Descriptive factors are summarized in Table 1. Because the long-term follow-up reports (6-9) consistently confirm the findings from the initial reports, only the initial results will be reviewed.

Table 1   Controlled Thrombolytic Mortality Trials

	GISSI-1	ISAM	AIMS	ISIS-2	ASSET
Agents	SK	SK	APSAC	SK	t-PA
No. pts.	11,806	1,741	1,258	17,187	5,011
Centers	176	38	39	417	52
Symptoms	<12 hr	<6 hr	<6 hr	<24 hr	<5 hr
ECG requirements	ST ↑	ST ↑	ST ↑	None	None
Age (years)	All	All	<70	All	≤75
ASA	No	Yes	No	Yes	No
Heparin	±	Yes (IV)	Yes (IV)	No	Yes (IV, 1 day)
Warfarin	No	Yes	Yes	No	No
Mortality					
Endpoint	14–21 days	21 days	30 days	35 days	30 days
Treatment	10.7%	6.3%	6.4%	9.2%	7.2%
Placebo	13.0%	7.1%	12.2%	12.0%	9.8%

Gruppo Italiano Per Lo Studio Della Streptochinasi Nell'Infarto Myocardico (GISSI-1)

The GISSI-1 trial (1) was an unblinded trial of intravenous streptokinase or standard therapy in 11,806 patients enrolled from 176 centers over 17 months. Patients had electrocardiographic (ECG) evidence of either ST-segment elevation or depression and symptoms of less than 12 hr duration. Of the patients admitted to the Italian CCUs during this period, 63% were excluded from the protocol: reasons included symptom duration greater than 12 hr (51%), streptokinase contraindications (21%), doubtful myocardial infarction (19%), and administrative complications (8%). Adjunctive drugs administered to these patients included antiplatelets (14%), heparin (62%), nitrates (37%), beta blockers (8%), and calcium blockers (48%). Hospital mortality (14–21 days) was reduced by 18% (10.7 versus 13.0%; $p = 0.0002$), with the greatest benefit seen in the first hour of symptoms (47% reduction) and a significant benefit seen up to 6 hr. A significant survival advantage was found for age < 65 years, anterior or multiple location infarct site, first infarction, and Killip I or II functional class. Conversely, no survival advantage was found for patients with age > 65 years, inferior infarct location, history of previous infarction, ST-segment depression, or Killip III or IV functional class.

Intravenous Streptokinase in Acute Myocardial Infarction (ISAM) Trial

The ISAM trial (2) was the first placebo-controlled double-blind randomized trial to enroll over 1000 patients. A total of 1741 patients from 38 centers were treated with streptokinase or placebo. Symptom duration was limited to 6 hr, and patients had to have ST-segment elevation. Patients over age 75 were excluded. Only 23% of the patients screened for the protocol were enrolled. Patients received aspirin, heparin, intravenous nitroglycerin, and warfarin. Either the large number of excluded patients or the most aggressive adjunctive therapy program of all the trials may have contributed to the low mortality found in the control group. There was an insignificant 11% reduction in 21-day mortality with streptokinase (6.3 versus 7.1%); patients treated within 3 hr had a 20% reduction in mortality (5.2 versus 6.5%).

APSAC Intervention Mortality Study (AIMS)

The AIMS trial (3) is the only double-blind, placebo-controlled trial that assessed anistreplase. The trial was stopped early after the second interim analysis showed survival benefit for treated patients. In the final report (8), 1258 patients from 39 centers had been enrolled. All had ECG evidence for ST-segment elevation and <6 hr of symptoms. Patients over age 70 years were excluded. Patients were treated with intravenous heparin, warfarin, and timolol (54%), but not aspirin. Thirty-day mortality was reduced by 50.5% (5.4 versus 12.1%; $p = 0.0006$). This excellent treatment result was probably exaggerated because of the premature study termination. Survival benefit was seen for all subgroups.

Second International Study of Infarct Survival (ISIS-2)

The ISIS-2 trial (4) was the largest randomized, placebo-controlled trial of thrombolytic treatment. A total of 17,187 patients from 417 hospitals were randomized between: (a) a 1-hr infusion of streptokinase; (b) 1 month of 160 mg/day aspirin; (c) both treatments; (d) neither treatment. Patients were eligible for treatment if they were within 24 hr of suspected myocardial infarction and the physician was uncertain whether treatment with streptokinase or with aspirin was indicated. ECG changes were not required. Significant reductions in 5-week vascular mortality were shown for both aspirin (9.4 versus 11.8%) and streptokinase (9.2 versus 12.0%). Importantly, the combination of both treatments had an additive effect (8.0 versus 13.2%). Additionally, survival benefit was shown in almost all subgroups.

Anglo-Scandinavian Study of Early Thrombolysis (ASSET)

The ASSET trial (5) is the only double-blind, placebo-controlled trial of alteplase. A total of 13,318 patients were screened to enroll 5011 (38%) patients in 52 centers within 5 hr of symptom onset. Reasons for exclusion included symptoms > 5 hr (74%) and age > 75 years (8%). There were no ECG requirements. Intravenous heparin was given for 21 hr, but aspirin was not used. One-month mortality was reduced by 26% (7.2 versus 9.8%); in patients with a confirmed diagnosis of myocardial infarction, mortality was reduced by 28% (9.4 versus 13.1%). Patients with later treatment or older age benefited.

RESULTS FROM SUBGROUP ANALYSES

The following review of subgroup data from the placebo-controlled thrombolytic trials has been organized to separate the results with streptokinase therapy (GISSI-1, ISIS-2) from the results with anistreplase (AIMS), streptokinase plus aspirin (ISIS-2), and alteplase (ASSET). The latter three treatment options produced superior benefit compared with streptokinase therapy alone, as can be seen by reviewing Tables 2–7. This subject has been reviewed by several other authors recently (10–12).

Symptom Duration

The greatest reduction in mortality occurs when thrombolytic therapy is initiated within the first hour of symptom onset. There was a 47% mortality reduction in the GISSI-1 trial and a 40% mortality reduction in the ISIS-2 trial for streptokinase therapy and a 56% mortality reduction in the ISIS-2 trial for streptokinase plus aspirin. Pooled results from the five controlled studies in patients treated within a 6-hr time limit demonstrate a mortality rate of 8.7%, a 27% mortality reduction (Fig. 1). Although this time limit has become a popular clinical convention, evidence exists supporting treatment in patients who present later than 6 hr. In a meta-analysis of six previous intravenous streptokinase trials, Yusuf et al. (13) found mortality reduction unrelated to symptom duration. Mortality rates for streptokinase and control groups were: 0–6 hr, 17 versus 20%; 6–12 hr, 18 versus 21%; >12 hr, 12 versus 22%. Reevaluation of the GISSI-1 trial reveals that the mortality reduction in patients treated with 1–3 hr of symptoms was 9.5 versus 11.1% compared with 12.6 versus 14.1% for patients with 6–9 hr of symptoms. The 6- to 9-hr results were statistically insignificant because of small sample size, although the absolute benefit was equivalent to patients with 1–3 hr of symptoms. No advantage was shown for symptom duration of 9–12 hr in the GISSI-1 trial, but in the ISIS-2 trial, significant mortality reduction was shown up to 24 hr. Preliminary results from the Estudio Multicentrico Estreptoquinasa Republica de America del Sur (EMERAS) trial (14) in almost 4000 patients, however, suggested only a trend toward survival benefit from streptokinase in patients treated from 7 to 12 hr (11.3 versus 12.8%), but no benefit in the group treated from 13 to 24 hr (11.0 versus 10.8%). More information regarding streptokinase therapy will be forthcoming from the ISIS-3 study. Results potentially could be

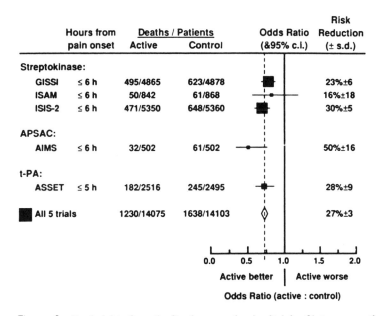

Figure 1   Pooled data from the five large randomized trials of intravenous thrombolysis showing a consistent mortality reduction of 27 ± 3% in the treated groups. (Reproduced with permission from Ref. 48.)

more positive in the Late Assessment of Thrombolytic Efficacy (LATE) trial, where alteplase is being studied in 5000 patients. Previous studies have suggested greater thrombolytic efficacy for alteplase relative to streptokinase in patients treated with symptom duration > 4 hr (15). In the recently completed TAMI-6 trial (16), a 64% patency rate was found in patients treated with TPA compared with 23% in placebo patients. Symptom duration ranged from 6 to 24 hr and angiography was performed a mean of 36 hr after symptom onset.

There are several possible explanations for survival benefit from thrombolytic therapy after the 3-hr time frame within which myocardial salvage is to be expected. First, it is difficult to clinically determine when occlusive thrombosis occurs; many patients have prodromal symptoms for minutes to hours, which may be included in an overestimate of ischemic time. Second, coronary thrombosis is a dynamic process, with dissolution and reformation of the occlusive thrombus resulting in intermittent reperfusion, which may prolong the potential for myocyte survival. Third, collateral circulation can also extend cell viability. Fourth, arterial patency has a favorable impact on left ventricular healing and remodeling independent of muscle salvage, which may lead to improvement in prognosis through "shape salvage" (17). Fifth, mural thrombus formation may be reduced (18).

Finally, electrical stability seems to be improved, potentially decreasing the risk for sudden death (19,20). Therefore, there are theoretical reasons to treat patients with > 6 hr of symptoms, and clinical trial data are supportive. From a practical standpoint, the best candidates appear to be patients with persistent ischemic chest pain and ST-segment elevation who present within 12 hr and have a low bleeding risk with ECG evidence of a large myocardial infarction.

Infarct Location

The controlled thrombolytic trials have consistently shown survival benefit for patients with anterior myocardial infarction where infarct size, mural thrombus formation, and electrical complications contributed to a 1-month mortality rate of approximately 18% in conventionally treated patients (Table 2). It has been more difficult to show a similar benefit in patients with inferior myocardial infarction, mostly because the control mortality is half that of anterior myocardial infarction. Early studies by Kennedy and colleagues (21,22) showed no survival benefit with streptokinase therapy, leading to the recommendation that treatment be reserved for patients with anterior myocardial infarction (23). Similar findings were observed in the GISSI-1 trial and the ISIS-2 trial. However, when aspirin was added to streptokinase, or when alteplase or anistreplase was used, statistically significant mortality differences were found (Table 2).

In addition to treatment strategy, another confounding factor has been that inferior infarction is a heterogeneous clinical entity with high-risk and low-risk patients, unlike anterior myocardial infarction, where risk is more consistent. For instance, mortality rates in inferior infarction associated with right ventricular infarction, third-degree atrioventricular block, or precordial ST-segment depression range from 8 to 20% (24). In the absence of those complications, mortality risk is less than 5%. Therefore, including low-risk patients, where treatment is unlikely to show benefit, dilutes the benefits seen in treating high-risk patients.

Therapeutic limitations in treating patients with inferior myocardial infarction include smaller infarct size with less ischemic muscle to potentially salvage, lower early patency rates in patients with right coronary artery lesions, higher reocclusion rates, and stimulation of the Bezold-Jarisch cardiodepressor-vasodepressor reflex (25). However, current data support treating patients without regard to infarct location.

Age

From 10 to 27% of patients are excluded from thrombolytic therapy because of advanced age (12). Ironically, although clinicians are more eager to treat younger patients because of the low risk for intracerebral hemorrhage, no trial has demonstrated treatment benefit for patients less than 50 years old. The major risk for death in younger patients is confined to the prehospital phase, with hospital mor-

Table 2 Mortality by Infarct Location

Study	Mortality rate				Mortality reduction	
	Treatment		Control			
	No.	%	No.	%	%	Lives saved/1000
Anterior myocardial infarction						
GISSI-1 (SK)	309/2134	14.5	403/2193	18.4	21	39
ISIS-2 (SK)	207/1835	11.3	329/1827	18.0	37	67
AIMS (APSAC)	29/294	9.9	51/292	17.5	43	76
ISIS-2 (SK/ASA)	92/918	10.0	185/898	20.6	51	106
Inferior myocardial infarction						
GISSI-1 (SK)	137/2009	6.8	145/2004	7.2	6	4
ISIS-2 (SK)	150/2076	7.2	185/2112	8.8	18	16
AIMS (APSAC)	11/329	3.3	26/335	7.8	58	45
ISIS-2 (SK/ASA)	69/1016	6.8	107/1047	10.2	33	34
ASSET (rt-PA)	47/753	6.3	74/754	9.8	36	35

Table 3   Mortality by Age

Study	Age (yrs)	Mortality rate				Mortality reduction	
		Treatment		Control			
		No.	%	No.	%	%	Lives saved/1000
GISSI-1 (SK)	<65	217/3824	5.7	291/3784	7.7	26	20
	65–75	240/1444	16.6	261/1442	18.1	8	15
	>75	171/592	28.9	206/623	33.1	13	42
ISIS-2 (SK)	<60	156/3864	4.2	224/3856	5.8	28	16
	60–69	320/3033	10.6	435/3023	14.4	26	38
	>70	309/1695	18.2	370/1716	21.6	16	34
AIMS (APSAC)	<60	15/372	4.0	23/379	6.1	34	21
	60–70	25/252	9.9	54/254	21.3	54	114
ISIS-2 (SK/ASA)	<60	71/1938	3.7	120/1924	6.2	40	25
	60–69	137/1500	9.1	245/1524	16.1	43	70
	>70	135/854	15.8	203/852	23.8	34	80
ASSET (rt-PA)	<55	29/748	3.8	33/745	4.4	14	6
	56–65	63/963	6.5	71/896	7.9	18	14
	66–75	90/827	10.8	140/852	16.4	34	56

tality rates less than 5%. In contrast, mortality risk increases in parallel with age, such that the greatest mortality risk, and the potential for greatest therapeutic benefit, is in the oldest patient (26). In the ISIS-2 trial, mortality was reduced from 37% to 20% in patients 80 years of age or older treated with streptokinase and aspirin. The treatment results by age from five trials are shown in Table 3. Because the risk of bleeding and stroke with therapy is increased in the elderly (27–29), emphasis on early treatment, large infarct size, and otherwise good general health may be appropriate. However, the potential to save more lives by treating elderly patients than can be saved by treating younger patients supports a more aggressive treatment posture in this high-risk group.

Gender

Women have higher mortality rates than men (30). Older age, more comorbid disease such as hypertension or diabetes mellitus, or later presentation has been used to explain this finding, but the observation remains somewhat controversial. In the four randomized trials that reported results by gender (Table 4), the pooled control mortality for men was 10.9% versus 17.2 for women. Thrombolytic therapy reduced the rates to 7.7% and 13.6%, respectively.

Electrocardiographic Criteria

The presence of ST-segment elevation is a universally accepted indication for thrombolytic therapy based on the results from the mortality trials. The number of leads exhibiting this change, however, is prognostically important. Results from the GISSI-1 study (31) demonstrated no survival benefit in small infarctions defined as those with ST-segment elevation in only two or three leads. Treatment benefit was shown for moderate infarction (four or five leads), large infarction, (six or seven leads), and extensive infarction (eight or nine leads) (Fig. 2).

Additional risk is also associated with the presence of ST-segment depression in reciprocal leads (32). Precordial ST-segment depression in inferior infarction increases both acute and chronic mortality risk 3–4 times, presumably because it reflects larger infarct size (33).

No treatment benefit was seen in GISSI-1 or ISIS-2 in patients who presented with only ST-segment depression. DeWood et al. (34) demonstrated that arterial patency was present in 74% of patients with non-Q-wave myocardial infarction studied within the first 24 hr, which suggests that nonocclusive thrombosis or spontaneous thrombolysis had occurred. Additionally, data from studies of thrombolytic therapy and unstable angina, where nonocclusive thrombus is present, have shown no treatment benefit (35). Thus, it appears that occlusive thrombosis needs to be present for thrombolytic therapy to be effective. One group of patients with thrombotic occlusion who exhibit ST-segment depression are those with nondominant circumflex disease, but mortality risk is low. High risk is pres-

Table 4   Mortality by Gender

| Study | Mortality rate | | | | Mortality reduction | |
| | Treatment | | Control | | | |
	No.	%	No.	%	%	Lives saved/1000
Men						
GISSI-1 (SK)	414/4703	8.8	497/4695	10.6	17	18
ISIS-2 (SK)	514/6519	7.9	719/6606	10.9	28	30
AIMS (APSAC)	34/514	6.6	56/516	10.9	39	43
ISIS-2 (SK/ASA)	218/3276	6.7	401/3342	12.0	44	53
ASSET (rt-PA)	132/1935	6.8	182/1928	9.4	28	26
Women						
GISSI-1 (SK)	214/1157	18.5	261/1156	22.6	18	41
ISIS-2 (SK)	269/2018	13.3	303/1927	15.7	15	24
AIMS (APSAC)	6/110	5.5	21/117	17.9	69	124
ISIS-2 (SK/ASA)	121/989	12.2	161/922	17.5	30	53
ASSET (rt-PA)	50/576	8.6	62/565	10.9	21	23

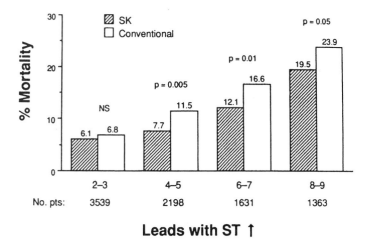

Leads with ST ↑

Figure 2   Comparison of the in-hospital mortality rate of patients with acute myocardial infarction in the GISSI study according to the electrocardiographically determined infarct size. (Reproduced with permission from Ref. 48.)

ent in patients with widespread ST-segment depression, which may represent left main or three-vessel disease. Results from the TIMI-3 trial and the ISIS-3 trial will hopefully clarify treatment strategies in this large subgroup of patients who constitute 30–40% of those who present with acute myocardial infarction.

Patients with ischemic chest pain and left bundle branch block may benefit from therapy. In the GISSI-1 trial, mortality was 8% with streptokinase versus 8.6% in controls. However, in the ISIS-2 trial, where control mortality was 28%, rates of 20% and 14% were associated with streptokinase and streptokinase plus aspirin therapy, respectively.

Finally, prior myocardial infarction increased mortality risk from 11% to 17% in GISSI-1, ISIS-2, and AIMS (Table 5). Although no mortality benefit was seen with treatment in the GISSI-1 trial, impressive benefit was shown in the other two trials.

Blood Pressure and Heart Rate

Many thrombolytic trials have excluded patients with hypertension because of the expectation that intracerebral hemorrhage rates would be increased. One uncontrolled preliminary report did show a significantly higher rate for transient pressures > 180 mmHg systolic or 120 mmHg diastolic (36). Similarly, results from the MITI trial have documented a 10% risk of stroke for systolic pressures over 200 mmHg (37). The ISIS-2 trial did show a survival benefit for patients with systolic pressures > 175 mmHg, but further definition of the pressures was not

Table 5   Mortality by Prior Myocardial Infarction History

| Study | Mortality rate | | | | Mortality reduction | |
| | Treatment | | Placebo | | | |
	No.	%	No.	%	%	Lives saved/1000
	No prior myocardial infarction					
GISSI-1 (SK)	468/4905	9.5	606/4926	12.3	23	28
ISIS-2 (SK)	587/6994	8.4	767/7049	10.9	23	25
AIMS (APSAC)	28/521	5.4	53/520	10.2	47	48
ISIS-2 (SK/ASA)	242/3502	6.9	433/3513	12.3	44	54
	Prior myocardial infarction					
GISSI-1 (SK)	157/927	16.9	147/889	16.5	-2	-4
ISIS-2 (SK)	190/1496	12.7	248/1442	17.2	26	45
AIMS (APSAC)	12/103	11.7	24/113	21.2	45	95
ISIS-2 (SK/ASA)	96/737	13.0	125/725	17.2	24	42

Table 6 Mortality by Blood Pressure

Study	Systolic BP	Mortality rate				Mortality reduction	
		Treatment		Control			
		No.	%	No.	%	%	Lives saved/1000
ISIS-2 (SK)	< 100	87/319	27.3	111/312	35.6	23	83
	100–124	297/2494	11.9	360/2531	14.2	16	23
	125–149	204/2901	7.0	294/2877	10.2	31	32
	150–174	168/2297	7.3	214/2307	9.3	22	20
	≥ 175	33/578	5.7	49/563	8.7	34	20
AIMS (APSAC)	≤ 100	9/59	15.3	15/66	22.7	33	74
	101–159	22/457	4.8	51/449	11.4	58	66
	≥ 160	9/105	8.6	11/116	9.5	9	9
ISIS-2 (SK/ASA)	≤ 180	45/158	28.5	58/157	36.9	23	84
	100–124	132/1238	10.7	209/1262	16.6	36	59
	125–149	89/1460	6.1	164/1430	11.5	47	54
	150–174	62/1146	5.4	114/1169	9.8	45	44
	≥ 175	14/289	4.8	22/280	7.9	39	31

offered. Important to the clinician, and underemphasized previously, is the inverse relationship between blood pressure and mortality (Table 6). Therefore, although survival benefit is present independent of blood pressure, the relative benefit decreases and the small risk of bleeding increases at higher pressure levels, suggesting that a higher threshold for treatment is reasonable if lower risk for benefit (inferior myocardial infarction, later presentation, male gender, younger age) or higher risk for bleeding (older age, lighter body weight) is present. Conversely, it appears that treatment is increasingly important with lower blood pressure measurements. Some clinicians choose to use alteplase or urokinase instead of streptokinase or anistreplase in hypotensive patients, but no difference in risk or benefit has been noted in the mortality trials. Despite thrombolytic therapy, mortality rates are greater than 10% when systolic blood pressure is under 125 mmHg.

No difference was seen in patients with heart rates under 60 beats/min versus 60–80 beats/min. Higher heart rates are associated with higher mortality rates and greater mortality reductions with treatment (Table 7).

Congestive Heart Failure and Cardiogenic Shock

Congestive heart failure or pulmonary edema was present in approximately 20% of patients in the GISSI-1 trial and the International Trial. Unfortunately, it does not appear that a clinically important survival benefit was achieved with thrombolytic therapy compared with control patients or even with the initial coronary care unit experience of Killip and Kimble 25 years ago (class I, 6%; class II, 17%; class III, 38%; class IV, 81%) (38). Even more disturbing is the fact that 1-year mortality rates in GISSI-1 Killip II or Killip III patients were 26.6 and 50.3%, respectively. Additionally, patients with cardiogenic shock have shown no mortality benefit with treatment compared with control patients or historical controls. These results are disappointing given the facts that thrombolytic therapy and successful reperfusion decrease infarct size, preserve left ventricular function, and improve survival in other subgroups. Further studies are needed to evaluate the possibility that conjunctive therapy with intra-aortic balloon counterpulsation, coronary angioplasty, or coronary bypass graft surgery might improve results in these patients.

Summary

A quick patient history, physical examination, and ECG analysis allow the clinician to evaluate the risks and benefits of thrombolytic intervention versus conventional care. High-risk patients (mortality > 10% despite thrombolytic therapy) are those with symptom duration greater than 3 hr, anterior infarct location, age > 65 years, female gender, ST-segment shifts in more than six leads, left bundle branch block, history of previous myocardial infarction, systolic blood pressure < 125 mmHg, heart rate > 100 beats/min, heart failure, cardiogenic shock, or diabetes

Table 7   Mortality by Heart Rate

Study	HR	Mortality rate						Mortality reduction	
		Treatment			Placebo				
		No.	%		No.	%		%	Lives saved/1000
ISIS-2 (SK)	< 80	346/4836	7.2		448/4778	9.4		23	22
	80–99	178/1663	10.7		219/1623	13.5		21	28
	≥ 100	152/1004	15.1		219/1013	21.6		30	65
AIMS (APSAC)	≤ 80	15/336	4.5		28/347	8.1		44	36
	80–99	16/216	7.4		35/225	15.6		53	82
	≥ 100	9/69	13.0		14/58	24.1		46	111
ISIS-2 (SK/ASA)	≤ 80	158/2421	6.5		250/2361	10.6		39	41
	80–99	74/796	9.3		124/808	15.3		39	60
	≥ 100	68/526	12.9		115/515	22.3		42	94

mellitus. It will be critically important to determine whether new thrombolytic regimens or additional adjunctive interventions can further improve the prognosis in these patients.

COMPARATIVE THROMBOLYTIC MORTALITY TRIALS

Three large-scale trials have assessed the relative efficacy of thrombolytic agents for mortality reduction. Two of these "megatrials" are completed and the results have been published, which include GISSI-2 (Gruppo Italiano per lo Studio della Sopravivenza Nell'Infarto Miocardico) and ISIS-3 (International Studies of Infarct Survival). A third trial, known as GUSTO (Global Utilization of Streptokinase and Tissue Plasminogen Activator for Occluded Coronary Arteries) is currently in progress. The algorithms for these trials are presented in Figures 3–5 and their overall design features in Table 8. These trials differ with respect to actual drug regimens tested, subcutaneous versus intravenous heparin randomization and utilization, time window of symptom duration for entry, and ECG inclusion criteria.

The GISSI-2/International t-PA/SK Trial

The GISSI-2 trial (39) was designed as a 12,000-patient trial using a composite endpoint of death and myocardial "injury." The International t-PA/SK trial (40) was an approximate 8000-patient extension of GISSI-2 to provide adequate statistical power for detecting differences in mortality. These data in aggregate (Fig. 6)

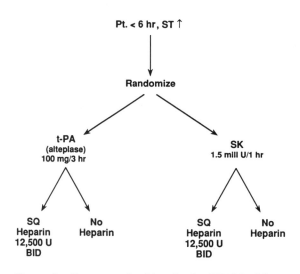

Figure 3   Treatment algorithm for the GISSI-2 trial.

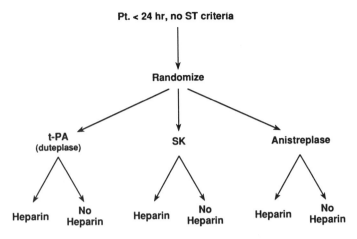

Figure 4   Treatment algorithm for the ISIS-3 trial.

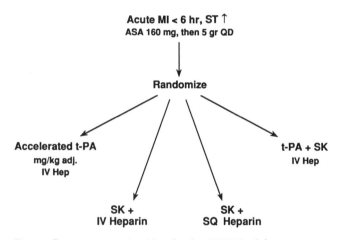

Figure 5   Treatment algorithm for the GUSTO trial.

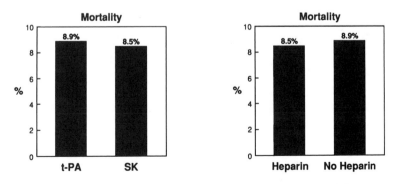

Figure 6   Mortality results in the GISSI-2/International t-PA/SK trial.

Table 8 Comparative Thrombolytic Trials to Assess Mortality Reduction

Trial	Total patients	Arms	Dose	Heparin	Entry criteria time limit	ST Elevation
GISSI-2/International	20,749	2	t-PA 100 mg/3 hr SK 1.5 mill U/1 hr	12,500 U SQ BID beginning 12 hr in 50% of patients	6 hr	Yes
ISIS-3	39,913	3	t-PA 0.6 MU/kg/4 hr SK 1.5 mill U/hr APSAC 30-mg bolus	12,500 U SQ BID beginning 4 hr in 50% of patients	24 hr	Not required
GUSTO	41,000[a]	4	t-PA 100 mg/90 min SK 1.5 mill U/1 hr t-PA 1 mg/kg/1 hr + SK 1.0 mill U/1 hr	In 3 arms: IV hep 5000-U bolus at start of therapy and 1000 U/hr × ≥48 hr adjusted to PTT, in SK arm with SQ hep, same as ISIS-3	6 hr	Yes

[a]Planned enrollment.

indicate that the thrombolytic agents, at the employed dose and treatment regimen, achieved an equivalent reduction of mortality. Streptokinase was associated with fewer strokes and more allergic reactions and transfusions compared with t-PA.

It is important to note that the heparin randomization in the GISSI-2 and International trials was to either subcutaneous heparin 12,500 U twice daily beginning 12 hr after thrombolysis or no heparin. As shown in Figure 6, there was no discernible mortality reduction. An interaction between streptokinase and subcutaneous heparin for reduction of mortality, not observed for t-PA and subcutaneous heparin, was noted in the GISSI-2 data set, but its significance is not well understood.

Third International Study of Infarct Survival (ISIS-3)

A major advance in our understanding of comparative thrombolytic agent therapy for reduction of mortality emanated from the ISIS-3 trial (41). In this study, there was a three-way comparison of thrombolytics, with the incorporation of anistreplase in one arm, the duteplase form of t-PA in another, and streptokinase as the reference arm. The randomization for heparin or no heparin involved the use of the same dose of calcium heparin as in GISSI-2 but the time of administration was 4 hr from start of thrombolytic therapy instead of 12 hr. Also, importantly, the ISIS-3 trial was a triple-placebo, triple-dummy controlled trial such that there was effective blinding of the patient and investigators as to the actual thrombolytic agent and to the heparin. Although this is a more difficult, cumbersome design, it is superior with respect to more complete, objective assessment compared with an "open" format.

In ISIS-3, as summarized in Figure 7, there was no difference in mortality rate between the three thrombolytic agents. There was, however, a higher stroke rate for t-PA and APSAC compared with streptokinase (Fig. 8). As in GISSI-2, an in-

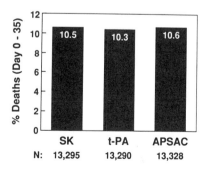

Figure 7   Mortality results in the ISIS-3 trial.

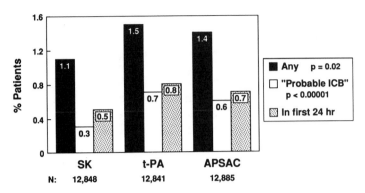

Figure 8   Stroke rate in the ISIS-3 trial. ICB = intracerebral bleed.

significant trend toward mortality reduction was associated with the use of subcutaneous heparin. When the GISSI-2/International t-PA/SK and ISIS-3 trials are combined, a statistically significant reduction in mortality and reinfarction were observed for subcutaneous heparin (Table 9), but there was an increase in bleeding complications. Nonrandomized data from approximately 3000 patients in ISIS-3 who received intravenous heparin (off protocol) suggested an even higher rate of overall stroke (2–2.5%) but a lower overall mortality (9.2%). The true benefit-to-risk ratio of intravenous heparin is controversial and needs to be established.

Table 9   Role of Subcutaneous Heparin per 1000 Patients Treated

		GISSI-2	ISIS-3
Advantages	Deaths	–4	–5
	Reinfarction	–1	–3
Disadvantages	Transfusion	+5	+3
	Intracerebral hemorrhage	+1	+2

ICH = intracerebral hemorrhage; GISSI = Gruppo Italiano per lo Studio della Sopravivenza nell'Infarto Miocardico; ISIS = International Studies of Infarct Survival; MI = myocardial infarction.
Source: Reprinted with permission from Topol (57).

The Global Utilization of Streptokinase and Tissue Plasminogen Activator for Occluded Coronary Arteries (GUSTO) Trial

New data have prompted the need for yet another large-scale comparative trial of thrombolytic agents. The basic objective in GUSTO is to determine whether rapid restoration of infarct artery patency or sustained patency or both are linked to improved survival compared with streptokinase and subcutaneous heparin administration. Improved ability to more rapidly achieve infarct artery patency has been suggested by the trials employing accelerated t-PA regimens. An enhanced predischarge patency rate has been demonstrated with the use of combination thrombolytic therapy and with intravenous heparin in trials with t-PA monotherapy.

Accelerated t-PA Dosing

The velocity of infarct artery recanalization has been increased by the front-loaded regimen developed by Neuhaus and colleagues (42). Three trials (42–44) have tested this regimen consisting of a 15-mg bolus, 50 mg over 30 min, and the subsequent 35 mg over the next 60 min. This is essentially the same as giving t-PA twice as fast as the conventional 3-hr regimen, but is further accentuated by administering 65% of the t-PA in the first 30 min. By 60 min into therapy in the three trials, infarct artery patency was approximately 75%, and by 90 min, it was 85% compared with previously documented patency rates at 90 min of approximately 70% for both t-PA and APSAC.

A legitimate concern about front-loaded t-PA and any thrombolytic regimen that appears to be more potent with respect to fibrinolysis is the potential for more serious bleeding. In reviewing the data from the completed trials with accelerated t-PA, including the recent TAMI-7 experience in 182 patients with several different accelerated regimens (45), excess bleeding has not been found. To date, the intracranial hemorrhage rate is 0.5% in 608 patients. In all these studies, daily oral aspirin was given and intravenous heparin was administered for at least the first 24–48 hr.

Combination Thrombolysis

With the use of combined fibrin-specific and nonspecific activators, reocclusion after successful thrombolysis has been approximately 5% (46,47). This incidence is substantially improved compared with prior studies of monotherapy in which a 12–25% incidence of reocclusion was quite common (48). Like accelerated t-PA, the increased thrombolytic potency has to date not been accompanied by an apparent excess of bleeding complications. Without reiterating all the data, it can be concluded that combination thrombolytic therapy with t-PA and SK or t-PA and UK, holds considerable promise as a key thromboprophylactic strategy (Chapter 13).

Heparin with Thrombolytics

There have been five randomized trials (49–53) involving the use of heparin with t-PA. Collectively, these trials indicate that early heparin therapy is required to sustain infarct artery patency after t-PA. Whereas intravenous heparin may not be important to achieve or facilitate initial patency (49) and administration does not appear to be necessary for more than 24 hr in uncomplicated patients (53), the data confirm a significant patency advantage with early intravenous heparinization after t-PA therapy. While this may also be the case with all other thrombolytic agents, there are no completed, controlled angiographic trials testing intravenous heparin with streptokinase or anistreplase. Importantly, the benefit of intravenous heparin compared with high-dose, subcutaneously administered heparin has not been assessed, but will be in GUSTO with streptokinase.

Thus, the rationale for the GUSTO trial stems directly from these three controversial areas. Using the strategies of rapid thrombolysis with accelerated t-PA, sustained thrombolysis with combination thrombolytics, and intravenous or subcutaneous heparin, the trial will address key, contemporary issues of optimal myocardial reperfusion therapy. It is currently ongoing in what will be a 15-country, four-continent, >700-hospital recruitment effort. The anticipated enrollment of 41,000 patients is expected to be completed by the end of 1992. In GUSTO, while there may be an increase in bleeding complications owing to more aggressive pharmacological therapy, it is hoped that an improved treatment strategy resulting in lower mortality than can be achieved with streptokinase and subcutaneous heparin will be identified.

ARE ALL THROMBOLYTICS "CREATED EQUAL"?

There has been considerable debate over the relative merits and disadvantages of one thrombolytic agent compared with another (54). Although there are distinct mechanistic differences between the agents and important differences in infarct artery patency (early and sustained rates), no trial to date has demonstrated a difference with respect to either left ventricular function (55) or mortality.

There are three possible ways to interpret the current lack of difference in mortality. First, there may indeed be a significant difference but it may be difficult to detect, particularly if adjunctive therapies, such as intravenous heparin, are important to coadminister. For example, a mortality reduction from 7.0 to 6.0%, a 15% decrease, would require a sample size of 20,000 patients with 80% power of detecting a difference between two thrombolytic agents. Clearly, the task of demonstrating an advantage of one thrombolytic agent or strategy over another is far more challenging, if indeed such advantage exists, compared with proving superiority over conventional or placebo therapy, because of the smaller mortality differences. Unless such trials are performed, however, it is impossible to assess whether all thrombolytic agents have equipotential of improving survival. More important, it will only be through such large-scale efforts that an improved pharmacological strategy can be unequivocally validated. Nevertheless, with the high attendant cost, obligatory time lag, and enormous effort and resource utilization for such "megatrials," it is hoped that eventually a clinical outcome index, with inclusion of several events besides mortality and reinfarction (55), will prove a useful substitute so that trials that require intake of 20,000–40,000 patients will not need to be routinely performed.

Second, it is possible that early infarct artery recanalization with relatively fibrin specific agents (e.g., t-PA, scu-PA) may be accompanied by a higher risk of reocclusion, negating the potential advantage of more timely myocardial reperfusion.

Third, it remains plausible that streptokinase has nonthrombolytic actions that make it uniquely advantageous in the setting of myocardial reperfusion. Such effects as viscosity reduction, scavenging free oxygen radicals, and collagen breakdown (48,56) are all potential theoretical special benefits of streptokinase.

Given the 9–10% mortality rate in all the therapeutic arms of the International and ISIS-3 trials, there is clearly room for further improvement in survival with reperfusion therapy. Although additional advances in developing more potent thrombolytic drugs will undoubtedly occur, the following chapters will focus on the potential benefits associated with adjunctive therapies.

REFERENCES

1. Gruppo Italiano per lo Studio della Streptochinasi nell'Infarto Miocardico (GISSI). Effectiveness of intravenous thrombolytic treatment in acute myocardial infarction. Lancet 1986; 1:397–402.
2. The ISAM Study Group. A prospective trial of Intravenous Streptokinase in Acute Myocardial infarction (ISAM). N Engl J Med 1986; 314:1465–71.
3. AIMS Trial Study Group. Effect of intravenous APSAC on mortality after acute myocardial infarction: preliminary report of a placebo-controlled clinical trial. Lancet 1988; 1:545–9.
4. ISIS-2 Collaborative Group. Randomized trial of intravenous streptokinase, oral aspirin, both or neither among 17187 cases of suspected acute myocardial infarction: ISIS-2. Lancet 1988; 2:349–60.
5. Wilcox RG, Olsson CG, Skene AM, et al. for the ASSET Study Group. Trial of tissue plasminogen activator for mortality reduction in acute myocardial infarction. Anglo-Scandinavian Study of Early Thrombolysis (ASSET). Lancet 1988; 2:525–30.
6. Gruppo Italiano per lo Studio della Streptochinasi nell'Infarto Miocardico (GISSI). Long-term effects of intravenous thrombolysis in acute myocardial infarction: final report of the GISSI study. Lancet 1987; 2:871–4.
7. Schroder R, Neuhaus K-L, Leizorovicz A, Linderer T, Tebbe U. A prospective placebo-controlled double-blind multicenter trial of intravenous streptokinase in acute

myocardial infarction (ISAM): long-term mortality and morbidity. J Am Coll Cardiol 1987; 9:197-203.

8. AIMS Trial Study Group. Long-term effects of intravenous anistreplase in acute myocardial infarction: final report of the AIMS study. Lancet 1990; 335:427-31.

9. Wilcox RG, von der Lippe G, Olsson CG, Jensen G, Skene AM, Hampton JR. Effects of alteplase in acute myocardial infarction: 6-month results from the ASSET study. Lancet 1990; 335:1175-8.

10. Guerci AD. Unresolved issues: treatment of elderly patients and patients with inferior infarction and non-ST-segment infarcts. Coronary Artery Dis 1990; 1:34-8.

11. Grines CL, DeMaria AN. Optimal utilization of thrombolytic therapy for acute myocardial infarction; concepts and controversies. J Am Coll Cardiol 1990; 16:223-31.

12. Muller DWM, Topol EJ. Selection of patients with acute myocardial infarction for thrombolytic therapy. Ann Intern Med 1990; 113:949-60.

13. Yusuf S, Collins R, Peto R, et al. Intravenous and intracoronary firbinolytic therapy in acute myocardial infarction: overview of results on mortality, reinfarction and side effects from 33 randomized controlled trials. Eur Heart J 1985; 6:556-85.

14. Paolasso E. EMERAS trial: results and discussion. Presented at the American College of Cardiology 40th Annual Scientific Session, Atlanta, GA, March 5, 1991.

15. Chesebro JH, Knatterud G, Roberts R, et al. Thrombolysis in Myocardial Infarction (TIMI) trial, phase 1: a comparison between intravenous tissue plasminogen activator and intravenous streptokinase: clinical findings through hospital discharge. Circulation 1987; 76:142-54.

16. Topol EJ, Ellis SG, Wall TC, et al. Does late reperfusion therapy for myocardial infarction improve left ventricular function? Preliminary results of the TAMI-6 randomized, controlled trial. J Am Coll Cardiol 1991; 17:45A (abstract).

17. Califf RM, Topol EJ, Gersh BJ. From myocardial salvage to patient salvage in acute myocardial infarction: the role of reperfusion therapy. J Am Coll Cardiol 1989; 14: 1382-8.

18. Eigler N, Maurer G, Shah PK. Effect of early systemic thrombolytic therapy on left ventricular mural thrombus formation in acute anterior myocardial infarction. Am J Cardiol 1984; 54:261-3.

19. Kersschot IE, Brugada P, Ramental M, et al. Effects of early reperfusion in acute myocardial infarction on arrhythmias induced by programmed stimulation: a prospective, randomized study. J Am Coll Cardiol 1986; 7:1234-42.

20. Sager PT, Perlmutter PA, Rosenfeld LE, McPherson CA, Wackers FJ, Batsford ZW. Electrophysiologic effects of thrombolytic therapy in patients with a transmural anterior myocardial infarction complicated by left ventricular aneurysm formation. J Am Coll Cardiol 1988; 12:19-24.

21. Kennedy JW, Ritchie JL, Davis KB, et al. Western Washington randomized trial of intracoronary streptokinase in acute myocardial infarction. N Engl J Med 1983; 309: 1477-82.

22. Kennedy JW, Martin GV, Davis KB, et al. The Western Washington intravenous streptokinase in acute myocardial infarction randomized trial. Circulation 1988; 77: 345-52.

23. Kennedy JW, Atkins JM, Goldstein S, et al. Recent changes in management of acute

myocardial infarction: implication for emergency care physicians. J Am Coll Cardiol 1988; 11:446-9.

24. Berger PB, Ryan TJ. Inferior myocardial infarction. High-risk subgroups. Circulation 1990; 81:401-11.

25. Bates ER. Reperfusion therapy in inferior myocardial infarction. J Am Coll Cardiol 1988; 12:44A-51A.

26. Sherry S, Marder VJ. Mistaken guidelines for thrombolytic therapy of acute myocardial infarction in the elderly. J Am Coll Cardiol 1991; 17:1237-8.

27. Anderson JL, Karagounis L, Allen A, Bradford MJ, Pryor TA. Age and systolic hypertension are risk factors for intracranial hemorrhage after thrombolysis. Circulation 1990; 82(Suppl III):III-431 (abstract).

28. Lew AS, Hod H, Cercek B, Shah PK, Ganz W. Mortality and morbidity rates of patients older and younger than 75 years with acute myocardial infarction treated with intravenous streptokinase. Am J Cardiol 1987; 59:1-5.

29. Chaitman BR, Thompson B, Wittry MD, et al. The use of tissue-type plasminogen activator for acute myocardial infarction in the elderly: results from Thrombolysis in Myocardial Infarction Phase I, open label studies and the Thrombolysis in Myocardial Infarction Phase II Pilot Study. J Am Coll Cardiol 1989; 14:1159-65.

30. Greenland P, Reicher-Reiss H, Goldbourt U, et al. In-hospital and 1-year mortality in 1,524 women after myocardial infarction. Comparison with 4,315 men. Circulation 1991; 83:484-91.

31. Mauri F, Gasparini M, Barbonaglia L, et al. Prognostic significance of the extent of myocardial injury in acute myocardial infarction treated by streptokinase (the GISSI trial). Am J Cardiol 1989; 63:1291-5.

32. Willems JL, Willems RJ, Willems GM, et al. Significance of initial ST segment elevation and depression for the management of thrombolytic therapy in acute myocardial infarction. Circulation 1990; 82:1147-58.

33. Bates ER, Clemmenson PM, Califf RM, et al. Precardial ST-segment depression predicts a worse prognosis in inferior infarction despite reperfusion therapy. J Am Coll Cardiol 1990; 16:1538-44.

34. DeWood MA, Stifter WF, Simpson CE, et al. Coronary arteriographic findings soon after non-Q-wave myocardial infarction. N Engl J Med 1986; 315:417-23.

35. Ambrose JA, Alexopolous D. Thrombolysis in unstable angina: will the beneficial effects of thrombolytic therapy in myocardial infarction apply to patients with unstable angina. J Am Coll Cardiol 1989; 13:1666-71.

36. Althouse R, Maynard C, Olsulfka M, Kennedy JW. Risk factors for hemorrhage and ischemic stroke in myocardial infarct patients treated with tissue plasminogen activator. J Am Coll Cardiol 1989; 13:153A (abstract).

37. Weaver WD, Martin JS, Litwin PE, et al. Clinical correlates of initial blood pressure in patients presenting with acute myocardial infarction. Circulation 1990; 82(Suppl III): III-431 (abstract).

38. Bates ER, Topol EJ. Limitations of reperfusion therapy for acute myocardial infarction complicated by congestive heart failure and cardiogenic shock. J Am Coll Cardiol 1991; 18:1077-84.

39. Gruppo Italiano Per Lo Studio Della Sopravivenza Nell'Infarto Miocardico. GISSI-2:

a factorial randomized trial of alteplase versus streptokinase and heparin versus no heparin among 12,490 patients with acute myocardial infarction. Lancet 1990; 336: 65–71.

40. The International Study Group. In-hospital mortality and clinical course of 20,891 patients with suspected acute myocardial infarction randomized between alteplase and streptokinase with or without heparin. Lancet 1990; 336:71–5.

41. Sleight P. ISIS-3 Trial: results of SK versus APSAC versus tPA. Presented at the American College of Cardiology 40th Annual Scientific Session, Atlanta, GA, March 5, 1991.

42. Neuhaus K, Feuerer W, Jeep-Tebbe S, et al. Improved thrombolysis with a modified dose regimen of recombinant tissue-type plasminogen activator. J Am Coll Cardiol 1989; 14:1566–9.

43. Carney R, Brandt T, Daley P, et al. Increased efficacy of rt-PA by more rapid administration: the RAAMI trial. Circulation 1990; 82:III-538 (abstract).

44. von Essen R, Vogt A, Roth M, Reib M, Tebbe U, Neuhaus KL. Early patency of infarct-related vessel after accelerated infusion of 100 mg rt-PA as compared to 30 mg APSAC: results of the TAPS study. Eur Heart J 1991; 12:30 (abstract).

45. Wall TC, Topol EJ, George BS, et al. The TAMI-7 trial of accelerated plasminogen activator dose regimens for coronary thrombolysis: preliminary data. Circulation 1990; 82(Suppl III):III-538 (abstract).

46. Califf RM, Topol EJ, Stack RS, et al. An evaluation of combination thrombolytic therapy and timing of cardiac catheterization in acute myocardial infarction: The TAMI 5 randomized trial. Circulation 1991; 83:1543–56.

47. Grines CL, Nissen SE, Booth DC, et al. A prospective, randomized trial comparing combination half dose tissue plasminogen activator with streptokinase to full dose tissue plasminogen activator. Circulation 1991; 84:540–49.

48. Topol EJ: Thrombolytic intervention. In Topol EJ, ed. Textbook of interventional cardiology. Philadelphia: Saunders, 1989, pp. 76–120.

49. Topol EJ, George BS, Kereiakes DJ, et al. A randomized controlled trial of intravenous tissue plasminogen activator and early intravenous heparin in acute myocardial infarction. Circulation 1989; 79:281–6.

50. Hsia J, Hamilton WP, Kleiman N, et al. A comparison between heparin and low-dose aspirin as adjunctive therapy with tissue plasminogen activator for acute myocardial infarction. N Engl J Med 1990; 323:1433–37.

51. Bleich SD, Nichols TC, Schumacher RR, et al. Effect of heparin on coronary arterial patency after thrombolysis with tissue plasminogen activator in acute myocardial infarction. Am J Cardiol 1990; 66:1412–7.

52. de Bono DP, Simoons ML, Tijssen J, et al. Early intravenous heparin enhances coronary patency after alteplase thrombolysis: results of a randomized double blind European Cooperative Study Group trial. Brit Heart J 1991 (in press).

53. Thompson PL, Aylward PE, Federman J, et al. A randomized comparison of intravenous heparin with oral aspirin and dipyridamole 24 hours after recombinant tissue-type plasminogen activator for acute myocardial infarction. Circulation 1991; 83: 1534–42.

54. Topol EJ, Califf RM. Tissue plasminogen activator: Why the backlash? J Am Coll Cardiol 1989; 13:1477-80.
55. Califf RM, Harrelson-Woodlief L, Topol EJ. Left ventricular ejection fraction may not be useful as an endpoint for thrombolytic therapy comparative trials. Circulation 1990; 82:1847-53.
56. Peuhkurinen KJ, Risteli L, Melkko JT, Linnaluoto M, Jounela A, Risteli J. Thrombolytic therapy with streptokinase stimulates collagen breakdown. Circulation 1991; 83:1969-75.

4

Complications of Thrombolytic Therapy

David C. Sane and Robert M. Califf
Duke University Medical Center, Durham, North Carolina

INTRODUCTION

The topic of complications of thrombolytic therapy must be approached in a carefully balanced manner. The many large and small trials completed and reported from a variety of medical care settings can give the practitioner a fairly complete picture of the general types and frequency of complications (Table 1). These complications can be divided conveniently into bleeding, allergic manifestations, hypotension, and myocardial rupture.

The extensive amount of available data allows us to now develop information about the characteristics of patients likely to develop specific complications. Thus, high- and low-risk individuals can be detected at the bedside. Unfortunately, simply assessing the likelihood of complications is not sufficient to exclude patients from treatment. The clinician should also have access to the same type of information about the probability of benefit. In fact, an emerging theme in the evaluation of thrombolytic therapy is that the same patients who are at highest risk of complication often also have greatest chance of benefit. This chapter presents a contemporary approach to assessing risk and benefit.

Table 1   Complications in 1000 Patients Treated with Thrombolytic
Therapy

1. Hemorrhage	
Systemic	
Invasive	150–300
Noninvasive	10–50
Intracranial	5
2. Anaphylaxis (SK, APSAC)	1
3. Other allergic complications (SK, APSAC)	15
4. Significant hypotension	20–40

HEMORRHAGIC COMPLICATIONS

Exclusion Criteria

The risk of severe hemorrhage can be reduced by careful attention to standard exclusion criteria (1). It is relatively easy to exclude patients with absolute contraindications to thrombolytic therapy, but the physician is more often faced with the decision of whether to exclude treatment based on one or more relative contraindications. Does the patient presenting with an acute anterior myocardial infarction (MI) and a history of a nonhemorrhagic stroke 2 years prior to admission present an unacceptable risk for thrombolysis? In the tertiary-care setting, direct angioplasty without thrombolysis (2) may be used in such cases, but the physician in the community must often make difficult clinical decisions without this option. A number of factors must be carefully weighed in making these decisions, including the estimated size of the infarction, the history of previous MI, the time interval to presentation, the patient's age, and the patient's general health and underlying medical problems.

Incidence

The reported incidences of hemorrhagic complications of thrombolytic therapy vary widely depending on the study design (invasive versus noninvasive) and the methods used for classifying bleeding outcomes. In a review of over 15,000 patients treated with streptokinase (SK) for acute MI, the incidence of major hemorrhage was 1% and of fatal hemorrhage 0.04% (3). The incidence of major hemorrhage was 15% in the invasive studies but only 0.8% in the noninvasive studies (3). In almost 2000 patients treated with rt-PA and subject to invasive procedure, the major bleeding rate was 12%, with 0.1% of hemorrhagic episodes being fatal (3).

Hemorrhagic complications were closely examined in the TAMI-1 study, which involved rt-PA administration with acute versus delayed angioplasty. In this population, the rate of significant clinically evident bleeding was 14%, the median drop in hematocrit was 11.4 points, and 31% of patients required transfusion of two units or more of packed erythrocytes (4). Invasive procedures, including coronary artery bypass grafting (CABG), angioplasty, and the insertion of an intra-aortic balloon pump, increased the risk of hemorrhage.

Thus, as many as one-third of patients undergoing invasive procedures during thrombolysis will have significant bleeding requiring transfusion, although life-threatening bleeding occurs in less than one in a thousand patients. If the patient is not subject to invasive procedures, the risk of major hemorrhage is 5% or less.

Clinical Risk Factors

Older age, lower body mass, and female sex are demographic risk factors for hemorrhage during thrombolytic therapy for acute MI (4). The risk attributable to female sex and lower body mass may be related to the higher level of thrombolytic agent achieved in these patients during fixed (weight-independent) dosing regimens. These risk factors are not strong enough to form the basis for absolute exclusion criteria, but should make the physician more vigilant, especially when other risk factors or relative contraindications are present.

By far the strongest clinical risk factors for hemorrhage are the invasive procedures that must often be performed in this setting. Cardiac catheterization, intra-aortic balloon pump insertion, and CABG performed within the first 24 hr all greatly increase the risk of hemorrhage (4). In addition to the surgical trauma itself, PTCA, intra-aortic balloon pumps, and cardiopulmonary bypass create quantitative and qualitative platelet defects and are accompanied by high-dose heparin administration.

Hematological Risk Factors

The hematological risk factors associated with hemorrhage have been most carefully examined for thrombolysis with rt-PA. Several studies have now shown that fibrinogen depletion, fibrinogen degradation product (FBDP) elevation, high rt-PA antigen levels, and prolonged bleeding time correlate with increased hemorrhagic risk (4-7) during rt-PA therapy. Fibrinogen depletion is much more pronounced with the nonspecific agents streptokinase, anistreplase, and urokinase than with rt-PA. Some studies (8,9) have shown a modest decrease in hemorrhage for rt-PA versus nonspecific agents, possibly on the basis of less fibrinogenolysis, although, in general, no appreciable differences are evident. FBDP elevation is directly proportional to fibrinogen depletion and is also more substantial with nonspecific agents. In addition to serving as a marker of the extent of fibrinogen depletion, FBDPs also have independent antiocoagulant activities. FBDPs inhibit fibrin polymerization and have antiplatelet effects.

Higher rt-PA antigen levels have been associated with excess hemorrhage (6). Higher rt-PA levels are likely to occur when standard (weight independent) dosing regimens are used, and this observation may explain the increased bleeding risk in women and patients with light body weights. Thrombolytic therapy is associated with biphasic effects on platelets with early stimulatory and delayed inhibitory actions (10). The stimulatory effects are believed to be partly responsible for reocclusion and primary thrombolytic failure. The numerous possible mechanisms for antiplatelet effects in this setting may contribute to hemorrhagic risk, however. In a small series of patients, a prolonged bleeding time (>9 min) was 69% sensitive and specific for spontaneous bleeding occurring after rt-PA administration (7).

Other Mechanisms

In addition to degrading fibrin (ogen) and platelet membrane components, plasmin has numerous other substrates. Factors V and VIII, important cofactors in thrombin generation, are degraded by plasmin (11). High-molecular-weight forms of von Willebrand factor are decreased by plasmin (12). Components of the extracellular matrix, such as fibronectin (13) and vitronectin (14), are degraded by plasmin, possibly accounting for the recent observation of increased vascular permeability during thrombolysis (15). The clinical relevance of these other effects of plasmin is unknown, but they possibly contribute to hemorrhagic risk.

Role of Heparin

Several studies have suggested that adjuvant therapy with heparin contributes to hemorrhagic risk during thrombolysis. In the ISIS-2 trial, for example, the excess hemorrhage in the SK-treated group was attributable to intravenous heparin administration (16). In the GISSI-2 trial, the patients who received subcutaneous heparin 12,500 units b.i.d. had a 1.64-fold (95% confidence interval 1.09-2.45) higher relative risk of hemorrhage than the no-heparin group (8). In addition to its anticoagulant activity, heparin may also contribute to hemorrhage by causing thrombocytopenia and by enhancing the fibrinolytic effect of plasminogen activators (17,18).

Recent studies have demonstrated that heparin prevents reocclusion after therapy with rt-PA (19,20). The efficacy of heparin in preventing reocclusion is directly proportional to the prolongation of the aPTT (21). Therefore, despite the fact that heparin contributes to hemorrhagic risk, its use in the thrombolytic setting is likely to expand until the efficacy and safety of alternate thrombin inhibitors have been assessed.

Therapy

Conservative Therapy

The majority of hemorrhagic episodes can be controlled by simple measures without transfusion therapy. Since most hemorrhage occurs at sites of vascular intervention, these should be inspected and manual pressure or sandbags applied to control oozing. About 4% of patients will need surgical intervention to control vascular bleeding at sites of cardiac catheterization (4). If the site of hemorrhage is unclear, stool guaiacs and gastric aspirates should be analyzed for blood. Retroperitoneal hemorrhages, which have been reported to complicate conventional heparin therapy, may be a cause of occult hemorrhage, particularly if femoral arterial access was used for catheterization.

If the bleeding is hemodynamically significant, thrombolytic agents, heparin, and antiplatelet agents should be discontinued. Since anistreplase is administered as a bolus, there is usually no chance to decrease the dose of this agent. Reversal of heparin with protamine should be considered if the bleeding is massive or intracranial, or if a bolus was recently administered. About 1 mg of protamine should be given for every 100 units of heparin administered within the preceding 4 hr. The patient should be carefully monitored during protamine infusion for uncommon but potentially life-threatening complications, including systemic hypotension, pulmonary hypertension, and anaphylaxis. Anaphylaxis occurs in 0.6–2% of patients and is more common in diabetics and other patients with prior exposure to protamine (22–25).

Transfusion Therapy

In a small number of patients, blood product transfusions may be required. These should be used recognizing the risks of transfusion in any patient and the unique risks accompanying the bleeding post-MI patient. The former risks include a variety of viral diseases (HIV, CMV, hepatitis) and allergic reactions. The risk of acquiring AIDS from screened blood is as high as 1:40,000 (26), and blood products derived from multiple donors (e.g., cryoprecipitate) carry additive risks. In addition to these risks, the patient administered thrombolytic therapy for an acute MI is also at risk for volume overload with pulmonary edema, exacerbation of bleeding (by repleting plasminogen), or the precipitation of rethrombosis (by correcting the hypocoagulable state).

If transfusion is necessary and the risks are acceptable, then cryoprecipitate is probably the best initial agent since it corrects hypofibrinogenemia as well as repleting factor VIII (27). Since fibrinogen depletion is most marked 3–5 hr after therapy, cryoprecipitate is most likely to be beneficial for bleeding at this time interval. The starting dose of cryoprecipitate (10 units) may need to be repeated because persistent plasminogen activator levels may produce fibrinogenolysis of the transfused product. For persistent bleeding, FFP followed by platelets is rec-

Table 2   Interventions for Hemorrhagic Episodes

Goal	Agent	Dose
1. Reverse heparin	Protamine	1 mg/100 units of heparin in past 4 hr
2. Replace RBC mass	Packed RBC	1 unit/g Hb reduction
3. Replace fibrinogen	Cryoprecipitate	10 units once or twice
4. Replace coagulation factors	FFP	1-2 units
5. Provide functional platelets	Platelets	10 units
6. Inhibit plasmin	Epsilon amino-caproic acid	5 g IV load, then 0.5-1.0 g/hr

ommended (Table 2). Platelet transfusions are most likely to be beneficial if the bleeding time is prolonged (>9 min). In cases of life-threatening bleeding that fail conservative measures, cryoprecipitate, and FFP, empirical platelet administration is warranted.

Antifibrinolytic Therapy

The administration of antifibrinolytic agents, epsilon aminocaproic acid (Amicar) and tranexamic acid (Cyclokapron), carries the risk of precipitating a coronary rethrombosis that would become resistant to repeat attempts at thrombolysis. Antifibrinolytic agents inhibit the actions of plasmin (28), preventing further fibrinogenolysis, but they do not correct the hypocoagulable state that is the immediate cause of hemorrhage. For these reasons, these agents should probably be reserved until conservative measures and transfusion products have failed to control the bleeding. They should be used concomitant with transfusion products in cases of intracranial bleeding, however, since the mortality of this event (25-70%) outweighs that of coronary rethrombosis. Antifibrinolytic therapy might also be considered earlier in the exsanguinating patient who is known to have failed thrombolysis and in whom no further attempts to achieve reperfusion are planned. Amicar is preferred to Cyclokapron because of its shorter half-life and potential for more rapid reversal of antifibrinolytic effects. A loading dose of 5 g followed by 0.5-1.0 g/hr should be used until bleeding is controlled.

Intracranial Hemorrhage

Intracranial hemorrhage (ICH) is the most devastating complication of thrombolytic therapy. Several mechanisms for ICH during thrombolysis have been pro-

Table 3   Proposed Mechanisms for ICH

---

1. Hypertension
2. Anticoagulant or antiplatelet effects
   A. Extensive fibrinogenolysis with elevation of FBDPs
   B. Supratherapeutic aPTT with heparin
   C. Aspirin
3. Fibrinolysis of physiological hemostatic plugs in cerebral vasculature
4. Hemorrhagic transformation of bland cerebral emboli
5. Abnormal cerebral vessels
   A. Age
   B. Hypertension
   C. Amyloidosis
   D. Congenital AVM (rare)

---

posed (Table 3). Although some patients have elevated blood pressure at the time of hemorrhage (29), and the risk of ICH may increase with higher systolic blood pressures (30), the relationship between hypertension and ICH is, at present, inconclusive. Many patients have no history of hypertension or elevated blood pressure during their hospital courses (31,32). Indeed, the mean blood pressure for patients with hemorrhagic CVAs was *lower* than that in a group with nonhemorrhagic CVA in the TAMI studies (32). Furthermore, the propensity for ICH to occur within the cortical and subcortical white matter and the relatively common multifocal occurrence are atypical for hypertensive bleeds (33) and represent a pattern more consistent with ICH associated with excessive anticoagulation. Hypertensive bleeds, in contrast, rarely affect the cortical white matter, involve the subcortical white matter in only 25% of cases, and show a predilection for other areas, such as the basal ganglia, thalamus, cerebellum, and pons (34). The report of decreased ICH with administration of metoprolol early after rt-PA therapy in the TIMI trial was postulated to be due to decreased blood pressure and/or decreased dP/dt (35). This beneficial effect was not observed, however, in the GISSI-2/International trial with atenolol (8). Thus, there is currently limited evidence for hypertension as a major proximal cause of ICH during thrombolytic therapy.

The anticoagulant effects common to all thrombolytic agents could also play a role in ICH. Excessive fibrinogenolysis with concomitant elevation in FBDPs creates a hypocoagulable state that has been correlated with risk of systemic hemorrhage (5,6). Low fibrinogen and high FBDPs have been noted in some patients with ICH (28,31). Other anticoagulant and antiplatelet effects of thrombolytic agents have not been studied for their association with either systemic or intracranial hemorrhage. The frequent use of heparin following thrombolytic therapy may contribute to ICH in some individuals. Heparin has been associated with excess systemic hemorrhage, even when administered subcutaneously (8). In the analysis by Kase and colleagues of six cases of ICH, all where heparinized and had prolonged aPTTs at the time of ICH (32). The anticoagulant effects of heparin may synergize with those of the thrombolytic agent. In addition, the majority of patients will have platelet defects due to aspirin, which is now standard therapy for an acute MI. None of the patients in Kase's study had received aspirin, and this agent did not increase ICH in the ISIS-2 trial (16,32). In summary, anticoagulant and antiplatelet effects probably contribute to the risk of ICH, but cannot alone explain the occurrence of this complication.

While some thrombolytic agents have relative fibrin specificity, none can differentiate between physiological and pathological fibrin. In other words, no currently available agents have thrombus specificity. This explanation has been offered for the majority of systemic hemorrhage associated with vascular interventions. ICH may also occur at the site of physiological fibrin plugs, but there have been no pathological findings to support this hypothesis. A history of cerebrovascular disease might contribute to the formation of the plasmin-susceptible fibrin plugs, but was not found to be associated with hemorrhagic CVAs in the TAMI studies (31). One cannot, of course, exclude a significant contribution of previous *silent* cerebrovascular events to the risk of ICH.

Overall, ICH represents less than 50% of all strokes that occur during thrombolytic therapy (Table 4; Ref. 31). The mural thrombi that occur over an infarcted ventricular wall are known sources of emboli, with the brain as a common embolic site. Bland cerebral infarcts remain the most common stroke occurring during a MI. With thrombolytic therapy, some of these may be transformed into hemorrhagic strokes. Furthermore, small cerebral emboli may produce clinically unrecognized infarcts associated with fibrin plugs that are lysed by plasminogen activation. Thus, both overt and silent bland infarcts may be transformed into hemorrhagic CVAs. Five of Kase's six patients had inferior MIs, which have

Table 4   Hemorrhagic (H) and Nonhemorrhagic (NH) Strokes During Thrombolytic Therapy

Study	No.	H	NH	Total
TIMI-2	2742	0.5%	0.7%	1.2%
ASSET	2525	0.3%	0.8%	1.1%
ECSG (#4,5)	355	1.0%	0.3%	1.3%
TAMI (#I,II,III)	708	0.6%	1.2%	1.8%

much lower detectable embolic rates than anterior MIs (32). This finding argues against, but does not exclude, embolic events as a substantial contributing factor to ICH.

All the factors mentioned above are common to the patient population who are candidates for thrombolytic therapy. While many of these factors may contribute to the risk of ICH, none alone seems to be an adequate explanation. The infrequent occurrence of this event suggests that patient-specific factors must be involved. The relatively common occurrence of hemorrhage at multiple sites (29,32) suggests that certain patients have abnormal cerebral vessels that place them at risk for ICH. Age and hypertension may produce cerebral vessels with increased susceptibility to hemorrhage. A history of hypertension may contribute to excess risk of ICH by contributing to diseased cerebral vessels, even if the association between acute elevations in blood pressure and ICH is weak. Several patients with ICH have had mild dementia, raising the possibility of cerebral amyloidosis as underlying etiology (32), but no pathological data support this hypothesis. Other diseases known to be associated with cerebrovascular disease, such as diabetes, do not seem to confer markedly increased risk of ICH (31). Thus, except for rare cases of major abnormalities, such as arteriovenous malformations (36), few data implicate cerebrovascular disease in the pathogenesis of ICH.

Patients with ICH are likely to have large (≥ 1 cm^2) lesions with midline shifts on computed tomography (CT) scans (31). They are more likely than patients with nonhemorrhagic CVAs to have depression of mental status (31). Headache, nausea, and vomiting are frequent initial symptoms (37) which may be incorrectly ascribed to nitrate effects or recurrent ischemia.

A common clinical problem is the occurrence of a new neurological change early in the course of thrombolytic therapy. If the change is nonfocal, particularly depressed consciousness, a detailed neurological examination is indicated. Many other aspects of acute MI care, especially pain medication or therapy for anxiety, can lead to depressed consciousness. The occurrence of a new focal neurological finding should prompt immediate discontinuation of antithrombotic therapy and an emergency CT scan. Assuming that a new focal deficit is due to an embolic event is unwise, because the progression of hemorrhagic stroke in this setting is often extremely rapid.

Besides having a low threshold for clinical suspicion, the management of ICH patients requires emergency CT scan and prompt reversal of anticoagulant effects. The plasminogen activator infusion should be discontinued and continued fibrin(ogen)olysis reversed with an antifibrinolytic agent (Amicar). Heparin should also be discontinued and systemic heparin reversed with protamine. Fibrinogen should be repleted with cyroprecipitate, and platelet administration should be considered.

Some ICH lesions, including subdural hematomas and space-occupying bleeds at surgically approachable sites (e.g., cerebellar ICH), may necessitate neurosurgical interventions (29,31,38). It is important to correct any anticoagulant and antiplatelet effects to prevent postsurgical rebleeding.

Future Directions

A variety of new pharmacological agents may soon improve the physician's ability to treat bleeding with thrombolytic therapy. Plasminogen activator inhibitor type 1 (PAI-1) inhibits rt-PA and urokinase (UK) rapidly and plasmin slowly. Human PAI-1 has recently been produced by recombinant DNA technology (39). In a rabbit model, the coadministration of rt-PA and aspirin prolongs the bleeding time and produces a bleeding tendency. The administration of active rPAI-1 reverses the prolonged bleeding time in this model (40). Aprotinin also reverses the prolongation of the bleeding time secondary to rt-PA in rabbits (41). Aprotinin, which inhibits plasmin and SK-plasmin, is also available as a recombinant protein, but because it is of bovine origin, antigenicity may limit its usefulness.

In a rabbit model, desmopressin (DDAVP) has been demonstrated to reverse the prolonged bleeding time associated with thrombolytic therapy (42). This agent deserves further studies in patients. DDAVP, rPAI-1, and aprotinin may be acceptable therapeutic options to some patients who would refuse blood transfusion products for religious or other reasons.

Since heparin has been implicated in excess hemorrhage during thrombolytic therapy, and since its efficacy in preventing reocclusion may be suboptimal, clinical trials with heparin substitutes are being initiated. Recombinant hirudin, hirudin-derived peptides, and Argatroban are direct, antithrombin III–independent thrombin inhibitors (43,44). These agents have the theoretical advantage of shorter half-lives and fewer interactions with platelets. Thus, their effects may be more rapidly reversed and thrombocytopenia may be less common. However, because they are also more potent antithrombins, they carry the hemorrhagic risk of any agent that interferes with physiological hemostasis. Future clinical trials with these agents in combination with plasminogen activators may help define the contribution of heparin to hemorrhage during thrombolytic therapy.

Since drugs with anticoagulant properties will continue to be important adjuvant agents in the successful treatment of myocardial infarction by thrombolysis, efforts to ensure safe levels of anticoagulation will continue. Devices that can rapidly measure prothrombin times, activated partial thromboplastin times, and global fibrinolysis parameters have undergone initial testing (45). With the ability to assess the physiological effects of antithrombotic therapy more rapidly and accurately, wide swings in anticoagulation, and the associated hemorrhagic risks, may be avoided.

Since most hemorrhage during thrombolysis is associated with vascular interventions, efforts will continue to reduce unnecessary procedures. The TAMI and TIMI studies have demonstrated that PTCA can be safely postponed in the majority of patients for 7–10 days following thrombolytic therapy. Efforts to noninvasively predict reperfusion using repetitive quantitative ECG analyses (46), CK-MM and CK-MB isoforms (47), and myoglobin determinations (48) may reduce the number of invasive procedures needed in this setting.

IMMUNOLOGICAL COMPLICATIONS

SK is a nonenzymatic protein produced by Group C beta-hemolytic streptococci (49). In contrast to urokinase and recombinant tissue plasminogen activator, which are proteins of human origin, SK is antigenic and has potential allergic complications. The overall rate of allergic complications of SK was reported to be 1.6% in the 5800 patients treated with the drug in the GISSI-1 trial (50), although rates as high as 28% have been reported in smaller studies (51,52).

The allergic complications of streptokinase can be divided into two broad categories: anaphylaxis and immune complex disease (Table 5). Anaphylaxis was reported to occur in 0.1% of the GISSI-1 patients treated with SK (50). Although rare, anaphylactic reactions can be life threatening, and they constitute a major additional stress to the critically ill patient with an acute MI. Sera from patients with SK-induced anaphylaxis have elevated levels of SK-specific IgE (53). A wheal-and-flare reaction occurring within 15 min of an intradermal injection of 100 IU of streptokinase has been correlated with the presence of elevated IgE anti-SK antibodies and has been recommended as a screening test for the patient at risk of anaphylaxis (54). This test has not been widely used, probably because of the overall low incidence of anaphylaxis and the desire to treat patients immediately after recognition of acute MI, without even a 15-min delay. Patients with no known prior exposure to SK have had anaphylaxis after the first dose (55), probably because of the widespread exposure to streptococcal organisms. Steroids administered prophylactically may not be successful in preventing anaphylaxis, especially if given immediately prior to SK infusion (54).

The symptoms of anaphylaxis may be especially difficult to recognize in the acute MI patient, being easily confused with cardiogenic shock, sudden death, and pulmonary edema. The treatment of anaphylaxis requires close attention to airway management, with intubation often required. Fluids should be administered copiously. The SK infusion should be discontinued and epinephrine 1:1000 at doses of 0.1–.5 ml injected subcutaneously. Intravenous or intratracheal epinephrine may precipitate ischemia and arrhythmias in this setting and should be used as a last resort. Intravenous aminophylline and steroids may also be helpful in ameliorating bronchospasm. Patients treated with beta blockers may be unresponsive to epinephrine and may therefore have a more protracted anaphylactic reaction (56).

In contrast to the immediate hypersensitivity reaction characteristic of anaphylaxis, patients may present 6–16 days following streptokinase therapy with a variety of constitutional symptoms and clinical findings similar to those seen in serum

Table 5 Allergic Reactions to Streptokinase

Type	Mediator	Skin tests	Clinical presentation	Comments
Anaphylaxis	IgE	Immediate wheal and flare	Hypotension/shock; bronchospasm; laryngeal edema; arrhythmias	Can occur without prior SK therapy
Immune complex disease	IgG/immune complexes	Delayed-type hypersensitivity	Fever; arthralgias; myalgias leukocytoclastic vasculitis; increased ESR; hematuria; elevated BUN and creatinine	Occurs 6–16 days after treatment; more common with previous SK exposure

Treatment
Anaphylaxis—maintain airway; fluids; epinephrine 0.1–0.5 ml of 1:1000 subcu; IV aminophylline; IV steroids
Immune complex disease—steroids

sickness (57–61). This more indolent course is probably an immune complex disease mediated by IgG-SK complexes (53). Patients with prior exposure to SK may be at increased risk for this complication (62). Manifestations include fever, arthralgias, leukocytoclastic vasculitis, and renal involvement (Table 5). Crescentic glomerulonephritis has been described and may respond to steroid therapy (63).

Since anisoylated plasminogen streptokinase activator complex (APSAC; anistreplase) contains streptokinase, it also has antigenicity and therefore the potential to lead to allergic complications. Preliminary studies indicate that, as expected, anistreplase has an allergic profile similar to that of SK (64). In a small study, 6 of 253 patients treated with anistreplase developed leukocytoclastic vasculitis (65). Since treatment with SK or anistreplase induces significant increases in anti-SK antibody titers, it is suggested that a patient be treated only once with these agents. In addition to the allergic risks of retreatment, these patients may have neutralizing antibodies that hinder effective thrombolysis. Recurrent acute MIs or other indications for thrombolytic therapy should be managed with tissue plasminogen activator or urokinase. Since the incidence of antibodies to rt-PA is only 0.18% (66), patients may be safely retreated with this plasminogen activator.

THROMBOEMBOLIC COMPLICATIONS

The lysis of preexistent thrombi in the left heart chambers or in aneurysms of the aorta or other large vessels has been reported to cause systemic thromboembolic events during thrombolytic therapy (67,68). For this reason, patients with mitral stenosis and atrial fibrillation, or other conditions associated with a high likelihood of left atrial thrombosis, have relative contraindications to thrombolytic therapy. The vegetations associated with subacute bacterial endocarditis may also embolize with fibrinolysis.

Failure to reperfuse the infarct-related artery may be a less obvious, but critically important, complication of fibrinolysis. Accumulating evidence points to paradoxical procoagulant activities of plasminogen activator therapy. Platelet activation has been described during therapy with SK and rt-PA (69,70). This activation may be due to direct platelet activtion by plasmin (71), to thrombin activity that is released from lysed thrombi (72), or to thrombin activity generated directly by plasminogen activators (73). Platelet activation with thrombus generation may also occur as a result of anti-SK antibodies (74). The direct plasminogen activator–induced prothrombotic state may in part be due to transient plasmin-mediated activation of factor V (75), a key cofactor in the pathway to thrombin generation. Another potential procoagulant process during thrombolysis is the direct cleavage of fibrinopeptides from fibrinogen by urokinase and rt-PA, creating fibrin-like molecules (76,77). All these prothrombotic mechanisms may contribute to the observed "ceiling" of reperfusion efficacy. Future studies with potent anticoagulants (e.g., direct thrombin inhibitors such as hirudin) may improve reperfusion rates and demonstrate that failure to reperfuse is partly a complication, rather than merely a limitation, of thrombolysis.

COMPLICATIONS IN SELECT SUBPOPULATIONS

Elderly Patients

The topic of age and complication rates of thrombolytic therapy has caused a great deal of clinical confusion. Early reports substantiated an expected outcome: elderly patients treated with thrombolytic therapy have a much higher bleeding complication rate than younger patients treated with thrombolytic therapy (4,78). Furthermore, elderly patients have a much higher mortality than younger patients (16,50,79). Despite the increased risk associated with older age, the best available data indicate that the absolute magnitude of mortality reduction with thrombolytic therapy is also greater in more elderly patients. Although the GISSI-1 study found no "statistically significant" benefit in patients aged 65–75, the estimated magnitude of the difference in the more elderly subgroup is compatible with the overall trend in the data (80). Other studies in the very elderly, in fact, found the greatest mortality benefit to occur in patients over age 75 (16).

Our interpretation of these data is that thrombolytic therapy fits the general model of medical intervention: the relative risk reduction is fairly constant across patients groups, including age groups; the absolute benefit in this model will always be greater in patients with a higher baseline risk without treatment. A 33% risk reduction in a young patient with an anterior MI will reduce the expected mortality from 9% to 6% (a 3% absolute risk reduction), while for an elderly patient, the risk of death is reduced from 27% to 18% (a 9% absolute risk reduction).

A reasonable clinical approach to the elderly patient is to assess the likelihood of benefit, taking into account the baseline risk and the likelihood of a complication and paying special attention to comorbid diseases likely to lead to impaired vascular integrity. Finally, in the very elderly, baseline functional status and patient preference should be carefully considered. Longer life in a dysfunctional state may not be desirable.

Patients Requiring Emergency CABG After Failed Thrombolysis and PTCA

Cardiopulmonary bypass decreases platelet count and function, is associated with increased endogenous fibrinolytic activity, and produces hemodilution of coagulation factors (81). Since thrombolytic therapy and cardiopulmonary bypass both may cause loss of platelet membrane glycoproteins IIb/IIa and Ib (81–83), platelet dysfunction may be especially significant in this setting. In addition to these effects, almost all patients are heparinized during cardiopulmonary bypass. For

Table 6 Bleeding with CABG Following Failed Thrombolysis

Ref.	n	No. patients requiring surgical reexploration; bleeding mechanism	Quantitative blood loss	Average transfusion requirements (units)		
84	24	1: mechanical 2: hemostatic defect	1457 ml total POB	PRBC	=	8.2
				FFP	=	8.0
				Platelets	=	11.0
85	32	2: mechanical 4: hemostatic defect	NR	PRBC	=	12.5
				FFP	=	8.7
				Cryo	=	1.2
				Platelets	=	0.9
86	24	1: mechanical 2: hemostatic defect	1202 ml/first 24 hr CTD	PRBC	=	5.6
				FFP	=	4.0
				Cryo	=	3.9
				Platelets	=	3.0

CTD = chest tube drainage; POB = postoperative bleeding; NR = not reported; PRBC = packed erythrocytes; FFP = fresh frozen plasma; cryo = cryoprecipitate.

these reasons, bypass grafting and other open heart surgeries are associated with significant blood loss, which may be increased if a plasminogen activator has recently been administered to the patient. Reexploration for perioperative bleeding complications has been reported in 13–19% of patients undergoing CABG after failed thrombolysis and PTCA (84–86; Table 6). About two-thirds of these bleeding complications have been due to hemostatic defects. At 3–5 days after the administration of thrombolytic therapy, CABG can be performed with no excess hemorrhage compared to elective cases (87–88).

Agents of potential usefulness in this setting include aprotinin, plasminogen activator inhibitor type 1, and epsilon amino caproic acid (EACA). Aprotinin inhibits both plasmin and SK-plasmin while PAI-1 directly inhibits rt-PA and UK. The availability of recombinant aprotinin and PAI-1 should facilitate future clinical trials with these agents in this setting. Since several studies now indicate that aprotinin reduces blood loss in the routine cardiopulmonary bypass patient (89–91), it may be the ideal agent for patients undergoing CABG after failed thrombolysis. Limited experience with EACA suggests that it will not be the best agent (92), but additional trials are indicated.

Complications in Patients with
Mistaken Diagnosis of MI

A major concern for the practitioner is the possibility of administering a thrombolytic agent to a patient who then has a complication in the face of a final diagnosis other than acute MI. The TAMI group has evaluated this problem in detail. Of 1387 consecutive patients entered into the TAMI studies with a diagnosis of acute MI, 20 (1.4%) did not have a final diagnosis of MI at discharge (93). The major reasons for misdiagnosis were unstable angina (five), early repolarization (five), old MI with persistent ST-segment elevation (one), left ventricular hypertrophy (one), acute pericarditis (two), vasospasm (three), and bundle branch block (one). No patients had acute aortic dissection. In this population, no significant bleeding complications occurred (95% CL = 0–3%).

A more sobering report from the ASSET group noted that when ST-segment elevation was not required as an entry criterion, 13 of 5005 patients (0.26%) had a final diagnosis of acute aortic dissection. In the rt-PA group, five aortic dissections were diagnosed in the first 24 hr and all were fatal (79).

From these two studies it appears that a requirement of ST-segment elevation on the electrocardiogram (ECG) for the institution of thrombolytic therapy will nearly eliminate the risk of catastrophic outcome due to inappropriate treatment of acute aortic dissection. However, it must also be considered that in the ASSET and ISIS-2 trials the *total* mortality was substantially lower in patients treated with thrombolytic therapy in the setting of bundle branch block (16,79). The *total* mortality was also lower, although not statistically significantly, in patients with normal ECGs on presentation.

Our approach to this issue is to advocate rapid treatment of patients with ST-segment elevation and compatible symptoms, but to urge more careful diagnostic evaluations (chest x-ray, echogram, angiogram) of patients with nondiagnostic ECGs. If the patient is treated as a medical emergency, the diagnostic workup should be completed in a reasonable time frame to permit therapeutic efficacy of thrombolytic therapy.

The Late Arrivers: Myocardial Rupture

Treatment of patients coming to diagnosis beyond 6 hr from symptom onset has been controversial. Several large-scale trials are currently underway specifically evaluating this population, but until these results are available, the best current data indicate a benefit of treatment at least out to 18 hr. The magnitude of this effect is less than in patients treated earlier, however. In addition, a recent meta-analysis indicated that a higher risk of myocardial rupture was present in patients treated later (94). The currently available clinical data suggest that the incidence of rupture is lower in patients treated earlier because of prevention of transmural extension of the infarction, whereas the more common transmural nature of infarction in patients treated later allows a tract for dissection of the myocardium by expanding intramyocardial hematoma. This increased risk does not mean that treatment should be withheld in these patients. The clinician should be alerted to the possibility of rupture, however, and in otherwise borderline cases, the lower magnitude of benefit should be considered.

OTHER COMPLICATIONS

Hypotension

There are several potential mechanisms for hypotension during thrombolytic therapy. Plasmin itself has hypotensive effects when infused in animals, owing to its stimulation of kallikrein production (95). Plasmin directly converts prekallikrein to kallikrein, which, in turn, converts high-molecular-weight kininogen to bradykinin, a potent hypotensive substance. Since bradykinin activity is destroyed by angiotensin-converting enzyme (96), the target of captopril and other ACE inhibitors, the hypotensive effects of plasmin could be exaggerated by these agents. Other mechanism for hypotension (Table 7) during thrombolysis include stimulation of the Bezold-Jarisch reflex (97), anaphylaxis, and reperfusion arrhythmias.

Lew et al. studied the hypotensive effect of 750,000 units of SK infused intravenously over 30 min in 98 patients (98). The systolic blood pressure fell an average of 35 mmHg and the diastolic declined by a mean of 20 mmHg. A fall of the systolic blood pressure to 90 mmHg or less occurred in 38% of patients. Faster rates of infusion were associated with more pronounced hypotension. Although the mean time to recovery of baseline blood pressure was only 9 min, several patients with severe left ventricular dysfunction had significant hypotension for more than an hour.

Since anistreplase is temporarily inactive, hypotension with this agent should theoretically be less severe, a prediction supported by some animal models (95). Nevertheless, hypotension is a common side effect of anistreplase therapy (99) and may be protracted because of the long half-life of anistreplase. In the AIMS

Table 7 Mechanisms of Hypotension During Thrombolytic Therapy

1. With bradycardia
   a. Reperfusion of inferoposterior MI (Bezold-Jarish reflex)
2. Without bradycardia
   a. Anaphylaxis (SK and anistreplase)
   b. Plasmin-mediated kallikrein and bradykinin production
   c. Reperfusion arrhythmias

study, patients who received anistreplase had lower mean blood pressures during the first 24 hr than did those who received placebo (100).

As expected from its greater plasmin production, SK therapy is associated with significantly greater hypotension than rt-PA administration. In the GISSI-2 trial (8), for example, 4.4% of SK-treated versus 2.0% of rt-PA-treated patients had significant hypotension.

Reperfusion Arrhythmias

Because of experience in animal models with rapid occlusion and reperfusion in which fatal ventricular arrhythmias are common, an excessive concern about reperfusion arrhythmias as a complication of thrombolytic therapy developed. In fact, individual cases of refractory arrhythmia at the time of reperfusion have been reported. However, detailed studies using Holter monitoring have failed to demonstrate a large difference in the occurrence of arrhythmia when patients achieving reperfusion have been compared with patients failing to achieve reperfusion (101,102). Furthermore, large trials have shown a reduction, rather than an increase, in the incidence of primary ventricular fibrillation in patients treated with thrombolytic therapy compared with conservative therapy. Any patient with expected acute myocardial infarction should be monitored and treated for arrhythmias, but the patient treated with thrombolytic therapy does not appear to be different in this regard.

REFERENCES

1. American College of Cardiology/American Heart Association Task Force on Assessment of Diagnostic and Therapeutic Cardiovascular Procedures. Guidelines for the early management of patients with acute myocardial infarction. J Am Coll Cardiol 1990; 16:249-92.

2. O'Keefe JH Jr, Rutherford BD, McConahay DR, Ligon RW, Johnson WL Jr, Giorgi LV, Crockett JE, McCallister BD, Conn RD, Gura GM Jr, Good TH, Steinhaus DM, Bateman TM, Shimshak TM, Hartzler GO. Early and late results of coronary angioplasty without antecedent thrombolytic therapy for acute myocardial infarction. Am J Cardiol 1989; 64:1221-30.

3. Fennerty AG, Levine MN, Hirsh J. Hemorrhagic complicatios of thrombolytic therapy in the treatment of myocardial infarction and venous thromboembolism Chest 1989; 95 (Suppl 2):88S-97S.

4. Califf RM, Topol EJ, George BS, Boswick JM, Abbottsmith C, Sigmon KN, Candela R, Masek R, Kereiakes D, O'Neill WW, Stack RS, Stump D. Hemorrhagic complications associated with the use of intravenous tissue plasminogen activator in treatment of acute myocardial infarction. Am J Med 1988; 85:353-9.

5. Rao AK, Pratt C, Berke A, Jaffe A, Ockene I, Schreiber TL, Bell WR, Knattrud G, Robertson TL, Terrin ML. Thrombolysis in Myocardial Infarction (TIMI) Trial-Phase I: hemorrhagic manifestations and changes in plasma fibrinogen and the

fibrinolytic system in patients treated with recombinant tissue plasminogen activator and streptokinase. J Am Coll Cardiol 1988; 11:1–11.

6. Stump DC, Califf RM, Topol EJ, Sigmon K, Thornton D, Masek R, Anderson L, Collen D, and the TAMI Study Group. Pharmacodynamics of thrombolysis with recombinant tissue-type plasminogen activator. Correlation with characteristics of and clinical outcomes in patients with acute myocardial infarction. Circulation 1989; 80:1222–30.

7. Gimple LW, Gold HK, Leinbach RC, Coller BS, Werner W, Yasuda T, Johns JA, Ziskind AA, Finkelstein D, Collen DC. Correlation between template bleeding times and spontaneous bleeding during treatment of acute myocardial infarction with recombinant tissue-type plasminogen activator. Circulation 1989; 80:581–8.

8. Gruppo Italiano per lo Studio della Sofravvivenza nell Infarto Miocardico. GISSI-2: a factorial randomized trial of alteplase versus streptokinase and heparin versus no heparin among 12,490 patients with acute myocardial infarction. Lancet 1990; 336:65–71.

9. The International Study Group. In hospital mortality and clinical course of 20891 patients with suspected acute myocardial infarction randomised between alteplase and streptokinase with or without heparin. Lancet 1990; 336(Part 1):71–5.

10. Coller BS. Platelets and thrombolytic therapy N Engl J Med 1990; 332:33–42.

11. Kane WH, Davie EW. Blood coagulation factors V and VIII: structural and functional similarities and their relationship to hemorrhagic and thrombotic disorders. Blood 1988; 71:539–55.

12. Hamilton KK, Fretto LJ, Grierson DS, McKee PA. Effects of plasmin on von Willebrand factor multimers. Degradation in vitro and stimulation of release in vivo. J Clin Invest 1985; 76:261–70.

13. Balian G, CLick EM, Crouch E, Davidson JM, Bornstein P. Isolation of a collagen-binding fragment from fibronectin and cold-insoluble globulin. J Biol Chem 1979; 254:1429–32.

14. Sane DC, Moser TL, Greenberg CS. Vitronectin proteolysis by plasmin results in loss of heparin binding activity. Fibrinolysis 1990; 4 (Suppl 3):65 (abstract).

15. Rudd MA, Johnstone M, George D, Loscalzo J. Vascular permeability is increased following thrombolytic therapy. Circulation 1990; 82:253 (abstract).

16. ISIS-2 (Second International Study of Infarct Survival) Collaborative Group. Randomized trial of intravenous streptokinase, oral aspirin, both, or neither among 17,187 cases of suspected acute myocardial infarction: ISIS-2. Lancet 1988; 2:349–60.

17. Andrade-Gordon P, Strickland S. Interaction of heparin with plasminogen activators and plasminogen: effects on the activation of plasminogen. Biochemistry 1986; 25:4033–40.

18. Edelberg JM, Pizzo SV. Kinetic analysis of the effects of heparin and lipoproteins on tissue plasminogen activator mediated plasminogen activation. Biochemistry 1990; 29:5906–11.

19. Bleich SD, Nichols T, Schumacher R, Cooke D, Tate D, Steiner C, Brinkman D. The role of heparin following coronary thrombolysis with tissue plasminogen activator (t-PA). Circulation 1989; 80(Suppl II): 113 (abstract).

20. Hsia J, Hamilton WP, Kleiman N, Roberts R, Chaitman BR, Ross AM. A comparison

between heparin and low-dose aspirin as adjunctive therapy with tissue plasminogen activator for acute myocardial infarction. N Engl J Med 1990; 232:1433-7.

21. De Bono. Presented at the American Heart Association meeting, Dallas, TX, November 1990.

22. Weiss ME, Nyhan D, Peng Z, Horrow JC, Lowenstein E, Hirshman C, Adkinson NF Jr. Association of protamine IgE and IgG antibodies with life-threatening reactions to intravenous protamine. N Engl J Med 1989; 320:886-92.

23. Weiler JM, Freiman P, Sharath MD, Metzgar WJ, Smith JM, Richerson HB, Ballas ZK, Halverson PC, Shulan DJ, Matsuo S, Wilson RL. Serious adverse reactions to protamine: are alternatives needed? J Allerg Clin Immunol 1985; 75:297-303.

24. Levy JH, Schwieger IM, Zaidan JR, Faraj BA, Weintraub WS. Evaluation of patients at risk for protamine reactions. J Thorac Cardiovasc Surg 1989; 98:200-4.

25. Stewart WJ, McSweency SM, Kellet MA, Faxon DP, Ryan TJ. Increased risk of severe protamine reactions in NPH insulin-dependent diabetics undergoing cardiac catheterization. Circulation 1984; 70:788-92.

26. Ward JW, Holmberg SD, Allen JR, Cohn DL, Critchley SE, Kleinman SH, Lenes BA, Ravenholt O, Davis JR, Quinn MG, Jaffe HW. Transmission of human immunodeficiency virus (HIV) by blood screened as negative for HIV antibody. N Engl J Med 1988; 318:473-8.

27. Sane DC, Califf RM, Topol EJ, Stump DC, Mark DB, Greenberg CS. Bleeding during thrombolytic therapy for acute myocardial infarction: mechanisms and management. Ann Intern Med 1989; 111:1010-22.

28. Verstraete M. Clinical application of inhibitors of fibrinolysis. Drugs 1985; 29:237-61.

29. Carlson SE, Aldrich MS, Greenberg HS, Topol EJ. Intracerebral hemorrhage complicating intravenous tissue plasminogen activator treatment. Arch Neurol 1988; 45:1070-3.

30. Weaver WD, Martin JS, Litwin PE, Eisenberg MS, Kudenchuk PJ, Ho MT, Hallstom AP, Cerqueira MD, Shaeffer SM, MITI Investigators. Clinical correlates of initial BP in patients presenting with acute myocardial infarction. Circulation 1990; 82:1709 (abstract).

31. O'Connor CM, Califf RM, Massey EW, Mark DB, Kereiakes DJ, Candela RJ, Abbottsmith C, George B, Stack RS, Aronson L, Mantell S, Topol E. Stroke and acute myocardial infarction in the thrombolytic era: clinical correlates and long-term prognosis. J Am Coll Cardiol 1990; 16:533-40.

32. Kase CS, O'Neal AM, Fisher M, Girgis GN, Ordia JI. Intracranial hemorrhage after use of tissue plasminogen activator for coronary thrombolysis. Ann Intern Med 1990; 112:17-21.

33. Sloan MA, Plotnick GD. Stroke complicating thrombolytic therapy of acute myocardial infarction. J Am Coll Cardiol 1990; 16:541-4.

34. Kase CS. Intracerebral hemorrhage: nonhypertensive causes. Stroke 1986; 17:590-5.

35. TIMI Study Group. Comparison of invasive and conservative strategies after treatment with intravenous tissue plasminogen activator in acute myocardial infarction: results of Thrombolysis in Myocardial Infarction (TIMI) Phase II Trial. N Engl J Med 1989; 320:618-27.

36. Proner J, Rosenblum BR, Rothman A. Ruptured arteriovenous malformation complicating thrombolytic therapy with tissue plasminogen activator. Arch Neurol 1990; 47:105-6.
37. O'Connor CM, Aldrich H, Massey EW, Uglietta J, Mark DB, Califf RM. Intracranial hemorrhage after thrombolytic therapy for acute myocardial infarction: clinical characteristics and in hospital outcome. J Am Coll Cardiol 1990; 15:213A (abstract).
38. Eleff SM, Borel C, Bell WR, Long DM. Acute management of intracranial hemorrhage inpatients receiving thrombolytic therapy: case reports. Neurosurgery 1990; 26:867-9.
39. Reilly TM, Seetharam R, Duke JL, David GL, Pierce SK, Walton HL, Kingsley D, Sisk WP. Purification and characterization of recombinant plasminogen activator inhibitor-1 from Escherichia coli. J Biol Chem 1990; 265:9570-4.
40. Vaughan DE, Declerck PJ, De Mol M, Collen D. Recombinant plasminogen activator inhibitor-1 reverses the bleeding tendency associated with the combined administration of tissue-type plasminogen activator and asprim in rabbits. J Clin Invest 1989; 84:586-91.
41. Clozel J-P, Banken L, Roux S. Aprotinin: an antidote for recombinant tissue-type plasminogen activator active in vivo. J Am Coll Cardiol 1990; 16:507-10.
42. Weinstein M, Johnstone M, Rudd MA, George D, Andrews T, Ware JA, Loscalzo J. Bleeding time is shortened in streptokinase-treated rabbits after DDAVP without an increase in von Willebrand factor. Blood 1989; 74:97a (abstract).
43. Markwardt F. Development of hirudin as an antithrombotic agent. Semin Thromb Hemostas 1989; 15:269-82.
44. Fitzgerald DJ, FitzGerald GA. Role of thrombin and thromboxane A2 in reocclusion following coronary thrombolysis with tissue-type plasminogen activator. Proc Natl Acad Sci USA 1989; 86:7585-9.
45. Sane DC, Gresalfi NJ, O'Mara L, Califf RM, Greenberg CS, Bovill E, Oberhardt BJ. A rapid new method for the assessment of coagulation and fibrinolysis parameters during thrombolytic therapy. Fibrinolysis 1990; 4 (Suppl 3): 36 (abstract).
46. Krucoff MW, Wagner NB, Pope JE, Mortara DM, Jackson YR, Bottner RK, Wagner GS, Kent KM. The portable programmable microprocessor-driven real-time 12-lead electrocardiographic monitor: a preliminary report of a new device for the noninvasive detection of successful reperfusion or silent coronary reocclusion. Am J Cardiol 1990; 65:143-8.
47. Christenson RH, Ohman EM, Clemmensen P, Grande P, Toffaletti J, Silverman LM, Vollmer RT, Wagner GS. Characteristics of creatine kinase-MB and MB isoforms in serum after reperfusion in acute myocardial infarction. Clin Chem 1989; 35:2179-85.
48. Ohman EM, Casey C, Bengtson JR, Pryor D, Tormey W, Horgan JH. Early detection of acute myocardial infarction: additional diagnostic information from serum concentrations of myoglobin in patients without ST elevation. Br Heart J 1990; 63:335-8.
49. Brogden RN, Speight TM, Avery GS. Streptokinase: a review of its clinical pharmacology, mechanism of action, and therapeutic uses. Drugs 1973; 5:57-445.
50. GISSI (Gruppo Italiano per lo studio della streptochinasi nell' infarto miocardico). Effectiveness of intravenous thrombolytic treatment in acute myocardial infarction. Lancet 1986; 1:397-401.

51. Thayer CF. Results of postmarketing surveillance program on streptokinase. Curr Ther Res 1981; 30:129-40.

52. McGrath KG, Zeffren B, Alexander J, Kaplan K, Patterson R. Allergic reactions to streptokinase consistent with anaphylactic or antigen-antibody complex-mediated damage. J Allerg Clin Immunol 1985; 76:453-7.

53. McGrath KG, Patterson R. Anaphylactic reactivity to streptokinase. JAMA 1984; 252:1314-7.

54. Dykewicz MS, McGrath KG, Davison R, Kaplan KJ, Patterson R. Identification of patients at risk for anaphylaxis due to streptokinase. Arch Intern Med 1986; 146:305-7.

55. Bednarczyk EM, Sherlock SC, Farah MG, Green JA. Anaphylactic reaction to strepto-kinase with first exposure: case report and review of the literature. Drug Intell Clin Pharm 1989; 23:869-72.

56. Jacobs RL, Rake GW Jr, Fournier DC, Chilton RJ, Culver WG, Beckmann CH. Poten-tiated anaphylaxis in patients with drug-induced beta-adrenergic blockade. J Allergy Clin Immunol 1981; 68:125-7.

57. McGrath KG, Zeffren B, Alexander J, Kaplan K, Patterson R. Allergic reactions to streptokinase consistent with anaphylactic or antigen-antibody complex mediated damage. J Allergy Clin Immunol 1985; 76:453-7.

58. Alexopoulos DK, Raine AEG, Cobbe SM. Serum sickness complicating intravenous streptokinase therapy in acute myocardial infarction. Eur Heart J 1984; 5:1010-2.

59. Totty WG, Romano T, Benian GM, Gilula LA, Sherman LA. Serum sickness follow-ing stroptokinase therapy. AJR 1982; 138:143-4.

60. Weatherbee TC, Esterbrooks DJ, Katz DA, Aronow WS, Kenik JG, Mohiuddin SM. Serum sickness following selective intracoronary streptokinase. Curr Ther Res 1984; 35:433-8.

61. Noel J, Rosenbaum LH, Gangadharan V, Stewart J, Galens G. Serum sickness like illness and leukocytoclastic vasculitis following intracoronary arterial streptokinase. Am Heart J 1987; 113:395-7.

62. McGrath K, Patterson R. Immunology of streptokinase in human subjects. Clin Exp Immunol 1985; 62:421-6.

63. Murray N, Lyons J, Chappell M. Crescentic glomerulonephritis: a possible complica-tion of streptokinase treatment for myocardial infarction. Br Heart J 1986; 56:483-5.

64. Johnson ES, Cregeen RJ. An interim report of the efficacy and safety of anisoylated plasminogen streptokinase activator complex. Drugs 1987; 33:298-311.

65. Bucknall C, Darley C, Flax J, Vincent R, Chamberlain D. Vasculitis complicating treatment with intravenous anisoylated plasminogen streptokinase activator complex in acute myocardial infarction. Br Heart J 1988; 59:9-11.

66. Reed Br, Chen AB, Tanswell P, Prince WS, Wert Rm Jr., Glaesle-Schwarz L, Grossbard E. Low incidence of antibodies to recombinant human tissue-type plas-minogen activator in treated patients. Thromb Haemostas 1990; 64:276-80.

67. Stafford PJ, Strachan CJL, Vincent R, Chamberlain DA. Multiple microemboli after disintegration of clot during thrombolysis for acute myocardial infarction. Br Med J 1989; 299:1310-2.

68. Zahger D, Weiss AT, Anner H, Waksman R. Systemic embolization following thrombolytic therapy for acute myocardial infarction. Chest 1990; 97:754-6.
69. Fitzgerald DJ, Catella F, Roy L, FitzGerald GA. Marked platelet activation in vivo after intravenous streptokinase in patients with acute myocardial infarction. Circulation 1988; 77:142-50.
70. Kerins DM, Roy L, FitzGerald GA, Fitzgerald DJ. Platelet and vascular function during coronary thrombolysis with tissue-type plasminogen activator. Circulation 1989; 80:1718-25.
71. Schafer AI, Maas AK, Ware JA, Johnson PC, Rittenhouse SE, Salzman EW. Platelet protein phosphorylation, elevation of cytosolic calcium and inositol phospholipid breakdown in platelet activation induced by plasmin. J Clin Invest 1986; 78:73-9.
72. Francis CW, Markham RE Jr, Barlow GH, Florack TM, Dobrzynski DM, Marder VJ. Thrombin activity of fibrin thrombi and soluble plasmic derivatives. J Lab Clin Med 1983; 102:220-30.
73. Eisenberg PR, Miletich JP. Induction of marked thrombin activity by pharmacologic concentrations of plasminogen activators in nonanticoagulated whole blood. Thromb Res 1989; 55:635-43.
74. Vaughan DE, Kirshenbaum JM, Loscalzo J. Streptokinase-induced, antibody-mediated platelet aggregation: a potential cause of clot propogation in vivo. J Am Coll Cardiol 1988; 11:1343-8.
75. Lee CD, Mann KG. Activation/inactivation of human factor V by plasmin. Blood 1989; 73:185-90.
76. Weitz JI, Leslie B. Urokinase has direct catalytic activity against fibrinogen and renders it less clottable by thrombin. J Clin Invest 1990; 86:203-12.
77. Weitz JI, Cruickshank MK, Thong B, Leslie B, Levine MN, Ginsberg J, Eckhardt T. Human tissue-type plasminogen activator releases fibrinopeptides A and B from fibrinogen. J Clin Invest 1988; 82:1700-7.
78. Lew AS, Hod H, Cercek B, Shah PK, Ganz W. Mortality and morbidity rates of patients older and younger than 75 years with acute myocardial infarction treated with intravenous streptokinase. Am J Cardiol 1978; 59:1-5.
79. Wilcox RG, Olsson CG, Skene AM, von der Lippe G, Jensen G, Hampton JR, ASSET Study Group. Trial of tissue plasminogen activator for mortality reduction in acute myocardial infarction: Anglo-Scandinavian Study of Early Thrombolysis (ASSET). Lancet 1988; 2:525-30.
80. Yusuf S, Sleight P, Held P, McMahon S. Routine medical management of acute myocardial infarction. Lessons from overviews of recent randomized controlled trials. Circulation 1990; 82(Suppl II):117-34.
81. Woodman RC, Harker LA. Bleeding complications associated with cardiopulmonary bypass. Blood 1990; 76:1680-97.
82. Stricker RB, Wong D, Shiu DT, Reyes PT, Shuman MA. Activation of plasminogen by tissue plasminogen activator in normal and thrombasthenic platelets: effect on surface proteins and platelet aggregation. Blood 1986; 68:275-80.
83. Adelman B, Michelson AD, Loscalzo J, Greenberg J, Handin RI. Plasmin effect on platelet glycoprotein Ib-von Willebrand factor interactions. Blood 1985; 65:32-40.
84. Skinner JR, Phillips SJ, Zeff RH, Kongtahworn C. Immediate coronary bypass fol-

lowing failed streptokinase infusion in evolving myocardial infarction. J Thorac Cardiovasc Surg 1984; 87:567-70.

85. Ferguson TB Jr, Muhlbaier LH, Salai DL, Wechsler AS. Coronary bypass grafting after failed elective and failed emergent percutaneous angioplasty. J Thorac Cardiovasc Surg 1988; 95:761-72.

86. Kereiakes DJ, Topol EJ, George BS, Abbottsmith CW, Stack RS, Candela RS, O'Neill WW, Martin LH, Califf RM. Emergency coronary artery bypass surgery preseves global and regional left ventricular function after intravenous tissue plasminogen activator therapy for acute myocardial infarction. J Am Coll Cardiol 1988; 11:899-907.

87. Wellens HA Jr, Schneider JA, Mikell FL, Moses HW, Dove JT, Batchelder JE, Taylor GJ. Early operative intervention after thrombolytic therapy for acute myocardial infarction. J Vasc Surg 1985; 2:186-91.

88. Anderson JL, Battistessa SA, Clayton PD, Cannon CY III, Askins JC, Nelson RM. Coronary bypass surgery early after thrombolytic therapy for acute myocardial infarction. Ann Thorac Surg 1986; 41:176-83.

89. Royston D, Bidstrup BP, Taylor KM, Sapsford RN. Effect of aprotinin on need for blood transfusion after repeat open-heart surgery. Lancet 1987; 2:1289-91.

90. van Oeveren W, Jansen NJ, Bidstrup BP, Royston D, Westaby S, Neuhof H, Wildevuur CR. Effects of aprotinin on hemostatic mechanisms during cardiopulmonary bypass. Ann Thorac Surg 1987; 44:640-5.

91. Alajmo F, calamai G, Perna AM, Melissano G, Pretelli P, Palmarini MF, Carbonneto F, Noferi D, Boddi V, Palminiello A. High dose aprotinin: hemostatic effects in open heart operations. Ann Thorac Surg 1989; 48:536-9.

92. Kates RA, Hill R, Reves JF. Reperfusion of acute myocardial infarction: role of anesthesia. In Reves JG, ed. Acute revascularization of the infarcted heart. Orlando, FL: Grune & Stratton, 1987:53.

93. Chapman GD, O'Connor CM, Kereiakes DJ, George BS, Candela RJ, Abbottsmith CW, Harrelson L, Ohman EM. Consequences of misdiagnosis of acute myocardial infarction leading top thrombolytic therapy: a multicenter expereience. JACC 1990; 15:227A (abstract).

94. Honan MB, Harrell FE, Jr., Reimer KA, Califf RM, Mark DB, Pryor DB, Hlatky MA. Cardiac rupture, mortality and the timing of thrombolytic therapy: a meta analysis. J Am Coll Cardiol 1990; 16:359-67.

95. Green J, Dupe RJ, Smith RAG, Harris GS, English PD. Comparison of the hypotensive effects of streptokinase-(human) plasmin activator complex and BRL 26921 (p-anisoylated streptokinase-plasminogen activator complex) in the dog after high dose, bolus administration. Thromb Res 1984; 36:29-36.

96. Adamski SW, Grega GJ. Contribution of kininase II to the waning of vascular actions of bradykinin. Am J Physiol 1988; 254:H1042-50.

97. Koren G, Weiss AT, Ben-David Y, Hasin Y, Luria MH, Gotsman MS. Bradycardia and hypotension following reperfusion with streptokinase (Bezold-Jarisch reflex): a sign of coronary thrombolysis and myocardial salvage. Am Heart J 1986; 112:468-71.

98. Lew AS, Laramee P, Cercek B, Shah PK, Ganz W. The hypotensive effect of intrave-

nous streptokinase in patients with acute myocardial infarction. Circulation 1985; 72:1321-6.

99. Munger MA, Forrence EA. Anistreplase: a new thrombolytic for the treatment of acute myocardioal infarction. Clin Pharm 1990; 9:530-40.

100. Fox KA. The safety of anistreplase from the placebo-controlled AIMS study. The AIMS Study Group. Clin Cardiol 1990; 13(Suppl 5): v22-6.

101. Miller FC, Krucoff MW, Satler LF, Green CE, Fletcher RD, Del Negro AA, Pearle DL, Kent KM, Rackley CE. Ventricular arrhythmias during reperfusion. Am Heart J 1986; 112:928-32.

102. Califf RM, O'Neil W, Stack RS, Aronson L, Mark DB, Mantell S, George BS, Candela RJ, Kereiakes DJ, Abbottsmith C, Topol EJ, and the TAMI study group. Failure of simple clinical measurements to preduct perfusion status after intravenous thrombolysis. Ann Intern Med 1988; 108:658-62.

II

ADJUNCTIVE PHARMACOTHERAPY

5

Nitroglycerin

Bodh I. Jugdutt

University of Alberta, Edmonton, Alberta, Canada

INTRODUCTION

Nitrates as Adjunctive Therapy to Thrombolysis

The advancement of thrombolytic therapy in the 1980s was inevitable in view of two major discoveries (1-9). First, it was noted that the thrombotic coronary occlusion that plays a central role in acute myocardial infarction (AMI) could undergo rapid spontaneous lysis, restoring antegrade flow in as many as 30% of patients (1-3). Second, it was demonstrated that early myocardial reperfusion with exogenous thrombolytic agents could salvage ventricular muscle and function (4-9). However, this dramatic result required that reperfusion be achieved within 2 hr of the onset of symptoms of AMI; otherwise myocardial stunning developed (10,11). Most hospitals are unsuccessful in mobilizing patients and doctors for such early recruitment and delivery of therapy. Even with such mechanisms in place, many patients fail to reperfuse (12) or develop early reocclusion (13) or postinfarction angina (14).

Although thrombolysis has become the primary therapy for AMI in the 1990s, a strong role exists for the concurrent use of nitrates. At least two arguments favor the use of nitrates as adjunctive therapy to thrombolysis. First, the efficacy of nitrates in the management of acute ischemic syndromes (15-17) has been established. Low-dose intravenous nitroglycerin has been used increasingly since the mid-1970s to relieve ischemic pain and to improve hemodynamics in AMI (Fig. 1) (18,19). In the 1980s, nitrates became recognized for their safety (20,21) and their ability to limit infarct size, infarct-related complications, and remodeling (20-23), and for their potential to improve survival (23,24). It is important to note that the beneficial effects of nitrates in AMI (Table 1) were reported in the prethrombolytic era and, therefore, usually in the presence of an occluded infarct-related artery and multivessel coronary artery disease. Thus, the benefits of nitrates can be expected whether or not thrombolytic therapy is successful.

Second, nitrates might widen the treatment window for thrombolytic therapy and "buy more time" until therapy can be applied. At the very least, combination therapy would be expected to provide the advantage of the beneficial effects of nitrates. In addition, other benefits can result. Thus, recent evidence suggests that concurrent nitrate and late reperfusion therapy (>4 hr) might result in early recovery of ventricular function (25). This contrasts with the late or no recovery of ventricular function with late reperfusion therapy alone (25). Whether adjunctive nitrate therapy can maintain patency of the infarct-related artery, prevent early reocclusion, or prevent postinfarction angina is not proven, but the potential for these benefits exist with their mechanisms of action.

Major Mechanisms for Nitrate Benefit

There are several mechanisms for nitrate action (Table 2). It was known for over a century that the principal cellular mechanism for the beneficial effect of nitrates in acute ischemic syndromes was vasodilatation due to vascular smooth muscle relaxation (26-28). In 1973, Needleman and Johnson (29) proposed that at the molecular level, exogenous nitrates interact with key sulfhydryl (SH) groups in specific nitrate receptors to trigger denitration and oxidation of the SH groups. In 1981, Ignarro et al. (30) proposed a cascade involving intracellular nitrate biotransformation, metabolic activation to nitric oxide (NO), S-nitrosothiol formation, guanylate cyclase activation, increased cyclic guanosine monophosphate (cGMP) formation, modified calcium ion (Ca^{2+}) traffic, and relaxation. In 1987, Palmer et al. (31) suggested that endothelial-derived relaxation factor (EDRF), a labile humoral agent thought to mediate the action of nitro vasodilators, might be NO. Thus, it appears that NO represents an "endogenous nitrate" that mediates vasodilatation. As EDRF is decreased in coronary atherosclerosis and acute ischemic syndromes (32,33), "exogenous nitrate" might supply EDRF and NO in those defective states. It is important to note that this exogenous nitrate-induced vasodilatation is independent of endothelium and is in fact more marked in the presence of denuded endothelium (34) or damaged endothelium (35).

A secondary mechanism for nitrate-induced relaxation is via the release of prostacyclin (PGl2) from endothelium (36). However, this endothelium-dependent release of PGl2 is blunted by endothelial damage in coronary atherosclerosis

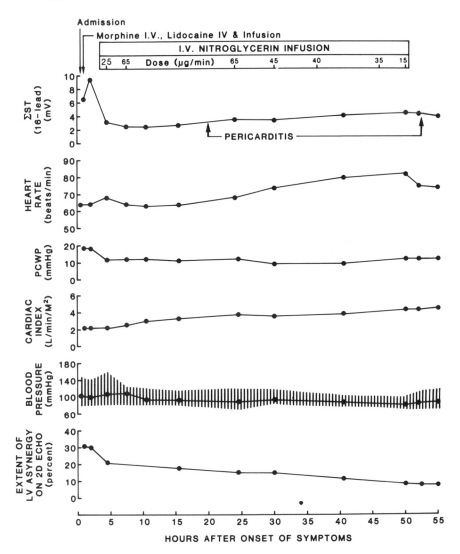

Figure 1 Typical changes with prolonged low-dose intravenous (I.V.) nitroglycerin therapy in a patient with anterior AMI. Prompt and persistent decreases in the sum of ST-segment elevation ($\sum$ST), pulmonary capillary wedge pressure (PCWP), and left ventricular asynergy on two-dimensional echocardiography (2D echo) were associated with a mild decrease in mean blood pressure and a mild increase in cardiac index.

Table 1   Beneficial Effects of Nitrates in AMI

1. Improved hemodynamics
2. Improved myocardial perfusion
3. Decreased ischemic injury and infarct size
4. Decreased ventricular remodeling
5. Improved regional and global ventricular performance
6. Decreased infarct-related complications
7. Improved survival

and acute ischemic syndromes. The loss of protective endothelium together with diminished EDRF and diminished PGl2 promotes platelet aggregation, the release of vasoactive substances such as thromboxane A2 and serotonin, and vasospasm (33,37–40). Biologically, EDRF and substances that release NO spontaneously cause a rise in platelet cGMP which suppresses the Ca^{2+} signal that precedes platelet activation, the release reaction, and aggregation (41). Organic nitrates, such as nitroglycerin, isosorbide dinitrate (ISDN), and isosorbide mononitrate (ISMN), which do not release NO spontaneously, are less effective in raising platelet cGMP (41). Nevertheless, antiplatelet and antithrombotic effects of exogenous nitrates have been demonstrated (42,43) and might play an important role in improving coronary perfusion in acute coronary syndromes and AMI.

Table 2   Mechanisms for Benefit by Nitrates in Acute Ischemic Syndromes and AMI

Decreased preload; increased venous capacitance
Decreased afterload and impedance
Increased collateral blood flow
Decreased coronary artery spasm
Increased diameter of epicardial arteries and stenoses
Increased endothelial-derived relaxation factor (EDRF) activity
Increased prostacyclin activity
Decreased platelet adhesiveness and platelet plugs
Increased coronary vein and lymphatic flow
Increased removal of noxious metabolites of ischemia
Decreased chamber size and wall stress
Decreased regional dilatation and infarct expansion
Decreased global dilatation and aneurysm formation
Improved regional and global ventricular performance

The main mechanism for nitrate benefit is vasodilatation (Table 2). It favorably modifies cellular energetics by tipping the supply-demand equation (19-22). First, it results in decreased myocardial oxygen demand via venodilatation, increased venous capacitance and venous pooling, decreased left ventricular (LV) preload, decreased LV size, and decreased wall tension and wall stress. A decrease in LV impedance and afterload further reduces wall stress and myocardial oxygen demand. Second, vasodilatation results in an increase in myocardial oxygen supply, via dilatation of epicardial conductance arteries, dilatation of stenoses, relief of coronary artery spasm, and an increase in collateral blood flow. The end result is relief of ischemic chest pain, decrease in ischemic injury and infarct size, salvage of LV geometry and function, and improved hemodynamics and LV performance (Table 1).

Nitrate Dose

The pharmacological fact that the effect of nitrates on different vascular beds is dose-related and nonuniform has important implications in therapy. The beneficial effects of nitrates in AMI (Table 1) are seen with low-dose therapy (20,23,25,43-58). With low-dose therapy, infusion rate is generally begun at 5 μg/min with increments of 5-10 μg/min every 5-10 min until the desired blood pressure endpoint or a dose of 200 μg/min is reached (Table 3). Low doses used in major trials of intravenous nitroglycerin in AMI are summarized in Table 4. High

Table 3   Typical Protocol for Low-Dose Intravenous Nitroglycerin

---

1. Can use standard IV set with infusion pump
2. Begin at 5 μg/min; increase by 5-10 μg/min every 5-10 min until the desired endpoint or a dose of 200 μg/min is reached
3. Titrate to desired hemodynamic endpoint: lower mean BP by
   10% in normotensives
   30% in hypertensives
   but not below 80 mmHg
4. Reassess if:
   systolic BP < 90 mmHg
   mean BP < 80 mmHg
   diastolic BP increases > 15 mmHg
   heart rate increases > 20% or drops < 50 bpm
5. Continue titration for at least 24 hr
6. Discontinue if hypotension; restart at 5 μg/min when safe
7. To stop, titrate down 5-10 μg/min every 5-10 min
8. Average dose range 30-140 μg/min

BP = blood pressure; IV = intravenous.

Table 4 Dose and Duration of Intravenous Nitroglycerin in AMI

Reference	Onset	Duration	Dose of titration regimen
Chiche (44)	24 hr	5–7 days	Begin 15 μg/min; increase to reduce SBP by 20 mmHg
Bussman (45)	<8 hr (mean 4.5) and >8 hr (mean 12.8)	48 hr	Begin 12.5 μg/min; increase to 100 μg/min to reduce PCWP by 10–30% and MBP no more than 10%
Flaherty (46)	<12 hr	48 hr	Begin 5 μg/min; increase to reduce MBP by 10%; keep SBP > 90 mmHg, HR > 50 bpm
Jugdutt (47)	<8 hr (mean 5.4)	48 hr	Begin 5 μg/min; increase to reduce MBP by 10%, not < 80 mmHg
Nelson(48)	<14 hr	90 min (ISDN)	Begin 50 μg/kg/hr; up to 200 μg/kg/hr to reduce MBP by 10 mmHg
Jaffe (49)	<12 hr	24 hr	Begin 10 μg/min, up to 200 μg/min to reduce SBP by 10% or to 95 mmHg, not < 90 mmHg; HR not < 50 bpm; HR increase not > 20
Lis (50)	<12 hr	48 hr	Begin 10 μg/min; increase to reduce SBP $\leq$ 30 in those with SBP > 135 mmHg, $\leq$15 in those with SBP 120–134 mmHg, and $\leq$5 in those with SBP 95–119 mmHg (average dose 35 $\pm$ 26 μg/min)
Jugdutt (23)	<12 hr (mean 5)	48 hr	Begin 5 μg/min; increase to decrease MBP by 10% in normotensive and 30% in hypertensive patients but not < 80 mmHg

HR = heart rate; ISDN = isosorbide dinitrate; MBP = mean blood pressure; PCWP = pulmonary capillary wedge pressure; SBP = systolic blood pressure.

dose refers to fixed dose infusions, often with no titration to a safe blood pressure endpoint, and average doses greater than 5 μg/kg/min, as often used in patients with congestive heart failure without AMI. Maximal venodilatation is achieved with very low doses of nitroglycerin and concentrations below 0.2 ng/ml (59). In the dog model, Bassenge and Stewart (60) showed that veins and coronary arteries dilate at very low doses (0.5 μg/kg/min), peripheral arteries at 10 times higher doses (5 μg/kg/min), and myocardial resistance vessels at 40 times higher doses (20 μg/kg/min). It is now clear that a decrease in LV impedance and profound LV unloading can be achieved by low doses of nitroglycerin before a detectable decrease in arm blood pressure develops in patients (61). Low-dose nitroglycerin also increased collateral blood flow in the dog model (55,56,62) and improved myocardial perfusion in patients with AMI (46). It also produced significant

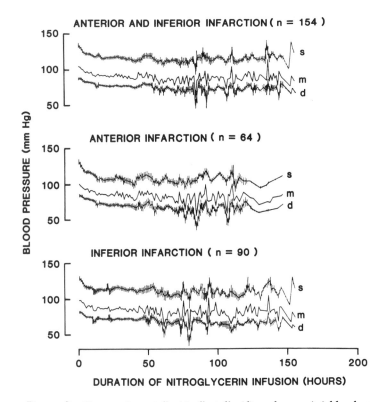

Figure 2 Changes in systolic (s), diastolic (d), and mean (m) blood pressure during prolonged low-dose nitroglycerin infusion therapy. Blood pressure was monitored by the spygmomanometer cuff method. [Data from 154 patients in the study by Jugdutt and Warnica (23), with permission.]

platelet antiaggregatory effects in patients with unstable angina and AMI (43). In contrast, high doses of nitrates produce excessive vasodilatation, increase the risk of lowering perfusion pressure (23,56), and consistently produce tolerance (63-66). The frequency of hemodynamic tolerance is, in fact, low with 48-hr low-dose nitroglycerin infusions in AMI and does not offset the benefits of therapy (67). Thus, "more nitroglycerin is not necessarily better" in AMI. Sustained decrease in blood pressure with low-dose therapy over more than 48 hr is illustrated in Figure 2.

HEMODYNAMICS

Preload Reduction and Filling Pressure

Nitrates produce marked lowering of preload and filling pressure. This effect prompted the initial use of intravenous nitroglycerin to unload the left ventricle and improve hemodynamics in patients with LV failure complicating AMI (19,68). The effect, referred to as an "internal phlebotomy," is primarily due to the dilatation of systemic and pulmonary veins (69). In early stages of AMI, limitation of ischemic injury might also contribute to the decrease in filling pressure (70). The dramatic fall in LV filling pressure occurs with low doses of nitroglycerin. Thus, Bussmann (71) measured a prompt decrease in LV filling pressure by as much as 40% within 5 min when mean arterial pressure fell only between 0 and 10%. Flaherty (19) and others (23,45-47) have emphasized that the degree of fall in LV filling pressure after nitroglycerin is directly proportional to the degree of elevation before nitroglycerin. All eight studies of low-dose nitroglycerin in AMI showed a decrease in LV filling pressure (23,44-50).

Afterload Reduction and the J-Curve Effect

In the presence of high blood pressure and afterload, high doses of nitroglycerin reduce blood pressure, afterload, and impedance to LV ejection (18,19,23). As a result, LV emptying is facilitated and stroke volume improves.

This favorable hemodynamic response is not seen in some patients with congestive heart failure and AMI, suggesting that there might be primary arteriolar receptor resistance (47,70,72-74). However, other factors might be operating, such as enhanced vasoconstrictor activity from excessive catecholamines, activation of the renin-angiotensin system, failure to dilate due to vessel wall edema, or impaired hepatic nitrate metabolism (74).

In early stages of AMI, reduction of afterload results in a decrease in ischemic injury (75,76). However, excessive reduction of afterload leads to a reduction of perfusion pressure, myocardial underperfusion, and increase in ischemic injury and infarct size (23,56,76). This "paradoxical J-curve effect" is not unique to nitrates. It is common to all vasodilators. It underscores the need for cautious administration (77,78) and further supports the use of low-dose nitroglycerin.

Cardiac Output

An inotropic effect of intravenous nitroglycerin was suggested by improvement in stroke volume, peak dp/dt, peak dp/dt/P, and flow in patients with coronary artery disease (79). In congestive heart failure, the cardiac output response depends on the baseline levels of cardiac output and preload (80). As the dose is increased, there is first a fall in filling pressure followed by a fall in arterial pressure, vascular resistance, and afterload. An increase in stroke volume might be counteracted by an excessive fall in preload. In AMI, cardiac output either improves (45,47,23) or is maintained (44,46,48–50) after low-dose nitroglycerin. Again, the response depends on the initial hemodynamic subset (46) and interrelated baseline factors, such as the level of hydration and preload, the dose and the degree of afterload reduction. In addition, the effects of nitroglycerin on ischemic injury and remodeling (20,21,23) influence the response.

MYOCARDIAL PERFUSION

Improved Antegrade Flow

Nitrates are unlikely to influence antegrade flow in the presence of a total thrombotic occlusion of the infarct-related artery. However, in the presence of subtotal thrombotic occlusion or a type II lesion (81,82), the ability of ntirates to dilate large coronary vessels and their spasmolytic, antiplatelet, and antithrombotic properties can potentially increase flow. Following thrombolytic therapy, these effects have the potential for preventing reocclusion, infarct extension, and ischemic syndromes such as postinfarction angina (14).

Improved Collateral Flow

Nitrates have the potential for increasing collateral blood flow, both in the presence and in the absence of a totally occluded infarct-related artery. They can dilate coronary artery stenoses in the same or adjacent beds, reverse coexisting coronary spasm, dilate intercoronary collateral channels, increase flow in intramural vessels secondary to decreased subendocardial compression as LV filling pressure is decreased, and cause a direct increase in intramural collateral flow. Increase in collateral flow with nitroglycerin has been demonstrated experimentally in the dog model (55,56,62,83). The latter effect is seen at low doses (55) and can be lost at high doses due to excessive nitrate-induced hypotension and reflex tachycardia (56). A large number of studies have shown that nitroglycerin causes a favorable redistribution of regional flow from nonischemic to ischemic areas (20,84). In AMI, Flaherty et al. (46) demonstrated that low-dose intravenous nitroglycerin therapy decreased thallium perfusion defect scores in patients who had small initial defects and prior history of chronic angina, suggesting the presence of preexisting collaterals. Although controversial, nitroglycerin has the potential for producing coronary steal (85).

An important experimental finding in the dog model is that collateral vessels opened by short-term nitroglycerin therapy in the setting of a total coronary artery occlusion may remain open after treatment is discontinued. Thus, Capurro et al. (62), using the radioactive microsphere method, showed that the increase in collateral flow found during nitroglycerin therapy between 10 and 70 min after coronary ligation was still present 4 hr later. Furthermore, the increase in collateral flow (measured by the same microsphere technique) during low-dose nitroglycerin therapy over 4–6 hr postocclusion was associated with myocardial salvage measured 2 days (55) and 7 days (56) later. Schaper and colleagues (86) demonstrated that collateral growth and development can occur over several days in canine and porcine hearts. In patients with AMI, collaterals might develop within 2 weeks (87).

In patients with thrombotic occlusion but prior chronic ischemic heart disease and abundant collaterals (86), nitrate-induced dilatation of collaterals can potentially increase nutrient flow to the ischemic risk zone and contribute to the removal of metabolic waste products during thrombolysis. In patients with an acute thrombotic occlusion but no prior history of chronic ischemic disease and poor collateral reserve (86,87), nitrate-induced dilatation might stimulate collateral growth and favorably influence outcome after acute thrombolytic therapy (23,25).

Thus, even if the infarct-related artery were to remain occluded, nitrate-induced collateral development can potentially protect the risk zone and prevent ischemia, infarct extension, and remodeling.

Inhibition of Platelet Aggregation and Thrombosis

The antiplatelet and antithrombotic effects of nitrates (42) have been demonstrated with low-dose intravenous nitroglycerin (1.2 μg/kg/min) during unstable angina and AMI (43). These effects of nitrates might potentially be of greater value during and after thrombolytic therapy. Thus, they might improve flow by blocking platelet aggregation, the release of vasoconstrictive compounds, platelet embolism, and occlusive changes in the infarct-related artery. Although nitrates are commonly used for treating ischemic episodes after AMI, there has been no trial to address the effect of these potential benefits on prognosis.

MYOCARDIAL SALVAGE

It is clear that low doses of nitrates produce maximal venodilatation, decrease LV size, decrease wall stress, decrease preload, and improve perfusion without marked decrease in blood pressure and afterload. These effects are adequate for limiting ischemic injury and infarct size (20). Higher doses to decrease blood pressure during an evolving AMI can potentially lower blood pressure below the critical level for myocardial perfusion and prove deleterious.

In the instrumented conscious dog model, the administration of low-dose intravenous nitroglycerin over the first 6 hr after coronary ligation to decrease the mean blood pressure by 10%, without letting it drop below 90 mmHg, resulted in a 54% decrease in LV filling pressure, more than 50% increase in collateral flow, and 51% decrease in infarct size (55). In that same study (55), the administration of methoxamine to counteract the small nitrate-induced decrease in blood pressure was associated with the same beneficial effects. It is therefore not necessary to ensure a decrease in blood pressure during early stages of nitroglycerin infusion to gain benefit during AMI.

In the same dog model, lowering of the mean blood pressure by more than 10% (range, 17–45%) to levels below an average of 83 mmHg (and down to 58 mmHg) abolished the beneficial effects on collateral flow and infarct size (56).

The risk of excessive hypotension and reflex tachycardia with high doses in AMI (72,77,78), or rapid bolus injection (72), or uncontrolled rapid absorption (88) has been recognized and favors the use of low-dose intravenous nitroglycerin in AMI (19,20). This nitroglycerin formulation is also preferred in AMI because of its rapid onset and offset of action. The regimen currently used at the author's institution is summarized in Table 3. This is similar to the recommendation published by the Task Force of the American Heart Association and American College of Cardiology in 1990 (17).

Ischemic Injury

Experimental (20,89) and clinical (23,45,47,70,72,77) studies with low-dose intravenous nitroglycerin therapy have consistently shown a decrease in ischemic injury. Bussmann et al. (76) showed that 3 mg/hr or 50 μg/min reduced ischemic injury, but 6 mg/hr or 100 μg/min produced tachycardia, hypotension, and less decrease in ST-segment elevation or an increase in ST-segment elevation. In a large randomized study with low-dose nitroglycerin averaging 45 μg/min (23), inadvertent hypotension (defined as mean blood pressure below 80 mmHg) developed in the first 12 hr of AMI in 9% of 154 patients and was associated with less reduction in ischemic injury.

Infarct Size

Low-dose intravenous nitroglycerin consistently reduced pathological infarct size in the dog model (55–58). In clinical studies, similar therapy reduced creatine kinase indexes of infarct size (23,45,47,49) and perfusion defect scores on thallium scintigraphy (46). Although some clinical studies suggested reduction of infarct size only in inferior AMI (46,49), both animal (55–58) and several clinical studies (23,45,47) indicate that the size of both anterior and inferior infarcts can be limited by low-dose intravenous nitroglycerin therapy.

Postinfarction Angina

Intravenous, oral, and other nitrate formulations have been suggested for postinfarction angina (14). There are no reported placebo-controlled, randomized, double-blind trials of nitrates in unstable angina pectoris. Intravenous nitroglycerin has been shown to be effective to "cool down" patients with unstable angina (16). Unlike in AMI, higher doses of nitroglycerin are tolerated in unstable angina and averaged 82 μg/min in one study (90). Intravenous ISDN, a longer-acting nitrate, has also been used effectively for unstable angina (91) but these patients did not have AMI.

Infarct Extension

This important postinfarction complication (92) was significantly reduced by 50% (from 22% to 11%, $p < 0.025$) with low-dose intravenous nitroglycerin therapy in a large randomized, placebo-controlled study (23). Flaherty et al. (46) found a similar effect with early therapy. Prolonged nitrate therapy after thrombolysis might also prevent this complication.

LEFT VENTRICULAR FUNCTION

Nitrates consistently decrease LV filling pressure, decrease right and LV volumes, and cause a favorable shift in the LV diastolic pressure-volume relation suggesting improvement in LV compliance and function (93). Low doses of nitroglycerin in AMI cause a leftward shift of the relation between stroke volume and LV filling pressure, suggesting improved LV function (47,88). However, the individual response in AMI depends on the initial coordinate position of the stroke output, the shape of the Frank-Starling curve (47,88), the initial preload and afterload (23,71), as well as the dose and timing of nitroglycerin therapy (23).

Regional LV Dysfunction and "Stunned" Myocardium

Low-dose intravenous nitroglycerin therapy in AMI has been shown to persistently decrease the extent of regional contractile or mechanical dysfunction measured by serial two-dimensional echocardiography (23,47).

In one study (25), the effect of low-dose therapy (average 45 μg/min) given before, during, and after coronary reperfusion with intracoronary streptokinase and/or angioplasty on LV function was investigated in patients with AMI. Therapy was continued for an average of 45 hr. Four randomly assigned treatment groups were studied: saline placebo, nitroglycerin alone, nitroglycerin plus reperfusion, and reperfusion alone. Serial measurements of LV function and geometry were made using serial two-dimensional echocardiography before and after therapy at 24 hr, 7 days, 6 weeks, 3 months, and 6 months. Although reperfusion was achieved late, between 2 and 6 hr after the onset of pain, there was a prompt and persistent decrease in LV regional mechanical dysfunction and an increase in global LV ejection fraction in groups receiving nitroglycerin. Importantly, these functional parameters did not improve with reperfusion alone or in palcebo controls. Thus, concomitant and prolonged low-dose nitroglycerin therapy might be effective in preventing myocardial stunning and persistent LV dysfunction after late reperfusion.

Global LV Ejection Fraction

Low-dose intravenous nitroglycerin during AMI results in prompt and persistent improvement in both regional and global LV ejection fraction (23,45–47,49). This beneficial effect of nitroglycerin was also noted after late reperfusion therapy in AMI (25).

REMODELING

Remodeling after AMI begins with acute infarct expansion (a stretching, thinning, and outward bulging of the infarct zone) and continues throughout the healing period after AMI, with late scar thinning (as a result of collagen compaction), aneurysm formation, global LV chamber dilatation, LV volume overload, hypertrophy of the noninfarct zone, and development of congestive heart failure (21,22,94,95).

Patients with marked acute infarct expansion are at high risk for cardiogenic shock, congestive heart failure, and death within the first month of AMI (92,97–99). The major determinants (21,22) of this early remodeling have been studied experimentally and include physical characteristics of the infarct (such as infarct size and transmurality), efficacy of the healing process, nutrient collateral flow, and mechanical deformation forces (preload, afterload, and wall stress). Patients with moderately large anterior AMI are at especially high risk for acute infarct expansion (92,97–99). Nitrates, therefore, have the potential for limiting remodeling by: (a) reducing preload, cavity size, wall stress, infarct size, infarct transmurality, and afterload (at higher doses) and (b) increasing collateral blood flow (21,22). Reperfusion, even late, limits infarct expansion and thinning (100), but only early reperfusion improves function (101).

Infarct Expansion and Thinning

Short-term acute administration of low-dose intravenous nitroglycerin over the first 6 hr of anterior AMI limited infarct expansion and thinning measured 7 days later in the dog model (57). In clinical studies, prolonged low-dose intravenous nitroglycerin therapy over 48 hr resulted in persistently decreased LV volume in anterior (23,47) and inferior (23) AMI for up to 1 year (23). In both these studies, limitation of LV enlargement was associated with improved LV performance (23,47). In the larger study (23), limitation of remodeling was manifested by: (a) limitation of LV enlargement with decreased LV internal diastolic dimension and LV volume; (b) attenuation of infarct expansion and thinning; (c) decreased frequency of the clinical infarct expansion syndrome (from 15% to 2%; $p < 0.0005$); (d) improved regional and global LV performance; (e) decreased infarct-related complications such as cardiogenic shock (from 15% to 5%; $p < 0.005$) and congestive heart failure; (f) decreased in-hospital mortality (from 26% to 14%; $p < 0.01$) and decreased one year mortality (from 31% to 21%; $p < 0.05$). In one study, late reperfusion alone was associated with attenuation of expansion and thinning without improvement in LV function (25). In contrast, late reperfusion combined with prolonged low-dose nitroglycerin therapy resulted in limitation of remodeling as well as a prompt and persistent improvement in LV function (25).

Aneurysm Formation

In patients with a first anterior Q-wave AMI, prolonged, long-term nitrate therapy, with low-dose intravenous nitroglycerin for the first 48 hr and buccal nitrate for the next 6 weeks, resulted in further limitation of remodeling, further improvement of LV function, prolonged limitation of LV dilatation, and decreased frequency of LV aneurysm formation (51–54). In these studies, an eccentric dosing schedule with an 8-hr nitrate-free interval was used to avoid tolerance. In the latest study (54), most patients received thrombolytic therapy with intravenous streptokinase or recombinant tissue-type plasminogen activator (rt-PA).

Cardiac Rupture

Rupture of the LV free wall or ventricular septum follows acute infarct expansion (92,96–99). No significant difference in the frequency of rupture could be demonstrated between nitrate and placebo groups in one large prethrombolytic clinical trial (23). However, in the dog model, nitrate therapy limited remodeling and raised the threshold at which the infarcted left ventricle ruptured as LV cavity pressure was increased using a balloon technique (58). In a recent study of cardiac rupture after thrombolysis, meta-analysis of 4692 deaths in 44,346 patients showed that early therapy decreased the risk of cardiac rupture but later therapy increased the risk (102). It is reasonable to expect that low-dose intravenous nitroglycerin therapy could reduce the frequency of cardiac rupture in both early and late thrombolytic groups.

PROGNOSIS

Morbidity: Heart Failure

Only two trials of prolonged low-dose intravenous nitroglycerin therapy over the first 48 hr after AMI reported on infarct-related complications (23,46).

In the first trial, Flaherty et al. (46) randomized 104 patients to therapy ($n = 56$) and placebo ($n = 48$). Initial analysis did not show differences in the endpoints. However, retrospective analysis revealed that the early-therapy subgroup (<10 hr after onset of symptoms) had a lower frequency of major infarct complications in the first 10 days. Prominent among these was new congestive heart failure (6% versus 30%). The frequency of infarct extension (12% versus 26%) and death (4% versus 19%) was also lower.

In the second trial (23), 310 patients were randomized to therapy ($n = 154$) and placebo ($n = 156$). Highly significant differences were found in all biological and clinical parameters shown in Table 1 (23). The functional Killip class scores over the first 10 days were significantly less ($p < 0.05$) in the therapy group. The New York Heart Association functional classes were also better in the nitrate group for up to 1 year of follow-up.

Arrhythmias

Nitroglycerin decreased infarct-related ventricular arrhythmias in experimental (103–105) and clinical (23,46) studies. This antiarrhythmic effect might be mediated via eicosanoids (105,106) and might be beneficial during reperfusion therapy.

LV Mural Thrombus

Only one study has prospectively assessed the frequency of LV thrombus using serial two-dimensional echocardiography (23). A highly significant 77% decrease in the frequency of LV thrombus was demonstrated with low-dose nitroglycerin therapy (5% versus 22%, $p < 0.0005$).

Table 5   Mortality in Major Trials of intravenous Nitroglycerin in AMI

Author/year	Follow-up	Nitrate deaths	Control deaths	$2p$
1. Chiche/1979	Hospital	3/50 (6%)	8/45 (18%)	NS
2. Bussmann/1981	18 months	4/31 (13%)	12/29 (41%)	<0.02
3. Flaherty/1983	3 months	11/56 (20%)	11/48 (23%)	NS
4. Jugdutt/1983	Hospital	1/11 (9%)	2/11 (18%)	NS
5. Nelson/1983	Hospital	0/14 (0%)	0/14 (0%)	NS
6. Jaffe/1983	Hospital	4/57 (7%)	2/57 (4%)	NS
7. Lis/1984	4 months	5/64 (8%)	10/76 (13%)	NS
8. Jugdutt/1988	3 months	24/154 (16%)	44/156 (28%)	<0.01
		52/437 (12%)	89/436 (20%)	<0.001

Mortality

There has not been one large trial on the effect of nitrates on mortality in AMI to date. Flaherty et al. (46) found a lower in-hospital mortality in the early subgroup (15% versus 39%, p = 0.003) on retrospective analysis. Jugdutt and Warnica (23) found a significant decrease in in-hospital deaths up to 38 days (14% versus 26%, $p < 0.01$), in deaths at 3 months (16% versus 28%, $p < 0.025$) and at 12 months (21% versus 31%, $p < 0.05$). The latter effect was mainly seen in the high-risk group of patients with anterior Q-wave AMI and the greatest topographic deterioration (23). The mortality from all individual clinical trials of intravenous nitroglycerin is summarized in Table 5. A meta-analysis of the pooled data from the trials of intravenous nitroglycerin and oral nitrates in AMI was performed by Yusuf et al. (24). The results indicated a 49% reduction in the odds of death of all trials with intravenous nitroglycerin (Fig. 3) and a 35% reduction in odds of death (2 $p < 0.001$) for all nitrate trials (24).

NITRATE DOSE AND TOLERANCE

Tolerance With High-Dose Nitrates

There is overwhelming evidence that tolerance develops during continuous high-dose nitrate therapy (26,27,63–66,107) and that a nitrate-free interval restores efficacy (63–66,107,108). However, such high doses are not recommended in AMI (17,30,23).

Nevertheless, tolerance has a molecular basis (109) and might be a problem when prolonged nitrate therapy is considered after AMI. Three mechanisms have

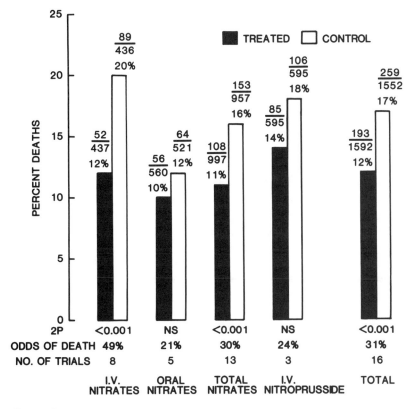

Figure 3   Summary of published randomized trials of nitrates and nitroprusside in AMI. [Modified from data by Yusuf et al. (24), with permission.]

been proposed: (a) sulfhydryl depletion; (b) vasoconstriction secondary to neuro-humoral activation; and (c) loss of hemodynamic efficacy due to expansion of in-travascular volume. All three mechanisms are probably operative in congestive heart failure (110).

Neurohumoral activation might not be significant in very early stages of AMI. Volume expansion and hemodilution was noted by Lis et al. (50) in patients with AMI. Reversal of tolerance after high-dose intravenous nitroglycerin (6.4 μg/kg/min) for 48 hr with N-acetyl cysteine supports the sulfhydryl hypothesis (107), although this effect was not confirmed by Dupuis et al. (110). However, N-acetyl cysteine does potentiate the effects of nitroglycerin and increase vascular sensitiv-ity (111). As in the case of nitrate dose, venous, coronary, and arterial beds show evidence of differential tolerance (112) as well as differential reversal by N-acetyl cysteine (113). Captopril, which has a sulfhydryl radical, failed to prevent tolerance after high doses of nitroglycerin (1.5 μg/kg/min) in patients with congestive heart failure (114).

Tolerance with Low-Dose Nitrates

Tolerance can be prevented by the use of the lowest effective dose, less frequent dosing, short-term formulations, eccentric dosing, and an adequate nitrate-free interval (65,66,108).

Tolerance with low-dose intravenous nitroglycerin therapy for the first 48 hr after AMI is rarely a problem (23,67). In the most recent study (67), partial tolerance developed in 24% of the 154 patients. This was only evident upon analysis of individual data but not when looking merely at group data (Fig. 2). It appeared early, requiring the dose to be increased within 11 ± 9 hr. Despite this evidence of tolerance on individual analysis, the average dose was 45 ± 34 μg/min and the dose range was 4–192 μg/min. Also in that study (23,67), group data indicated lasting beneficial effects on multiple endpoints (Table 1). However, when infusions were stopped, blood pressure and LV volumes increased for the entire group but not in the tolerant group (23,67).

ADVERSE EFFECTS

Hypotension

Increased sensitivity is a more important problem than tolerance with low-dose intravenous nitroglycerin in AMI (23). Increased sensitivity is common in patients with hypovolemia, inferior wall infarction, right ventricular infarction syndrome (23), or advanced age (115). In a recent study (23), 15 patients (10%) developed a mean blood pressure below 80 mmHg within 30 min and 11 had inferior AMI. Eleven patients (7%) needed a dose less than 6 μg/min to maintain the target blood pressure, and 10 had inferior AMI. Of 14 patients (9%) whose mean blood pressure fell below the target between 3 and 12 hr, 9 had inferior AMI. In those 14 patients, the mean blood pressure averaged 75 ± 4 mmHg and the dose averaged only 25 ± 4 μg/min (range, 10–35 μg/min). Infarct size in these patients was larger than in those with mean blood pressure persistently above 80 mmHg.

In two other studies with low-dose nitroglycerin in AMI, Jaffe et al. (49) found hypotension in 14% and tachycardia in 20% of patients, and Flaherty et al. (46) had to discontinue the infusion in 9% and slow it down in 11% due to hypotension.

In patients undergoing thrombolysis with streptokinase or rt-PA, low-dose intravenous nitroglycerin therapy has not been associated with any increased risk of hypotension at the author's institution to date (25,54; unpublished data). Nitroglycerin infusion is begun after admission and continued for 48 hr, without interruption during thrombolytic therapy, although downward titration of the dose is often required.

Side Effects

Other side effects, such as sinus bradycardia and headache, were uncommon with low-dose intravenous nitroglycerin therapy (23,44–50).

CONCLUDING COMMENTS

There is no compelling reason why patients with AMI who are given thrombolytic therapy should not receive low-dose intravenous nitroglycerin therapy for the first 48 hr. The multiple benefits of low-dose intravenous nitroglycerin therapy in AMI have been demonstrated in eight randomized clinical trials (23,44–50). There are no reports of any adverse reactions in studies where the combination of low-dose intravenous nitroglycerin and thrombolytic therapy was used (25,54). One study suggested that the combination might widen the window for thrombolytic therapy (25). Thus, low-dose nitroglycerin should be started as early as possible after AMI. In practice, the infusion can be started in the emergency room before the patient is wheeled to the coronary care unit. In addition, thrombolytic therapy with streptokinase or rt-PA can be initiated and given concurrently without risk of hypotension. The nitroglycerin infusion should then be continued for 48 hr. However, the need for individual dose titration in AMI should be emphasized. Down-titration of the dose of intravenous nitroglycerin might be necessary when it is being given together with a thrombolytic agent. Higher doses of intravenous nitroglycerin might be better tolerated during postinfarction angina (14). Whether long-term nitrate therapy with a longer-acting formulation should be started after 48 hr of intravenous nitrate therapy is still the subject of ongoing clinical research. Recent small, randomized studies indicate that eccentric dosing of buccal and oral nitrates to allow a nitrate-free interval (51–54) might be effective as long-term therapy after AMI to further limit remodeling. Sustained-release isosorbide-5-mononitrate is currently under investigation for limitation of postinfarction remodeling and has been suggested to cause less tolerance. All nitrate formulations (including sublingual, topical, aerosolized, and intravenous nitroglycerin) are effective in controlling angina after AMI. Although a nitrate-free interval might reduce nitrate tolerance with chronic therapy, there are no data on increased morbidity from ischemic events due to nitrate tolerance or the nitrate-free interval during chronic nitrate therapy after AMI. The need for protection from silent ischemia during nitrate tolerance or the nitrate-free interval remains unresolved.

ACKNOWLEDGMENT

The author thanks Catherine Jugdutt for secretarial support and typing.

REFERENCES

1. DeWood MA, Spores J, Notske R, Mouser LT, Burroughs R, Golden MS, Lang HT. Prevalence of total coronary occlusion during the early hours of transmural myocardial infarction. N Engl J Med 1980; 303:897-902.

2. Bertrand ME, Lefebvre JM, Laisne CL, Rousseau MF, Carre AG, LeKieffre JP. Coronary angiography in acute transmural myocardial infarction. Am Heart J 1979; 97:61-9.

3. Davies MJ, Thomas A. Thrombosis and acute coronary artery lesions in sudden cardiac ischemic death. N Engl J Med 1984; 310:1137-40.

4. The I.S.A.M. Study Group. A prospective trial of Intravenous Streptokinase in Acute Myocardial Infarction (I.S.A.M.): mortality, morbidity and infarct size at 21 days. N Engl J Med 1986; 314:1465-71.

5. Yusuf S, Collins, R, Peto R, Furberg C, Stampfer MJ, Goldhaber SZ, Hennekens CH. Intravenous and intracoronary fibrinolytic therapy in acute myocardial infarction: overview of results on mortality, reinfarction and side-effects from 33 randomized controlled trials. Eur Heart J 1985; 6:556-85.

6. Simoons ML, Serruys PW, van den Brand M, Res J, Verheugt FWA, Krauss XH, Remme WJ, Bar F, de Zwaan C, van der Laarse A, Vermeer F, Lubsen J. Early thrombolysis in actue myocardial infarction: limitation of infarct size and improved survival. J Am Coll Cardiol 1986; 7:717-28.

7. Gruppo Italiano per lo Studio della Streptochinasi nell´Infarto Miocardico. Long-term effects of intravenous thrombolysis in acute myocardial infarction: Final report of the GISSI study. Lancet 1987; 2:871-74.

8. ISIS 2 Collaborative Group. Randomized trial of intravenous streptokinase, oral aspirin, both, or neither among 17,987 cases of suspected acute myocardial infarction: ISIS 2. Lancet 1988; 2:349-60.

9. Kennedy JW, Ritchie JL, Davis KB, Fritz JK. Western Washington randomized trial of intracoronary streptokinase in acute myocardial infarction. N Engl J Med 1983; 309:1477-82.

10. Braunwald E, Kloner RA. The stunned myocardium: prolonged, postischemic ventricular dysfunction. Circulation 1982; 66:1146-49.

11. Braunwald E. Myocardial reperfusion, limitation of infarct size, reduction of left ventricular dysfunction, and improved survival—should the paradigm be expanded? Circulation 1989; 79:441-4.

12. Verstraete M, Arnold AER, Brower RW, Collen D, de Bono DP, de Zwaan C, Erbel R, Hillis WS, Lennane RJ, Lubsen J, Mathey D, Reid DS, Rutsch W, Schartl M, Schofer J, Serruys PW, Simoons ML, Uebis R, Vahanian A, Verheugt FWA, von Essen R. Acute coronary thrombolysis with recombinant human tissue-type plasminogen activator: initial patency and influence of maintained infusion on reocclusion rate. Am J Cardiol 1987; 60:231-7.

13. Johns JA, Gold HK, Leinbach RC, Yasuda T, Gimple LW, Werner W, Finkelstein D, Newell J, Ziskind AA, Collen D. Prevention of coronary artery reocclusion and reduction in late coronary artery stenosis after thrombolytic therapy in patients with acute myocardial infarction. A randomized study of maintenance infusion of recombinant human tissue-type plasminogen activator. Circulation 1988; 78:546-56.

14. Becker RC, Gore JM, Alpert JS. Postinfarction unstable angina. Pathophysiologic basis for current treatment modalities. Cardiology 1989; 76:144-57.

15. Abrams J. Current concepts: nitroglycerin and long-acting nitrates. N Engl J Med 1980; 302:1234-37.

16. Conti CR. Use of nitrates in unstable angina pectoris. Am J Cardiol 1987; 60:31H-34H.

17. Gunnar RM, Fisch C. Special Report: ACC/AHA Guidelines for the early management of patients with acute myocardial infarction. Circulation 1990; 82:664-707.

18. Flaherty JT, Reid PR, Kelly DT, Taylor DR, Weisfeldt ML, Pitt B. Intravenous nitroglycerin in acute myocardial infarction. Circulation 1975; 51:132-9.

19. Flaherty JT. Intravenous nitroglycerin in acute myocardial infarction. Cardiovasc Rev Rep 1990; 11:46-52.

20. Jugdutt BI. Intravenous nitroglycerin infusion in acute myocardial infarction: myocardial salvage. Cardiovasc Rev Rep 1984; 5:1145-63.

21. Michorowski BL, Senaratne MPJ, Jugdutt BI. Myocardial infarct expansion. Cardiovasc Rev Rep 1987; 8:42-7.

22. Michorowski BL, Senaratne MPJ, Jugdutt BI. Deterring myocardial infarct expansion. Cardiovasc Rev Rep 1987; 8:55-62.

23. Jugdutt BI, Warnica JW. Intravenous nitroglycerin therapy to limit myocardial infarct size, expansion and complications. Effect of timing, dosage and infarct location. Circulation 1988; 78:906-19.

24. Yusuf S, Collins R, MacMahon S, Peto S. Effect of intravenous nitrates on mortality in acute myocardial infarction: an overview of the randomized trials. Lancet 1988; 1:1088-92.

25. Tymchak WJ, Michorowski BL, Burton JR, Jugdutt BI. Preservation of left ventricular function and topography with combined reperfusion and intravenous nitroglycerin in acute myocardial infarction. J Am Coll Cardiol 1988; 11:90A (abstract).

26. Brunton TL. On the use of nitrite of amyl in angina pectoris. Lancet 1967; 2:97-8.

27. Murell W. Nitroglycerin as a remedy for angina pectoris. Lancet 1879; 1:80-1,113-5, 115-22,225-7.

28. Hay M. The chemical nature and physiological action of nitroglycerine. Practitioner 1883; 30:422-33.

29. Needleman P, Johnson EM Jr. Mechanism of tolerance development to organic nitrates. J Pharmacol Exp Ther 1973; 184:709-15.

30. Ignarro LJ, Lippton H, Edwards JC, Baricos WH, Hyman AL, Kadowitz PJ, Gruetter CA. Mechanism of vascular smooth muscle relaxation by organic nitrates, nitroprusside and nitric oxide: evidence for the involvement of S-nitrosothiols as active intermediates. J Pharmacol Exp Ther 1981; 218:739-49.

31. Palmer RMJ, Ferrige AG, Moncada S. Nitric oxide release accounts for the biological activity of endothelium-derived relaxing factor. Nature 1987; 327:524-6.

32. Bassenge E, Busse R. Endothelial modulation of coronary tone. Prog Cardiovasc Dis 1988; 30:349-80.

33. Vanhoutte PM, Shimokawa H. Endothelium-derived relaxing factor and coronary vasospasm. Circulation 1989; 80:1-9.

34. Freiman PC, Mitchell GG, Heistad DD, Armstrong ML, Harrison DG. Atherosclerosis impairs endothelium-dependent vascular relaxation to acetylcholine and thrombin in primates. Circ Res 1986; 58:783-9.

35. Rafflenbeul W, Bassenge E, Lichtlen PR. Competition between endothelium- and nitroglycerin-induced coronary vasodilatation. Circulation 1988; 78(Suppl II):II-455 (abstract).

36. Trimarco B, Cuoculo A, Van Dorne D, Ricciardelli B, Volpe M, DeSimone A, Condorelli M. Late phase of nitroglycerin-induced coronary vasodilatation blunted by inhibition of prostaglandin synthesis. Circulation 1985; 71:840-8.

37. Gorlin R, Fuster V, Ambrose JA. Anatomic-physiologic link between acute coronary syndromes. Circulation 1986; 74:6-9.

38. Busse R, Luckoff A, Bassenge E. Endothelium-derived relaxant factor inhibits platelet activation. Naunyn-Schmiedebergs Arch Pharmacol 1987; 336:566-71.

39. Hirsh PD, Hillis LD, Campbell WB, Firth BG, Willerson JT. Release of prostaglandins and thromboxane into the coronary circulation in patients with ischemic heart disease. N Engl J Med 1981; 304:685-91.

40. Smitherman TC, Milam M, Woo J, Willerston JT, Frengel LP. Elevated beta thromboglobulin in peripheral venous blood of patients with acute myocardial ischemia: direct evidence of enhanced platelet reactivity in vivo. Am J Cardiol 1981; 48:395-402.

41. Pohl U, Busse R, Bassenge E. EDRF-induced augmentation of cGMP levels in platelets passing through the coronary vascular bed. Circulation 1988; 78(Suppl II):II-182 (abstract).

42. Lam JYT, Chesebro JH, Fuster V. Platelets, vasoconstriction and nitroglycerin during arterial wall injury. Circulation 1988; 78:712-6.

43. Diodati J, Theroux P, Latour JG, Lacoste L, Lam JYT, Waters D. Effects of nitroglycerin at therapeutic doses on platelet aggregation in unstable angina pectoris and acute myocardial infarction. Am J Cardiol 1990; 66:683-8.

44. Chiche P, Baligadoo SJ, Derrida JP. A randomized trial of prolonged nitroglycerin infusion in acute myocardial infarction (Abstract). Circulation 1979; 59 & 60(Suppl II):11-164.

45. Bussmann WD, Passek D, Seidel W, Kaltenbach M. Reduction of CK and CK-MB indexes of infarct size by intravenous nitroglycerin. Circulation 1981; 63:615-22.

46. Flaherty JT, Becker LC, Bulkley BH, Weiss JL, Gerstenblith G, Kallman CH, Silverman KJ, Wei JY, Pitt B, Weisfeldt ML. A randomized prospective trial of intravenous nitroglycerin in patients with acute myocardial infarction. Circulation 1983; 68:576-88.

47. Jugdutt BI, Sussex BA, Warnica JW, Rossall RE. Persistent reduction in left ventricular asynergy in patients with acute myocardial infarction by intravenous infusion of nitroglycerin. Circulation 1983; 68:1264-73.

48. Nelson GIC, Silke B, Ahuya RC, Hussain M, Taylor SH. Haemodynamic advantages

of isosorbide dinitrate over frusemide in acute heart-failure following myocardial infarction. Lancet 1983; 1:730-3.

49. Jaffe AS, Geltman EM, Tiefenbrunn AJ, Ambos HD, Strauss HD, Sobel BE, Roberts R. Reduction of infarct size in patients with inferior infarction with intravenous glyceryl trinitrate. A randomized study. Br Heart J 1983; 49:452-60.

50. Lis Y, Bennett D, Lambert G, Robson D. A preliminary double-blind study of IV nitroglycerin in acute myocardial infarction. Intensive Care Med 1984; 10:179-84.

51. Michorowski BL, Tymchak WJ, Jugdutt BI. Improved left ventricular function and topography by prolonged nitroglycerin therapy after acute myocardial infarction. Circulation 1987; 76(Suppl IV):IV-128 (abstract).

52. Jugdutt BI, Neiman JC, Michorowski BL, Tymchak WJ, Genge TJ, Fitzpatrick LK. Persistent improvement in left ventricular geometry and function by prolonged nitroglycerin therapy after anterior transmural acute myocardial infarction. J Am Coll Cardiol 1990; 15:214A (abstract).

53. Humen DP, McCormick L, Jugdutt BI. Chronic reduction in left ventricular volumes at rest and exercise in patients treated with nitroglycerin following anterior MI. J Am Coll Cardiol 1989; 13:25A (abstract).

54. Jugdutt BI, Tymchak W, Humen D, Gulamhusein S, Hales M. Prolonged nitroglycerin versus captopril therapy on remodeling after transmural myocardial infarction. Circulation 1990; 82(Suppl III):III-442 (abstract).

55. Jugdutt BI, Becker LC, Hutchins GM, Bulkley BH, Reid PR, Kallman CH. Effect of intravenous nitroglycerin on collateral blood flow and infarct size in the conscious dog. Circulation 1981; 63:17-28.

56. Jugdutt BI. Myocardial salvage by intravenous nitroglycerin in conscious dogs: Loss of beneficial effect with marked nitroglycerin-induced hypotension. Circulation 1983; 68:673-84.

57. Jugdutt BI. Delayed effects of early infarct-limiting therapies on healing after myocardial infarction. Circulation 1985; 72:907-14.

58. Jugdutt BI. Effect of nitroglycerin and ibuprofen on left ventricular topography and rupture threshold during healing after myocardial infarction in the dog. Can J Physiol Pharmacol 1988; 66:385-95.

59. Imhof PR, Ott B, Frankhauser P, Chu LC, Hodler J. Difference in nitroglycerin dose-response in the venous and arterial beds. Eur J Clin Pharmacol 1980; 18:455-60.

60. Bassenge E, Stewart DJ. Effects of nitrates in various vascular sections and regions. Z Kardiol 1986; 75(Suppl 3):1-7.

61. Kelly RP, Gibbs HH, O'Rourke MF, Daley JE, Mang K, Morgan JJ, Avolio AP. Nitroglycerin has more favorable effects on left ventricular afterload than apparent from measurement of pressure in a peripheral artery. Eur Heart J 1990; 11:138-44.

62. Capurro NL, Kent KM, Smith HJ, Aamodt R, Epstein SE. Acute coronary occlusion: Prolonged increase in collateral flow following brief administration of nitroglycerin and methoxamine. Am J Cardiol 1977; 39:679-83.

63. Schwartz AM. The cause, relief and prevention of headache arising from contact with dynamite. N Engl J Med 1946; 235:541-4.

64. McGuinness BW, Harris EL. "Monday head." An interesting occupational disorder. Br Med J 1961; 2:745-7.

65. Abrams J. Tolerance to organic nitrates. Circulation 1986; 74:1181-5.
66. Parker JO. Nitrate tolerance. Am J Cardiol 1987; 60:44H-8H.
67. Jugdutt BI, Warnica JW. Tolerance with low dose intravenous nitroglycerin therapy in acute myocardial infarction. Am J Cardiol 1989; 64:581-7.
68. Armstrong PW, Walker DC, Burton JR, Parker JO. Vasodilator therapy in acute myocardial infarction: A comparison of sodium nitroprusside and nitroglycerin. Circulation 1975; 52:1118-22.
69. Ferrer MI, Bradley SE, Wheeler HO, Enson Y, Prersig R, Brickner PW, Conroy RJ, Harvey RM. Some effects of nitroglycerin upon the splanchnic, pulmonary and systemic circulations. Circulation 1966; 33:357-73.
70. Flaherty JT, Come PC, Baird MG, Rouleau J, Taylor DR, Weisfeldt ML, Greene HL, Becker LC, Pitt B. Effects of intravenous nitroglycerin on left ventricular function and ST segment changes in acute myocardial infarction. Br Heart J 1976; 38:612-21.
71. Bussmann WD. Nitroglycerin in the treatment of acute myocardial infarction. Acta Med Scand 1981; 210:165-75.
72. Come PC, Flaherty JT, Weisfeldt M, Green L, Becker LC, Pitt B. Reversal of the beneficial effects of intravenous nitroglycerin in patients with acute myocardial infarction by phenylephrine. N Engl J Med 1975; 293:1003-7.
73. Armstrong PW, Moffat JA, Marks GS. Arterial-venous nitroglycerin gradient during intravenous infusion in man. Circulation 1982; 66:1273-6.
74. Ribner HS, Bresnahan D, Hsieh AM, Silverman R, Tommaso C, Coath A, Askenazi J. Acute hemodynamic responses to vasodilator therapy in congestive heart failure. Prog Cardiovasc Dis 1982; 25:1-42.
75. Maroko PR, Kjekshus JK, Sobel BE, Watanabe T, Covell JW, Ross J Jr, Braunwald E. Factors influencing infarct size following experimental coronary artery occlusions. Circulation 1971; 43:67-82.
76. Bussmann WD, Schofer H, Kurita H, Ganz W. Nitroglycerin in acute myocardial infarction. X. Effect of small and large doses of I.V. nitroglycerin on ST-segment deviation: experimental and clinical results. Clin Cardiol 1979; 2:106-12.
77. Prodger SH, Ayman D. Harmful effects of nitroglycerin: with special reference to coronary thrombosis. Am J Med Sci 1932; 184:480-91.
78. Friedberg CK. Acute coronary occlusion and myocardial infarction. In Friedberg CK, ed. Diseases of the heart. 3rd ed. Philadelphia: Saunders, 1966:913-4.
79. Strauer BE. Ventricular function and coronary hemodynamics after intravenous nitroglycerin in coronary artery disease. Am Heart J 1978; 95:210-19.
80. Franciosa JA, Blank RC, Cohn JN. Nitrate effects on cardiac output and left ventricular outflow resistance in chronic congestive heart failure. Am J Med 1978; 64:207-13.
81. Ambrose JA, Hjemdahl-Monsen CE, Borrico S, Gorlin R, Fuster V. Angiographic demonstration of a common link between unstable angina pectoris and non-Q-wave acute myocardial infarction. Am J Cardiol 1988; 61:244-7.
82. Forrester JF, Litvak F, Grundfest W, Hickey A. A perspective of coronary disease seen through the arteries of living man. Circulation 1987; 75:505-13.
83. Marcho P, Vatner SF. Effects of nitroglycerin and nitroprusside on large and small coronary vessels in conscious dogs. Circulation 1981; 64:1101-7.

84. Horwitz LD, Gorlin R, Taylor WJ, Kemp HG. Effects of nitroglycerin on regional myocardial blood flow in coronary artery disease. J Clin Invest 1971; 50:1578-84.

85. Gross GJ, Warltier DC. Intracoronary versus intravenous nitroglycerin on the transmural distribution of coronary blood flow. Cardiovasc Res 1977; 11:499-506.

86. Schaper W, Sharma HS, Quinkler W, Markert T, Wunsch M, Schaper J. Molecular biologic concepts of coronary anastomoses. J Am Coll Cardiol 1990; 15:513-8.

87. Schwartz H, Leiboff RH, Bren GB, Wasserman AG, Katz RJ, Varghese PJ, Sokil AB, Ross AM. Temporal evolution of the human coronary collateral circulation after myocardial infarction. J Am Coll Cardiol 1984; 4:1088-93.

88. Williams DO, Amsterdam EA, Mason DT. Hemodynamic effects of nitroglycerin in acute myocardial infarction: decrease in ventricular preload at the expense of cardiac output. Circulation 1975; 51:421-7.

89. Chiarello M, Gold HK, Leinbach RC, Davis MA, Maroko PR. Comparison between the effects of nitroprusside and nitroglycerin on ischemic injury during acute myocardial infarction. Circulation 1976; 54:766-73.

90. Curfman GD, Heinsimer JA, Lozner EC, Fung HL. Intravenous nitroglycerin in the treatment of spontaneous angina pectoris: a prospective, randomized trial. Circulation 1983; 67:276-82.

91. Distante A, Maseri A, Severi S, Bragini A, Cherchia S. Management of vasospastic angina at rest with continuous infusion of isosorbide dinitrate. Am J Cardiol 1979; 44:533-9.

92. Hutchins GM, Bulkley BH. Infarct expansion versus extention: Two different complications of acute myocardial infarction. Am J Cardiol 1978; 41:1127-32.

93. Ludbrook PA, Byrne JD, Kurnick PB, McKnight RC. Influence of reduction of preload and afterload by nitroglycerin on left ventricular diastolic pressure-volume relations and relaxation in man. Circulation 1977; 56:937-43.

94. Jugdutt BI, Amy RW. Healing after myocardial infarction in the dog: Changes in infarct hydroxyproline and topography. J Am Coll Cardiol 1986; 7:91-102.

95. Pfeffer MA, Braunwald E. Ventricular remodeling after myocardial infarction. Experimental observations and clinical implications. Circulation 1990; 81:1161-72.

96. Eaton LW, Weiss JL, Bulkley BH, Garrison JB, Weisfeldt ML. Regional cardiac dilatation after acute myocardial infarction. N Engl J Med 1979; 300:57-62.

97. Jugdutt BI, Michorowski BL. Role of infarct expansion in rupture of the ventricular septum after acute myocardial infarction: A two-dimensional echocardiographic study. Clin Cardiol 1987; 10:641-52.

98. Jugdutt BI, Basualdo CA. Myocardial infarct expansion during indomethacin or ibuprofen therapy for symptomatic post-infarction pericarditis. Influence of other pharmacologic agents during early remodeling. Can J Cardiol 1989; 5:211-21.

99. Jugdutt BI. Identification of patients prone to infarct expansion by the degree of regional shape distortion on an early two-dimensional echocardiogram after myocardial infarction. A prospective study. Clin Cardiol 1990; 12:28-40.

100. Hochman JS, Choo H. Limitation of myocardial salvage. Circulation 1987; 75:299-306.

101. Touchstone DA, Beller GA, Nygaard TW, Tedesco C, Kaul S. Effects of successful intravenous reperfusion therapy on regional myocardial function and geometry in hu-

mans: A tomographic assessment using two-dimensional echocardiography. J Am Coll Cardiol 1989; 13:1506-13.

102. Honan MB, Harrell FE, Reimer KA, Califf RM, Mark DB, Pryor DB, Hlatky MA. Cardiac rupture, mortality and timing of thrombolytic therapy: a meta-analysis. J Am Coll Cardiol 1990; 16:359-67.

103. Borer JS, Kent KM, Goldstein RE, Epstein SE. Nitroglycerin-induced reduction in the incidence of spontaneous ventricular fibrillation during coronary occlusion in the dog. Am J Cardiol 1974; 33:517-20.

104. Kent KW, Smith ER, Redwood DR, Epstein SE. Beneficial electrophysiologic effects of nitroglycerin during acute myocardial infarction. Am J Cardiol 1974; 33:513-6.

105. Jugdutt BI. Effect of PGE_1, PGE_2, and PGI_2 on ventricular arrhythmias during myocardial infarction in conscious dogs: Relation to infarct size. Prostaglandins Med 1981; 7:431-55.

106. Morcillio E, Reid PR, Dubin N, Ghodgaonkar R, Pitt B. Myocardial prostaglandin E release by nitroglycerin and modification by indomethacin. Am J Cardiol 1980; 45: 53-7.

107. Packer M, Lee WH, Kessler PD, Gottlieb SS, Medina N, Yushak M. Prevention and reversal of nitrate tolerance in patients with congestive heart failure. N Engl J Med 1987; 317:799-804.

108. Thadani U, Prasad R, Hamilton SF, Voyles W, Doyle R, Karpow S, Reder R, Teague SM. Usefulness of twice-daily isosorbide-5-mononitrate in preventing development of tolerance in angina pectoris. Am J Cardiol 1987; 60:477-82.

109. Fung HL, Chong S, Kowaluk E. Mechanisms of nitrate action and vascular tolerance. Eur Heart J 1989; 10(Suppl A):2-6.

110. Dupuis J, Lalonde G, Lemieux R, Rouleau JL. Tolerance to intravenous nitroglycerin in patients with congestive heart failure: Role of increased intravascular volume, neurohumoral activation and lack of prevention with N-acetylcysteine. J Am Coll Cardiol 1990; 16:923-31.

111. Horowitz JD, Antman EM, Lorell BH, Barry WH, Smith TW. Potentiation of the cardiovascular effects of nitroglycerin by *N*-acetylcysteine. Circulation 1983; 68:1247-53.

112. Stewart DJ, Elsner D, Sommer O, Holtz J, Bassenge E. Altered spectrum of nitroglycerin action in long-term treatment: nitroglycerin-specific venous tolerance with maintenance of arterial vasodepressor potency. Circulation 1986; 74:573-82.

113. Munzel T, Holtz J, Mulsch A, Stewart DJ, Bassenge E. Nitrate tolerance in epicardial arteries or in the venous system is not reversed by N-acetylcysteine in vivo, but tolerance-independent interactions exist. Circulation 1989; 79:188-97.

114. Dupuis C, Lalonde G, Bichet D, Rouleau JL. Captopril does not prevent nitroglycerin tolerance in heart failure. Can J Cardiol 1990; 6:281-6.

115. Alpert JS. Nitrate therapy in the elderly. Am J Cardiol 1990; 65:23J-7J.

6

Beta-Blockers as Adjunctive Therapy in Acute Myocardial Infarction

Koon K. Teo
University of Alberta Hospital, Edmonton, Alberta, Canada

INTRODUCTION

Large randomized, controlled clinical trials conducted over the last two decades have shown convincingly that use of beta-adrenergic blocking agents (beta-blockers) in patients after acute myocardial infarction produces medically worthwhile reductions in mortality and major morbidity (1). At present, data are available from at least 70 randomized controlled clinical trials of beta-blockers involving over 53,000 patients. Among these trials of beta-blocker therapy in acute myocardial infarction, only two, which included nearly 2000 patients, have been carried out during the thrombolytic era (2,3); one trial studied patients who were primarily enrolled into a trial of thrombolytic/reperfusion therapy (2), while in the other, some patients might have received thrombolytic therapy as routine therapy (3). At present, three important questions exist regarding the use of beta-blockers during and following myocardial infarction. First, how soon and for how long after acute myocardial infarction should beta-blocker treatment be administered? Second, are properties found in some agents (e.g., intrinsic sympathomimetic property) beneficial or harmful? Third, has the effectiveness of beta-blocker therapy and the need for such therapy been substantially altered by the advent of effective thrombolytic treatment?

In this chapter, these issues will be discussed using data from randomized controlled clinical trials. Further, insights that can be obtained from some of these trials as to the mechanisms of benefit due to beta-blockade will be discussed. It is inevitable that, because of the large number of trials available, some results *may appear* to be inconsistent. Some of these apparent inconsistencies are due to study design and lack of adequate statistical power to detect a real, but moderate effect. Still, the busy clinician needs to know data which are reliable and applicable to clinical practice. Therefore, in order to avoid selection or systematic biases, the data from all these trials will be examined, irrespective of the results. Conclusions are based on both the results of the individual trials and an overview of all the available randomized controlled trials of beta-blockers, so that, in addition to avoiding selection and systematic biases, there will be adequate statistical power to reliably detect or exclude moderate-sized effects of the order of 15–25% changes in risk. The rationale, methodology, and limitations for conducting such overviews from different trials have been described previously (1,4).

PHARMACOLOGICAL PROPERTIES OF BETA-BLOCKERS

Since the pioneering work of Langley (5) and Ahlquist (6), much has been learned about the pharmacological properties of these agents. These drugs competitively and in a dose-dependent fashion inhibit the binding of catecholamines to beta-adrenergic receptors found on the tissue cell membrane. Lands et al. (7) further subclassified these receptors into beta$_1$-receptors (found in cardiac, intestinal, and adipose tissues) and beta$_2$-receptors (found in bronchial and vascular smooth muscle). Commonly used beta-blockers can be classified as beta$_1$ or "cardioselective" if the agent preferentially interacts with beta$_1$-receptors or "noncardioselective" if it interacts with both subtypes of receptors. Metoprolol and atenolol are examples of cardioselective beta$_1$-blockers. Propranolol, timolol, and pindolol are examples of noncardioselective beta-blockers (8) (Table 1). It has been suggested that cardioselective beta-blockers may be safer in asthmatic patients, but in practice this property does not appear to confer any additional advantage for the asthmatic patient, in whom these agents should be used cautiously.

Intrinsic sympathomimetic activity (ISA) is a property of some beta-blockers (e.g., pindolol, alprinolol, and acebutalol), which paradoxically retain a degree of agonist activity with respect to the same beta-adrenergic receptors (8) (Table 1). There is no good evidence that these beta-blockers with ISA are inherently safer in patients at risk from beta-blockade (e.g., asthmatics) than in those without. Whether they confer additional benefit or harm in patients after myocardial infarction will be discussed later.

With respect to pharmacokinetics, some beta-blockers are lipid-soluble (e.g., propranolol, metoprolol and pindolol). This property enhances intestinal absorption and metabolism by the liver, leading to a relatively short plasma half-life. Water-soluble beta-blockers (e.g., timolol, atenolol) are less readily absorbed and less extensively metabolized by the liver (Table 1). Water-soluble beta-blockers

Table 1   Pharmacological Properties of Beta-Blockers in Clinical Use

Drug	Cardioselectivity	ISA	Membrane stabilizing	Lipid solubility[a]
Acebutolol	+	+	+	Moderate
Alprenolol	-	+	+	?
Atenolol	+	-	-	Weak
Metoprolol	+	-	-	Moderate
Nadolol	-	-	-	Weak
Oxprenolol	-	+	+	Moderate
Pindolol	-	+	+	Moderate
Propranolol	-	-	+	High
Sotolol	-	-	-	Weak
Timolol	-	-	-	Weak

[a]Agents with weak lipid solubility are highly soluble in water, and vice versa.
ISA = intrinsic sympathomimetic activity; + = present; - = absent; ? = not available.

have a longer plasma half-life. These agents do not cross the blood-brain barrier as easily as fat-soluble agents. Such differences in properties are unlikely to result in differing efficacy of beta-blockade therapy but may be important in development of certain side effects.

Previously, beta-blockers had not been used because of serious concerns about properties that could potentially cause harm in patients after acute myocardial infarction. Chief among these concerns was the negative inotropic effect, which presumably could easily tip an already weakened heart into failure or exacerbate existing cardiac failure. Concern that beta-blockade might cause severe atrioventricular block by its action on the conduction system has been expressed.

However, certain properties of beta-blockers could be potentially beneficial in ischemic heart disease. These agents reduce heart rate, blood pressure, and myocardial contractility, thus reducing workload and myocardial oxygen consumption. Theoretically, the resultant reduction in wall stress may be expected to prevent myocardial rupture during acute myocardial infarction. During acute myocardial ischemia, administration of a beta-blocker results in a favorable redistribution of the coronary blood from the epicardium to the more ischemic endocardial region (9). In a recent thrombolytic trial (2), the observation that patients given a beta-blocker following thrombolytic therapy were less likely to develop cerebral hemorrhage gave rise to the interesting hypothesis that this beneficial effect may be brought about by decreased disruption of the hemostatic plug. If confirmed by further investigation, this beneficial effect will be of particular value with the increasing use of thrombolytic agents.

Animal experiments have shown that direct cathecholamine-induced myocardial necrosis that occurs during periods of intense sympathetic stimulation, such as during acute myocardial infarction, may be prevented by beta-blockade. These experiments have also shown that, by inhibiting cathecholamine-induced lipolysis during acute ischemia, the levels of circulating free fatty acids are reduced, shifting myocardial metabolism to glucose utilization, which requires less oxygen (10). Finally administration of beta-blockers before coronary ligation reduces infarct size and raises the threshold for ventricular fibrillation.

These theoretical considerations and experimental results suggest that patients with acute myocardial infarction can benefit from beta-blockade therapy. However, only clinical investigations in humans could determine whether the balance between the potentially harmful and beneficial effects of beta-blockers would translate into overall clinical benefit.

TRIALS OF BETA-BLOCKERS AFTER ACUTE MYOCARDIAL INFARCTION

Short-Term Trials of Early Intervention

In the mid-1960s to early 1970s, a number of small trials of beta-blockers given orally on admission, usually within 24 hr but up to 72 hr after onset of symptoms, were carried out. Duration of treatment varied from 2 days to 4 weeks. None of these 22 trials, reviewed by Yusuf et al. (1), showed significant beneficial or harmful effects. Overall, when the results were pooled by an overview (Table 2), a 7% nonsignificant reduction in mortality in favor of beta-blockers was suggested, but with a 95% confidence interval of 26% reduction to 18% excess mortality, a harmful effect could not be ruled out. In retrospect, these trials, involving a total of 1900 patients allocated to active treatment and 1711 to controls, were too small to detect a significant difference reliably, if one were present. More important, concern was expressed that oral administration was associated with a considerable delay before full beta-blockade could be achieved. This delay might be critical because it is during the first few hours after onset of symptoms that myocardial cell injury and death occur, the infarction becomes completed, and dangerous arrhythmias such as ventricular fibrillation frequently occur. Such time delay could be overcome by administering the agent intravenously.

Therefore, starting in the 1970s, a series of beta-blocker trials, in which the first dose of the agent was given intravenously followed by oral administration, were conducted (1). These early-intervention trials started treatment soon after onset of myocardial infarction. At least 26 trials have been carried out. Twenty-three trials were short-term, lasting from 3 min to 4 weeks (1). The other three trials were long-term studies (1 year each in two trials and 3 months in one) (11-13). Mortality was designated as one of the main endpoints in only a few of the short-term trials (1). In the majority of the studies, the effect of beta-blockade on infarct size

Table 2 Early Short-Term Intervention with Beta-Blockers: Effect on Mortality

	Deaths/patients (*n*)		Odds reduction	
Trials	Active	Control	(%)	95% CI
Oral treatment only				
22 small trials (1)	165/1900	165/1711	-7	-26% to +18%
Intravenous followed by oral treatment[a]				
26 small trials (1)	117/2901	126/2830	-9	-30% to +17%
MIAMI (14)[b]	79/2877	93/2901	-15	-37% to +15%
ISIS-1 (15)	317/8037	367/7990	-15*	-27% to -1%
TIMI-IIB (2)[c]	17/696	17/694	0	-49% to +93%
Total[a]	530/14,511 (3.7%)	603/14,415 (4.2%)	-13**	-23% to -2%

[a]All available data on 0- to 7-day mortality from trials that started with intravenous followed by oral treatment.
[b]MIAMI trial, 15-day mortality: 123/2877 for active group and 142/2901 for controls; odds reduction: 13%; 95% CI -32% to +11%; p = NS.
[c]TIMI-IIB, 6-day mortality.
95% CI = 95% confidence interval; - = reduction; + = excess mortality.
*$p < 0.05$.
**$p < 0.02$.

was the primary endpoint. Other endpoints of interest were arrhythmias, hemodynamic function, and pain relief. Mortality was the primary endpoint in all three long-term studies. In most studies treatment was started within 24 hr of onset of symptoms, and the initial intravenous dose (e.g., 5–10 mg propranolol, 5–10 mg atenolol, or 10–15 mg metoprolol) was followed by oral treatment for varying durations.

Altogether, data on 7-day mortality are available from these 26 small trials, which allocated 2901 patients to beta-blockade and 2830 patients to control treatment (Table 2). Collectively, 117 patients assigned to beta-blockers died, compared to 126 deaths for those assigned to control. This represents a reduction in odds of death of 9% with a 95% confidence interval ranging from 30% reduction to 17% increase in odds of death. This result is almost identical to that of the oral beta-blocker trials, i.e., a small non-significant reduction in mortality in patients treated with early beta-blockade.

Two large multicenter beta-blocker trials were subsequently carried out to further investigate the effect of early intervention on mortality. The first was the Metoprolol in Acute Myocardial Infarction (MIAMI) trial (14), which recruited nearly 6000 patients, 2877 to metoprolol and 2901 to placebo (Table 2). The primary endpoint of this study was to determine whether short-term mortality, defined as death within 15 days after acute myocardial infarction, could be reduced by early intervention with metoprolol. There were 123 deaths (4.3%) in the metoprolol group and 142 deaths (4.9%) in the placebo group. The 13% reduction in 15-day mortality in the active treatment group was not statistically significant (p = 0.29). The 95% confidence interval ranged from 32% reduction to 11% increase in odds of death. The 7-day mortality in this trial happened to be lower than in other trials, and although there was a 15% (95% confidence interval of 37% reduction to 16% increase in odds of death) reduction in mortality in the beta-blocker–treated group, this also did not reach statistical significance.

In the much larger First International Study of Infarct Survival (ISIS-1) (Table 2) there were 317 vascular deaths (3.9%) within 7 days in 8037 patients allocated to beta-blocker, compared to 367 vascular deaths (4.6%) in 7990 patients allocated to placebo (15). There was a 15% reduction in mortality (95% confidence interval ranged from 27% to 1% reductions in odds of death), which was statistically significant in favor of atenolol, the beta-blocker used in the study (p < 0.05).

In a substudy of the Thrombolysis in Myocardial Infarction Phase II Trial (TIMI-IIB), 1390 patients were randomized to receive metoprolol (696 patients) or placebo (694 patients) following thrombolytic therapy with tissue plasminogen activator (t-PA) (2). This TIMI-II substudy had insufficient power to detect a difference in mortality between the two groups, which turned out to be the same (17 deaths during the first 6 days) in both groups (Table 2).

Overall, 530 of 14,511 patients (3.7%) allocated beta-blockers and 603 of 14,415 control patients (4.2%) died within 7 days of starting treatment (Table 2). When the 7-day mortalities of all 29 early-intervention trials of intravenous followed by oral therapy are combined by an overview, there is a 13% reduction in mortality (95% confidence interval ranged from 23% to 2% reduction in odds of death, p < 0.02), in favor of beta-blockade.

Mechanisms of Benefit

In both the ISIS-1 and MIAMI trials, it had been observed that almost all the differences in mortality occurred in days 0–1. However, Yusuf et al. pointed out that this apparent appreciable effect on mortality found mainly in days 0–1 was not strongly supported when the aggregate of data from the other randomized intravenous beta-blocker trials was considered (15). Most of the mortality following myocardial infarction also occurs during this early acute phase, and there have been some fears that the development of serious adverse effects from use of beta-blockers early postinfarction (e.g., cardiac failure) may adversely affect this mortality. The data-derived hypothesis that the beneficial effect of treatment is also predominantly seen during this early period is probably useful in allaying such fears.

Although the mechanisms for early mortality reduction by beta-blockade are

Table 3   Early Short-Term Intervention with Beta-Blockers: Effects on Nonmortality Endpoints

Endpoints	Events/patients (n)		Odds reduction (%)	95% CI
	Active	Control		
Ventricular fibrillation	306/13,909	355/13,654	−15*	−29% to −1%
Reinfarction	308/11,021	371/11,070	−18**	−30% to −4%
Infarction prevented[a]	658/2,286	765/2,420	−13***	−22% to 0%

[a]Development of definite myocardial infarction prevented, probably due to early treatment with beta-blocker.
95% CI = 95% confidence interval; − = reduction in favor of beta-blockers. For these nonmortality endpoints, data are not available from all trials and the pooled results should be interpreted cautiously.
*$p < 0.01$.
**$p < 0.02$.
***$p < 0.05$.

not entirely clear, a number of observations from these trials may suggest how such benefits can occur. Experimentally, it has been shown that beta-blockers are protective in development of ventricular fibrillation during acute myocardial infarction (16). Several trials have reported a reduction in ventricular fibrillation in patients assigned to beta-blockade (17–19). Overall, the available data from 27 trials (Table 3) suggest a 15% significant ($p < 0.01$) reduction in ventricular fibrillation (15). However, as most patients with ventricular fibrillation did survive after defibrillation, this reduction in ventricular fibrillation alone cannot explain the reduction in mortality.

A retrospective analysis of the ISIS-1 results suggests that the early benefit is chiefly due to the lower number of deaths from myocardial rupture and, to a lesser extent, to the fewer episodes of fatal ventricular fibrillation in the atenolol group (20). A similar trend has been observed in the MIAMI trial and in another large metoprolol trial (14). Data on the mode of death are not available from the other small trials. This possibility of a reduction in myocardial rupture remains an interesting hypothesis.

Data on major morbidity suggest that beta-blockers reduce reinfarction and infarct extension. Examination of the data on reinfarction (or on infarct extension in three small trials) during the first 7 days after infarction (available on about 22,000 patients) indicates that reinfarction occurred in 308 of 11,021 patients (2.8%) treated with beta-blockers, while 371 of 11,070 patients (3.4%) in the control group has reinfarction (15). This represents an 18% reduction in odds of reinfarction in favor of the beta-blocker group (95% confidence interval ranged from 4% to 30% reduction, $p < 0.02$) (Table 3).

Before the widespread use of thrombolytic agents, infarct size was usually estimated indirectly by measurement of serum enzyme levels. Enzyme release is reduced 20–30% by intravenous beta-blockade administered within 12 hr after
onset of symptoms (21). Taken together with other indices of infarct size, such as
electrocardiographic ST-segment changes, there is reasonable evidence that infarct size is reduced by early beta-blockade. Reductions in infarct size may lead to
prevention of transmural necrosis and myocardial rupture.

A number of placebo-controlled trials have shown that early use of beta-blockers can reduce ischemic pain (22–24). This pain relief correlates with the time
course and magnitude of the reduction in blood pressure and heart rate, suggesting
that this benefit may be produced by a reduction in oxygen demand. Reduction in
oxygen demand may also be operative in preventing the development of myocardial infarction if treatment is started early in some patients. In five trials, specific
data are available on patients without definite electrocardiographic evidence of
myocardial infarction when treatment was started (14,15,18,25,26). These patients received treatment early in the course of the infarction process, and development of a definite myocardial infarction was prevented in some. Overall, of 2286
patients assigned to beta-blockade, 658 (28.8%) developed an infarct compared to
765 of 2420 patients (31.6%) who are assigned placebo. This reduction of 13% is
statistically significant ($p < 0.05$) (Table 3). However, this conclusion has to be
interpreted cautiously because of absence of data from several trials.

Long-Term Trials

Unlike the short-term early intervention trials of beta-blockers after myocardial
infarction, which examined a number of intermediate endpoints such as infarct
size, arrhythmia, and pain relief, the long-term trials primarily examined the effects of treatment on mortality. Initial assessment of results in these trials suggested a degree of inconsistency. While some of these trial results were statistically
significant in favor of beta-blockers on their own, most were not. This discrepancy could possibly be due to differences among the various beta-blockers studied, but is more likely due to inadequate sample sizes and differences in trial populations.

Altogether, at least 26 trials involving more than 24,000 patients have been
conducted (Table 4) (27). In 17 of these trials, which included about 19,700 patients, treatment was started days to weeks after the myocardial infarction and
continued long-term (1,15). In eight other trials, treatment was started early and
continued long-term (1). Data on short-term mortality in some of these eight trials
have been included in the short-term early intervention results reported above. In
the majority of these trials follow-up was for 1 year or more. In one trial, follow-
up was for 3 months (13) and in another from 3 to 9 months (28). A recent trial of
about 600 patients studied the effects of beta-blockade on high-risk patients who

Table 4   Late Long-Term Intervention with Beta-Blockers: Effect on Mortality

Trials	Deaths/patients (n)		Odds reduction (%)	95% CI
	Active	Control		
25 trials (21)	917/12,140	1,090/11,551	-22*	-29% to +15%
APSI (3)	17/298	34/309	-50**	-71% to -11%
Total*	934/12,438 (7.5%)	1,124/11,860 (9.5%)	-23***	-30% to -16%

All available mortality from 26 randomized controlled trials on late long-term intervention with beta-blockers; 95% CI = 95% confidence interval; - = reduction; + = excess mortality.
*$p < 0.0001$.
**$p < 0.02$.
***$p < 0.00001$.

were enrolled on average 10.5 days after onset of the infarction and followed for over 300 days (3).

In five of these trials, patients showed significant reductions in mortality on their own (3,12,13,29,30). A favorable trend, however, was demonstrated by most of the other trials. In the Norwegian timolol trial, 98 of 945 patients (10%) allocated beta-blockade therapy died compared to 152 deaths (16%) in 939 patients in the control group ($p < 0.002$) during a follow-up of 1–3 years (29). In the Beta-blocker Heart Attack trial (BHAT), there were 138 deaths in 1916 patients (7%) on treatment with propranolol and 188 deaths in 1921 controls (10%) during a median treatment period of 2 years ($p = 0.004$) (30). Similarly, in the metoprolol trial by Salathia et al., 27 of 391 patients (7%) in the active treatment group and 43 of 364 patients (12%) in the placebo group died ($p < 0.02$) during 1 year of follow-up (12). Hjalmarson et al. reported comparable results in their trial, in which there were 22 deaths in 680 patients (3%) given metoprolol compared to 39 deaths in 674 patients (6%) given placebo during 3 months of treatment ($p < 0.02$) (13). In the recent trial of acebutolol in high-risk patients after myocardial infarction, there were 17 deaths in 298 acebutolol-treated patients (6%) and 34 deaths in the placebo group of 309 patients (11%) following treatment averaging 300 days. The reduction in mortality was statistically significant ($p < 0.02$) (3).

In total, in these 26 long-term trials of beta-blocker enrolling over 24,000 patients, there were 934 deaths in 12,438 patients (7.5%) allocated to beta-blockers compared to 1124 deaths in 11,860 patients (9.5%) in the control group (27) (Table 4). Overall, the reduction in mortality is 23% in favor of beta-blockers (95% confidence interval ranging from 16% to 30% reduction in mortality). This 23% reduction in mortality is highly statistically significant ($p < 0.0001$) with a

Table 5   Late Long-Term Intervention with Beta-Blockers: Effects on Endpoints Other than All-Cause Mortality

Endpoints	Events/patients (n)		Odds reduction (%)	95% CI
	Active	Control		
Sudden death	289/8,028	401/7712	-32***	-42% to -21%
Nonsudden death	336/8,115	356/7704	-12*	-24% to +3%
Nonfatal reinfarction	565/10,089	729/9720	-27**	-35% to -19%

– = reduction in favor of beta-blockers; + = excess mortality. 95% CI = 95% confidence interval.
*p not significant.
**$p < 0.0001$.
***$p < 0.00001$.

narrow 95% confidence interval of about one-sixth to one-third reduction in odds of death (27).

Other Beneficial Effects in Long-Term Beta-Blocker Trials

Although total mortality is the primary endpoint in the long-term beta-blocker trials and data are available from all trials, other important endpoints, such as sudden and nonsudden deaths and nonfatal reinfarction, have been reported in most trials. Sufficient numbers of such endpoints are available to allow a reasonably reliable overview.

Most long-term beta-blocker trials have classified deaths into "sudden" (presumably due to arrhythmia or cardiac rupture) and "nonsudden" (presumably nonarrhythmic, including a few noncardiovascular deaths), based on the time to death from onset of symptoms. The definition of sudden deaths has not been uniform and includes "instantaneous," "under 1 hr," "within 2 hr of symptoms," and "under 24 hr." Overall, about half of all deaths had been classified as "sudden" under this general classification. Of the data available on 15,800 patients, sudden deaths have been reduced significantly by 32% (3.6% in beta-blocker–treated patients and 5.2% in control patients, 95% confidence interval in reductions of 21–42%, $p < 0.00001$) (Table 5) (1). A trend toward a reduction in nonsudden deaths was also suggested (12% reduction, 95% confidence interval ranging from 24% reduction to 3% excess mortality, p = NS) (Table 5) (1). This analysis of the data according to modes of death requires careful interpretation because of the nonuniform definition of sudden death. These data cannot be accepted as reliably as those on total mortality. However, the reduction in sudden death of about one-third, with 95% confidence limits of about one-fifth to two-fifths, suggests a very large treatment effect. It can only be speculated that a number of mechanisms of benefit, such as anti-ischemic and antiarrhythmic effects and a reduction in cardiac rupture, are operative in producing this decrease in sudden death.

Similarly, data on nonfatal reinfarction have not been reported by all the long-term trials, but a sufficient number did so. The available data on over 20,000 patients indicate that long-term treatment with beta-blockers reduces reinfarction significantly by 27% (5.6% of patients on beta-blockers had reinfarction, compared to 7.5% in control patients, 95% confidence interval of 19–35% reductions, $p < 0.0001$) (Table 5). These results are similar to results of the trials of short-term intravenous beta-blocker therapy. This suggests that anti-ischemic mechanisms that are operative during the acute phase of myocardial infarction and reduce reinfarction short-term are likely to be effective during long-term therapy.

Influence of Ancillary Properties

Intrinsic sympathomimetic activity (ISA) has been associated with some inconsistency in the interpretation of the results of some long-term trials of beta-blockers. In an earlier overview of such trials, it had been noted that beta-blockers without ISA (metoprolol, atenolol, propranolol, sotolol, and timolol) were associated with significant reductions in odds of death by 31% (95% confidence interval ranged from 21% to 39% reductions, $p < 0.0001$) (1) (Table 6). Conversely, although agents with ISA (alprenolol, oxprenolol, pindolol) were associated with reductions in odds of death to some degree, the results were not statistically significant (10% reduction in mortality, 95% confidence interval ranged from 23% reduction to 5% excess mortality, p = NS) (Table 6) (1). Moreover, the difference between the 31% reduction in mortality in agents without ISA and the 10% reduction in those with ISA was statistically significant ($p < 0.01$). This led to speculation that there may be important differences between the two classes of beta-blockers that could somehow influence the protective effect of beta-blockers. However, two later trials showing consistent beneficial effects have subsequently been published (3,31) (Table 6). Overall, the 17% reduction in mortality (95% confidence interval ranging from 4% to 28% reductions) in agents with ISA is statistically significant ($p < 0.02$). The 95% confidence interval overlaps closely those without ISA, suggesting similar protective benefits are conferred by both groups (Table 6). A recent suggestion that these beta-blockers with ISA may confer additional benefits because they appear to cause no or little disturbance in blood cholesterol levels, unlike those without ISA, is an interesting hypothesis that may lead to increased use of these agents in some quarters. To be certain of real benefit, this hypothesis needs further testing.

The finding that beta-blockers with and without ISA similarly confer beneficial effects is consistent with the view that the several other known ancillary properties of beta-blockers do not appear to assert a material influence on the

Table 6   Long-Term Intervention with Beta-Blockers: Influence of ISA on Mortality

Trials	Deaths/patients (n) Active	Control	Odds reduction (%)	95% CI
Beta-blockers without ISA				
13 trials (1)	469/6204	604/5753	-31****	-39% to -21%
Beta-blockers with ISA				
11 earlier trials (1)	358/4248	382/4107	-10*	-23% to +5%
Schwartz (31)	11/485	29/488	-61***	-79% to -26%
APSI (3)	17/298	34/309	-50**	-72% to -11%
Total[a]	386/5021 (7.7%)	445/4904 (9.1%)	-17**	-28% to -4%

[a]Total for beta-blockers with ISA. Note that the 95% confidence interval for beta-blockers with and without ISA overlap considerably. See text for further discussion.
ISA = intrinsic sympathomimetic activity; 95% CI = 95% confidence interval; - = reduction; + = excess mortality.
*p not significant.
**p < 0.02.
***p < 0.01.
****p < 0.0001.

cardioprotective effects of these agents as a class. There is little evidence that the cardioselectivity or membrane-stabilizing properties of an agent have any substantial influence on its effect on mortality (1).

Patient Subgroups—High Risk Versus Low Risk

It is clearly established that beta-blocker therapy is beneficial in patients who have survived acute myocardial infarction. However, it is also obvious that practicing physicians have a great interest in knowing reliably whether specific subgroups of patients would benefit more from treatment than others. Post hoc subgroup analyses have suggested that certain characteristics may be associated with a particular benefit from beta-blockers, but most often these subgroup findings have not been confirmed in the majority of trials (11,32–35), illustrating the important principle that analyses of subgroups that have not been defined a priori and properly powered are unlikely to be reliable and can be misleading.

To overcome this deficit, the Beta-Blocker Pooling Project (BBPP) investigators recently published some data collected from nine long-term secondary prevention trials to determine whether there were subsets of postinfarction patients who might benefit to a greater or lesser extent than the average patient population

(36). Data collection and analysis were conducted in a novel way. Briefly, raw data from all nine trials were pooled in a previously agreed and defined protocol, including definition of subgroups, standardization of data collection, and statistical methods. The primary endpoint was total 1-year mortality. A total of 13,679 patients (6973 on beta-blockers, 6706 on placebo) were included. Overall, 374 patients on beta-blockade and 461 control patients died at 1 year. The difference in mortality was 24% (95% confidence interval of 13–34% reduction) in favor of beta-blocker therapy ($p < 0.0001$). These results are in close agreement with the results of the larger overview discussed earlier.

Patients at "high risk" were those who, prior to their qualifying myocardial infarction, had a history of myocardial infarction, angina pectoris, hypertension, treatment with digitalis, or mechanical or electrical complications, and they had a higher-than-average mortality. In these "high risk" subgroups, there were marked reductions in all causes of mortality in the beta-blocker patients compared to the corresponding controls. The reductions in mortality were greater than the overall reduction from the combined data and the findings were consistent across all trials. Benefits were also gained by "lower risk" subgroups (36). These findings have to be regarded with a degree of caution because of the retrospective nature of the analyses, but the results do indicate that on average, individuals from each subgroup tend to derive some benefit from beta-blocker therapy, with the high-risk patients appearing to derive at least as much, if not greater, benefit. Conversely, there are no particular subgroups in which treatment with beta-blocker is worse than placebo.

A recent trial has been specifically designed to investigate the effect of beta-blocker therapy on a subset of high-risk patients (expected mortality >20% during the first year of myocardial infarction) defined according to a registry maintained by the investigators prior to the trial(3). To be eligible for enrollment, patients had to have at least six "secondary risk factors," including at least one of the following "major risk factors" before index event—history of dyspnea on mild exertion, documented atrial fibrillation, ventricular fibrillation, ventricular tachycardia, overt heart failure, or sinus tachycardia; during index event—reinfarction or angina pectoris before the eighth day. Although there was a statistically significant reduction in mortality by 50% in the beta-blocker group (95% confidence interval ranging from 11% to 72% reduction, $p < 0.05$) (Table 6) after an average 318 days of treatment, the 1-year total mortality at 12% in the control group had been much lower than expected. This trial was stopped following an interim analysis (3). While the stated reason for stopping was that the study population was in fact different (lower projected risk) from that originally planned, the possibility that the magnitude of benefit may be somewhat overestimated because the study was prematurely stopped at a time when there was strong evidence of benefit could not be excluded.

Nevertheless, the data from this study suggesting that patients with high risk following acute myocardial infarction will benefit from beta-blocker therapy are corroborated by similar findings from other studies, such as the BBPP (36), MIAMI (14), and timolol studies (29). These benefits, which may be as large as, if not larger than, the overall effect, translate into prevention of substantially more deaths in absolute numbers when high-risk patients are treated. Such high-risk patients should be treated unless there are specific contraindications. Although it can be argued that patients at low risk of death will derive less benefit, these patients form a substantial majority of postinfarction patients, so a considerable number of deaths will be prevented when absolute numbers are considered. Furthermore, the risk-benefit profile of beta-blockers in these patients is so favorable that it is medically worthwhile to treat them unless there are contraindications.

ADVERSE EFFECTS

Adverse effects of beta-blocker therapy can be divided into two types. First are those which involve a certain degree of discomfort, such as cold extremities, hypotension, fatigue, and central nervous system (CNS) symptoms, which may be ameliorated by dosage adjustment or change to another agent. Second are those other more serious adverse effects, such as heart failure, bradycardia, and conduction disturbances, which may require medication withdrawal, with or without temporary supportive measures. Information on adverse effects has not been uniformly collected and reported in all trials. Further, those studies which reported such adverse effects varied in the definition of even common side effects. For these reasons, information is not as reliable as that on the main endpoints.

The BHAT group has described in detail the adverse effect profile of propranolol (37) (Table 7). The reported data indicate that there are small excesses in adverse effects, particularly those which are relatively minor. These can probably be alleviated by the use of an alternative agent such as a beta$_1$ cardioselective agent to minimize respiratory or peripheral circulatory symptoms or a hydrophilic agent to reduce CNS side effects.

Overall, the incidence of heart failure was slightly, but not significantly, higher in active treatment patients (17.5%) than in controls (16.8%, p = NS) when treatment was started intravenously (1). This small excess was also seen in long-term trials (overall, 5.9% in beta-blocker patients and 5.4% in controls, $p < 0.05$). Data from ISIS-1, the largest of the short-term beta-blocker trials, are not available, but the use of various treatments for heart failure, such as diuretics, nitrates, and digoxin, did not differ in treated and control patients (15). Some trials have reported the incidence of cardiogenic shock. With early treatment, orally or intravenously, the incidence of cardiogenic shock was 3.2% in patients allocated beta-blocker and 3.0% in controls (1). In ISIS-1, 5% of patients on atenolol needed in-hospital use of inotropic agents, compared to 3.4% among controls

Table 7   Side Effects of Prolonged Treatment with Propranolol[a]

	Patients with complaints at any time during the trial (%)		
	Propranolol (*n* = 1916)	Placebo (*n* = 1921)	Difference
Shortness of breath	66.8	65.5	1.3
Bronchospasm	31.3	27.0	4.3
Cold hands, feet	10.0	7.7	2.3
Diarrhea	5.5	3.6	1.9
Tiredness	66.8	62.1	4.7
Reduced sexual activity	43.2	42.0	1.2
Depression	40.7	39.8	0.9
Nightmares	39.7	36.9	2.8
Faintness	28.7	26.6	2.1
Insomnia	21.1	18.8	2.3
Blacking out	9.1	10.3	−1.2
Hallucinations	5.9	4.5	1.4

[a]The average duration of follow-up was about 2 years, at 3-month intervals. Symptoms were recorded at any time during follow-up. Although the occurrence of side effects appears to be more frequent in the propranolol-treated patients, patients on placebo reported similar side effects almost as frequently.

Source: Data from the Beta-blocker Heart Attack Trial (BHAT) (30,37), adapted in present form by Yusuf et al. (1).

(15). This difference was noted mainly during the first day of treatment. Interestingly, there was no difference in mortality in those patients who required inotropic support and received atenolol and those who received placebo. It has been suggested that most episodes of hypotension were reversible and did not have a permanent deleterious effect.

There is a concern that beta-blockers may produce serious atrioventricular conduction disturbances because of the beta-blocking effect on the atrioventricular node and may increase the risk of heart block. However, no clear excess was apparent in an overview of data from the limited number of trials that reported the frequency of heart block (4.3% among patients treated with beta-blockers, 4.2% among controls) (1).

Bradycardia has been regarded as either a beneficial or an adverse effect depending, respectively, on whether symptoms improve or develop as a result of the treatment. In most patients, any excessive bradycardia and hypotension are adequately managed by stopping the beta-blocker without any further active treatment, but when this is necessary, atropine or a beta1-agonist may be required. The data available are too limited to indicate reliably whether an excess of symptomatic hypotension requiring active treatment has occurred (1).

Overall, the development of adverse effects as a result of treatment has to be assessed against the development of heart failure and atrioventricular conduction disturbances due to the disease process itself, both acute and chronic. Also, the information on adverse effects has not been uniformly and systematically collected and reported, and adverse effects have not been uniformly defined. The data therefore should be interpreted cautiously. This should not be interpreted that adverse effects are not to be taken seriously, as they occur, by and large, in patients not likely to have serious contraindications for beta-blocker therapy. It is to be noted also that in some of the trials, up to 50% of patients with acute myocardial infarction had been excluded because of such obvious contraindications to beta-blockade therapy as heart failure, chronic lung disease, high degree of conduction disturbances, hypotention, and bradycardia.

BETA-BLOCKADE AS ADJUNCTIVE THERAPY WITH THROMBOLYTIC TREATMENT

With the clear evidence of benefit from recent randomized trials of thrombolytic therapy (38–42), this treatment has become routine in patients with acute myocardial infarction. On the other hand, the efficacy of beta-blockers following acute myocardial infarction was evaluated before the common use of thrombolytic agents. An important question therefore is whether or not the use of beta-blockers is likely to be useful in conjunction with thrombolytic therapy (43).

One point of view is that the value of these drugs may have been altered substantially by prior thrombolytic therapy, so that all previous information is not relevant. An extreme example of this view is that patients have gained all they are expected to with the use of thrombolytic therapy, that adding a beta-blocker is not likely to confer additional benefits, and that the potential for adverse effects due to the beta-blocker therefore does not justify its use.

Another view is that this is not necessarily the case. While there may be differences in the degree of benefit or harm produced by a beta-blocker when used with or without a thrombolytic agent, it is unlikely that the effects of the beta-blocker are nullified or reversed in the former situation. Ideally, large trials would be needed to reevaluate beta-blocker therapy in conjunction with the thrombolytic agent to resolve this issue. However, this ideal is unlikely to be attainable in view of the clear evidence of benefit demonstrated with both classes of agents. We are then left with three complementary approaches in drawing a reasonable conclusion regarding the use of beta-blockers.

First, large trials testing combination therapies should be evaluated. For example, the Second International Study of Infarct Survival (ISIS-2), employed a 2 × 2 factorial design evaluating the effects of placebo, aspirin, and streptokinase (40). No similar trial has been conducted with a beta-blocker and thrombolytic therapy.

Second, when an agent, such as a beta-blocker, is already known to be of benefit, one can examine whether the effects of thrombolytic therapy are modified in a subset of patients receiving the beta-blocker compared to those not receiving it. In a substudy of the Thrombolysis in Myocardial Infarction Phase II Trial (TIMI-IIB), 1390 patients were randomized to receive beta-blocker or placebo following thrombolytic therapy with tissue plasminogen activator (2). In this trial early intravenous metoprolol was followed by oral treatment. Although this study did not have sufficient power to detect plausible differences in mortality, there were fewer nonfatal reinfarctions and recurrent ischemic episodes in the beta-blocker-treated group compared to the control group during the first 6 days. The fatal plus nonfatal reinfarction rate in the metoprolol group was 18/696 (2.6%) in the metoprolol group and 31/694 (4.5%) in the control group ($p < 0.06$), and the nonfatal reinfarction rates in the two groups were 16/696 (2.4%) and 31/694 (4.5%), respectively, ($p < 0.02$). This result is consistent with trials conducted prior to the widespread use of thrombolytic therapy, which have been reviewed previously and summarized in this chapter.

The third course is to extrapolate from the older data based on whether or not the mechanisms by which beta-blockers are thought to produce benefits have been changed dramatically by the use of thrombolytic therapy. The presumed mechanism of benefit from thrombolytic therapy (coronary recanalization) leaves a number of pathways that could lead to an adverse outcome unaffected or worsened. For example, following thrombolytic therapy, a significant number of patients suffer early death from cardiac rupture, reinfarction, or potentially lethal arrhythmias (44). Additional approaches to reducing oxygen demand, decreasing wall stress, and preventing reperfusion damage may lead to further reduction in mortality and morbidity. Beta-blockers have been shown to reduce cardiac rupture, reinfarction, and arrhythmias, probably by reducing ischemia and myocardial wall stress. Based on the known mechanisms of death and morbidity that are prevented by beta-blockers and the limited amount of data indicating further benefit among patients who have previously received thrombolytic therapy, it appears that the benefits from beta-blockers are likely to accrue whether or not previous thrombolytic therapy is used. Addition of a beta-blocker concomitantly with or soon after the thrombolytic therapy can therefore be expected to reduce mortality and morbidity.

WHO TO TREAT AND WHAT OTHER AGENTS TO USE?

From the trials of beta-blockers, there is no evidence that any subgroup of patients will receive more or less than the average observed benefit. Depending on the baseline risk, the absolute gain (in the number of lives saved, etc.) will be quite different. For example, a larger number of patients at low risk of death, e.g., inferior infarct patients, will have to be treated to save one life than patients at high risk, e.g., those with large anterior infarct. The problem is that, while a decision whether or not to treat has to be made early after the infarction phase, much of the risk stratification cannot be done until after this acute phase. However, the cost of early intervention with beta-blockade is quite modest, so the cost-benefit ratio is highly favorable even if all patients without contraindication are treated (45,46). In one cost analysis, it has been estimated that the cost of saving an additional life by the use of beta-blockers intravenously followed by oral therapy for 7 days is about $1250 and that if the potential savings from reductions or prevention in reinfarctions and cardiac arrests were included, the use of beta-blockers could result in a net saving in costs to the health care system (45). This contrasts markedly with the cost of thrombolytic agents. In a similar cost analysis, the cost of saving an additional life has been estimated to be thousands to tens of thousands of dollars, depending on the patient's baseline risk and the thrombolytic agent used (47).

The mechanisms of action of aspirin and nitrates, which have been shown to be beneficial in acute myocardial infarction, are different from those of beta-blockers and thrombolytic agents. There are no reasons to expect negative interactions among these agents. It is possible that beta-blockers and intravenous nitrates may prevent some cardiac ruptures. The combination of a beta-blocker and a nitrate is well tolerated and may be expected to be complementary, especially in patients with large infarct size and tachycardia. Therefore, it is quite likely that the combination of a thrombolytic agent, a beta-blocker, and a nitrate, in addition to aspirin, will lead to maximum benefit.

While the data clearly support the use of beta-blockers during the early phase of myocardial infarction, there are no data to indicate whether they are of benefit when used beyond the 1- to 2-year average duration of most long-term trials. It has been suggested that perhaps, based on the trial results, treatment need not be continued after the mortality curves stop diverging. The interpretation is that no further gains can be expected with further therapy. However, it has been suggested that this interpretation may not be correct. For example, after the mortality curves diverge initially, the treated groups will contain some high-risk patients whose early deaths have been prevented. If the curves continue to remain parallel, this might indicate that there is some continuing protection with treatment. Therefore, in the absence of a large clinical trial and based on the mechanisms of benefit in secondary prevention, one reasonable approach is to continue with the beta-blocker therapy unless there are contraindications.

REFERENCES

1. Yusuf S, Peto R, Lewis J, Sleight P. Beta-blockade during and after myocardial infarction: An overview of the randomized trials. Prog Cardiovasc Dis 1985; 17:335-71.

2. The TIMI Study Group. Comparison of invasive and conservative strategies after treatment with intravenous tissue plasminogen activator in acute myocardial infarction: results of the thrombolysis in myocardial infarction (TIMI) phase II trial. N Engl J Med 1989; 320:618-27.

3. Boissel JP, Leizorovicz A, Picolet H, Peyrieux JC for the APSI Investigators. Secondary prevention after high-risk acute myocardial infarction with low-dose acebutolol. Am J Cardiol 1990; 66:251-60.

4. Early Breast Cancer Trialists' Collaborative Group. Effects of adjuvant tamoxifen and of cytotoxic therapy on mortality in early breast cancer: an overview of 61 randomized trials among 28,896 women. N Engl J Med 1988; 319:1681-92.

5. Langley JN. On the reaction of cells and of nerve endings to certain poisons: chiefly as regards the reaction of striated muscles to nicotine and to curare. J Physiol (Lond) 1905; 33:374-413.

6. Ahlquist RP. A study of the adrenotropic receptors. Am J Physiol 1948; 153:586-99.

7. Lands AM, Arnold A, McAuliff JP, et al. Differentiation of receptor systems activated by sympathomimetic amines. Nature 1967; 214:597-8.

8. Conolly ME, Kersting F, Dollery CT. The clinical pharmacology of beta-adrenoceptor-blocking drugs. Prog Cardiovasc Dis 1976; 19:203-34.

9. Pitt B, Craven P. Effect of propranolol on regional myocardial blood flow in acute ischemia. Cardiovasc Res 1970; 4:176-9.

10. Opie LH, Thomas M. Propranolol and experimental myocardial infarction: substrate effects. Postgrad Med J 1976; 52(Suppl 4):124-32.

11. Anderson MP, Bechsgaard P, Frederiksen J, et al. Effect of alprenolol on morality among patients with definite or suspected acute myocardial infarction: preliminary results. Lancet 1979; 2:865-8.

12. Salathia KS, Barber JM, McIlmoyle EL, et al. Very early intervention with metoprolol in suspected acute myocardial infarction. Eur Heart J 1985; 6:190-8.

13. Hjalmarson A, Elmfeldt D, Herlitz J, et al. Effect on mortality of metoprolol in acute myocardial infarction: a double-blind randomized trial. Lancet 1981; 2:823-7.

14. The MIAMI Trial Research Group. Metoprolol in Acute Myocardial Infarction (MIAMI). A randomized placebo-controlled international trial. Eur Heart J 1985; 6: 199-226.

15. ISIS-1 (First International Study of Infarct Survival) Collaborative Group. A randomized trial of intravenous atenolol among 16,027 cases of suspected myocardial infarction. Lancet 1986; 2:57-66.

16. Kan MI, Hamilton JT, Manning GW. Protective effect of beta-adrenoceptor blockade in experimental coronary occlusion in conscious dogs. Am J Cardiol 1972; 30:832-7.

17. Ryden L, Arniego R, Arnman KI, et al. A double-blind trial of metoprolol in acute myocardial infarction: effects on ventricular tachycardia. N Engl J Med 1983; 308: 614-8.

18. Yusuf S, Sleight P, Rossi PRF, et al. Reduction in infarct size, arrhythmias, chest pain, and morbidity by early intravenous beta-blockade in suspected acute myocardial infarction. Circulation 1983; 67(Suppl I):32-41.

19. Norris RM, Barnaby P, Brown MA, Geary G, Clarke ED, Logan RL, Sharpe DN. Pre-

vention of ventricular fibrillation during acute myocardial infarction by intravenous propranolol. Lancet 1984; 2:883-6.

20.   ISIS-1 (First International Study of Infarct Survival) Collaborative Group. Possible mechanisms for the early mortality reduction produced by beta-blockade started early in acute myocardial infarction. Lancet 1988; 1:921-3.

21.   Held PH, Teo KK, Yusuf S. Effects of beta-blockers, calcium channel blockers, and nitrates in acute myocardial infarction and unstable angina pectoris. In: Topol EJ, ed. Textbook of interventional cardiology. Philadelphia: Saunders, 1990:49-65.

22.   Richterova A, Herlitz J, Holmberg S, et al. Goteborg Metoprolol Trial: effects on chest pain. Am J Cardiol 1984; 53:32D-36D.

23.   Ramsdale DR, Faragher EB, Bennett DH, et al. Ischemic pain relief in patients with acute myocardial infarction by intravenous atenolol. Am Heart J 1982; 103:459-67.

24.   International Collaborative Study Group. Reduction of infarct size with the early use of timolol in acute myocardial infarction. N Engl J Med 1984; 310:9-15.

25.   Norris RM, Sammel NL, Clarke E, Smith WM. Protective effect of propranolol in threatened myocardial infarction. Lancet 1978; 2:907-9.

26.   Herlitz J, Emanuelsson H, Swedberg K, Vedin A, Waldenstrom A, Waldenstrom J, Hjalmarson A. Goteborg Metoprolol Trial. Enzyme-estimated infarct size. Am J Cardiol 1984; 53:15D-21D.

27.   Teo K, Yusuf S, Furberg C. Effect of antiarrhythmic drug therapy on mortality following myocardial infarction. Circulation 1990; 82:111-197 (abstract).

28.   Baber NS, Evans DW, Howitt G, et al. Multicentre post-infarction trial of propranolol in 49 hospitals in the United Kingdom, Italy and Yugoslavia. Br Heart J 1980; 44: 96-100.

29.   Norweigian Multicenter Study Group. Timolol-induced reduction in mortality and reinfarction in patients surviving acute myocardial infarction. N Engl J Med 1981; 304:801-7.

30.   Beta-Blocker Heart attack Trial Research Group. A randomized trial of propranolol in patients with acute myocardial infarction. I. Mortality results. JAMA 1982; 247: 1707-14.

31.   Schwartz PJ, Motolese M, Pollavini G, Malliani A, Bartorelli C, Zanchetti A, and the Sudden Death Italian Prevention Group. Surgical and pharmacological antiadrenergic interventions in the prevention of sudden death after a first myocardial infarction. Circulation 1985; 72(Suppl III):III-358 (abstract).

32.   Multicentre International Study Group. Improvement in prognosis of myocardial infarction by long-term beta-adrenoceptor blockade using practolol. Br Med J 1975; 3:735-40.

33.   Hawkins CM, Richardson DW, Vokonas PS, for the BHAT Research Group. Effects of propranolol in reducing mortality in older myocardial infarction patients. The beta-blocker heart attack trial experience. Circulation 1983; 67(Suppl I):94-7.

34.   Gunderson T for the Norwegian Multicentre Study Group. Influence of heart size on mortality and reinfarction in patients treated with timolol after myocardial infarction. Br Heart J 1985; 50:135-9.

35.   Furberg CD, Byington RP for the BHAT Research Group. What do subgroup analyses

reveal about differential responses to beta-blocker therapy? The beta-blocker heart attack trial experience. Circulation 1983; 67(Suppl I):98-101.

36. The Beta-Blocker Pooling Project Research Group. The Beta-Blocker Pooling Project (BBPP): subgroup findings from randomized trials in postinfarction patients. Eur Heart J 1988; 9:8-16.

37. Beta-Blocker Heart Attack Trial Research Group. A randomized trial of propranolol in patients with acute myocardial infarction. II. Morbidity results. JAMA 1983; 250: 2814-9.

38. Yusuf S, Wittes J, Friedman L. Overview of results of randomized clinical trials in heart disease. JAMA 1988; 260:2088-93.

39. Gruppo Italiano per lo Studio della Streptochinasi nell'Infarto Miocardico (GISSI). Effectiveness of intravenous thrombolytic treatment in acute myocardial infarction. Lancet 1986; 1:397-402.

40. ISIS-2 (Second International Study of Infarct Survival) Collaborative Group. Randomized trial of intravenous streptokinase, oral aspirin, both or neither among 17,187 cases of suspected acute myocardial infarction. Lancet 1988; 2:349-60.

41. Gruppo Italiano per lo Studio della Sopravvivenza nell'Infarto Miocardico. GISSI-2: a factorial randomized trial of alteplase versus streptokinase and heparin versus no heparin among 12,490 patients with acute myocardial infarction. Lancet 1990; 336: 65-71.

42. Held PH, Teo KK, Yusuf S. Effects of tissue-type plasminogen activator and anisoylated plasminogen streptokinase activator complex on mortality in acute myocardial infarction. Circulation 1990; 82:1668-74.

43. Teo KK, Yusuf S. Selecting adjunctive treatments for use with thrombolysis in acute myocardial infarction. Primary Cardiol 1990; 16:27-40.

44. Yusuf S, Sleight P, Held P, McMahon S. Routine medical management of acute myocardial infarction: lessons from overviews of recent randomized controlled trials. Circulation 1990; 82(Suppl II):117-34.

45. Teo KK, Held P, Yusuf S. Economic advantage of using aspirin, intravenous nitrates and beta-blockers in myocardial infarction. Clin Invest Med 1990; 13:C65 (abstract).

46. Goldman L, Sia STB, Cook EF, Rutherford JD, Weinstein MD. Cost and effectiveness of routine therapy with long-term beta-adrenergic antagonists after acute myocardial infarction. N Engl J Med 1988; 319:152-7.

47. Teo KK, Held P, Yusuf S. Comparative cost effectiveness of thrombolytic therapy in myocardial infarction. Clin Invest Med 1990; 13:C65 (abstract).

7

Calcium Channel Blockers in the Treatment of Acute Myocardial Infarction

Gabriel B. Habib
VA Medical Center and Baylor College of Medicine, Houston, Texas

Robert Roberts
Baylor College of Medicine and Methodist Hospital, Houston, Texas

INTRODUCTION

In the last decade, calcium antagonists have gained widespread acceptance in the management of cardiovascular disease. Their efficacy in the treatment of hypertension and angina pectoris is well established and their role in patients recovering from myocardial infarction has gradually evolved but remains the subject of some investigation. In this chapter, we will review the role of calcium antagonists as adjunctive therapy in patients recovering from myocardial infarction.

CLINICAL PHARMACOLOGY OF CALCIUM ANTAGONISTS

The basic action of calcium antagonists, both in the myocardium and in vascular smooth muscle, is inhibition of the slow inward calcium current carried by the voltage-dependent, receptor-operated channels (1–3). In the myocardium, this inhibition may reduce calcium release from the sarcoplasmic reticulum and have a negative inotropic action. In vascular smooth muscle, inhibition of the receptor-operated channels causes vasodilatation. Fortunately, cardiac muscle is much less sensitive than vascular smooth muscle to calcium antagonists.

   Calcium antagonists are derived from three distinct classes of compounds, namely the dihydropyridines (nifedipine), the diphenylalamines (verapamil), and the benzothiazepines (diltiazem), which have in common an affinity for the calcium channel protein. However, although all three classes of compounds are characterized by their affinity for the calcium channel protein, they have quite distinct binding sites on the protein, and in fact, diltiazem was recently shown to increase the affinity of the protein for nifedipine as opposed to being the expected competitive antagonist. Many other properties are also different. Diltiazem and verapamil reduce the heart rate, whereas nifedipine increases it. The systemic vasodilator effect of nifedipine is more pronounced in normotensive individuals than that of diltiazem or verapamil, although all three are quite effective in patients with hypertension. It is recommended that they not be grouped together but be considered separate drugs.

Calcium antagonists decrease the spontaneous discharge rate of isolated sinoatrial nodal tissue and decrease atrioventricular conduction. Recently, diltiazem, but not nicardipine, was found to abolish norepinephrine release at the terminal sympathetic neuron (4). This may explain the widely different pharmacological effects of various calcium antagonists in intact animals and in humans. Activation of the sympathetic nervous system in response to a fall in blood pressure induced by nifedipine is unopposed. However, the fall in blood pressure induced by diltiazem is not associated with increased sympathetic tone due to inhibition of norepinephrine release by diltiazem. The net result is an increase in circulating catecholamines and heart rate in patients treated with dihydropyri-dines (nifedipine) (5) and a decrease in heart rate with verapamil or diltiazem. The increased sympathetic tone and resultant increase in heart rate associated with the dihydropyridines may have potentially detrimental effects in patients recovering from myocardial infarction, as will be discussed later.

Calcium antagonists have been developed as therapeutic agents primarily for their vasodilator action. Calcium antagonists induce vasodilatation in the small sphincter arterioles and inhibit vasomotor tone in larger coronary vessels. In contrast to nitroglycerin, which has essentially no effect on regulatory arterioles, calcium antagonists increase total coronary flow 50–100% over that of normal levels and in areas of myocardial ischemia increase subendocardial flow (6,7). This is in marked contrast to nitroglycerin, which acts primarily on the larger coronary vessels. Nitroglycerin does not increase total coronary flow under normal resting conditions or during myocardial ischemia, but redistributes flow to the subendocardial region of the ischemic area (8). Thus, calcium antagonists are less likely than nitrates to cause coronary steal, a phenomenon mediated by an increase in blood flow to normal myocardial tissue with a concomitant reduction in blood flow to ischemic areas. The beneficial effect of calcium antagonists on myocardial ischemia relates to their improved balance between myocardial oxygen demand and supply, which, in the case of the rate-lowering calcium antagonists, is a combination of increased supply and decreased demand. In addition to these functions, calcium antagonists may be cardioprotective by enhancing cell viability, possibly through the inhibition of calcium influx. Increased intracellular calcium clearly accompanies cell death, but the causal relationship between intracellular calcium overload and cell death has not been demonstrated conclusively. Experimental studies have shown calcium antagonists to limit infarct size and to be cardioprotective, particularly in the case of diltiazem and to a lesser extent for verapamil and nifedipine (7,9). Most recently, in one clinical study with a small sample size, diltiazem was shown to limit infarct size in patients with acute myocardial infarction, infarct size being estimated from thallium-201 scans (10). This study alone is not adequate to confirm or recommend that diltiazem be used for limitation of infarct size. In the experimental studies with diltiazem as with other calcium antagonists, cardioprotective effects were demonstrated only if the drug was given prophylactically. Another possible mechanism to be concerned with in humans for diltiazem, verapamil, and nifedipine is their inhibition of platelet aggregation. The inhibitory effect of diltiazem on platelet aggregation has been shown in both in vitro and in vivo studies and is additive with the effect of low-dose aspirin (11-14). The concentration of diltiazem required for platelet inhibition is very high, and whether diltiazem exerts a significant antiplatelet effect with clinical doses remains controversial. Inhibition of platelet aggregation by calcium antagonists has a rational basis since calcium is the common pathway whereby platelets are activated.

Recently, calcium antagonists have been shown in experimentally induced atherosclerosis in rabbits and primates to inhibit development of atherosclerosis. This has now been demonstrated in several experimental studies (15-17) and was recently confirmed in humans in two large clinical trials with nifedipine (18) and nicardipine (19). In both studies, there was an inhibition of the development of new coronary atherosclerotic lesions assessed by quantitative coronary angiography but no effect on existing lesions. Surprisingly, more cardiac deaths occurred in patients treated with nifedipine in one clinical trial (18) and more myocardial infarctions occurred in patients treated with nucardipine in the second trial (19). These findings have significant implications for the treatment of ischemic heart disease, particularly in patients with angina and hypertension. While the mechanism of this protection from atherosclerosis is still unknown, it is not due to lipid-lowering effect but may instead be mediated by the antioxidant action of calcium antagonists (20).

CALCIUM ANTAGONISTS AND THEIR ROLE IN ACUTE MYOCARDIAL INFARCTION

Beta-blockers decrease the incidence of myocardial ischemia and sudden cardiac death, presumably by decreasing myocardial oxygen demand and risk for ventricular fibrillation. Beta-blockers have been effective in the prevention of recurrent ischemia, reinfarction, and death in patients recovering from myocardial infarction. Since beta-blockers decrease myocardial oxygen demand primarily by reducing heart rate, it was thought that calcium antagonists, by increasing coronary blood flow, would complement the effect of beta-blockers and represent a major addition to the therapeutic armamentarium in the management of myocardial infarction and recurrent ischemia. It was also hoped that finally there would be an agent that would increase coronary flow rather than simply decrease myocardial oxygen demand. The experimental data referred to earlier, together with the benefit demonstrated in angina and transient myocardial ischemia, suggested that calcium antagonists might play a major role in the therapy of myocardial infarction. Subsequently, multiple studies were performed to assess the role of calcium antagonists in patients with acute myocardial infarction. The major endpoints were infarct size, recurrent ischemia, reinfarction, and death. Since there appear to be significant differences among the three major classes of calcium antagonists, each will be discussed separately, beginning with nifedipine.

CLINICAL TRIALS WITH NIFEDIPINE

There have been 10 randomized, prospective, double-blind, placebo-controlled clinical trials assessing the effect of nifedipine on infarct size, left ventricular function, reinfarction, or survival in patients with acute myocardial infarction or unstable angina. Salient features of these 10 studies, which enrolled 9866 patients, are compared in Table 1. Three large multicenter trials (21–23) were designed to evaluate the effect of nifedipine as secondary preventive therapy for survivors of acute Q-wave myocardial infarction. Mortality was the primary endpoint of these three trials. A total of 8140 patients were randomized and followed for 1–10 months. Combined results of these three trials showed mortality was increased in nifedipine-treated patients by 11%. Two of these trials were prematurely terminated owing to inconclusive outcome or excessive deaths in the nifedipine-treated group. Five other trials (24–28) were designed specifically to evaluate the effect of nifedipine on limitation of infarct size as estimated by cumulative plasma MB creatine kinase (CK) release. A total of 1079 patients were randomized, and the results showed infarct size increased by 1–32%. Two other clinical trials (29,30) were designed to evaluate the effect of nifedipine on prevention of recurrent ischemia, reinfarction, or left ventricular function. Neither of these trials showed any benefit with nifedipine therapy. These 10 clinical trials of nifedipine therapy in patients with acute myocardial infarction or unstable angina will be reviewed next.

Table 1   Endpoints of Nifedipine Clinical Trials

Study	# Randomized pts (sample size)	Primary endpoint	Time from onset (hr)	Daily nifedipine dose (mg)
NAMIS (1984)	171	Progression	4.6	120
Norwegian (1985)	227	Infarct size (MB CK)	5.5	50/40
TRENT (1986)	4491	1 mo mortality	<8 (68%)	40
HINT (1986)	515	Recurrent ischemia or reinfarction (48 hr)		60
SPRINT-I (1986)	2276	10 mo mortality, reinfarction	7–21 days	30
Irish (Dublin) (1986)	98	Infarct size (MB CK)	3.3	40
SPRINT-II (1988)	1373	6 mo mortality, reinfarction	<3 (75%)	60
Belfast (1988)	434	Infarct size (MB CK) and hospital mortality	1.85	60
Johns Hopkins (1988)	132	LVEF, IS (TI^{210})	8	120
Erbel (1988)	149	Infarct size (MB CK)	2.7	60
Total	9866			

IS = infarct size.

Trial of Early Nifedipine in Acute Myocardial Infarction: TRENT

TRENT, a double-blind, placebo-controlled trial (21), was designed to assess the effect of nifedipine (10 mg four times daily for 4 weeks) on mortality at 1 month in patients with suspected myocardial infarction. Among 4491 patients enrolled, acute myocardial infarction was confirmed in 75% regardless of treatment allocation. In 4801 excluded patients, 1-month mortality was 18.2%, including a 26.8% mortality rate in those with confirmed myocardial infarction. In the nifedipine and placebo groups, 1-month mortality rates were 6.7% and 6.8%, respectively. Among enrolled patients with confirmed myocardial infarction, 1-month mortality rates were similar in the nifedipine and placebo groups. TRENT was prematurely terminated because benefit from nifedipine could not be demonstrated.

The Secondary Prevention Reinfarction Israeli Nifedipine Trial: SPRINT-I

SPRINT-I, a double-blind, placebo-controlled trial (22), was conducted in 14 Israeli hospitals. It was designed to determine whether chronic administration of nifedipine, 10 mg three times daily, starting 7–21 days after acute myocardial infarction, results in a reduction in 1-year mortality or nonfatal reinfarction. Patients surviving a recent Q-wave myocardial infarction were randomized to nifedipine or placebo and followed up for 12 months. Mortality rates and incidence of nonfatal reinfarction in patients treated with nifedipine were the same as in patients receiving placebo. Subgroups analysis revealed no difference in mortality or reinfarction between nifedipine- and placebo-treated patients in any prospectively defined subgroups. The study was terminated on the basis of no difference in clinical outcome, possibly because of too low a dose of nifedipine.

The Secondary Prevention Reinfarction Israeli Nifedipine Trial: SPRINT-II

SPRINT-II (23) was designed to determine whether nifedipine titrated up to 60 mg daily decreased mortality and nonfatal reinfarction in high-risk survivors of acute myocardial infarction, between the ages of 50 and 79 years. High-risk indicators were anterior infarction, recurrent infarction, history of angina or hypertension, and maximal serum LDH level at least three times normal. Of 2050 eligible patients with suspected myocardial infarction with a systolic blood pressure > 90 mmHg, 1373 patients were enrolled and followed up for 6 months. Nifedipine was administered within 3 hr of hospital admission in 75% of all patients and within 3–48 hr in the remainder. Among the 828 final participants, there was no significant difference in 6-month mortality (9.3% versus 9.3%) or nonfatal reinfarction (5% versus 3.5%) in patients treated with nifedipine and placebo, respectively. However, when data from all randomized patients were analyzed, an excess mortality was noted in the nifedipine-treated patients compared to the placebo group (15.8% versus 12.6%). This excess mortality was primarily due to a higher mortality in the first 6 days of treatment with nifedipine (7% versus 4.2%). This increased mortality occurred primarily in patients with systolic blood pressure ≤ 100 mmHg, suggesting that the unfavorable effect of nifedipine may be due to its hypotensive effect. Accordingly, SPRINT-II was prematurely terminated.

Nifedipine Therapy for Threatened and Acute Myocardial Infarction: NAMIS

NAMIS was a multicenter, double-blind, placebo-controlled study (24) designed to assess the effect of early administration of nifedipine (20 mg every 4 hr for 14 days) on progression of threatened myocardial infarction and on infarct size. Patients were eligible for participation if they had chest pain longer than 45 min without Q waves within 6 hr of randomization. A total of 171 of 243 eligible patients were enrolled and received nifedipine (89 patients) or placebo (92 patients) for 14 days. Mean time from onset of symptoms to treatment with nifedipine was 4.6 hr. Among 171 enrolled patients, 105 had threatened myocardial infarction and 66 had acute myocardial infarction at the time of randomization.

Progression to acute myocardial infarction was documented in 75% of 105 patients with threatened myocardial infarction, regardless of whether the patients received placebo or nifedipine. Furthermore, enzymatic estimates of infarct size were similar among nifedipine- and placebo-treated patients with threatened myocardial infarction who progressed to acute myocardial infarction and in patients with acute myocardial infarction at randomization. The 2-week mortality, a secondary endpoint, was significantly higher for nifedipine-treated patients (7.9% versus 0%). However, the 6-month mortality did not differ significantly (10.1% versus 8.5%). Thus, nifedipine failed to prevent acute myocardial infarction or to limit the extent of myocardial necrosis even when given prophylactically in patients with threatened myocardial infarction. The lack of effect of nifedipine on infarct size was ascribed to the increase in heart rate.

The Norwegian Nifedipine Multicenter Trial

In the Norwegian Nifedipine Trial (25), 227 patients with suspected myocardial infarction were randomized within 12 hr of onset of symptoms to nifedipine (112 patients) or placebo (115 patients). In contrast to NAMIS, the Norwegian Nifedipine Trial involved a lower dose of nifedipine (10 mg five times daily for 2 days followed by 10 mg four times daily for 6 weeks), and the mean delay from onset of symptoms to treatment was 5.5 hr.

A total of 885 patients with suspected Q-wave myocardial infarction were screened. Of 623 eligible patients, 157 were enrolled and acute myocardial infarction was confirmed in 74 patients on nifedipine and in 83 patients on placebo. Thus, progression to acute myocardial infarction was documented in 66% and 72% of nifedipine- and placebo-treated patients, respectively. Infarct size, the primary endpoint, was similar in nifedipine- and placebo-treated patients. Among 47 patients treated within 3 hr of onset of symptoms, there was a 33% increase in infarct size in nifedipine-treated patients compared with placebo.

The Irish Studies

Two double-blind, placebo-controlled, single-center trials, the Belfast (26) and Dublin (27) studies, addressed the issue of myocardial salvage with very early administration of sublingual nifedipine in patients with suspected myocardial infarction (Table 1). Both trials succeeded in initiating nifedipine within 6 hr of onset of myocardial infarction, with most patients receiving treatment within 2–3 hr. Infarct size estimated from plasma MB CK was the primary endpoint in both trials.

In the Belfast study (26), 434 patients with suspected myocardial infarction were randomized to receive nifedipine (217) or placebo (217). An initial dose of 10 mg of nifedipine was given sublingually at a median time of 111 min after onset of chest pain. Enzymatic estimates of infarct size and peak plasma MB CK activity were not significantly different in the nifedipine and placebo groups. Time from onset of chest pain to peak plasma MB CK activity was also similar in the nifedipine and placebo groups.

Clinical outcome variables, namely, frequency of ventricular fibrillation during the initial 48 hr, pulmonary edema, reinfarction, cardiogenic shock, and mortality during hospitalization, were similar in the nifedipine and placebo groups. In summary, very early administration of sublingual nifedipine (median delay to treatment of 111 min) did not limit infarct size or decrease complications of myocardial infarction.

A similarly designed clinical trial was performed in Dublin (27). In 98 randomized patients the mean time from onset of chest pain to treatment was 3.3 hr in both nifedipine and placebo groups. Infarct size estimated by plasma MB CK activity in 78% of patients with confirmed myocardial infarction was similar in nifedipine and placebo groups. The observed 8.4% increase in infarct size was not statistically significant; neither was the slightly higher mortality in the patients receiving nifedipine.

German Trial

The unique feature of this study published by Erbel et al. in 1988 (28) is the use of sublingual and intracoronary nifedipine in the very early phase of myocardial infarction as adjunctive therapy to streptokinase. A total of 149 patients with acute myocardial infarction were randomized in this double-blind, placebo-controlled study to receive sublingual and intracoronary nifedipine during and after reperfusion with streptokinase (74 patients) or placebo (75 patients). All patients received intravenous and intracoronary streptokinase. Percutaneous transluminal coronary angioplasty was performed in 55% of patients treated with nifedipine and in 60% of the placebo group. Mean delay from onset of symptoms to treatment with sublingual nifedipine and intravenous streptokinase was 2.7 hr. Reperfusion was successfully achieved with streptokinase and coronary angioplasty in 61 of 74 nifedipine-treated patients (82%) and 71 of 75 placebo patients (95%). Neither infarct size measured by MB CK release nor global or regional left ventricular function measured by gated cardiac blood pool scanning showed any evidence of myocardial salvage in patients treated with nifedipine. Moreover, mortality rates were slightly, but not significantly, higher in nifedipine-treated patients (13% versus 8%) and the reocclusion rate was the same in nifedipine and placebo-treated patients. These results suggest that nifedipine treatment following reperfusion does not limit infarct size or reduce mortality.

The Holland Interuniversity Nifedipine/Metoprolol Trial: HINT

This was a prospective, multicenter, double-blind, placebo-controlled trial (29) designed to evaluate the effect of nifedipine, metoprolol, or both on recurrent myocardial infarction and ischemia in patients with unstable angina pectoris. Among 537 randomized patients, 177 patients were pretreated with a beta-blocker whereas 338 others were not. The overall incidence of both myocardial infarction and recurrent ischemia was lowest in metoprolol-treated patients (28%) and highest in nifedipine-treated patients (47%). In patients pretreated with a beta-blocker, the incidence of recurrent ischemia and infarction was lower in the nifedipine-treated patients compared with the placebo group (30% versus 51%). However, in the majority of patients (338 patients) not previously treated with a beta-blocker, nifedipine monotherapy was associated with a higher incidence of recurrent ischemia and infarction (47%), compared with metoprolol-treated patients (28%) and the placebo group (37%). Thus, in patients with unstable angina, the combination of nifedipine and metoprolol provided no advantage over metoprolol alone, whereas nifedipine monotherapy was clearly detrimental. The study also suggested that nifedipine, if used in patients with unstable angina, should be combined with a beta-blocker. HINT was prematurely terminated because of the worse outcome of patients treated with nifedipine alone.

The Johns Hopkins Study

This was a double-blind, randomized, placebo-controlled, single-center trial (30) designed to assess the effect of nifedipine (40–120 mg daily for 6 weeks) on left ventricular function and infarct size in patients with low-risk acute myocardial infarction of less than 12 hr duration. Low-risk acute myocardial infarction was defined by an initial left ventricular ejection fraction greater than 35% and Killip class I or II. Treatment was started about 8 hr after onset of symptoms and continued for 6 weeks. Global and regional left ventricular systolic function was assessed by gated blood pool scanning obtained before and 10 days after initiation of therapy with nifedipine (64 patients) or placebo (68 patients). Infarct size was estimated by quantitative thallium-201 perfusion scintigraphy.

Global left ventricular ejection fraction, both before and 10 days after treatment, was similar in the nifedipine (53% and 54%) and placebo groups (55% and 52%), respectively. Pretreatment thallium defect scores were also similar in the nifedipine and placebo groups. Thus, nifedipine does not decrease infarct size or improve left ventricular function in patients with low-risk myocardial infarction.

The Eisenberg Trial

This small trial (31) was specifically designed to evaluate the effect of nifedipine on recurrent chest pain and reinfarction over a 13-day follow-up period in 50 patients with non-Q-wave myocardial infarction randomly allocated to nifedipine, 20-30 mg every 6 hr or placebo. Recurrent chest pain, the primary endpoint, occurred in 52% of patients treated with nifedipine and 48% of the placebo patients. There was no difference in the frequency of chest pain or reinfarction between the two groups.

CLINICAL TRIALS WITH VERAPAMIL

Compared with the extensive experience with nifedipine, few clinical trials have been performed to assess the safety and efficacy of verapamil in patients with acute myocardial infarction. To date, five clinical trials involving a total of 3341 patients have been conducted in Denmark, Germany, and England. Unfortunately, three of these trials were either open-label or single-blind. The only two double-blind, prospective, randomized, placebo-controlled trials were published by the Danish Study Group on Verapamil in Myocardial Infarction (DAVIT-I and DAVIT-II).

Hansen's Verapamil in Acute Myocardial Infarction Study

This trial (32) was an open-label pilot study of the safety and efficacy of verapamil, 0.1 mg/kg intravenously followed by 360 mg orally per day, in 61 patients with acute myocardial infarction. The duration of follow-up was 6 months. Patients in the verapamil group had a three- to fourfold greater incidence of sino-atrial block and second- or third-degree atrioventricular block. The incidence of infarction and death was similar in verapamil- and placebo-treated patients; however, the study was flawed by the high dropout rate in the verapamil group.

The Danish Study Group on Verapamil in Myocardial Infarction: DAVIT-I

This study (33) was a double-blind, randomized, placebo-controlled multicenter trial in which patients randomized to the verapamil group received 0.1 mg/kg verapamil intravenously followed by 360 mg per day orally and were followed for 6 months (Table 2). A total of 1436 patients were enrolled, with 717 patients in the verapamil group and 719 patients in the placebo group. Unfortunately, 303 patients in the verapamil group and 246 patients in the placebo group were withdrawn from the study before the 6-month period was completed. Cardiac failure developed in 187 verapamil-treated patients and in 142 placebo patients, whereas

Table 2   Verapamil in Myocardial Infarction Trials: Study Design

	Davit-I	Davit-II
Sample size	3498	1775
Treatment	Verapamil, 0.1 mg/kg IV, then 120 mg p.o. t.i.d.	Verapamil 120 mg p.o. t.i.d.
Delay to treatment	0.5–12 hr (median 4 hr)	7–15 days (mean 9 days)
Primary endpoints	Mortality and reinfarction	Mortality First major event[a]
Duration of follow-up	6 months	18 months

[a]First major event was defined as death or reinfarction.

second- or third-degree atrioventricular block developed in 115 verapamil-treated patients versus 50 placebo patients. Interestingly, intermittent atrial fibrillation was significantly reduced in the verapamil-treated group. At 2- and 6-month follow-up, the prevalence of cardiac failure was similar in both groups. The mortality rates in the verapamil- and placebo-treated groups were similar during the 6-month follow-up period (12.8% versus 13.9%), as was the reinfarction rate (7% versus 8.3%) (Table 3). A major drawback was the high withdrawal rate (42%) in the verapamil-treated patients.

The Thuesen Trial

In 1983, Thuesen et al. (34) reported the results of a double-blind, placebo-controlled trial involving 54 verapamil-treated and 46 placebo-treated patients with acute myocardial infarction. Verapamil was given intravenously (0.1 mg/kg) and then orally (360 mg/day). The mean time to treatment was 12 hr in verapamil-treated patients and in the placebo group. There was also no difference in cumulated CK release. However, failure of verapamil to limit infarct size in this study may be due to inappropriate delay in initiating treatment with verapamil.

The Bussmann Trial

In 1984, Bussman et al. (35) reported the results of a prospective, nonblinded clinical study of intravenous verapamil, 5–10 mg/hr for 48 hr, in 54 patients with acute myocardial infarction. Infarct size estimated by plasma MB CK activity was smaller in the verapamil-treated patients, but since this was not a placebo-controlled trial, the results were not persuasive.

Table 3   Verapamil in Myocardial Infarction Trials

	DAVIT-I			DAVIT-II		
	Verapamil	Placebo	p	Verapamil	Placebo	p
Mortality[a] all randomized patients	12.8	13.9	NS	11.1	13.8	NS
Reinfarction[a] all randomized patients	7	8.3	NS	10.4	14.4	0.04
Mortality, no heart failure	N/A			7.7	11.8	0.02
Mortality, heart failure[b]	N/A			17.9	17.5	NS
First major event,[c] no heart failure	N/A			14.6	19.7	0.01
First major event,[c] heart failure	N/A			24.9	24.9	NS

[a]All values are expressed as mean (%).
[b]Heart failure in DAVIT-II trial was defined as heart failure not stabilizing while receiving furosemide ≥ 160 mg/day.
[c]First major event in DAVIT-II trial was defined as death or reinfarction during follow-up after the index infarction.

The Danish Study Group on Verapamil in Myocardial Infarction: DAVIT-II

This double-blind, placebo-controlled multicenter clinical trial (36) was designed to evaluate the effect of verapamil, 360 mg/day, administered 7–15 days after an acute myocardial infarction on mortality and reinfarction over 18 months (Table 2). A total of 1775 patients with acute myocardial infarction were randomized to oral verapamil (120 mg t.i.d.) or placebo. Baseline clinical characteristics were similar in both groups. Mean time from chest pain to treatment was 9 days. Treatment was stopped permanently in 486 verapamil-treated patients and in 516 placebo patients. The most common reasons for discontinuation of treatment were: angina pectoris, death, second- or third-degree atrioventricular block, unwillingness to continue, and heart failure. Thus, 486 (55.4%) and 516 (57.5%) patients were alive and on treatment at the end of the study period in the verapamil and placebo groups, respectively. There was a statistically insignificant reduction in total mortality (11.1% versus 13.8%), but a statistically significant reduction in the combined endpoint of death and nonfatal reinfarction (18% versus 21.6%) in verapamil-treated patients compared with the placebo group (Table 3). Reinfarction rate was also reduced significantly from 13.2% to 11%. In patients with heart failure, mortality and reinfarction rates were similar in the verapamil and placebo groups. However, in patients without heart failure, mortality was significantly reduced from 11.8% to 7.7%, cardiac events (death and nonfatal reinfarction) from 19.7% to 14.6%, and reinfarction alone from 12.7% to 9.4%.

CLINICAL TRIALS WITH DILTIAZEM

There are only three clinical studies assessing the effect of diltiazem on infarct size (10), reinfarction (37), and mortality (38). These three clinical trials comprise a total of 3074 patients with confirmed acute myocardial infarction and are substantially different in trial design, study population, objectives, and endpoints. Results from these trials have led to the recommendation that diltiazem be used for prevention of reinfarction after non-Q-wave infarction. In view of this indication, a brief discussion of non-Q-wave infarction will follow prior to the discussion of the role of diltiazem.

Non-Q-Wave Infarction

The term "subendocardial" implies that myocardial damage is restricted to the endocardium, but since the damage frequently extends into the mid- and epicardial layers, this term has been changed to non-Q-wave infarction. On the electrocardiogram (ECG), subendocardial infarction is manifested as ST-T changes without the development of Q waves. Thus, it is diagnosed in patients with chest pain, ECG changes without Q waves, and elevated plasma MB CK activity. Transmural infarction is associated with the development of Q waves and today is more appropriately termed Q-wave infarction. It was recognized in the 1970s that non-Q-wave infarction was associated with relatively low in-hospital mortality and complication rates. However, in long-term (2–3 years) follow-up studies the mortality rate was the same in Q-wave and non-Q-wave infarction. The overall 1-month mortality in patients with non-Q-wave infarction based on a pool of 3751 patients was 10.2% compared with 19.9% in 11,400 patients with Q-wave infarction (39). The difference is statistically significant. Analysis of pooled data on long-term follow-up studies of 3346 patients with non-Q-wave infarction and 7641 patients with Q-wave infarction showed a slightly, but significantly, higher long-term mortality in patients with non-Q-wave myocardial infarction (31.2% versus 26.3%) (40).

In an attempt to explain this difference in short- and long-term prognosis, a prospective study (41) was performed with plasma MB CK activity assayed every 4 hr for the first 72 hr and every 12 hr subsequently for 14 days in 200 consecutive patients admitted with acute myocardial infarction (1979–1980). Concomitantly, clinical and ECG status was monitored and recorded daily throughout hospitalization in an attempt to correlate enzymatic evidence of reinfarction with chest pain and ST-T wave changes on ECG. Reinfarction was confirmed by a reelevation of

Table 4   Clinical Outcome Variables in Q-Wave Versus Non-Q-Wave Myocardial Infarction: Results of Pooled Data

Endpoint of study	Duration of follow-up	QMI (% death or reinfarction)	NQMI (% death or reinfarction)	p
Short-term mortality (25 studies)	5–30 days	11,400 (19.9)	3,751 (10.2)	<0.0001
Long-term mortality (22 studies)	6–96 months	7,641 (26.3)	3,346 (31.2)	<0.001
Reinfarction (14 studies)	Up to 44 months	4,095 (5.7)	1,201 (15.7)	<0.001
Peak CK level (12 studies)		(1,167)	(538)	<0.001

Source: Adapted from Gibson (39).

MB CK activity above 15 IU/liter after decline of values to baseline or to <8 IU/liter. Reinfarction was confirmed in 17% (35 patients) of all patients with acute myocardial infarction. Among 58 patients with non-Q-wave infarction, 25 had reinfarction (43%), compared with only 10 of 124 patients with Q-wave infarction (8%). Reinfarction was associated with chest pain in 90% and with ST-T wave changes in 80%. Patients who experienced reinfarction exhibited a deterioration of left ventricular ejection fraction from 56 to 34%. Analysis of the ECG and the serial radionuclide ventriculograms confirmed the site of reinfarction to be the same as the initial myocardial infarction in 86% of patients. The hospital mortality in patients with non-Q-wave infarction without reinfarction was 7%, compared with 16% in patients with reinfarction.

Following this report, 13 clinical studies published from 1981 to 1986 confirmed the higher incidence of reinfarction in patients with non-Q-wave infarction. Pooled data reported by Gibson (39) on 1201 patients with non-Q-wave infarction and 4095 patients with Q-wave infarction showed a threefold higher reinfarction rate (Table 4) in patients with non-Q-wave infarction. Patients with non-Q-wave infarction are more vulnerable to recurrent myocardial injury in the same territory; thus cumulative myocardial necrosis results from repetitive episodes of infarction, which lead to a decrease in left ventricular function and increased risk for death. In a prospective study (42) of 350 consecutive patients with acute myocardial infarction followed for 9 months, 125 of whom had non-Q-wave infarction, 57 patients (16%) died during the first 3 weeks after the index infarction. Three-week mortality was 23% with Q-wave infarction and 10% with non-Q-wave infarction ($p < 0.01$). Most of the deaths among patients with Q-wave infarction occurred early, whereas mortality remained substantial during follow-up among patients with non-Q-wave infarction. At the end of the 9-month follow-up, mortality in both groups was similar (30% for Q-wave infarction and 27% for non-Q-wave infarction). The most distinctive finding was the substantially higher 21-day mortality among patients with non-Q-wave infarction with recurrent infarction compared with those without reinfarction (23% versus 8%). Overall mortality at the end of the 9-month follow-up period in patients with non-Q-wave infarction was higher in the 64 patients with non-Q-wave infarction and reinfarction than in the 61 patients without such a recurrence (34% versus 23%). Statistical analysis of clinical data indicated that reinfarction was the single most powerful predictor of 1-year mortality (43). In the patients with non-Q-wave infarction, 1-year mortality was about fourfold greater in the presence of reinfarction.

The most recent data on non-Q-wave infarction comes from the Diltiazem Reinfarction Study (43) (DRS) which analyzed the 1-year follow-up data on 576 patients, of whom 515 survived. In-hospital (14 day) reinfarction was an independent predictor of early mortality, but it was not independently associated with late mortality, thus confirming earlier reports indicating that most of the excess deaths in patients with non-Q-wave infarction occurred early after the index infarction. Analysis of the data reflected a different natural history for patients with Q-wave and non-Q-wave infarction. The vulnerable period for Q-wave infarction lasted only 6–12 weeks, whereas in non-Q-wave infarction it continued for several months, albeit being more intense in the first 3 months. The distinct natural history of Q-wave and non-Q-wave infarction is shown in Figure 1. Thus, the explanation for the paradox between the early low mortality and the subsequent long-term mortality of non-Q-wave infarction versus Q-wave infarction is the increased and prolonged vulnerability of non-Q-wave infarction to subsequent repeated episodes of infarction. The potential benefit of early prophylactic therapy to prevent reinfarction in patients with non-Q-wave infarction is obvious. This benefit was demonstrated using diltiazem in the DRS and MDPIT trials, which will be discussed in detail in the next section.

The importance of this prophylactic treatment is further emphasized by the increasing prevalence of non-Q-wave infarction. In 1987, Goldberg et al. (44), after surveying 16 community hospitals in western Massachusetts, showed a steady increase in the prevalence of non-Q-wave myocardial infarction from 28% in 1975 to 42.6% in 1981. The most recent figures suggest that the prevalence of non-Q-wave myocardial infarction in 1991 is around 50%. This increased prevalence probably relates to the widespread use of thrombolytic therapy, bypass surgery, coronary angioplasty, and other therapies. It is now well established that patients treated successfully with early thrombolytic therapy are more likely to evolve non-Q-wave infarction, and the most common type of infarction after cardiac surgery by far is non-Q-wave infarction (45).

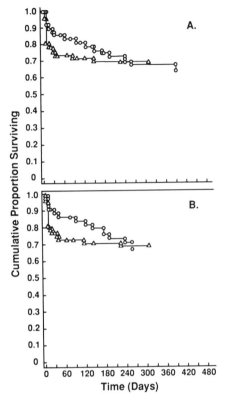

Figure 1   Survival of 225 patients with Q-wave infarction (triangles) and of 125 patients with non-Q-wave infarction (circles). (A) Data from all patients; (B) patients without a prior myocardial infarction. Patients with prior infarction were excluded from the analysis. [Reproduced with permission of American Heart Association from Marmor et al. (42).]

Diltiazem Reinfarction Study (1986)

The DRS (37) was a placebo-controlled, randomized, double-blind, multicenter trial of 576 patients with non-Q-wave myocardial infarction. The primary endpoint was reinfarction occurring during the subsequent 14 days, defined as an increase of 50% or more in plasma MB CK activity above the preceding baseline level. The MB CK activity was measured at 12-hr intervals throughout the study period or every 8 hr if reinfarction was suspected. Secondary endpoints were postinfarction angina and refractory postinfarction angina, the latter defined as angina requiring treatment with some other form of therapy within the 14 days of randomization.

Baseline clinical characteristics were comparable in the diltiazem-treated patients (287) and the placebo group (289). At 14 days, the cumulative reinfarction rate was 12.9% in the placebo group and 6.3% in the diltiazem group. This 51% reduction in the reinfarction rate was statistically significant ($p < 0.029$, 90% confidence interval of +7% to 67%). A total of 38 of 42 patients (90%) who had reinfarction had clinical or ECG manifestations.

Secondary endpoints, namely, recurrent chest pain, refractory postinfarction angina, and total mortality, were also reported. Refractory angina occurred in 30 patients, 20 in the placebo group and 10 in the diltiazem group. The cumulated lifetable rate of refractory angina was 6.9% in the placebo group and 3.5% in the diltiazem group, reflecting a 50% reduction in the incidence of refractory postinfarction angina in the diltiazem-treated patients. There was also a 28% reduction in the incidence of angina associated with ECG changes. All-cause mortality was 3.1% in the placebo group and 3.8% in the diltiazem group.

Diltiazem up to 360 mg/day was well tolerated despite concomitant use of beta-blockers in 61% of the diltiazem-treated patients. There were no differences between placebo and diltiazem groups in the occurrence of left ventricular failure, cardiogenic shock, high-grade atrioventricular block, asystole, severe bradycardia, or hypotension. These results indicate that diltiazem, 90 mg every 6 hr, started 48–72 hr after the onset of non-Q-wave infarction, is safe and effective pharmacological therapy in preventing reinfarction. The consistent reduction in the three prognostically important clinical endpoints, namely, reinfarction, angina associated with ST-T wave changes, and medically refractory angina, together with the safety of diltiazem, provided strong data for advocating diltiazem treatment routinely in patients with non-Q-wave infarction. However, since this trial was for only 14 days, it remained to be determined whether diltiazem would be effective in preventing reinfarction long-term and whether it would prolong survival. These questions were addressed in a long-term trial, MDPIT.

The Multicenter Diltiazem Postinfarction Trial: MDPIT

The Multicenter Diltiazem Postinfarction Trial (38) (MDPIT) was a double-blind, placebo-controlled, prospective, randomized clinical trial conducted in 23 clinical centers (19 in the United States and four in Canada). This trial was designed to determine whether long-term therapy with diltiazem in patients surviving myocardial infarction would reduce mortality and reinfarction. Unlike the Diltiazem Reinfarction study (DRS), MDPIT enrolled 2466 patients with Q-wave or non-Q-wave myocardial infarction, and diltiazem was given 60 mg four times per day initiated 3–15 days after onset of infarction and continued for up to 52 months (mean follow-up was 25 months), with a minimum follow-up of 12 months.

The overall mortality was similar in both groups (13.5%), most of which (75%) was due to cardiac causes. Cardiac events (death and reinfarction) occurred in 202 diltiazem- and 226 placebo-treated patients, respectively. This 11% reduction in cardiac deaths or nonfatal reinfarction was not statistically significant ($p = 0.26$). Subset analysis of 12 prospectively preselected variables identified a significant ($p = 0.004$) bidirectional interaction between diltiazem treatment and presence of pulmonary congestion. A total of 1909 patients without pulmonary congestion (80% of study population) treated with diltiazem experienced a 23% lower cumulative rate of cardiac events; whereas of the remaining patients with pulmonary congestion (20%), those receiving diltiazem had a higher cumulative rate of death. Analysis of cardiac events was performed in a subgroup of 634 patients with non-Q-wave myocardial infarction. Overall, there were 46 cardiac deaths and 62 nonfatal reinfarctions during the 25-month follow-up. The cumulative 1-year cardiac event rate was 15% in the placebo group (388) and 9% in the diltiazem group (296). This 40% reduction in 1-year cardiac event rate was statistically significant ($p = 0.0296$). At the end of 4.5 years, the cumulative reduction in cardiac events remained at 34%. Analysis for an interaction between diltiazem and pulmonary congestion in the non-Q-wave infarction group showed the same results as for Q-wave infarction; namely, 19% of the patients had pulmonary congestion in this group and, diltiazem was associated with a higher mortality. The beneficial effect in the remaining patients receiving diltiazem was enhanced to a 60% reduction in death and reinfarction. These findings confirmed the results of the DRS study, which had showed a 51% reduction in reinfarction in patients with non-Q-wave infarction treated with diltiazem. In view of these results, the Joint AHA/ACC Task Force (46) recommended diltiazem be used routinely in patients with non-Q-wave infarction for at least 1 year in patients without a contraindication, such as cardiac failure with pulmonary congestion.

CONSENSUS AND RECOMMENDATIONS OF CALCIUM BLOCKERS IN PATIENTS SURVIVING MYOCARDIAL INFARCTION

The extensive trials studying nifedipine in patients with acute myocardial infarction, postmyocardial infarction, or unstable angina have provided some definitive conclusions: (a) Acute administration of nifedipine in patients with evolving infarction is contraindicated for limitation of infarct size, prolongation of life, or prevention of early reinfarction. The results indicate that at best, one would expect no effect and at worst, there may be a deleterious effect. (b) Nifedipine, as monotherapy, is contraindicated in patients with unstable angina and, if used, must be used in conjunction with a beta-blocker or some other agent that decreases the heart rate.

Diltiazem was shown to increase mortality in patients recovering from myocardial infarction with pulmonary congestion, but in patients recovering from myocardial infarction without pulmonary congestion, particularly patients recov-

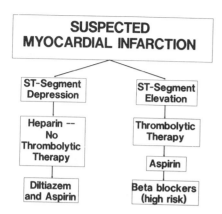

Figure 2   Schematic diagram illustrating the recommended approach to patients with acute myocardial infarction depending on the presence of ST-segment depression or elevation on the admission electrocardiogram.

ering from non-Q-wave infarction, there was a significant reduction in the incidence of reinfarction and angina, which was maintained for at least 4.5 years. These results led to the Joint AHA/ACC Task Force to recommend the routine treatment of diltiazem in patients recovering from non-Q-wave infarction for at least 1 year. Thus, routine prophylactic therapy of diltiazem up to 360 mg/day is recommended in patients recovering from non-Q-wave infarction to be initiated within 48 hr from onset of symptoms and be continued for at least 1 year. It is of some interest that beta-blockers have been shown in several trials, including BHAT, ISIS-1, Norwegian Timolol Trial, and MIAMI study, not to be effective in reducing reinfarction and death in patients recovering from non-Q-wave infarction. It is also of interest that in three trials of thrombolytic therapy (GISSI-1, GISSI-2, and ISIS-2) patients with ST-segment depression (70–80% of patients with non-Q-wave infarction present with ST depression) exhibited no benefit from thrombolytic therapy. Thus, the only proven therapy for non-Q-wave infarction is diltiazem since neither angioplasty nor surgery has been evaluated. Nevertheless, in a retrospective analysis (47) aspirin was shown to be effective in reducing cardiac death and reinfarction in patients with non-Q-wave infarction. In the scheme presented in Figure 2 we are recommending aspirin on that basis plus the beneficial effect observed for aspirin on cardiac events in other clinical trials. Diltiazem can be used safely in combination with beta-blockers, nifedipine, and verapamil; however, the latter combination should be used with caution since both drugs can induce bradycardia.

Verapamil has also been shown in DAVIT-II to reduce the combined incidence of death and reinfarction. The reduction in death as a single endpoint was not statistically significant; however, statistical significance was reached when both endpoints were combined. Verapamil, in DAVIT-II, was associated with a 17% reduction in death and nonfatal reinfarction compared to placebo over 18 months, whereas diltiazem, in MDPIT, was associated with a reduction in the same cardiac events of 40% at 1 year and 34% after 4.5 years. Thus, it appears that diltiazem is more effective; however, the claim can only be substantiated by a trial in which the two drugs are compared in the same general patient population. The side effect profile of diltiazem appears safer than that of verapamil. In making a recommendation of the specific use and application of verapamil in the patient surviving non-Q-wave myocardial infarction, however, it is somewhat more complex. It is well recognized in multiple trials that beta-blockers are associated with a 25% reduction on average in the incidence of death and reinfarction following Q-wave infarction. It is also well documented, as indicated earlier, that the effect in patients with non-Q-wave infarction is minimal, if any, from beta-blockers. Given these statistics, then, one would not recommend verapamil as primary therapy post-myocardial infarction in patients recovering from Q-wave infarction. On the other hand, since we do not have a prospective trial specifically designed to assess the effect of verapamil in non-Q-wave infarction or even a retrospective analysis of its effect in non-Q-wave infarction, it is difficult at this time to recommend verapamil as first-line therapy for treatment of the patient surviving myocardial infarction. Nevertheless, it is reasonable, given the available data, to consider verapamil as appropriate therapy in patients following non-Q-wave infarction should there be a contraindication to diltiazem. One should be extremely cautious about using verapamil in conjunction with diltiazem or beta-blockers in patients recovering from non-Q-wave infarction.

REFERENCES

1. Fleckenstein A. Calcium antagonism in heart and smooth muscle. New York: Wiley, 1983:272-9.
2. Henry PD, Perez JE. Clinical pharmacology of calcium antagonists. In Conti CR, ed. Cardiac drug therapy. Philadelphia: Davis, 1984:93-109.
3. Chaffman M, Brogden RN. Diltiazem: a review of its pharmacological properties and therapeutic efficacy. Drugs 1985; 29:387-454.
4. Jayakody RL, Kappagoda CT, Senaratne MPJ. Effect of calcium antagonists on adrenergic mechanisms in canine saphenous veins. J Physiol 1986; 372:25-39.
5. Schwartz A, Grupp G, Millard RW. Calcium channel blockers: possible mechanisms of protective effects on the ischemic myocardium. In Weiss GB, ed. New perspectives on calcium antagonists. Bethesda, MD: American Physiological Society, 1981:191-210.
6. Roberts R, Jaffe AS, Henry PD, Sobel BE. Nifedipine and acute myocardial infarction. Hertz 1981; 6:90-97.

7. Henry PD, Shuchleib R, Borda LJ, Roberts R, Williamson JR, Sobel BE. Effects of nifedipine on myocardial perfusion and ischemia in dogs. Circ Res 1978; 43:372-80.

8. Fukuyama T, Schechtman KB, Roberts R. The effects of intravenous nitroglycerin on hemodynamics, coronary blood flow and morphologically and enzymatically estimated infarct size in conscious dogs. Circulation 1990; 62:1227-38.

9. Selwyn PA, Welman E, Fox K, Horlock P, Pratt J, Klein M. The effects of nifedipine on acute experimental ischemia and infarction in dogs. Circ Res 1977; 44:16-23.

10. Zannard F, Amor M, Karcher G, Maurin P, Ethevenot G, Sabag C, Bertrand A, Pernot C, Gilgenkrantz J-M. Effect of diltiazem on myocardial infarction size estimated by enzyme release, serial thallium-201 single-photon emission computed tomography and radionuclide angiography. Am J Cardiol 1988; 61:1172-7.

11. Altman R, Seazziota A, Dujoune C. Diltiazem potentiates the inhibitory effect of aspirin on platelet aggregation. Clin Pharmacol Ther 1988; 44:320-5.

12. Westwick J, Mark G, Powling MJ, Kakkar VV. Diltiazem, the cardiac slow channel calcium antagonist, is a potent, selective and competitive inhibitor of platelet activating factor (PAF) on human platelets. Thromb Haemost 1983; 50:42.

13. Ring ME, Corrigan JJ, Fenster PE. Antiplatelet effects of oral diltiazem, propranolol and their combination. Br J Clin Pharmacol 1987; 24:615-20.

14. Fristchka E, Kribben A, Distler A, Philipp T. Inhibition of aggregation and calcium influx of human platelets by nitrendipine. J Cardiovasc Pharmacol 1987; 9:S85-S89.

15. Henry PD. Calcium channel blockers and atherosclerosis. J Cardiovasc Pharmacol 1990; 16:I-512-I-515.

16. Henry PD, Bentley KI. Suppression of atherogenesis in cholesterol-fed rabbit treated with nifedipine. J Clin Invest 1981; 68:1366-9.

17. Habib JB, Bossaller C, Wells S, Williams C, Morrisett JD, Henry PD. Preservation of endothelium-dependent vascular relaxation in cholesterol-fed rabbit by treatment with the calcium blocker PN 200110. Circ Res 1986; 58:305-9.

18. Lichten PR, Hugenholtz PG, Rafflenbeul W, Hecker H, Jost S. Retardation of angiographic progression of coronary artery disease by nifedipine: results of the International Nifedipine Trial on Antiatherosclerotic Therapy (INTACT). Lancet 1990; 335: 1109-13.

19. Waters D, Lesperance J, Francetich M, Causey D, Theroux P, Chiang YK, Hudon G, Lemarbre L, Reitman M, Joyal M, Gosselin G, Dyrda I, Macer J, Havel, RJ. A controlled clinical trial to assess the effect of a calcium channel blocker on the progression of coronary atherosclerosis. Circulation 1990; 82:1940-53.

20. Kugiyama K, Kerns SA, Morrisett JD, Roberts R, Henry PD. Impairment of endothelium-dependent arterial relaxation by lysolecithin in modified low-density lipoproteins. Nature 1990; 344:160-2.

21. Wilcox RG, Hampton RF, Banks DC, Birkhead JS, Brooksby IAB, Burns-Cox CJ, Haye MJ, Joy MD, Malcolm AD, Mather HG, Rowley JM. Trial of early nifedipine in acute myocardial infarction: the Trent study. Br Heart J 1986; 293:1204-8.

22. Neufeld HN. Calcium antagonist in secondary prevention after acute myocardial infarction: the secondary prevention reinfarction nifedipine trial (SPRINT). Eur Heart J 1986; 7(Suppl B):51-2.

23. The Israeli SPRINT Study Group. Secondary prevention reinfarction Israeli nifedi-

pine trial (SPRINT): a randomized intervention trial of nifedipine in patients with acute myocardial infarction. Eur Heart J 1988; 9:354-64.

24. Muller JE, Morrison J, Stone PH, Rude RE, Rosner B, Roberts R, Pearle DL, Turi ZG, Schneider JF, Serfas DH, Tate C, Scheiner E, Sobel BE, Hennekens CH, Braunwald E. Nifedipine therapy for patients with threatened and acute myocardial infarction: a randomized, double-blind, placebo-controlled comparison. Circulation 1984; 69: 740-7.

25. Sirnes PA, Overskeid K, Pedersen TR, Bathen J, Drienes A, Froland GS, Kjekshus JK, Landmark K, Rokseth R, Sirnes KE, Sundoy A, Torjussen BR, Westlund KM, Wik BA. Evolution of infarct size during the early use of nifedipine in patients with acute myocardial infarction: The Norwegian Nifedipine Multicenter Trial. Circulation 1984; 70:638-44.

26. Walker CJE, MacKenzie G, Adgey AAJ. Effect of nifedipine on enzymatically estimated infarct size in the early phase of acute myocardial infarction. Br Heart J 1988; 59:403-10.

27. Branagan JP, Walsh K, Kelly P, Collins WC, McCafferty D, Walsh MJ. Effect of early treatment with nifedipine in suspected acute myocardial infarction. Eur Heart J 1986; 7:859-65.

28. Erbel R, Pop T, Meinertz T, Olshausen KV, Treese N, Henrichs KJ, Schuster CJ, Rupprecht HJ, Schllurmann W, Meyer J. Combination of calcium channel blocker and thrombolytic therapy in acute myocardial infarction. Am Heart J 1988; 115:529-38.

29. The Holland Interuniversity Nifedipine/Metoprolol Trial (HINT) Research Group. Early treatment of unstable angina in the coronary care unit: a randomized, double blind, placebo controlled comparison of recurrent ischaemia in patients treated with nifedipine or metoprolol or both. Br Heart J 1986; 56:400-13.

30. Gottlieb SO, Becker LC, Weiss JL, Shapiro EP, Chandra NC, Flaherty JT, Gottlieb SH, Ouyang P, Mellits ED, Towsend SN. Nifedipine in acute myocardial infarction: an assessment of left ventricular function, infarct size, and infarct expansion. A double-blind, randomized, placebo-controlled trial. Br Heart J 1988; 59:411-8.

31. Eisenberg PR, Lee RG, Biello DR, Geltman EM, Jaffe AS. Chest pain after nontransmural infarction: the absence of remediable coronary vasospasm. Am Heart J 1985; 110:515-21.

32. Hanen JF, Sigurd B, Mellemgaard K, Lyngbye J. Verapamil in acute myocardial infarction. Dan Med Bull 1980; 27:105-9.

33. The Danish Study Group on Nerapamil in Myocardial Infarction. Verapamil in acute myocardial infarction. Eur Heart J 1984; 5:516-28.

34. Thuesen L, Jorgensen JR, Kvistgaard HJ, Sorensen JA, Vaeth M, Jensen EB, Jensen JJ, Hagerup L. Effect of verapamil on enzyme release after early intravenous administration in acute myocardial infarction: double blind randomised trial. Br Med J 1983; 286:1107-8.

35. Bussmann W-D, Seher W, Gruengras M. Reduction of creatine kinase and creatine kinase-MB indexes of infarct size by intravenous verapamil. Am J Cardiol 1984; 54: 1224-30.

36. The Danish Study Group on Verapamil in Myocardial Infarction. Effect of verapamil

on mortality and major events after acute myocardial infarction (The Danish Verapamil Infarction Trial II, DAVIT-II). Am J Cardiol 1990; 66:779-85.

37. Gibson RS, Boden WE, Theroux P, Strass HD, Pratt CM, Gheorghiae M, Capone RJ, Young PM, Schechtman K, Perryman MB, Roberts R, and the Diltiazem Reinfarction Study Research Group. Diltiazem and reinfarction in patients with non-Q-wave myocardial infarction: results of a double-blind, randomized, multicenter trial. N Engl J Med 1986; 315:423-9.

38. The Multicenter Diltiazem Postinfarction Trial Research Group. The effect of diltiazem on mortality and reinfarction after myocardial infarction. N Engl J Med 1988; 319:385-92.

39. Gibson RS. Non-Q-wave myocardial infarction: diagnosis, prognosis, and management. Curr Probl Cardiol 1988; 13:1-72.

40. Roberts R. Recognition, diagnosis, and prognosis of early reinfarction: the role of calcium-channel blockers. Circulation 1987; 75(Suppl V):V-139-V-147.

41. Marmor A, Sobel BE, Roberts R. Factors presaging early recurrent myocardial infarction ("extension"). Am J Cardiol 1981; 48:603-10.

42. Marmor A, Geltman EM, Schechtman K, Sobel BE, Roberts R. Recurrent myocardial infarction: clinical predictors and prognostic implications. Circulation 1982; 66: 415-21.

43. Schechtman KB, Capone RJ, Kleiger RE, Gibson RS, Schwartz DJ, Roberts R, Boden WE, and the Diltiazem Reinfarction Study Group. Differential risk patterns associated with three-month as compared to three to twelve month mortality and reinfarction after non-Q-wave myocardial infarction. J Am Coll Cardiol 1990; 15:940-7.

44. Goldberg RJ, Gore JM, Alpert JS, et al. Non-Q-wave myocardial infarction: Recent changes in occurrence and prognosis—a community wide perspective. Am Heart J 1987; 113:273.

45. Roberts B. Thrombolysis and its sequelae: calcium antagonists as potential adjunctive therapy. Circulation 1989; 80:IV-93-IV-101.

46. ACC/AHA Task Force Report. Guidelines for the early management of patients with acute myocardial infarction: a report of the American College of Cardiology/American Heart Association Task Force on assessment of diagnosis and therapeutic cardiovascular procedures. J Am Coll Cardio 1990; 16:249-92.

47. Klimt CR, Knatterud GL, Stamler J, Meier P, and the Investigator Group. Persantine-aspirin reinfarction study. Part II: Secondary coronary prevention with persantine and aspirin. J Am Coll Cardiol 1986; 7:251-69.

8

Aspirin Therapy of Acute Myocardial Infarction

Charles H. Hennekens
*Harvard Medical School and Brigham and
Women's Hospital, Boston, Massachusetts*

INTRODUCTION

Of the options currently available in the treatment of acute myocardial infarction (MI), the administration of oral aspirin is perhaps the simplest and least expensive therapy with demonstrated clinical benefit. The evidence concerning the efficacy of aspirin in the treatment of acute evolving MI forms an important part of the totality of evidence that demonstrates clear benefits of aspirin on cardiovascular disease in various categories of patients (1).

As regards aspirin's general medical utility, precursors to the modern synthesized drug have been used to treat human disease for more than 2000 years. Hippocrates gave patients an extract produced from the bark of white willow trees to relieve aches and pains. Unbeknown to the father of medicine in the fifth century B. C., willow bark extract contains salicin, whose synthesized analog, acetylsalicylic acid, would, in the 20th century, become the most widely used drug in the world. Aspirin was synthesized in 1899 by the German chemist Felix Hoffman, who is said to have been motivated in part by humanitarian efforts to find an effective pain reliever for his father, who suffered from disabling arthritis.

Despite its widespread use, it was not until the 1970s that the potential for low-dose aspirin to reduce risks of cardiovascular disease was first demonstrated. Sir John Vane, who later received the Nobel Prize for his work, demonstrated that in platelets, small amounts of aspirin irreversibly acetylate the active site of cyclooxygenase, which is required for the production of thromboxane A2, a powerful promoter of platelet aggregation (2). Higher doses provided no additional benefit, and far higher doses were postulated to reverse this tendency due to activation of vessel wall enzymes.

Further evidence suggesting the possibility of beneficial effects of aspirin has emerged over the last 20 years from observational epidemiological studies, which have suggested that aspirin may reduce risks of cardiovascular disease by about 20% (3, 4). Such reductions in a common and serious disease can have both a clinical and public health impact. However, unlike basic research, epidemiology is crude and inexact since observations on free-living humans can rarely take place under the rigidly controlled conditions possible in the laboratory. When we search for 20–30% effects, the size of uncontrolled confounding present in case-control and cohort study designs might easily be as large as the magnitude of the benefits or risks we are trying to detect. As a result, the most reliable study design for detecting such small to moderate effects is a randomized trial of sufficiently large sample size (5).

ASPIRIN IN ACUTE MI

Randomized trial data concerning aspirin in acute MI from the Second International Study of Infarct Survival (ISIS-2) are quite conclusive (6). There was one earlier randomized trial of aspirin in acute MI (7), but the sample size was small and the protocol involved administration of just a single tablet.

In ISIS-2, 417 hospitals in 17 different countries randomized 17,187 patients with suspected acute MI to assess the effects of intravenous streptokinase and oral aspirin. Utilizing a placebo-controlled, 2×2 factorial design, the trial randomly assigned subjects to either a 1-hr infusion of streptokinase (1.5 million units), 1 month of daily aspirin (160 mg), both active treatments, or neither treatment. Patients were eligible if they were thought to be within 24 hr of the onset of symptoms of suspected MI and to have no clear indication for, or contraindication to, streptokinase or aspirin.

Five weeks after randomization, there were 804 vascular deaths in the group allocated to aspirin and 1016 among those receiving aspirin placebo (Table 1), yielding a highly significant 23% reduction in risk among those taking aspirin. This reduction was very similar to that seen for streptokinase (SK), which was associated with a statistically significant 25% reduction in 5-week vascular mortality. The group receiving both active agents experienced a highly significant 42% reduction in 5-week vascular mortality, suggesting that the effects of aspirin and streptokinase are largely additive. Further, for those treated within 6 hr of onset of symptoms, the mortality reduction was over 50%. As expected, SK-treated patients fared better when therapy was initiated earlier, but benefits persisted for those randomized up to 24 hr. In contrast, the 23% mortality reduction among as-

Table 1   Results from the Second International Study of Infarct Survival (ISIS-2): Events in the First 5 Weeks After Suspected MI

Endpoint	Aspirin (160 mg/day for 1 month) (N = 8587)	Placebo (1 tablet/day for 1 month) (N = 8600)	Reduction (% ± SD)
Nonfatal reinfarction	83	170	50 ± 9
Nonfatal stroke	27	51	46 ± 17
Total cardiovascular mortality	804	1016	23 ± 4
Any vascular event	914	1237	23 ± 4

pirin takers was present regardless of the interval from onset of symptoms to initiation of therapy.

As regards nonfatal vascular events, there were 83 nonfatal reinfarctions in the aspirin group compared with 170 among those on placebo, yielding a 50% reduction from aspirin. A similar reduction of 46% was seen for nonfatal stroke, where there were 27 in the aspirin group compared with 51 among those assigned placebo. Both reductions were statistically significant and were also present for fatal reinfarction and stroke. For all important vascular events (a category that included nonfatal MI, nonfatal stroke, and total vascular death), there were 914 in the aspirin group and 1237 in the placebo group, yielding a 23% reduction in the aspirin group. There were no differences between the groups receiving aspirin and aspirin placebo in the incidence of major bleeding requiring transfusion or cardiac rupture. There was a small benefit of aspirin on cardiac arrest and a slight increase in minor bleeding not requiring transfusion.

SECONDARY PREVENTION TRIALS

In secondary prevention among survivors of previous cardiovascular events, a total of 25 randomized trials have been completed of various antiplatelet agents, including aspirin, dipyridamole (Persantine), or sulfinpyrazone (Anturane), either alone or in combination. The study populations for these trials included a total of approximately 29,000 individuals, 18,000 with a history of myocardial infarction (10 trials), 9000 with a history of stroke or transient ischemic attack (13 trials), and 2000 with unstable angina (two trials). While the majority of these individual trials reported findings compatible with benefits of aspirin, usually most were far too small to yield statistically stable results. In such circumstances, one method to diminish the play of chance is to perform an overview in which the results of the trials are considered in aggregate. An overview of these trials has been conducted

Table 2 Overview of 25 Trials of Antiplatelet Therapy in the Secondary Prevention of Cardiovascular Disease

Endpoint	All (25 trials)	Cerebrovascular (13 trials)	MI (10 trials)	Unstable angina (2 trials)
Nonfatal MI	32 ± 5	35 ± 12	31 ± 5	35 ± 17
Nonfatal stroke	27 ± 6	22 ± 7	42 ± 11	—[a]
Total cardiovascular death	15 ± 4	15 ± 7	13 ± 5	37 ± 19
Important vascular event	25 ± 3	22 ± 5	22 ± 4	36 ± 13

[a] Too few events reported to permit assessment of effect of aspirin.
Patients with prior vascular disease at entry into therapy. Figures represent reduction in risk (percentage ± SD) among those assigned antiplatelet therapy.

and yielded statistically reliable estimates of the benefits of aspirin in secondary prevention (8) (Table 2).

The endpoints analyzed in the overview were nonfatal MI, nonfatal stroke, total cardiovascular death, and total important vascular events. There was a 32% reduction in subsequent MI associated with antiplatelet therapy. For nonfatal stroke, there was a 27% decrease in risk, and for total vascular mortality, the reduction was 15%. Finally, for the combined endpoint of important vascular events, the overview demonstrated a 25% decrease. All these reductions were statistically significant.

When the trials are considered separately according to patient entry criteria, the trials of survivors of MI demonstrated statistically significant decreases in risk of 31% for nonfatal reinfarction, 42% for nonfatal stroke, 13% for vascular death, and 22% for any vascular event. The trials of patients with cerebrovascular disease demonstrated statistically significant reductions of 35% for MI, 22% for subsequent nonfatal stroke, 15% for vascular death, and 22% for any vascular event. Finally, for unstable angina, there were statistically significant decreases of 35% in nonfatal MI, 37% in vascular death, and 35% in any vascular event, but too few strokes to provide meaningful data.

Because there was no obvious large difference between the effects of antiplatelet therapy in the different types of trials, information from all 25 trials was combined to provide both direct and indirect comparisons of the effects of the three different types of antiplatelet therapy that were tested. Each type was significantly better than no treatment, and there were no significant differences between the three main types. In particular, these trials provide no good evidence that dipyridamole plus aspirin is any more effective than aspirin alone. Further, there was no evidence that doses of 1.0–1.5 g of aspirin daily were any more effective in avoiding cardiovascular events than a lower dose of 0.3 g, or one standard aspirin tablet, per day. This observation is pharmacologically plausible, in that doses even lower than 0.3 g/day would have produced virtually complete inhibition of cyclooxygenase-dependent platelet aggregation (9). At present, however, direct evidence on the effects of aspirin in doses lower and less frequent than 0.3 g/day is not available from these trials of secondary prevention.

PRIMARY PREVENTION TRIALS

Two randomized trials of aspirin in primary prevention have been completed, both among male physicians (10, 11). The U. S. trial (10) randomized 22,071 male physicians, aged 40–84, and tested 325 mg aspirin on alternate days, utilizing a double-blind, placebo-controlled, 2×2 factorial design, which allowed independent testing of the effects of beta-carotene supplementation on risks of cancer. The aspirin component of the trial was terminated early, based on the emergence of a statistically extreme benefit on occurrence of a first MI. Aspirin takers had a 44% reduction in risk of MI, with significant benefits on fatal and nonfatal events ($p <$ 0.00001). For all important vascular events, there was a statistically significant 18% reduction in the aspirin group ($p < 0.01$). As regards stroke and total vascular death, there were insufficient numbers of these events to allow for meaningful inferences.

The British Doctors' Trial (11) randomized 5139 male physicians, aged 50–78, and tested a daily dose of 500 mg aspirin, with the control group simply asked to avoid aspirin or any aspirin-containing compounds. The subjects were aware of their assignment, but the investigators remained blinded. In the British trial, there were no significant differences for nonfatal MI, nonfatal stroke, vascular death, or all important vascular events.

Because the U. S. trial was so much larger, an overview of the U. S. and British trials (12) demonstrated a highly significant 32% reduction in risk of nonfatal MI (Table 3). For stroke and vascular death, even with the two trials considered together, there were too few endpoints from which to draw firm conclusions. The available data showed a nonsignificant 18% apparent increase in nonfatal stroke and a nonsignificant 5% reduction in cardiovascular mortality. However, the wide confidence limits around these estimates indicate that the present data on primary prevention of stroke and cardiovascular death are insufficient upon which to draw meaningful inferences.

Table 3   Aspirin in Primary Prevention: U. S. Physicians' Health Study and British Doctors' Trial

Endpoint	U. S. Physicians' Health Study	British Doctors' Trial	Overview
Nonfatal MI	39 ± 9	3 ± 19	32 ± 8
Nonfatal stroke	↑19 ± 15	↑13 ± 24	↑18 ± 13
Total cardiovascular death	2 ± 15	7 ± 14	5 ± 10
Any vascular event	18 ± 7	4 ± 12	13 ± 6

Figures represent reduction in risk (percentage ± SD) among those assigned aspirin.

↑ = nonsignificant increased risk of stroke among aspirin-allocated subjects.

CLINICAL IMPLICATIONS

Over the past several years, considerable evidence has accumulated on the role of aspirin in reducing risks of cardiovascular disease. In acute MI, there is conclusive evidence that aspirin therapy started within 24 hr of the onset of symptoms of MI will reduce subsequent mortality.

Less certain, however, is the best dose, frequency of administration, or rate of release of aspirin or other platelet-active agents for achieving the optimal net benefit on reinfarction, stroke, and vascular death. To address this question, basic research findings are needed to determine the optimal regimen for controlling thromboxane while also sparing prostacyclin and minimizing the occurrence of side effects. The importance of prostacyclin sparing could also be further elucidated. In addition, clinical research is necessary to determine the optimal loading dose during evolving MI to achieve the most rapid clinical antithrombotic effect. It may be, for example, that a dose of at least 160 mg might be optimal during evolving MI, even though lower daily doses are able to completely inhibit platelet cyclooxygenase after a few days.

As regards the application of current knowledge to clinical practice, as is the case with thrombolytic therapy, aspirin is currently not being given to many acute MI patients for whom the drug is probably indicated. Indeed, because of aspirin's clear benefit and very low risk of side effects in acute MI, further research might now consider whether emergency medical technicians should administer aspirin to patients with suspected evolving MI, or even whether it might be prudent for individuals with such symptoms to self-medicate themselves. A major concern in such situations is that symptoms suggestive of MI may, in fact, reflect some gastrointestinal or other bleeding problem for which aspirin might even be contraindicated. Further investigations may be able to determine whether there are net benefits from use of aspirin in suspected acute MI by paramedics and the general public.

Despite the remaining unanswered questions, clear evidence now exists that aspirin therapy, administered in acute care facilities, confers a conclusive and clinically important benefit in most patients evolving an MI. Indeed, treatment of 100 acute MI patients with 1 month of aspirin can preclude approximately two deaths and one nonfatal event (6). Continuation of low-dose aspirin for 1 or 2 years could preclude another two deaths and three nonfatal events, making the total avoided by early and late MI treatment equal to four fatal and four nonfatal events (6). In other patient categories, there is also now strong evidence of aspirin's efficacy. Specifically, among those with a prior MI, unstable angina pectoris, stroke, or TIA, aspirin reduces the risk of subsequent cardiovascular events. For primary prevention, prophylactic aspirin therapy should be considered for those whose risk of a first MI is sufficiently high to warrant the possible adverse effects of long-term administration of the drug.

As with all emerging therapies for acute MI, the potential benefits of aspirin should be viewed in the context of current knowledge about modification of cardiovascular risk factors. For example, as regards blood cholesterol, a 10% decrease corresponds to a roughly 20–30% reduction in risks of cardiovascular disease (13). For blood pressure, a 5–6 mm decrease in diastolic pressure among those with mild-to-moderate hypertension appears to lower risks of coronary heart disease by 14% and stroke by 42% (14). Finally, cessation of cigarette smoking results in an approximately 50% decrease in coronary heart disease, perhaps even within a matter of months (15). Thus, aspirin should be viewed as an adjunct, not an alternative, to control or elimination of other cardiovascular risk factors, and should be prescribed only by a physician or other primary health care provider based on an individual clinical judgment. If used in this manner aspirin will reduce cardiovascular morbidity and mortality in a wide variety of patient settings, but especially during evolving MI.

ACKNOWLEDGMENT

I am indebted to Michael Jonas for expert editorial assistance.

REFERENCES

1. Hennekens CH, Buring JE, Sandercock P, Collins R, Peto R. Aspirin and other antiplatelet agents in the secondary and primary prevention of cardiovascular disease. Circulation 1989; 80:749–56.
2. Moncada S, Vane JR. Arachidonic acid metabolites and the interactions between platelets and blood-vessel walls. N Eng J Med 1979; 300:1142–7.

3. Hennekens CH, Karlson LK, Rosner B. A case-control study of regular aspirin use and coronary deaths. Circulation 1978; 58:35-8.

4. Hammond EC, Garfinkel L. Aspirin and coronary heart disease: findings of a prospective study. Br Med J 1975; 2:269-71.

5. Hennekens CH, Buring JE. Epidemiology in medicine. Boston: Little Brown, 1987.

6. ISIS-2 (Second International Study of Infarct Survival) Collaborative Group. Randomized trial of intravenous streptokinase, oral aspirin, both, or neither among 17,187 cases of suspected acute myocardial infarction: ISIS-2. Lancet 1988; 2:349-60.

7. Elwood PC, Williams WO. A randomized controlled trial of aspirin in the prevention of early mortality in myocardial infarction. J R Coll Gen Pract 1979; 29:413-6.

8. Antiplatelet Trialists' Collaboration. Secondary prevention of vascular disease by prolonged anti-platelet therapy. Br Med J 1988; 296:320-32.

9. Stampfer MJ, Jakubowski JA, Deykin D, Schafer AI, Willett WC, Hennekens CH. Effect of alternate day regular and enteric coated aspirin on platelet aggregation, bleeding time, and thromboxane A_2 levels in bleeding-time blood. Am J Med 1986; 81:400-5.

10. Steering Committee of the Physicians' Health Study Research Group. Final report on the aspirin component of the ongoing Physicians' Health Study. N Engl J Med 1989; 321:129-35.

11. Peto R, Gray R, Collins R, Wheatley K, Hennekens C, Jamrozik K, Warlow C, Hafner B, Thompson E, Gilliland J, Doll R. Randomized trial of prophylactic daily aspirin in British male doctors. Br Med J 1988; 296:313-6.

12. Hennekens CH, Peto R, Hutchison, GB, Doll R. An overview of the British and American aspirin studies. N Engl J Med 1988; 318:923-4.

13. Peto R, Yusuf S, Collins R. Cholesterol-lowering trial results in their epidemiologic context. Circulation 1985; 72(Suppl III):451 (abstract).

14. Hebert PR, Fiebach NH, Eberlein KA, Taylor JO, Hennekens CH The community-based randomized trials of pharmacologic treatment of mild-to-moderate hypertension. Am J Epidemiol 1988; 127:581-90.

15. Hennekens CH, Buring JE, Mayrent S. Smoking, aging and coronary heart disease. In Bosse R., ed. Smoking and aging, Lexington, MA: D. C. Heath, 1984, pp. 95-115.

9

Newer Antiplatelet Agents in Acute Myocardial Infarction

Joseph Loscalzo
Brigham and Women's Hospital, Brockton/West Roxbury
VA Medical Center, and Harvard Medical School,
Boston, Massachusetts

Ari Ezratty
Brigham and Women's Hospital, Boston, Massachusetts

INTRODUCTION

Antiplatelet therapy has been the focus of much research in the treatment and prevention of ischemic heart disease. Early pathological studies by Haerem in 1972 revealed platelet aggregates in up to 50% of patients suffering sudden ischemic death [1]. In 1974, Elwood and colleagues observed that regular aspirin use was associated with a decreased incidence of acute myocardial infarction (AMI) [2]. These studies provided the impetus for many basic and clinical trials of a wide array of antiplatelet agents aimed at blocking the different events that lead to platelet activation and aggregation.

The fact that platelets play a critical role in the pathogenesis of unstable coronary syndromes—unstable angina, acute myocardial infarction, and sudden death —has also been shown by several recent pathological, angiographic, and clinical studies. Davies and colleagues demonstrated the presence of platelet thrombi in segments of myocardium distal to ruptured atheromatous plaques in patients dying suddenly [3,4]. Coronary angiographic analyses revealed that patients with AMI and unstable angina are more likely to have intraluminal filling defects and irregular (type 2) lesions consistent with thrombosis compared to patients with chronic stable angina [5]. Finally, coronary angioscopic studies revealed complex atherosclerotic plaque and thrombi in patients with unstable angina, but not in those with stable angina [6].

Several studies have examined the use of aspirin as a means of primary and secondary prevention of ischemic heart disease. The Physician's Health Study [7], the VA Cooperative Study [8], the Canadian Multicenter Trial [9], and the Montreal Heart Institute Trial by Theroux and colleagues [10] all demonstrated marked decreases in mortality in patients treated with aspirin compared to placebo. Moreover, a more recent meta-analysis of 25 trials involving over 29,000 patients revealed that antiplatelet therapy reduces vascular mortality by 15%, recurrent myocardial infarction by 25%, and unstable angina by 36% [11]. These data, coupled with the recently recognized role of platelets in attenuating the temporal benefits of, and promoting reocclusion following, thrombolytic therapy [12], have served as the impetus for further studies using agents with novel mechanisms of platelet inhibition. Before we discuss these new antiplatelet agents, it is important to review the molecular mechanisms of platelet adhesion and aggregation.

MECHANISMS OF PLATELET ACTIVATION AND AGGREGATION

The unstimulated platelet circulates as a flattened disk. Its surface membrane consists of an outer coat (glycocalyx), which contains glycoproteins, and an inner phospholipid bilayer. The glycoproteins can be separated by size using polyacrylamide gel electrophoresis (Table 1). These surface glycoproteins mediate platelet adhesion to the subendothelium and platelet aggregation responses. Platelets also contain two internal membrane systems that facilitate secretion of granules during

Table 1   Platelet Surface Glycoprotein Receptors and Ligands

Glycoprotein	Ligand
GP Ia/IIa	Collagen
GP Ib/IIa	Fibronectin
GP Ic/IIa	Laminin
GP Ib/IXa	von Willebrand factor
GPIIb/IIIa	Fibrinogen, Fibronectin vitronectin, thrombospondin, von Willebrand factor
GP IV	Thrombospondin, collagen
GP V	Thrombin

Table 2   Platelet Granule Contents and Their Functions

	Action
Alpha granules	
Thrombospondin	Binds to fibrinogen, collagen
Fibronectin	
Platelet factor IV	Competes with antithrombin III, possible cytokine for megakaryocytes
Tissue growth factor-beta	Stimulates smooth muscle cell proliferation
Fibroblast growth factor	Promotes vessel wall repair
Platelet-derived growth factor	Promotes smooth muscle cell proliferation
Beta thromboglobulin	Useful marker of aggregation, function unknown
Dense bodies	
ADP, serotonin, calcium	Agonists of platelet aggregation

activation, some of the constituents of which support additional platelet recruitment to the growing platelet thrombus. Important products contained within platelet granules (alpha granules and dense bodies) are listed in Table 2.

The sequence of primary hemostasis and thrombosis begins with platelet adhesion to the subendothelium of damaged vessel walls. Platelet adhesion requires multimers of von Willebrand factor, which are synthesized by endothelial cells and which bind to glycoprotein Ib/(IX) on the platelet surface. Thrombospondin, fibronectin, and other adhesive proteins are also available in the subendothelial layer for binding to platelet glycoproteins. The exposure of platelets to collagen and thrombin activates platelets, which leads to release of platelet contents such as thromboxane A2, prostaglandin endoperoxides, platelet activating factor (PAF), and ADP, all of which increase platelet aggregation responses. Simultaneously, platelet binding to collagen and thrombin activates the enzyme phospholipase C, which catalyzes the formation of diacylglycerol (DAG) and inositol triphosphate (IP3), two key intermediates in platelet activation.

DAG activates protein kinase C, which catalyzes the phosphorylation of proteins involved in the secretion of granule contents. IP3 is a potent platelet agonist and a calcium ionophore. An increase in intracellular calcium concentration activates phospholipase A2, which liberates arachidonic acid from membrane phospholipid pools. Arachidonic acid is oxidized within the platelet by one of two pathways. The first involves cyclooxygenase as the rate-limiting (and initial) enzymatic step, which yields prostaglandin endoperoxides and, ultimately, through the action of thromboxane synthetase, thromboxane A2. This prostanoid is a potent vasoconstrictor and platelet agonist, which can recruit additional platelets to the aggregate and induce additional release of platelet granule contents. The second pathway involves lipoxygenase and yields hydroxy-eicosatetraenoic acid (HETE), which is of unclear functional significance in platelets, but which in leukocytes is a precursor of leukotrienes. The binding of thromboxane A2 to its receptor on the platelet surface effects an increase in intracellular calcium and a decrease in cyclic AMP, thereby promoting platelet aggregation.

Once platelets are activated, several events occur almost simultaneously. The platelet undergoes a shape change, which increases its surface area and facilitates adhesion, granule secretion, and aggregation. After the events of platelet adhesion and activation have occurred, a calcium-dependent conformational change in the glycoprotein IIb/IIIa complex is induced. This promotes the binding of the bivalent fibrinogen molecule to the IIb/IIIa receptor, which results in the aggregation of platelets. The IIb/IIIa receptor is unique in that it is capable of binding fibrinogen, fibronectin, thrombospondin, vitronectin, and von Willebrand factor, all of which contain the tripeptide sequence Arg-Gly-Asp (RGD). RGD represents a consensus sequence critical for ligand binding to this receptor. In addition, fibrinogen binds to glycoprotein IIb/IIIa through a dodecapeptide site on the carboxy-terminus of the gamma chain. Fibrinogen binding to platelet glycoprotein IIb/IIIa is commonly viewed as the final pathway leading to platelet aggregation.

To expand this paradigm further, we must consider the endothelial effectors that impair platelet aggregation. Endothelial cells can influence the platelet aggregation response by their release of prostacyclin (PGI2) and prostaglandin E1 (PGE1), tissue-type plasminogen activator (t-PA), and endothelium-derived relaxing factor (EDRF). The platelet inhibitory prostaglandins increase intracellular cyclic AMP and thereby inhibit platelet aggregation and promote disaggregation, while EDRF operates through a cyclic GMP-dependent mechanism to achieve the same ends. A mechanism by which endogenous t-PA disaggregates platelets may be through selective proteolysis of platelet-bound fibrinogen by plasmin [12].

It is clear that the sequence of events leading to platelet aggregation is extraordinarily complex. However, it is also readily apparent that many novel approaches to inhibiting platelet function are possible within the context of these complex molecular interactions. Until recently, the list of available antiplatelet agents has been limited to aspirin, with its documented efficacy in the primary and secondary prevention of ischemic heart disease, and several other agents without clearly proven value. In the last 5 years, however, numerous agents have been introduced that operate at virtually every step leading to platelet adhesion and aggregation (Table 3). These include: cyclooxygenase inhibitors, prostacyclin analogs, thromboxane receptor antagonists, thromboxane synthetase inhibitors, phosphodiesterase inhibitors, serotonin receptor antagonists, fibrinogen receptor antagonists, von Willebrand factor receptor antagonists, ticlopidine, synthetic thrombin inhibitors, and organic nitrates, which are increasingly being recognized as impor-

Table 3   Inhibitors of Platelet Responses and Sites of Action

Class	Inhibitor	Site of action
Cyclooxygenase inhibitors	ASA, sulfinpyrazone,	Cyclooxygenase
Prostacyclin analogs	PGI$_2$, Iloprost, PGE$_1$	Cyclic AMP
Thrombozane receptor antagonists	Sultatroban, SQ29548,	Thromboxane A$_2$
Thromboxane synthetase inhibitors	CGS13080	Thromboxane A$_2$
Phosphodiesterase inhibitors	Dipyridamole	Cyclic AMP
Serotonin receptor antagonists	Ketanserin	Serotonin
Fibrinogen receptor angatonists	RGD peptides, 7E3, 10E5	Glycoprotein IIb/IIIa
von Willebrand factor receptor antagonists	Aurin-tricarboxylic acid	Glycoprotein Ib/IX
Ticlopidine	Ticlopidine	?
Thrombin inhibitors	Argatroban, hirudin, PPACK heparin	Thrombin
Nitrates	Nitroglycerin, nitroprusside	Cyclic GMP

tant platelet inhibitors. These classes of agents, their mechanism(s) of action, and the results of basic and clinical trials involving them will now be presented.

ANTIPLATELET AGENTS AND CORONARY THROMBOSIS

Experimental Data

Cyclooxygenase Inhibitors

The best studied of all antiplatelet agents is the class of cyclooxygenase inhibitors. Cyclooxygenase catalyzes the conversion of arachidonic acid to prostaglandin endoperoxides, which can then be converted to thromboxane A$_2$ in platelets. This class of agents includes aspirin, an irreversible inhibitor of cyclooxygenase, and sulfinpyrazone and nonsteroidal anti-inflammatory agents such as ibuprofen, which are reversible inhibitors of cyclooxygenase. Aspirin is discussed in Chapter 8.

Prostacyclin and Analogs

Prostacyclin (PGI$_2$) is produced by endothelial cells from prostanoid endoperoxides utilizing the enzyme prostacyclin synthetase. PGI$_2$ inhibits platelet aggrega-

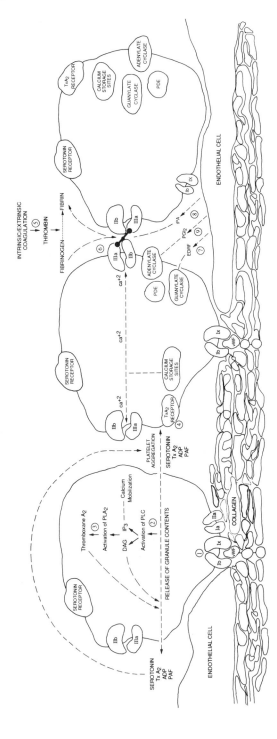

Figure 1   (1) Platelet adhesion to subendothelium; GP Ib/IX, wVF dependent. (2) Platelet activation leads to release of granule contents, activation of phospholipase C (PLC). (3) PLC yields DAG and IP₃, which ultimately yield thromboxane A₂ (TxA₂). (4) TxA₂ binds to receptor on platelets inducing conformational change in GP IIb/IIIa; calcium, cAMP dependent. (5) Intrinsic and extrinsic pathways of coagulation yield thrombin, fibrin. (6) GP IIb/IIIa binds bivalent fibrinogen inducing platelet aggregation. (7) Endothelial cells release EDRF, which inhibits platelet aggregation; cGMP dependent. (8) Endothelial cells release t-PA, which converts plasminogen to plasmin and promotes fibrinolysis and platelet disaggregation. (9) Endothelial cells release PGI₂, which inhibits platelet aggregation; cAMP dependent.

tion by effecting an increase in intracellular cyclic AMP. Early reports [13,14] demonstrated numerous protective effects of PGI2 in models of ischemia, such as vasodilatation, decreased oxygen consumption, reduction in the release of lysosomal enzymes, and, perhaps, limitation of infarct size.

Nicolini and colleagues have reported the effects of Iloprost in t-PA–induced thrombolysis using a canine model of thrombolysis [15]. Surprisingly, the results of this trial demonstrated in animals treated with this PGI2 analog an increase in the time to lysis, a decrease in the duration of reperfusion, and increased reocclusion rates compared with control animals (t-PA alone). In addition, plasma t-PA levels were 30% lower in Iloprost-treated animals compared to control. The mechanism by which Iloprost decreased the thrombolytic potential of t-PA may be multifactorial. Increased hepatic blood flow may increase the rate of metabolism of t-PA and thereby decrease its plasma concentration [16]. Alternatively, Iloprost may produce a coronary steal phenomenon and effectively decrease the amount of t-PA delivered to the site of thrombosis [16]. Thus, at the present time, any beneficial effects of PGI2 and its analogs in combination with thrombolytic therapy remain unproven.

Prostaglandin E1 (PGE2) acts in a similar fashion to PGI2. It produces platelet disaggregation by increasing intraplatelet cyclic AMP and has also been shown to stabilize neutrophilic lysosomes and to produce vasodilatation.

Thromboxane A2 Receptor Antagonists

The mechanism of reocclusion after thrombolysis is probably multifactorial. Although it has been well documented that in vivo thrombosis and platelet aggregation are associated with release of platelet products such as thromboxane A2, it has only recently been shown that thromboxane A2 is released following thrombolytic therapy [17] as well. This release is likely caused by platelet activation in response to thrombin and/or plasmin at sites of ruptured atherosclerotic plaque. To address specifically this issue and possibly enhance the effect of thrombolytic agents, efforts have been directed at antagonism of the thromboxane receptor.

Shebuski and colleagues investigated effects of the thromboxane receptor antagonist sulatroban on t-PA–induced thrombolysis and reocclusion rates in a canine model [18]. Sulatroban blocks thromboxane A2-induced platelet aggregation and prevents thromboxane A2-mediated vasoconstriction. In this trial, sulatroban produced dose-related improvements in time to lysis and reocclusion rates. In animals treated with the highest dose ($10\,\mu g/kg$) plus t-PA, reocclusion occurred in only 11%, which compared favorably with control (t-PA alone), in which 83% reoccluded. Therefore, this study suggests that inhibition of thromboxane A2-mediated platelet aggregation may be important in enhancing the effects of thrombolytic agents. The combination of SQ29548, another thromboxane A2 receptor antagonist, with ketanserin, a serotonin receptor blocker, has been demonstrated to be superior to either agent alone in preventing reocclusion after t-PA in the canine model studied [19]. Thus, reocclusion after thrombolytic therapy is a complex process, as is the platelet's role in this process; platelet inhibition may need to be approached with several agents having different mechanisms of action for optimal therapeutic benefits.

Thromboxane Synthetase Inhibitors

Whereas thromboxane receptor antagonists may be beneficial by limiting the direct effects of thromboxane A_2 produced during thrombolysis, thromboxane synthetase inhibitors may potentially be more advantageous in that by blocking the synthesis of thromboxane A_2 altogether, the endoperoxide pool may be shunted toward the synthesis of prostacyclin. CGS 13080, a thromboxane synthetase inhibitor, effectively blocks the synthesis of thromboxane A_2 and has been shown to increase the production of prostacyclin as evidenced by the appearance of the latter's metabolites in urine and serum [20]. Consequently, prostacyclin may exert its antiplatelet and vasodilator effects. Mickelson et al. reported the effects of CGS 13080 on streptokinase-induced thrombolysis in a canine model [21]. Results demonstrated a decrease in the reocclusion rate and an improvement in coronary blood flow in animals treated with CGS 13080 plus streptokinase compared with controls (streptokinase alone).

Phosphodiesterase Inhibitors

Compounds that increase the concentration of cyclic AMP inhibit platelet aggregation irrespective of the agonist used. Phosphodiesterase is an enzyme that degrades cyclic AMP to $5'$-AMP, and therefore, its inhibition results in the intracellular accumulation of cyclic AMP. Dipyridamole inhibits phosphodiesterase and has been used widely in combination with cyclooxygenase inhibitors in the treatment of patients with ischemic heart disease. Dipyridamole may stimulate PGI_2 release, inhibit thromboxane A_2 formation, block the uptake of adenosine into erythrocytes producing cyclic AMP for platelet inhibition, and exert synergistic effects with aspirin [22].

Serotonin Receptor Antagonists

Evidence has accumulated that platelets possess cell-surface receptors for serotonin, and that serotonin is a potent inducer of platelet aggregation in whole blood and platelet-rich plasma [23]. In addition, it has been shown that antagonists to the serotonin receptor abolish cyclic flow variations that are dependent on recurrent platelet thrombus formation in vivo [24,25]. Interestingly verapamil, a calcium channel antagonist, has also been shown to inhibit serotonin-induced platelet aggregation [24,26]. Ashton and colleagues demonstrated that ketanserin, a serotonin receptor antagonist, prevented cyclic flow variations in 8 of 10 dogs [27]. The results were similar to those using two different thromboxane receptor antagonists. The effect of combined administration of serotonin and thromboxane receptor antagonists on the incidence of reocclusion flowing thrombolysis was investigated by Golino and colleagues [28]. The combination of ketanserin and SQ29548, a thromboxane A_2 receptor antagonist, abolished cyclic flow variations and prevented reocclusion, whereas either single agent alone, as well as heparin, was ineffective in this regard. Thus, combination therapy directed at different effector sites in the platelet activation sequence may prove beneficial in addressing the problem of reocclusion.

Fibrinogen Receptor Antagonists

RGD-Containing Peptides. The final common pathway of platelet aggregation is the binding of fibrinogen to platelet glycoprotein IIb/IIIa. The tripeptide sequence Arg-Gly-Asp (RGD) is contained in all ligands that bind to this receptor and occurs twice in the fibrinogen molecule. Fibrinogen also binds to platelets via a dodecapeptide sequence on its carboxyterminal gamma chain. Several synthetic, as well as purified, naturally occurring proteins containing RGD peptides are currently being investigated as a means of antagonizing the binding of fibrinogen to its platelet receptor.

Bitistatin is an 83-amino acid peptide that contains the RGD sequence at residues 64-66. It is derived from the venom of the viper *Bitis arietans* and is similar to two other snake venom peptides, trigramin and echistatin [29]. In experimental studies, bitistatin exhibited dose-responsive inhibition of ex vivo platelet aggregation, as well as inhibition of platelet-dependent cyclic flow variations. Similar inhibitory potential toward the IIb/IIIa receptor has been observed with monoclonal antibodies (vide infra) directed at this receptor [30].

A recent trial examined the effects of bitistatin on the incidence of reperfusion and rate of reocclusion flowing administration of t-PA in a canine model of thrombolysis [31]. The results revealed that a combination of heparin, bitistatin, and t-PA was superior to any single agent or combination of agents in improving the time to and incidence of reperfusion. Reocclusion occurred in 22% of animals in this group compared to 83% in any other group tested. In all groups that received bitistatin, platelet aggregation responses to ADP were inhibited. Platelet inhibition was reflected in a marked prolongation of bleeding time, which, importantly, was reversible within 3 hr of therapy.

Trigramin is a naturally occurring peptide of 72 amino acids purified from the venom of *Trimeresurus granieneus* [32]. Interestingly, it shares homologous sequences with collagen, laminin, and von Willebrand factor and has been shown to antagonize the binding of von Willebrand factor and fibrinogen to glycoprotein IIb/IIIa. The potential for blocking both platelet adhesion and aggregation may prove of clinical value; however, further studies are clearly warranted to test the clinical efficacy of this unique agent.

Monoclonal Antibodies to Glycoprotein IIb/IIIa.   Recently, monoclonal antibodies directed at the IIb/IIIa receptor have been introduced as another means of antagonizing fibrinogen binding and platelet aggregation. These agents are potent inhibitors of platelet aggregation to all agonists. Both 7E3 and 10E5 (two different antibodies that have been most actively studied) abolished periodic thrombus formation and cyclic flow variations and protected against the restoration of these phenomena upon further exposure to platelet agonists or intimal damage [33]. These effects, however, occurred at the expense of marked, irreversible prolongation of bleeding time.

   A trial that examined the effects of 7E3 as an adjunct to thrombolysis with t-PA in canine model of coronary thrombolysis was recently reported [34]. Results revealed more rapid reperfusion and prevention of reocclusion in all dogs treated with the highest dose of 7E3 (0.8 mg/kg) and t-PA (0.45 mg/kg). At successively lower doses of antibody (0.1–0.6 mg/kg), the effects on reocclusion rates were less predictable. Importantly, dogs treated with 7E3 at the higher doses (0.6–0.8 mg/kg) displayed up to fourfold increases in bleeding time. In a similar trial [35], the effects of 7E3 (0.8 mg/kg) were compared with those of aspirin, dipyridamole, and t-PA alone. Reocclusion was prevented in all dogs treated with 7E3. This outcome compared favorably with all other treatment strategies in which reocclusion occurred predictably. The safety of 7E3 when administered in conjunction with t-PA, full-dose heparin, and aspirin was investigated in a study of 10 healthy rhesus monkeys [36]. No untoward effects or evidence of hemorrhage was noted at postmortem analysis, although a relatively low dose of 7E3 was used (0.3 mg/kg). Thus, monoclonal antibodies to glycoprotein IIb/IIIa offer a potent new strategy for platelet inhibition that is, unfortunately, complicated by their profound effects on bleeding time. Future trials may identify an optimal dosing scheme for this potent class of agents.

von Willebrand Factor Inhibitors

The activation of platelets at sites of severe arterial narrowing is probably attributable to several factors, one of which is shear stress. Recent studies have shown that shear stress–induced platelet aggregation is dependent on the presence of large multimers of von Willebrand factor that can bind to platelet glycoproteins Ib(/IX) and IIb/IIIa. The origin of these von Willebrand multimers has been postulated to be (dysfunctional) endothelial cells presumably in the vicinity of atherosclerotic plaque. Interestingly, shear stress–induced platelet aggregation has been shown to occur independent of fibrinogen and arachidonic acid.

   Phillips and co-workers have shown that aurin tricarboxylic acid, a triphenylmethyl dye compound, inhibits von Willebrand–dependent platelet agglutination and adhesion by binding to von Willebrand factor [37]. This binding prevents the interaction between von Willebrand factor and glycoprotein Ib(/IX) and thereby inhibits platelet adhesion. The effect of aurin tricarboxylic acid on platelet-dependent cyclic flow variations in a canine model of coronary stenosis was also recently examined [38]. Aurin tricarboxylic acid produced dose-responsive inhibition of cyclic flow variations in all animals tested without any observed effect on hemodynamics or hemostatic parameters. Thus, antagonists of von Willebrand factor may be useful platelet inhibitors under conditions of high shear.

Ticlopidine

Ticlopidine is a thienopyridine derivative that has been studied extensively in western Europe. It is available in oral form, 80–90% of which is absorbed in the proximal gut with peak plasma levels within 1–3 hr of ingestion. The inhibitory effects of ticlopidine appear approximately 24–48 hr after ingestion of a 500-mg dose, which suggests that metabolites may be active inhibitors of platelet function. Toxicity with ticlopidine includes neutropenia in 1%, gastrointestinal upset in 5%, and skin reactions in 1.9% of patients [39]. Although many clinical trials have demonstrated the platelet inhibitory effect of this compound, its mechanism of action remains unclear. Ticlopidine inhibits primary and secondary platelet aggregation in response to ADP, PAF, and collagen, and some investigators have suggested that it may function as an ADP receptor antagonist. The absence of platelet inhibition in response to arachidonic acid implies that it is acting independent of cyclooxygenase. The combination of aspirin and ticlopidine inhibits platelet aggregation by ADP, collagen, PAF, and arachidonic acid, with a consequent decrease in beta-thromboglobulin, but only at the expense of marked elevation in bleeding times [39].

Thrombin Inhibitors

The exposure of tissue factor in the subendothelial layers activates the coagulation system through the generation of thrombin, which, in addition to converting fibrinogen to fibrin, is an important platelet agonist. Because reocclusion following thrombolysis and angioplasty occurs in up to 30% of patients despite treatment with heparin [40], several new, selective thrombin inhibitors are being evaluated as alternative forms of therapy.

Argatroban, a synthetic, competitive thrombin inhibitor, has been demonstrated to be more potent than heparin in the acceleration of thrombolysis and the prevention of reocclusion [41]. In normal volunteers, argatroban prolonged thrombin times and partial thromboplastin times without any significant effect on bleeding time unless aspirin was administered, as well [42]. Yasuda and colleagues investigated the effects of argatroban compared with those of intravenous aspirin or the monoclonal antibody against the platelet fibrinogen receptor 7E3 in a canine model of thrombosis [43]. Not surprisingly, dogs treated with a combination of the thrombin inhibitor and aspirin had the shortest times to lysis after t-PA and the lowest rate of reocclusion compared to any agent alone. This benefit was associated with threefold, reversible prolongation of template bleeding time, which compared favorably with that of 7E3-treated dogs, in which the bleeding time was markedly and irreversibly prolonged.

Recombinant hirudin is another specific thrombin inhibitor, initially derived from the medicinal leech and more recently available as a recombinant product. Hirudin prevents thrombin (and fibrin) formation by blocking the activation of factors V and VIII and also prevents fibrin stabilization by impairing activation of factor XIII, the cross-linking enzyme. Hirudin also inhibits thromin-induce platelet aggregation. Although clinical data on use of this agent are sparse, one in vivo study demonstrated that hirudin is superior to heparin in reducing the deposition of platelets and fibrinogen at sites of deep arterial injury [44].

D-phenylanalyl-L-prolyl-1-arginyl-chloromethyl ketone (PPACK) is a relatively nonspecific, irreversible serine protease active-site inhibtor which, because it inhibits thrombin, has also been shown to decrease the deposition of platelets and fibrinogen on arterial grafts in animals [45,46]. In contrast to hirudin, however, PPACK's lack of absolute specificity may limit its ultimate use.

Nitrates

Organic nitrates have been one of the mainstays of therapy for unstable coronary syndromes syndromes, although the mechanism(s) by which they exert their beneficial effects remains controversial. It is well known that nitrates relax vascular smooth muscle, producing vasodilatation in coronary, systemic arterial, and venous circulations, thereby decreasing preload and afterload and, as a consequence, myocardial oxygen requirements [47]. Organic nitrates also have potent antiplatelet effects that have been recognized for over 20 years; however, the role that the antithrombotic effects of nitrates play in alleviating myocardial ischemia in unstable coronary syndromes has only recently begun to be appreciated. Organic nitrates have been shown to inhibit platelet aggregation by producing an increase in intracellular cyclic GMP, probably by way of the formation of S-nitrosothiols, which are potent activators of guanylate cyclase [47].

By 1980, the antiplatelet effects of nitroglycerin, nitroprusside, and isosorbide dinitrate were established in in vitro studies by several groups [48,49]. Mellion and colleagues demonstrated that nitric oxide inhibits platelet aggregation in association with an elevation in platelet cyclic GMP [50]. Loscalzo subsequently showed that the sulfhydryl donor N-acetylcysteine potentiates the inhibition of platelet aggregation by nitrates, and that platelet inhibition is preceded by a rise in cyclic GMP [51]. Folts and colleagues [52] have recently shown that organic nitrates inhibit periodic platelet thrombus formation in their canine model of platelet-dependent cyclic flow variations. Thus, there is substantive evidence of an antiplatelet effect of nitrates. The mechanism by which nitrates produce platelet inhibition is dependent on cyclic GMP and is mechanistically similar to that in vascular smooth muscle.

Clinical Data

Although numerous new classes of antiplatelet agents have been introduced in the last 5 years, the clinician's choices remain limited. Data from clinical trials in humans are lacking for most of these agents, and those for which data are available are often controversial. Several clinical trials exist in which the results suggest indisputable benefits of platelet inhibition with aspirin; therefore, aspirin treatment is incorporated into our current standard of routine patient care. Thus, new platelet inhibitors will need to be at least as effective as aspirin prior to gaining acceptance.

Two major trials have documented the beneficial effects of sulfinpyrazone in patients with ischemic heart disease. In the Anturane Reinfarction Trial (ART), a 50% reduction in 1-year cardiac mortality as well as a 75% reduction in sudden death were noted in those taking sulfinpyrazone compared with placebo [53]. These data were reproduced in an Italian cohort (ARIS) [54]. Finally, inasmuch as preliminary data using indobufen, a reversible cyclooxygenase inhibitor, as an antiplatelet agent in patients undergoing coronary bypass surgery are promising when compared with aspirin therapy [55], the utility of efficacy and safety of reversible inhibition of cyclooxygenase should be addressed in acute coronary syndromes.

Several trials exist in which the data demonstrate a beneficial effect of prostacyclin analogs, but one of insufficient magnitude to alter our therapeutic approach at this time. Also, use of these agents has been limited by nausea and systemic hypotension [56–58]. Sharma and colleagues examined the effects of prostaglandin E_1 in combination with intracoronary streptokinase in 14 patients with acute myocardial infarction [57]. The results demonstrated improvement in the rate of and time to reperfusion. In addition, the dose of streptokinase needed to produce reperfusion was lower in the PGE_1-treated patients. Thus, PGE_1 is a potentially effective antiplatelet agent and the widespread use of which will depend on further randomized investigation. Topol et al. [58] studied the intravenous combination of rt-PA and Iloprost in 25 patients. Compared with rt-PA alone, combination therapy did not improve infarct artery patency or left ventricular function.

Similarly, the monoclonal antibody inhibitor of the platelet fibrinogen glycoprotein IIb/IIIa receptor 7E3 has not been fully evaluated on a clinical level at this time. Recently, Gold and colleagues reported phase I human trial data of this monoclonal antibody in 16 patients with unstable angina [59]. Preliminary data revealed that 7E3 produced dose-dependent prolongation of bleeding time and near-complete inhibition of platelet aggregation to ADP that persisted for up to 72 hr. These effects apparently correlated with angina-free periods. In addition, platelet counts decreased almost 20% without evidence of any hemorrhagic episodes. Clearly, further studies will be necessary to characterize the dose-response relationships in humans and the effects of 7E3 on hemostatic parameters when combined with existing treatment strategies (aspirin and thrombolytic therapy). Although potentially beneficial effects have been ascribed to dipyridamole, an independent, positive clinical effect has never been documented. Two major studies have investigated the efficacy of dipyridamole in the secondary prevention of acute myocardial infarction. In the PARIS I study, 2026 patients who had survived a myocardial infarction were randomized to aspirin plus dipyridamole, aspirin alone, or placebo [60]. The results after 41 months follow-up revealed no statistical difference in event rates between the treatment groups. In the PARIS-II trial [61], aspirin plus dipyridamole therapy resulted in a 24% reduction in coronary events compared to placebo. Thus, the current data do not support the use of dipyridamole as a useful antiplatelet agent in ischemic heart disease.

Few clinical trials have addressed the use of ticlopidine in unstable coronary syndromes [62,63]. In the largest trial [63], 652 patients with unstable angina were randomized to receive conventional therapy with nitrates, beta-blockers, and calcium blockers, or with ticlopidine, 500 mg/day, plus conventional therapy. After a 6-month follow-up, a 46% risk reduction of vascular death and nonfatal myocardial infarction was noted for patients treated with ticlopidine; however, despite these promising findings, it is important to note that at the time of this trial patients with unstable angina were not routinely treated with aspirin. Another study examined the use of ticlopidine in 43 patients with acute myocardial infarction [62]. Platelet survival times were decreased in patients treated with placebo compared to those taking ticlopidine; however, owing to the very small sample size, no definitive statement could be made regarding event rates.

Two large clinical trials were designed to investigate the role of ticlopidine in patients with transient ischemic attack and stroke [64,65]. The results demonstrated modest improvement in event rates when compared with aspirin or placebo therapy. These studies provided the impetus for further investigations with ticlopidine in patients with unstable coronary syndromes.

The clinical effects of nitrates in patients with unstable coronary syndromes have been well documented; however, few trials mention the antiplatelet properties that may have contributed to the observed clinical results. In vitro and in vivo studies have demonstrated the platelet inhibitory effect of organic nitrate compounds, but this effect had not been confirmed in patients until recently. DeCaterina and colleagues first demonstrated the antiplatelet effects of isosorbide dinitrate in 22 healthy volunteers [66]. Diodati and colleagues demonstrated that intravenous nitroglycerin in therapeutic doses inhibited platelets in patients with unstable angina and acute myocardial infarction [67]. Hackett and colleagues observed that intermittent coronary occlusion occurs frequently in patients early in the course of myocardial infarction [68]. The administration of intracoronary isosorbide dinitrate during arteriography restored coronary artery patency. The authors postulate that a mechanism involving vasospasm superimposed on the culprit lysing thrombus to explain the prompt relief of reocclusion induced by nitrates. None of the observed effects were attributed to an antiplatelet effect of nitrates. However, in retrospect, it seems plausible that at least part of the effect was mediated by the inhibition of platelet-dependent cyclic flow variations by nitrates. Finally, Yusuf and colleagues reported an analysis of 10 trials that investigated the role of intravenous nitrates on mortality in acute myocardial infarction [69]. Taken together, a 35% reduction in mortality could be attributed to the use of nitrates. In light of previous survival data with other antiplatelet agents, it would not be surprising if this improvement in mortality were entirely the result of the antiplatelet effects of nitrates. However, without direct evidence for this mechanism, one can only assume that both the vasodilatory and platelet inhibitory actions of nitrates may equally contribute to the observed clinical response.

CONCLUSION

The role of platelets in the pathophysiology of unstable angina and AMI has been established. Aspirin and thrombolytic therapy are now part of standard care in AMI, providing documented improvement in patient survival. However, in response to thrombolysis, activation of platelets may attenuate the lytic response and induce reocclusion. Thus, current studies have focused on the development of more potent and selective antiplatelet agents to be used alone or adjunctively in the treatment of acute coronary syndromes.

Although numerous agents of virtually every possible mechanistic class have been introduced recently, very few are currently being tested in human clinical trials. Cyclooxygenase inhibitors, clearly the most studied of all antiplatelet agents, have documented efficacy in treating unstable coronary syndromes. Preliminary data suggest that reversibility of platelet inhibition may be desirable, but this remains inadequately studied. Prostacyclin analogs inhibit platelet aggregation and produce vasodilatation. Early trials raise the possibility that their use in conjunction with thrombolytic therapy may not be beneficial. Both thromboxane A2 antagonists and thromboxane synthestase inhibitors improve time to lysis and decrease reocclusion rates after thrombolytic therapy, while thromboxane synthetase inhibitors also allow prostanoid endoperoxides to be shunted to the synthesis of prostacyclin. The clinical benefit of this mechanism is as yet unproven. Phosphodiesterase inhibitors exert numerous experimental effects on platelet function, which have not translated into a positive clinical response. Serotonin receptor antagonists have not been studied extensively in human trials, but their nonselective nature and their potential for systemic side effects limit their use.

Fibrinogen receptor antagonists, including the reversible RGD-containing peptides and irreversible monoclonal antibodies to the IIb/IIIa receptor, enhance time to lysis and decrease rates of reocclusion at the expense of elevated bleeding times. Clinical trials in conjunction with aspirin and thrombolytic agents will need to assess the hemorrhagic risk involved with varying doses of these potent agents. Aurin tricarboxylic acid inhibits platelet adhesion and aggregation at sites of high shear rate without any adverse effects identified as yet in early animal trials. Ticlopidine may be useful antiplatelet agent; however, data from previous trials thus far published are not useful in our assessment of this agent because these studies were performed prior to the routine use of aspirin. Selective thrombin inhibitors inhibit platelet aggregation, improves rates of lysis and reocclusion when combined with aspirin, and may decrease the deposition of fibrinogen and platelets at sites of arterial injury. Finally, nitrates exert both vasodilatory and platelet inhibitory effects mediated by increases in cyclic GMP. The precise contribution of each mechanism to be observed clinical response is still controversial. Clearly, many more clinical trials are needed to increase our understanding of the most relevant mechanism(s) of platelet inhibition so that we may develop an agent or group of agents with optimal clinical actions and minimal adverse effects.

ACKNOWLEDGMENTS

This work was supported in part by NIH grants HL40411 and HL43344, by a National Grant-in-Aid from the American Heart Association with funds contributed in part by the Massachusetts Affiliate, and by a Merit Review Award from the U.S. Veterans Administration. Dr. Loscalzo is the recipient of a Research Career Development Award from the National Institutes of Health (KO4 HL02273). Dr. Ezratty is a cardiology fellow at the Brigham and Women's Hospital.

REFERENCES

1. Haerem JD. Platelet aggregates in intramyocardial vessels of patients dying suddenly and unexpectedly of coronary artery disease. Atherosclerosis 1972; 15:199-213.
2. Elwood PC, Cochrane AL, Burr ML, Sweetman PM, Williams G, Welsby E, Hughes SJ, Renton R. A randomized controlled trial of acetylsalicylic acid in the secondary prevention of mortality from myocardial infarction. Br Med J 1974; 1:436-40.
3. Davies MJ, Thomas AC, Knapman PA, Hangartner R. Intramyocardial platelet aggregation in patients with unstable angina suffering sudden ischemic cardiac death. Circulation 1986; 73:418-27.
4. Davies MJ. A macro and micro view of coronary vascular insult in ischemic heart disease. Circulation 1990; (Suppl. II):II-38-46.
5. Ambrose JA, Winters S, Stern A, Eng A, Teicholz LE, Gorlin R, Fuster V. Angiographic morphology and pathogenesis of unstable angina. J Am Coll Cardiol. 1985; 5: 629-38.

6. Sherman CT, Litvack F, Grundfest W, Lee M, Hickey A, Chaux A, Kass R, Blanche C, Matloff J, Morgenstern L, Ganz W, Swan H, Forrester J. Coronary angioscopy in patients with unstable angina pectoris. N Engl J Med 1986; 315:913-19.

7. The Steering Committee of the Physicians' Health Study Research Group. Preliminary report: findings from the aspirin component of the ongoing Physicians Health Study. N Engl J Med 1988; 318:262-4.

8. Lewis HD, Davis JW, Archibald DG, Steinke W, Smitherman T, Doherty J. Protective effects of aspirin against acute myocardial infarction and death in men with unstable angina. N Engl J Med 1983; 309:396-403.

9. Cairns JA, Gent M, Singer J, Finnie K, Frogalt G, Hoder D, Jablonsky G, Kostuk W, Melendez L, Myers M, Sackett D, Sealey B, Tanser P. Aspirin, sulfinpyrazone or both in unstable angina. Results of a Canadian multicenter trial. N Engl J Med 1986 312: 1369-75.

10. Theroux P, Ouimet H, McCans J, Latour J, Joly P, Levy G, Pelletier E, Pharm B, Juneau M, Stasiak J, DeGuise P, Pelletier G, Rinzler D, Pharm B, Waters D. Aspirin, heparin or both to treat acute unstable angina. N Engl J Med 1988; 319:1105-11.

11. Antiplatelet Trialists Collaboration. Secondary prevention of vascular disease by prolonged antiplatelet treatment. Br Med J 1988; 296:213-19.

12. Loscalzo J. The role of platelets in thrombolysis. J Vasc Med Biol 1989; 1:213-9.

13. Lefer AM, Ogletree ML, Smith JB. Prostacyclin: a potentially valuable agent for preserving myocardial tissue in acute myocardial ischemia. Science 1978; 200:52-4.

14. Melin JA, Becker LC. Salvage of ischemic myocardium by prostacyclin during experimental myocardial infarction. J Am Coll Cardiol 1983; 2:279-88.

15. Nicolini FA, Mehta JL, Nichols WW, Saldeen T, Grant M. Prostacyclin analogue iloprost decreases thrombolytic potential of tissue-type plasminogen activator in canine coronary thrombosis. Circulation 1990; 81:1115-22.

16. Hassan S, Pickles H. Epoprostenol (prostacyclin, PGl_2) increases apparent liver blood flow in man. Prostaglandins Leikotrienes Med 1983; 10:449-54.

17. Fitzgerald DJ, Catella F, Roy F, FirzGerald G. Marked platelet activation in vivo after intravenous streptokinase in patients with acute myocardial infarction. Circulation 1988; 77:142-50.

18. Shebuski RJ, Smith JM, Storer BL, Granett J, Bugelski P. Influence of selective endoperoxide/thromboxane A_2 receptor antagonist, with sulatroban on lysis time and reocclusion rate after tissue plasminogen activator-induced coronary thrombolysis in the dog. J Pharmacol Exp Ther 1988; 246:790-6.

19. Ashton JH, Ogletree ML, Michel IM, Golino P, McNatt J, Taylor A, Raheja S, Schmitz J, Buja L, Campbell W, Willerson J. Cooperative mediation of serotonin S_2 and thromboxane A_2. Prostaglandin H2 receptor activation of cyclic flow variations in dogs with severe coronary artery stenosis. Circulation 1987; 76:952-60.

20. MacNab MW, Foltz EL, Graves BS, Rinehart RK, Tripp SL, Feliciano NR, Sen S. The effects of a new thromboxane synthetase inhibitor, CGS 13080, in man. J Clin Pharm 1984; 24:76-83.

21. Mickelson JK, Simpson PJ, Mennen TG, Gallas G, Lucchesi B. Thromboxane synthetase inhibition with CGS 13080 improves coronary blood flow after streptodinase-induced thrombolysis. Am Heart J 1987; 113:1345-52.

22. Fitzgerald DA. Dipyridamole. N Engl J Med 1987; 316:1247-56.

23. Declerck F, Xhonneux B, Leysen J, Janssen P. Evidence for function 5-HT2 receptor sites on human blood platelets. Biochem Pharm 1984; 33:2807-11.

24. Bevan J, Heptinstall S. Effects of combinations of 5-hydroxytryptamine receptor antagonists on 5-HT-induced human platelet aggregation. Arch Pharm 1986; 334: 341-5.

25. Folts JD, Gallagher K, Rowe GG. Blood flow reductions in stenosed canine coronary arteries: vasospasm or platelet aggregation? Circulation 1982; 65:248-56.

26. Glusa E, Bevon J, Heptinstall S. Verapamil is a potent inhibitor of 5-HT-induced platelet aggregation. Thromb Res 1989; 55:239-45.

27. Ashton JH, Benedict CR, Fitzgerald C, Raheja S, Taylor A, Campbell W, Buja L, Willerson J. Serotonin as a mediator of cyclic flow variations in stenosed coronary arteries. Circulation 1988; 78:701-11.

28. Golino P, Buja LM, Ashton JH, Kulkarni P, Taylor A, Willerson J. Effect of thromboxane and serotonin receptor antagonists on intracoronary platelet deposition in dogs with experimentally stenosed canine coronary arteries. Circulation 1986; 73: 572-78.

29. Gan ZR, Gould RJ, Jacobs JW, Friedman P, Polokoff M. A potent platelet aggregation inhibitor from the venom of the viper, *Echis carinatus*. J Biol Chem 1988; 263: 19827-32.

30. Shebuski RJ, Ramjit DR, Bencen GH, Polokoff M. Characterization and platelet inhibitory activity of bitistatin, a potent RGD containing peptide from the viper, *Bitis arietans*. J Biol Chem 1989; 264:21550-6.

31. Shebuski RJ, Stabilito IJ, Sitko GR. Acceleration of recombinant tissue-type plasminogen activator-induced thrombolysis and prevention of reocclusion by the combination of heparin and the Arg-Gly-ASP containing peptide bitistatin in a canine model of coronary thrombosis. Circulation 1990; 82:169-77.

32. Huang T, Holt JC, Kirby EP, Niewiarowski S. Trigramin: Primary structure and its inhibition of von Willebrand factor binding to glycoprotein IIb/IIIa complex on human platelets. Biochem 1989; 28:661-6.

33 Coller B, Folts JD, Smith SR, Scudder L, Jordon R. Abolition of in vivo platelet thrombus formation in primates with monoclonal antibodies to the platelet GP IIb / IIIa antibody in a canine preparation. Circulation 1988; 77:1766-74.

34. Gold HK, Coller BS, Yasuda T, Saito T, Fallon J, Guerrero L, Leinbach R, Ziskind A, Collen D. Rapid and sustained coronary artery recanalization with combined bolus injection of recombinant tissue-type plasminogen activator and monoclonal antiplatelet GP IIb/IIIa antibody in a canine preparation. Circulation 1988 77:670-7.

35. Yasuda T, Gold HK, Fallon JT, Leinbach R, Guerrero J, Scudder L, Kanke M, Shealy D, Ross M, Collen D, Coller B. Monoclonal antibody against the platelet glycoprotein IIb/IIIa receptor prevents coronary artery reocclusion after perfusion with recombinant tissue-type plasminogen activator in dogs. J Clin Invest 1988; 81:1284-91.

36. Iuliucci FD, Treacy G, Cornell S, Berger HF. Potent anti-thrombotic activity and safety of antiplatelet monoclonal antibody 7E3 Fab combined with thrombolytic and anticoagulant drugs. Circulation 1990; 82:III-602.

37. Phillips MD, Moake JL, Nolasco L, Turner N. Aurin tricarboxylic acid: a novel inhibi-

tor of the association of von Willebrand factor and platelets. Blood 1988; 72: 1898-1903.

38. Strony J, Phillips M, Brands D, Moake J, Adelman B. Aurin tricarboxylic acid in a canine model of coronary artery thrombosis. Circulation 1990; 81:1106-14.

39. Saltiel E, Ward A. Ticlopidine, a review of its pharmacodynamic and pharmacokinetic properties, and therapeutic efficacy in platelet-dependent disease states. Drugs 1987; 34:222-62.

40. Topol EJ, Morris DC, Smalling RW, Schumacher RR, Taylor CR, Nishikawa A, Lieberman HA, Collen D, Tufte ME, Grossbard EB. A multicenter, randomized placebo controlled trial of a new form of intravenous recombinant tissue-type plasminogen activator in acute myocardial infarction. J Am Coll Cardiol 1987; 9: 1205-13.

41. Jang IK, Gold HK, Ziskind AA, Leinback R, Fallon J, Collen D. Prevention of platelet-rich arterial thrombosis by selective thrombin inhibition. Circulation 1990; 81: 219-25.

42. Clarke R, Fitzgerald DJ. The human pharmacology of argatroban, a specific thrombin inhibitor. Circulation 1990; 82(4):III-603, 2394 (abstract).

43. Yasuda T, Gold HK, Yaoita H, Leinbach R, Guerrero J, Jang I, Holt R, Fallon J, Collen D. Comparative effects of aspirin, a synthetic inhibitor and a monoclonal antiplatelet glycoprotein IIb/IIIa antibody on coronary artery reperfusion, reocclusion and bleeding with recombinant tissue-type plasminogen activator in a canine preparation. J Am Coll Cardiol 1990; 16:714-24.

44. Heras M, Chesebro JH, Penny WJ, Bailey K, Badimon L, Fuster V. Effects of thrombin inhibition on the development of acute platelet thrombus deposition during angioplasty in pigs. Heparin versus recombinant hirudin, a specific thrombin inhibitor. Circulation 1989; 79:657-65.

45. Greco NJ, Tenner TE, Narendra TN, Jamieson GA. PPACK-thrombin inhibits thrombin-induced platelet aggregation and cytoplasmic acidification but does not inhibit platelet shape change. Blood 1990; 75:1983-90.

46. Hanson SR, Harker LA. Interruption of acute platelet dependent thrombosis by the synthetic antithrombin D-phenylalany-L-prolyl-L-arginyl chloromethylketone. Proc Natl Acad Sci USA 1988; 85:3184.

47. Ignarro LJ, Lippton H, Edwards J, Baricos W, Lyman A, Kadowitz P. Mechanisms of vascular smooth muscle relaxation by organic nitrates, nitrites, nitroprussides, and nitric oxide: evidence for the involvement of S-nitrosothiols as activator intermediates. J Pharm Exp Ther 1981; 218:739-41.

48. Gerzer R, Karrenbroke B, Siess W, Hiem JM. Direct comparison of the effects of nitroprusside, sin 1, and various nitrates in platelet aggregation and soluble guanylate cyclase activity. Throm Res 1988; 52:11-21.

49. Gruetter CA, Gruetter DY, Lyon JE, Kadowitz PJ, Ignarro LJ. Relationship between cyclic guanosine 3'-5' monophosphate formation and relaxation of coronary arterial smooth muscle by glyceryl trinitrate, nitroprusside, nitrite and nitric oxide: effects of methylene blue and methemoglobin. J Pharm Exp Ther 1981; 219:181-6.

50. Mellion BT, Ignarro LJ, Myers CB, Ohlstein EH, Ballot BA. Inhibition of platelet aggregation by S-nitrosothiols. Heme-dependent activation of soluble guanylate cyclase and stimulation of cyclic GMP accumulation. Mol Pharm 1983; 23:653-64.

51. Loscalzo J. *N*-acetylcysteine potentiates inhibition of platelet aggregation by nitroglycerin. J Clin Invest 1985; 76:703–8.
52. Folts JD, Stamler J, Loscalzo L. *N*-acetylcysteine potentiates IV nitroglycerin in inhibitory periodic platelet thrombus formation in stenosed dog coronary arteries. J Am Coll Cardiol 1989; 13:145a.
53. The Anturane Reinfarction Trial Research Group. Sulfinpyrazone in the prevention of cardiac death after myocardial infarction: the Anturane Reinfarction Trial. N Engl J Med 1978; 298:289–95.
54. The Anturane Reinfarction Trial Research Group. Sulfinpyrazone in the prevention of sudden death after myocardial infarction. N Engl J Med 1988; 302:5, 250–6.
55. Rovelli F, Campolo L, Cataldo G, deGaetano G, Lavezzari M, Mannucci PM, Marubini E, Montoro C, Orzan F, Pellegrini A. Indobufen versus aspirin plus dipyridamole after coronary artery bypass surgery. Effects on patency one year after surgery. Circulation 1990; 82:III-507.
56. Swedberg K, Held P, Wadenvik H, Kutti J. Central hemodynamic and antiplatelet effects of Iloprost—a new prostacyclin analogue—in acute myocardial infarction in man. Eur Heart J 1987; 8:362–8.
57. Sharma B, Wyeth RP, Gimenez HJ, Franciosa J. Intracoronary prostaglandin E_1 plus streptoinanse in acute myocardial infarction. Am J Cardiol 1986; 58:1161–6.
58. Topol EJ, Ellis S, Califf RM, George BS, Stump DC, Bates ER, Nabel EG, Walton JR, Candela RJ, Leek L, Kline EM, Pitt B. Combined tissue-type plasminogen actirator and prostacyclin therapy for acute myocardial infarction. J Am Coll Cardiol 14: 877–84.
59. Gold HK, Gimple LW, Yasuda T, Leinbach RS, Werner W, Holt R, Jordan R, Berper H, Collen D, Coller BS. Pharmacodynamic study of F(ab)₂ fragments of murine-monodonal antibody 7E3 directed against human platelet glycoprotein IIb/IIIa in patients with unstable angina pectosis. J Clin Invest 1990; 86:651–9.
60. The Persantine-Aspirin Reinfarction Study Research Group. Persantine and aspirin in coronary heart disease. Circulation 1980; 62:449–61.
61. Klimt CR, Knatterud GL, Stamler J, Meier P. Persantine-aspirin reinfarction study. Part II. Secondary coronary prevention with persantine and aspirin. J Am Coll Cardiol 1986; 7:251–69.
62. Knudson J, Kjoller E, Skagen K, Gormsen J. The effect of ticlopidine on platelet functions in acute myocardial infarction, a double blind controlled trial. Thrombo Hemost 1985; 53:332–6.
63. Balsano F, Rizzon P, Violi F, Scrutinio D, Cimminiello C, Aguglia F, Pasotti C, Ruddelli G, and the Studio della Ticlopidina nell'Angina Instable Group. Antiplatelet treatment with ticlopidine in unstabe angina, a controlled multicenter clinical trial. Circulation 1990; 82:17–26.
64. Gent M, Easton DJ, Hachiniski VC, Panak E, Sicurella J, Blakely J, Ellis D, Harbison J, Roberts R, Turpie A. The Canadian American Ticlopidine Study in thromboembolic stroke. Lancet 1989; 2:1215–20.
65. Haas WK, Easton DJ, Adams HP, Pryse-Phillips W, Malony B, Anderson S, Kamm B for the ticlopidine Aspirin Stroke Study Group. A randomized trial comparing ticlopi-

dine with aspirin for the prevention of stroke in high risk patients. N Engl J Med 1989; 321:501-7.

66. DeCaterina R, Giannessi D, Crea F, Chierchia S, Bernini W, Gazzetti P, L'Abatte A. Inhibition of platelet function by injectable isosorbide dinitrate. Am J Cardiol 1984; 53:1683-7.

67. Diodati J, Theroux P, Latour JG, LaCoste L, Lam JT, Waters D. Effects of nitroglycerin at therapeutic doses on platelet aggregation in unstable angina pectoris and acute MI. Am J Cardiol 1990; 66:683-8.

68. Hackett D, Davies G, Chierchia S, Maseri A. Intermittent coronary occlusion in acute MI. Value of combined thrombolytic and vasodilator therapy. N Engl J Med 1987; 317(17):1055-9.

69. Yusuf S, MacMahon S, Collins L, Peto R. Effect of intravenous nitrates on mortality in MI: an overview of the randomized trials. Lancet 1988; 1088-92.

10

The Role of Heparin in the Management of Acute Myocardial Infarction

Allan M. Ross

George Washington University, Washington, D.C.

INTRODUCTION

Our understanding of the role of heparin in the treatment of acute myocardial infarction has, over the past decades, gone through similar gyrations as has that of other agents active in the coagulation-thrombolysis-anticoagulation scheme (i.e., warfarin, plasminogen activators, and antiplatelets). These gyrations are accounted for by the erroneous transient discounting of the major role of thrombus in atherosclerotic heart disease, and specifically in acute myocardial infarction, on the basis of limited autopsy information tabulated in the 1960s (1).

Persistent investigators who reconfirmed the central role of thrombosis (2,3) redirected interest in all coagulation system active agents, including, of course, heparin. This potent anticoagulant obviously got its name from the liver, owing to the fact that the first crude extracts of the substance came from that organ (and cardiac tissue as well), having been identified by a medical student (McLean) working in the laboratory of Howell in Baltimore in 1915 (4). Although it clearly exists naturally in humans, the minute heparin circulating levels appreciable are of uncertain importance in maintaining coagulation homeostasis in health. Heparin is actually a family of compounds of varying molecular weights whose anticoagulant properties are due to their strong electronegative charge.

When administered in pharmacological doses, heparin complexes with natively occurring antithrombin-3 (AT-III), which then binds and inactivates thrombin. Additionally, heparin exerts anticoagulant activity by inhibiting the activation of thromboplastin.

The route of administration and dose of heparin powerfully affect its efficiency as an anticoagulant by laboratory measurement (e.g., partial thromboplastin time, PTT, or activated clotting time, ACT). Heparin is by no means bound exclusively to AT-III. Other binding sites exist, particularly on vascular endothelial cells and some white blood cells. Heparin bound to these other receptors produces no anticoagulant effects. When a large bolus of the agent is administered via the intravenous route, followed by a continuous infusion, the nonanticoagulant receptors quickly become saturated and additional molecules accomplish the intended pharmacological effect of enhancing AT-III activity, which in turn leads to inactivation of thrombin. Heparin in such a circumstance has a substantial half-life, approximately 30–60 min, with ultimate clearance being renal.

In marked contrast, low-dose heparin, specifically slowly released heparin, as occurs if the agent is given subcutaneously, results in extensive extraction by the saturable endothelial cell clearance mechanism; achieved heparin blood concentrations are low and measures of anticoagulation demonstrate subtherapeutic levels (5) in a majority of patients even when doses of 12,500–15,000 units are given subcutaneously twice daily (6). Furthermore, when the subcutaneous route is selected, even in the minority of patients who achieve therapeutic PTT values (1 1/2 to 2× control), this effect is slow to occur, taking many hours (7).

As an antithrombin potentiator, heparin acts predominantly by preventing new or recurrent clot formation, having little effect on existing thrombus. Inhibition of clinically evident new thrombosis correlates strongly with the degree to which PTT is rendered prolonged. This relationship of heparin's measured anticoagulant adequacy to the frequency of adverse thromboembolic endpoints has been carefully examined. Basu et al. (8), in an attempt to prevent recurrence of deep-vein thrombosis and embolism, heparinized 157 patients. In 90 of these, PTT was prolonged to >50 sec, and none suffered recurrence, whereas among patients in the subtherapeutic range, recurrence was seen in 8%.

In a confirmatory trial of heparin to prevent second episodes of venous thromboembolism, Hull et al. (6) observed recurrence in 25% of 53 patients whose heparin dose was insufficient to prolong the PTT to 1.5 times control, but in only 2% (1 of 62 patients) with therapeutic levels of anticoagulation (Fig. 1).

These reports demonstrate a considerably greater need for PTT prolongation to avoid recurrences than appears to be necessary as primary prophylaxis against venous thrombosis de novo, since trials in general surgical or orthopedic surgery patients show substantially reduced thrombosis incidence with less intensive therapy (i.e., 3500–5000 units subcutaneously every 8 or 12 hr) (9). This variable dose requirement in different settings fits well with the observation that already existing thrombus exerts a powerful prothrombotic influence. As will be discussed

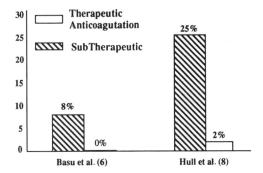

Figure 1   The importance of fully therapeutic (1 1/2 to 2× control PTT) heparin anticoagulation on prevention of recurrent thromboembolism.

subsequently, thrombin released during clot lysis is a particularly strong procoagulant stimulant.

HEPARIN TREATMENT OF MYOCARDIAL INFARCTION

Published information on this topic falls into three broad categories: (a) early studies of heparin after myocardial infarction to lower all causes of morbidity and mortality, (b) heparin in the treatment or prevention of left ventricular mural thrombosis, and (c) the recent studies of heparin adjunctive to thrombolytic therapy to prevent reocclusion/reinfarction.

Early Heparin Studies

The studies of heparin after myocardial infarction in the prethrombolytic era, in retrospect, were probably undersized to show significant benefit. Presumably this treatment's mechanisms of action (as monotherapy) would be: reduction in rethrombosis–reinfarction after spontaneous lysis; reduced clot propagation and consequently reduced infarct extension; and less pulmonary and systemic thromboembolic morbidity and mortality. As these endpoints are less numerous than the rate of reclosure and reinfarction after plasminogen activator therapy, the sample size of published investigations allows for a very large beta error.

The Medical Research Council (10) trial of nearly 1500 patients showed a 16% reduction, in heparin-treated patients, of combined mortality and reinfarction compared with controls (31% versus 26%). This difference was not statistically significant, although reductions by two-thirds of pulmonary embolism and one-half of strokes was significant.

Initial intravenous heparin followed by high-dose subcutaneous administration was investigated in a 1136-patient placebo-controlled trial at the Bronx Municipal Hospital (11). Modest reductions were seen among treated patients in mortality (21% versus 15%, a 28% decline), reinfarction, pulmonary embolism, and stroke, but none of statistically significant magnitude. Finally, the smallest of these early studies, the Veterans Administration Cooperative Study (12) of 999 men, showed similar trends in favor of heparin in all the above-mentioned endpoints. It is of some interest to note that the magnitude of benefit for early post–myocardial infarction heparin therapy in these reports is highly analogous to the favorable results with aspirin alone, described decades later by the International Study of Infarct Survival (ISIS-2) investigators (13); i.e., heparin reduced mortality by 20–25% even when given without a plasminogen activator.

Heparin to Prevent Left Ventricular Mural Thrombus After Myocardial Infarction

Development of a mural thrombus detectable by echo cardiography is a well-recognized complication of infarction, particularly anterior infarction of sufficient magnitude to effect substantial apical contractile dysfunction or frank aneurysm. Numerous studies have been undertaken to define the frequency of this complication and/or to assess the impact of anticoagulant prophylaxis. Several smaller studies (30–60 patients) describe an ambient incidence of mural thrombus of 25–50% and a variably successful reduction in this rate with diverse heparin (and warfarin) regimens (14–16).

Two large studies are considerably instructive on the issue, the Studio Sulla Calciparina Nell'Angina e Nella Trombosi Ventricolare Nell'Infarto (SCATI) study (17) of 200 patients and the report by Turpie et al. on 221 patients (7). The SCATI protocol randomized acute anterior wall myocardial infarction patients presenting for treatment within 24 hr of infarct pain onset to heparin therapy or to the control group. Heparin was administered starting as an immediate intravenous bolus of 2000 units followed by subcutaneous heparin, 12,500 units 9 hr later and every 12 hr thereafter until hospital discharge. Additionally, patients arriving early (within 6 hr of pain onset) received thrombolytic therapy (streptokinase) whereas those beyond 6 hr from the start of pain were not given a plasminogen activator. The endpoint was left ventricular mural thrombus detected by 2-D echo gram at the time of hospital discharge. In the heparin group the incidence was 17.7% (19/107) versus 36.6% (34/93) in the controls ($p < 0.01$).

The study by Turpie and his associates compared (by random assignment) the efficacy of high-dose (12,500 units every 12 hr) versus low-dose (5000 units every 12 hr) heparin for 10 days in attempted prophylaxis against mural thrombi in acute anterior myocardial infarction patients. Thrombus was identified by echo on the 10th postinfarction day and was found in 10 of 95 (11%) high-dose heparin patients compared with 28 of 88 (32%) treated with the lower-dose heparin regimen ($p < 0.001$).

A supportable conclusion from these reports would be that heparin anticoagulation is effective in reducing intracavitary thrombosis and that this efficacy appears to increase with higher doses.

Heparin as an Adjunct to Thrombolytic Therapy

In the 1990s considerable controversy has been generated regarding the use of heparin to prevent rethrombosis after reperfusion. Actually, the frequency of rethrombosis has been imprecisely quantified. It has been well established, however, that powerful stimuli for recurrent thrombosis exist locally when a coronary thrombus undergoes dissolution. Obviously, one reason is that the underlying cause of the initial occlusion, i.e., a flow-limiting stenosis and ruptured plaque cap which stimulated thrombosis originally, is not affected by the plasminogen activators. Of perhaps equal importance is the observation that lysis per se is a stimulant for new clot formation. Studies by Owen et al. (18) and Gulba et al. (19) established that administering any of the plasminogen activators results in a rise of circulating fibrinopeptide A (released when fibrinogen is converted to fibrin). The mechanism has in part been worked out and is explained by the pivotal role of thrombin. At the time of an initial clot formation, excess thrombin is bound within the accumulating thrombus. When local plasmin concentration (intrinsic or pharmacologically induced) acts to dissolve that thrombus, entrapped excess thrombin is released to catalyze a new round of fibrinogen to fibrin conversion, and to activate circulating platelets as well. It might, therefore, be expected that the greatest risk of postlytic reocclusion might exist rather early after coronary patency is first restored.

Such a temporal pattern has now been observed. From a qualitative point of view, angiographic observations (20) have shown cyclical patterns of clot lysis and clot formation soon after administration of effective activators. The early events are schematized in Figure 2. Lysis and rethrombosis are occurring simultaneously. If the rate of the former predominates (as in this example), patency is restored and persists. Alternatively, in up to 20% of patients, immediate rethrombosis factors predominate and persistent patency is not achieved.

The actual frequency of transient reperfusion followed by immediate or subsequent reocclusion in plasminogen activator-treated myocardial infarction patients is not specifically known. A wide range has been reported from 0 to nearly 50% (21-27). To fully characterize this phenomenon, one would need, in a cohort of several hundred patients, to perform an extended sequence of posttreatment follow-up angiograms. Figure 3 describes the patency status of seven hypothetical infarct patients treated with a plasminogen activator. The patency status is in constant flux, with vessels opening, closing, and reopening across a given time span.

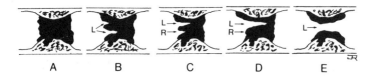

Figure 2   The initial stages of thrombolysis are characterized by competing forces of lysis (L) and rethrombosis (R). Local rethrombosis is stimulated by release of thrombin from dissolving clot plus the underlying obstruction, placque cap rupture, stasis, etc. In this hypothetical example, lysis overshadows rethrombosis and patency is restored.

Typical clinical trials require an angiogram only once or twice in such a period and, therefore, provide a snapshot of only one of two points of an active continuum. Furthermore, the activator dosing and, importantly, the adjunctive anticoagulant regimen employed strongly influence the phenomena observed.

Perhaps the most enlightening clinical description of reocclusion, its timing and its endpoint impact, is the recently published summary from the series of Thrombolysis and Angioplasty in Myocardial Infarction (TAMI) trials. Ohman et al. (28) reported on 810 patients who had 90-minute angiograms and a follow-up study either for recurrent signs and symptoms or routinely prior to discharge. The overall reocclusion rate in this cohort treated with different activators and heparin regimens was 12%. Importantly, the peak frequency of reclosure was very early,

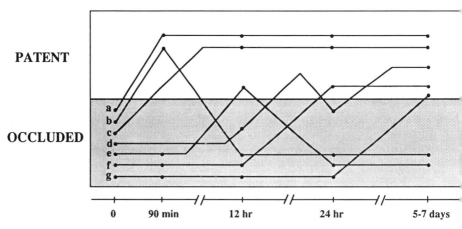

Figure 3   Patency is not an all-or-none phenomenon. Rather it is a continuum of reperfusion and reocclusion over time as schematized by seven hypothetical patients (a-f). Angiography at only one point in time inadequately characterizes the outcome of therapy.

i.e., in the first postthrombolysis day. Patients who had reocclusion had a nearly threefold higher in-hospital mortality rate compared with those whose coronary patency persisted (11% versus 4%; $p < 0.01$).

Given the role of thrombin in the reocclusion process, the antithrombin heparin has been used empirically from the beginning of the current "thrombolytic era." In reports from most North American reperfusion experiences, heparinization has been by intravenous bolus followed by continuous intravenous infusion. Clinicians have reported a correlation between anticoagulation adequacy and the likelihood of recurrent ischemic symptoms after thrombolysis. In a study by Kaplan et al. (29), the frequency of poststreptokinase recurrent ischemia was shown to correlate strongly with inadequate heparinization. Recurrent events, presumably indicative of rethrombosis, occurred up to 4 times more often in patients with a subtherapeutic PTT than in those with fully effective heparinization.

Clinicians and clinical investigators in Europe have not widely adopted treatment strategies incorporating full and early intravenous anticoagulation. Specifically, the results of the important ISIS–2 trial (13) encouraged the notion that antiplatelet therapy with aspirin might be adequate postlytic management, since, in that trial, 160 mg of aspirin (ASA) (as monotherapy) reduced 5-week mortality as much as streptokinase (SK) did, and the combination (SK plus ASA) produced additive benefit (presumably combining reperfusion with prevention of reocclusion). This trend toward the use of ASA with SK spawned further examination of the need for heparin when thrombolysis was accomplished with other activators. Earlier investigations on reocclusion prevention in rt-PA–treated patients had been inconclusive. Johns et al. (30) compared reocclusion risk after rt-PA–induced coronary thrombolysis among patients randomized to intravenous heparin or to a prolonged rt-PA infusion (an additional 4 hr) as the strategy to prevent recurrent thrombus. In this 52-patient investigation, reocclusion occurred in 19% of the heparin group and none of the prolonged rt-PA infusion group. Their conclusion was that heparin was inadequate rethrombosis prophylaxis, but the opposite results were then shown in a larger European Cooperative Study group trial (31).

The European group randomized 81 infarct patients, after a 90-min rt-PA thrombolytic regimen, to either 6 hr of intravenous heparin or an additional 6 hr of rt-PA. Reocclusion was infrequent in both groups (6% and 5%, respectively), and the authors concluded that heparin was adequate adjunctive therapy.

HEPARIN AND TISSUE PLASMINOGEN ACTIVATOR

Synergism

Laboratory studies have established that heparin appears to increase the rate at which clot dissolution occurs in the presence of rt-PA and other activators. Cercek et al. (32) measured the change in weight of a thrombus influenced by rt-PA and found greater dissolution over an equal period of time if heparin was added to the model. This observation is consistent with true synergism but may also be explained by prevention of new clot formation while the old clot is undergoing lysis.

The question of rt-PA/heparin synergism has also been examined in a clinical trial. Topol et al. (33) compared the success rate of achieving 90-min patency with an rt-PA infusion alone versus the combination of rt-PA and simultaneous intravenous heparin. In this relatively small study (134 patients), the 90-min patency rate was the same, 79%, in both groups, suggesting that at least in the initial phase of plasmin action, synergism is not operative in the clinical setting. This observation may also have contributed to the notion that anticoagulation with or after thrombolysis might not be essential, particularly if early aspirin therapy is administered.

Subsequent Patency

Against a background of these various observations, three recent studies more specifically examined the requirement for heparin with rt-PA. The Heparin-Aspirin Reperfusion Trial (HART) (34) randomized 205 rt-PA–treated acute infarct patients to receive either 80 mg of concomitant aspirin chewed and swallowed at the start of therapy, and then daily, or an immediate 5000-unit intravenous heparin bolus, followed by a week of intravenous heparin infusion, aimed at maintaining the PTT $\geq$ 1.5 times control. Initial coronary angiography was performed between 7 and 24 hr after treatment had started. The mean time to this coronary study was 18 hr after treatment onset, presumably encompassing the period of greatest early reocclusion risk. The group receiving heparin had a patency rate of 82%, not dissimilar from other observations in similarly treated patients at this time interval (35). Patients in whom aspirin was substituted for heparin had only a 52% patency rate at the same time point. Given the previously mentioned results of the TAMI-3 study showing a 79% 90-min patency for rt-PA without heparin, it seems reasonable to hypothesize that in HART, heparin did prevent, but aspirin failed to prevent a high rate of reocclusion (30%) sometime between 90 min and 18 hr post–rt-PA infusion onset. This study also examined late reocclusion by repeating angiography at the end of a week in patients with patent arteries on the first day. In the aspirin group, late reocclusion was 5%; in the heparin-treated patients, 12% (p = NS). This aspect of the trial could be taken to indicate that beyond the first postlytic day, aspirin may, in fact, suffice as a reocclusion prevention measure. However, it should be noted that few ASA group patients remained at risk beyond 18 hr owing to the high early reocclusion rate. The cohorts, while apparently comparable at the start of treatment, had diverged by 24 hr.

Some criticism of this study has been raised regarding the dose of aspirin utilized, 80 mg. This dose had been selected by the TIMI trial as adequate to suppress

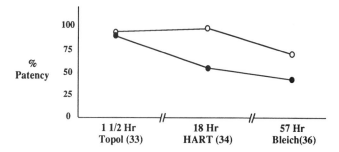

Figure 4   The effect of early intravenous heparin on initial patency and apparent reocclusion after rt-PA reperfusion. At 90 min, 79% of infarct arteries are patent with or without anticoagulation. Thereafter, heparinized patients (open circles) show very superior patency rates (at 18 and 57 hr) compared with a randomized nonheparin cohort (closed circles).

platelet aggregation. However, the speed of achieving this effect may be dose dependent. The dose of aspirin selected in the ISIS-2 trial was 160 mg.

A second rt-PA/heparin study was performed by Bleich et al. (36), differing from HART in that one group received heparin but the controls were not given ASA. Furthermore, the mean time from rt-PA infusion onset to patency-determining angiography was 57 hr. Patency for rt-PA, plus heparin, was 71%; for rt-PA without heparin, 44% (Fig. 4).

The largest of this triad of studies was the sixth of the European Cooperative Study Group (37). They randomized 687 rt-PA–treated myocardial infarction patients to aspirin alone or aspirin plus intravenous heparin. The aspirin dose was large, 250–300 mg, intravenously or orally. In the heparin group, although PTTs were generally recorded, the dose, by protocol, was not increased if subtherapeutic values were obtained. Furthermore, patency-determining angiograms were quite delayed, performed 3–5 days after the beginning of treatment. Patency with heparin was shown to be 83%; without heparin, it was 75% ($p < 0.01$). The results in the heparin group are quite consistent with those of the other trials. The relatively high rate of patent arteries in the aspirin group may relate to the high dose of this agent. Alternatively, the prolonged time to angiography may have influenced the finding since, at the approach of 1 week post–myocardial infarction, patency rates tend to be similar in all patients regardless of treatment owing to eventual spontaneous recanalization (38). Particularly interesting are the patency correlations to measured PTTs in this study. Whereas mean patency in the heparin group, as stated, was 83%, it may be dichotomized by adequacy of anticoagulation. For patients with recorded PTT values in the therapeutic range, patency was 93%. For those with subtherapeutic PTT (inadequate heparin dosing), it was only 77% (38).

A reasonable conclusion from these investigations is that therapeutic levels of anticoagulation accomplished with early intravenous heparin preserve rt-PA-induced coronary patency. Aspirin at low doses is ineffective in accomplishing this goal, although at high doses it may exert an increased effect.

Duration of Intravenous Heparin

Only one study of significant sample size has considered the duration of intravenous heparin after rt-PA-induced thrombolysis. The Australian National Heart Foundation Trial (39) treated 202 patients with rt-PA and intravenous heparin. After 24 hr they were randomized to continue on intravenous heparin for a week or be switched to oral aspirin and dipyridamole. Coronary angiograms at the end of the week revealed equivalent patency, 80% in both groups. Seemingly, this information conforms to the notion that the most important time for thrombin inhibition after rt-PA lysis is the first 12–24 hr. It should also be noted, however, as discussed above, that when coronary angiography is done late after myocardial infarction, i.e., 7–10 days, fairly high patency is seen for all thrombolytic-anticoagulant regimens, even in patients who receive no plasminogen activator at any time!

Subcutaneous Heparin

Although this combination has been used in large mortality trials, no patency or reocclusion studies are available for consideration. Given what has been described above, regarding the general effects of subcutaneous heparin and the European Cooperative Group's correlation of patency to PTT prolongation, one might hypothesize that the subcutaneous route of heparin administration would not be ideal in rt-PA-treated patients.

HEPARIN AND OTHER ACTIVATORS

Saruplase, or scu-PA (single-chain urokinase-like plasminogen activator, also referred to as pro-urokinase), is another human protein–derived recombinant thrombolytic, which shares essential properties with rt-PA (short-acting, relatively fibrin specific, etc.). A heparin–no heparin patency comparison has now been performed with this agent, although the coronary angiogram was rather early (6–12 hr) (40). The results were very similar to those seen with rt-PA. Patency for saruplase plus intravenous heparin was 81% compared with 60% for saruplase without heparin ($p < 0.02$).

No angiography-based studies specifically comparing streptokinase or anistreplase with and without heparin have been reported. One might speculate, based on longer half-life, fibrinogen depletion, and high drug-induced fibrin (and fibrinogen) degradation products (FDPs, themselves "anticoagulant"), that the need for early intravenous heparin with these agents may be less than with rt-PA or saru-plase. Such a hypothesis, however remains to be proven. There is, however, some indirect evidence that the clinical outcome in streptokinase-treated patients is superior when heparin is coadministered. A specific interrogation of this issue was undertaken in the SCATI trial (17). Streptokinase-treated infarct patients randomized to a small (2000 unit) intravenous bolus followed by subcutaneous heparin had a lower in-hospital mortality rate (10/218, 5%) than those randomized to no heparin (19/215, 9%; $p < 0.05$). In the ISIS-2 trial (13), nonrandomized use of heparin with SK was reported to the coordinating center and shown to be associated with a lower 5-week mortality rate (6.7% with intravenous heparin, 7.4% with subcutaneous heparin) compared with an 8.5% mortality rate in those receiving no heparin at all.

In the Gruppo Italiano per Lo Studio Della Sopravvivenza Nell'Infarto Miocardico (GISSI-2) trial (ostensibly a comparison of SK and rt-PA in acute myocardial infarction patients), heparin was given subcutaneously in half the 20,000 patients but only after a 12-hr delay (41). No impact was observed for this anticoagulant strategy among patients who received rt-PA as their allocated activator, or for the total cohort receiving SK. Of interest, however, SK-treated patients who survived at least 12 hr (long enough to start the delayed heparin regimen) had a lower subsequent mortality rate if given subcutaneous heparin (5%) than those in whom the anticoagulant was omitted (6.2%, $p < 0.01$). This could be construed as supporting the notion that the initial systemic anticoagulant effects of SK allow for a heparin benefit despite the considerable period of time before onset of the agent's action can be expected to occur.

HEPARIN AND BLEEDING RISK

Although a modest increase in hemorrhagic complications has been shown in early (prethrombolytic) trials of heparin, greater concerns exist regarding anticoagulation in patients receiving plasminogen activators. Substantial data on this subject have become available but need to be considered differently for small studies and large trials, and also separately for investigations incorporating invasive procedures (arterial punctures) and those without such interventions.

Small studies from only one or a few institutions tend to have detailed case-reporting requirements and dedicated clinical research personnel. Possibly, for these reasons, all complications tend to be more commonly reported than in the very large studies done in dozens or hundreds of centers with only brief reporting requirements.

For example, the Thrombolysis in Myocardial Infarction (TIMI-1) trial (27) was small (13 centers), utilized the services of dedicated research nurse coordinators, and required angiographic procedures: among 113 patients receiving rt-PA and intravenous heparin, the major bleeding rate (requiring≥2 units of blood transfusion) was 25%, and the minor bleeding rate (mostly hematomas at arterial puncture sites) was 66%. In marked contrast was the large Anglo-Scandinavian Study of Early Thrombolysis (ASSET) trial (42), which also administered rt-PA and intravenous heparin, but to 2512 patients in 52 hospitals and required no angiography: major bleeding was reported as 1.2% and minor bleeding, 5.5%!

The best information on the plasminogen activator–heparin combination bleeding risk derives from trials in which patients were randomized to heparin and no-heparin groups. For rt-PA (as a prototype of relatively fibrin-specific agents), these trials are HART (34), Bleich (36), GISSI-2 (41), and ISIS-3 (43). For SK (as an example of a systemic lytic agent), the relevant trials are SCATI (17), GISSI-2 (41), and ISIS-3 (43). In the HART trial (34), there were 14/106 (13%) patients who had bleeding episodes in the rt-PA + heparin (intravenous) treated cohort and 10/99 (10%) in the rt-PA + aspirin group (p = NS). There was only one episode of intracerebral bleeding in the trial (a no-heparin patient), suggesting a very modest hemorrhagic risk.

In contrast, a higher frequency was cited in the study by Bleich et al., which listed hemorrhagic complications by category: "minor," "major," and "severe." The rates among those receiving intravenous heparin with rt-PA were 52%, 10%, and 2%, respectively, whereas those randomized to no heparin suffered minor bleeds in 36% and major events in 2%.

In the SCATI study, with myocardial infarction patients randomized to a heparin or control group, serious bleeding was seen almost exclusively in patients who received SK and the early intravenous plus delayed subcutaneous heparin. The frequency among 360 heparinized patients of retroperitoneal and intracerebral bleeds was one patient each; gastrointestinal bleeding was observed in two, cutaneous hematoma in three, and other "minor" bleeds in nine patients. Thus, the overall bleeding rate was 16/360, or 4.4%; however, 142 of these 360 did not receive SK and hence the real denominator is lower and the bleeding rate, therefore, somewhat higher. In nonheparinized patients, the total bleeding rate was two patients (0.6%), both gastrointestinal in origin.

The two recent largest trials, GISSI-2 and ISIS-3, provide the most information on the subject, despite rather brief reporting requirements. These studies, however, only shed light on the adverse effects of the delayed subcutaneous use of heparin.

The GISSI trial was reported separately for the Italian component and the International extension (44), both delaying by 12 hr the use of heparin (12,500 units subcutaneously twice daily). The Italian report does not separate heparin and non-heparin patients according to their assigned plasminogen activator. There were no differences, based on the heparin/no-heparin randomization in hemorrhagic or total strokes. Major hemorrhage was 1% with heparin, 0.6% without, while minor bleeds were seen in 9.6% and 5.3% respectively.

The report from the International collaborators gives complications for the entire combined cohort of nearly 21,000 patients, stratified by activator. Concerning strokes, hemorrhagic or otherwise, the four subgroups (SK with and without heparin and rt-PA with or without heparin) were all clustered within a narrow range, with variation never exceeding 3 per thousand. Other major bleeding was 0.8% for rt-PA with heparin, 0.5% without; for streptokinase it was 1.2% with heparin and 0.6% without.

The greatest controversy over the adverse effects of heparin added to a plasminogen activator was generated at the March 1991 American College of Cardiology Annual Scientific Sessions, where the preliminary results of ISIS-3 were presented. This study of more than 40,000 patients contained six major subgroups: treatment with SK, anistreplase, or duteplase (a tissue-type plasminogen activator) each with and without subcutaneous heparin delayed 4 hr from the start of lytic therapy and given as 12,000 units twice daily. The precise numbers cannot be considered final at this time, but major bleeding requiring transfusion was increased from 0.8% to 1.1% by the addition of heparin, and "probable" cerebral bleeding increased from 0.4% to 0.6%.

Acting in the other direction, heparin decreased recurrent infarction from 3.6% to 3.3% and decreased all causes of hospital mortality from 7.5% to 7.0% ($p < 0.03$). Hence, on balance, the largest studies, which used delayed subcutaneous heparin, appear to show a small favorable net effect for anticoagulation.

Overall, one can deduce that aggressive thrombolytic plus heparin strategies used in protocols requiring arterial puncture increase minor bleeding substantially but that major bleeding is augmented by the order of 1 or 2%. Delayed subcutaneous heparin does produce fewer such episodes. Perhaps most important, the most severe bleeding complication, i.e., intracerebral bleeds, seems augmented by heparin use only by a magnitude of one to three patients per thousand and is fully offset by an overall mortality reduction of equal or greater magnitude.

CONCLUSIONS

The goals of reperfusion therapy in acute myocardial infarction are to establish and then preserve coronary patency. While the evidence supporting the role of heparin's antithrombin activity in initial lysis is inconclusive, studies clearly demonstrate a substantial benefit for use of the agent to prevent recurrent thrombosis. This is particularly evident when relatively fibrin-specific plasminogen activators (rt-PA and pro-urokinase) are utilized. The need for early heparin to maintain patency when established by the more systemic activators (SK, APSAC) is less well established although, by inference, one can postulate a significant benefit for heparin administration in this setting as well.

The risk of recurrent thrombosis is greatest early after thrombolysis. Hence, logic dictates early intense anticoagulation. The effectiveness of the adjunct is directly related to the degree with which clotting parameters are prolonged (particularly PTT). High-dose intravenous heparinization is substantially more effective than use of the drug subcutaneously.

Finally, although a modest increase in hemorrhagic complications must be expected when an anticoagulant is added to a thrombolytic, such bleeding episodes tend to be minor and do not contribute as substantially to long-term morbidity as they do to overall benefit.

REFERENCES

1. Roberts WC, Buja LM. The frequency and significance of coronary arterial thrombi and other observations in fatal acute myocardial infarction: a study of 107 necroscopy patients. Am J Med 1972; 52:425-43.
2. Davies M, Woolf N, Robertson WB. Pathology of acute myocardial infarction with particular reference to occlusive coronary thrombi. Br Heart J 1976; 38:659-54.
3. DeWood MA, Spores J, Notske R, et al. Prevalence of total coronary occlusion during the early hours of transmural myocardial infarction. N Engl J Med 1980; 303:897-902.
4. McLean J. The thromboplastic action of cephalin. Am J Physiol 1916; 41:250-7.
5. Boneu B, Caranobe C, Sie P. Pharmacokinetics of heparin and low molecular weight heparin. In Hirsh J, ed. Bailliere's clinical haematology: antithrombotic therapy. London: Bailliere Tindall, 1990; 531-44.
6. Hull RD, Raskob GE, Rosenbloom D, et al. Heparin for 5 days as compared with 10 days in the initial treatment of proximal venous thrombosis. N Engl J Med 1990; 322:1260-4.
7. Turpie AGG, Robinson JG, Doyle DJ, et al. Comparison of high-dose with low-dose subcutaneous heparin to prevent left ventricular mural thrombosis in patients with acute transmural anterior myocardial infarction. N Engl J Med 1989; 320:352.
8. Basu D, Gallus A, Hirsh J, Cade J. A prospective study of the value of monitoring heparin treatment with the activated partial thromboplastin time. N Engl J Med 1972; 287:324-7.
9. Collins R, Scrimgeour A, Yusuf S, Peto R. Reduction in fatal pulmonary embolism and venous thrombosis by perioperative administration of subcutaneous heparin: overview of results of randomized trials in general, orthopedic, and urologic surgery. N Engl J Med 1988; 318:1162-73.
10. Working Party on Anticoagulant Therapy in Coronary Thrombosis to the Medical Research Council. Assessment of short-term anticoagulant administration after cardiac infarction. Br Med J 1969; 1:335-42.
11. Drapkin A, Merskey C. Anticoagulant therapy after acute myocardial infarction, relation of therapeutic benefit to patient's age, sex, and severity of infarction. JAMA 1972; 222:541-8.
12. Ebert RV. (Chairman, Executive Committee, Veteran's Administration Collaborative Study). Anticoagulants in acute myocardial infarction, results of a cooperative clinical trial. JAMA 1973; 225:724-9.

13. Second International Study of Infarct Survival (ISIS-2) Collaborative Group. Randomised trial of intravenous streptokinase, oral aspirin, both or neither among 17,187 cases of suspected acute myocardial infarction: ISIS-2. Lancet 1988; 2:349-60.

14. Nordrehaug HE, Johannessen KA, Von der Lippe G. Usefulness of high-dose anticoagulants in preventing left ventricular thrombus in acute myocardial infarction. Am J Cardiol, 1985; 55:1491-3.

15. Gueret P, Dubourg O, Ferrier A, et al. Effects of full-dose heparin anticoagulation on the development of left ventricular thrombosis in acute transmural myocardial infarction. J Am Coll Cardiol 1986; 8:419-26.

16. Arvan S, Boscha K. Prophylactic anticoagulation for left ventricular thrombi after acute myocardial infarction: a prospective randomized trial. Am Heart J 1987; 113:688-93.

17. Studio Sulla Calciparina Nell'Angina e Nella Trombosi Ventricolare Nell'Infarto Group (SCATI). Randomised controlled trial of subcutaneous calcium-heparin in acute myocardial infarction. Lancet. 1989; 2:182-6.

18. Owen J, Friedman KD, Grossman BA, et al. Thrombolytic therapy with tissue plasminogen activator or streptokinase induces transient thrombin activity. Blood 1988; 72:616-20.

19. Gulba DC, Barthels M, Westhoff-Bleck M, et al. Increased thrombin levels during thrombolytic therapy in acute myocardial infarction, relevance for the success of therapy. Circulation 1991; 83:937-44.

20. Hackett D, Davies G, Chierchia S, Maseri A. Intermittent Coronary occlusion in acute myocardial infarction, value of combined thrombolytic and vasodilator therapy. N Engl J Med 1987; 317:1055-9.

21. Merx W, Dorr R, Rentrop R, et al. Evaluation of the effectiveness of intracoronary streptokinase infusion in myocardial infarction: postprocedure management and hospital course in 204 patients. Am Heart J 1981; 102:1181.

22. Serruys PW, Wijns W, van den Brand M, et al. Is transluminal coronary angioplasty mandatory after successful thrombolysis? Br Heart J 1983; 50:257.

23. Urban PL, Cowley M, Goldberg S, et al. Intracoronary thrombolysis in acute myocardial infarction: clinical course following successful myocardial reperfusion. Am Heart J 1984; 108:873.

24. Ferguson DW, White CW, Schwartz JL, et al. Influence of baseline ejection fraction and success of thrombolysis on mortality and ventricular function after acute myocardial infarction. Am J Cardiol 1984; 54:705.

25. Anderson JL, Marshall HW, Bray BE, et al. A randomized trial of intracoronary streptokinase in the treatment of acute myocardial infarction. N Engl J Med 1983; 308:1305.

26. Leiboff RH, Katz RJ, Wasserman AG, et al. A randomized, angiographically controlled trial of intracoronary streptokinase in acute myocardial infarction. Am J Cardiol 1984; 53:404.

27. Chesebro JH, Knatterud G, Roberts R, et al. Thrombolysis in myocardial infarction (TIMI) Trial, phase I: A comparison between intravenous tissue plasminogen activator and intravenous streptokinase. Circulation 1987; 76:142.

28. Ohman EM, Califf RM, Topol EJ, et al. Consequences of reocclusion after successful reperfusion therapy in acute myocardial infarction. Circulation 1990; 82:781-91.

29. Kaplan K, Davison R, Parker M, et al. Role of heparin after intravenous thrombolytic therapy for acute myocardial infarction. Am J Cardiol, 1987; 59:241-4.

30. Johns JA, Gold HK, Leinbach RC, et al. Prevention of coronary artery reocclusion and reduction in late coronary artery stenosis after thrombolytic therapy in patients with acute myocardial infarction, a randomized study of maintenance infusion of recombinant human tissue-type plasminogen activator. Circulation 1988; 78:546-56.

31. Verstraete M, Bernard R, Bory M, et. al. (European Cooperative Study Group). Randomized trial of intravenous recombinant tissue-type plasminogen activator versus intravenous streptokinase in acute myocardial infarction. Lancet, 1985; 1:842-7.

32. Cercek B, Lew AS, Hod H, et. al. Enhancement of thrombolysis with tissue-type plasminogen activator by pretreatment with heparin. Circulation 1986; 74:583.

33. Topol EJ, George BS, Kereiakes DJ, et al. A randomized controlled trial of intravenous tissue plasminogen activator and early intravenous heparin in acute myocardial infarction. Circulation 79:281-6 (1989).

34. Hsia J, Hamilton WP, Kleiman N, et al. A comparison between heparin and low-dose aspirin as adjunctive therapy with tissue plasminogen activator for acute myocardial infarction. N Engl J Med 1990; 323:1433-7.

35. The TIMI Research Group. Immediate vs. delayed catheterization and angioplasty following thrombolytic therapy for acute myocardial infarction, TIMI IIA results. JAMA 1988; 260:2849-58.

36. Bleich SD, Nichols TC, Schumacher RR, et. al. Effect of heparin on coronary arterial patency after thrombolysis with tissue plasminogen activator in acute myocardial infarction. Am J Cardiol 1990; 66:1412-7.

37. European Cooperative Study Group. A randomized trial of heparin versus placebo after rt-PA induced thrombolysis. Presented at the 12th Congress of European Cardiologists. Stockholm, Sweden, September. 1990.

38. Verstraete M. Personal communication.

39. Thompson PL, Aylward PE, Federman J, et al. (National Heart Foundation of Australia Coronary Thrombolysis Group). A randomized comparison of intravenous heparin with oral aspirin and dipyridamole 24 hours after recombinant tissue-type plasminogen activator for acute myocardial infarction. Circulation 1991; 83:1534-42.

40. Tebbe U. A randomized trial of heparin versus placebo after pro-urokinase induced thrombolysis. Presented at the George Washington University 6th International Workshop on Thrombolysis and Interventional Therapy in Acute Myocardial Infarction, Dallas, Texas, November 1990.

41. Gruppo Italiano per Lo Studio Della Sopravvivenza Nell'Infarto Miocardico. GISSI-2: a factorial randomised trial of alteplase versus streptokinase and heparin versus no heparin among 12,490 patients with acute myocardial infarction. Lancet 1990; 336:65-70.

42. Wilcox RG, Olsson CG, Skene AM, et al., for the ASSET Study Group. Trial of tissue plasminogen activator for mortality reduction in acute myocardial infarction. Anglo-Scandinavian Study of Early Thrombolysis (ASSET). Lancet 1988; 2:525-30.

43. Sleight P. Preliminary outcome data, ISIS-3. Presented at the American College of Cardiology Annual Scientific Meeting, Atlanta, Georgia, March 1991.
44. The International Study Group. In-hospital mortality and clinical course of 20,891 patients with suspected acute myocardial infarction randomized between alteplase and streptokinase with or without heparin. Lancet 1990; 336:71-5.

11

Antithrombin Agents' Emerging Role as an Adjuvant Therapy in Acute Myocardial Infarction

John H. Ip and Douglas Israel
Mount Sinai Medical Center, New York, New York

Valentin Fuster
Harvard Medical School and Massachusetts General Hospital, Boston, Massachusetts

INTRODUCTION

The goal of thrombolytic therapy is to restore myocardial perfusion in the shortest possible time to prevent and limit myocardial necrosis. The ideal thrombolytic regimen should produce the highest rate of reperfusion and the lowest incidence of bleeding and rethrombosis. However, with the use of current therapeutic approaches and infusion protocols, the reperfusion rates are often less than 80% and reocclusion rates may exceed 15% (1,2). Consequently, different therapeutic regimens have been investigated to accelerate recanalization and prevent reocclusion. These include the use of combination thrombolytic therapy (3), anticoagulants (4–8), and potent antiplatelet agents, such as monoclonal antibodies for the GP IIb/IIIa platelet receptor and thromboxane A2 antagonists (Table 1) (1,9). The potential roles of these new strategies are discussed elsewhere in this book. In this chapter, we will focus on (a) the central role of thrombin and altered hemorrheology in the pathophysiology of reocclusion following thrombolysis and (b) the emerging antithrombin agents and their potential clinical roles as adjuvant therapeutic agents in the treatment of acute myocardial infarction.

Table 1 Antithrombotic Agents

Antithrombotic agents	Shear rate		Enhances thrombolysis	Decreases reocclusion	Bleeding time	Platelet antibodies
	High	Low				
Heparin	+	++	+	+	++	+
Aspirin	++	+	±	+	+	++
Antithrombins (Hep/ASA/No)	++	++	++	++	+	++
AntiGPIIb/IIIa (HepNo)	++	+	++	++	±	±
TXA$_2$–S$_2$ receptor	++	?	++?	++?	+	++
TXA$_2$ Synth-receptor (Hep)						

++, very favorable; +, favorable; ±, less favorable.

PATHOPHYSIOLOGY OF REOCCLUSION AFTER THROMBOLYSIS (Figs. 1,2)

The incidence of rethrombosis following coronary thrombolysis may be as high as 15-20% (1,2). To date, three main contributing factors for the development of rethrombosis have been identified, (a) shear stress associated with persistence of luminal stenosis and residual thrombus, (b) the thrombogenic stimulus caused by residual thrombus, and (c) the generation of thrombin and activation of platelets during thrombolysis.

Shear Stress

Shear stress is a measure of the difference in blood velocity between the center of the vessel and along the wall. To investigate the altered hemorrheology seen with significant coronary stenosis, we have developed a computed-assisted nuclear scintigraphic method using an extracorporeal perfusion chamber in which different vessel wall substrate can be exposed to flowing blood at different shear stress (10). Using stripped tunica media as the exposure substrate, we demonstrated a marked increment in platelet deposition when higher degrees of stenosis were used. The reason for this phenomenon is that, in a system with mild obstruction to flow, the shear stress is low. However, with higher degrees of stenosis, the shear stress is markedly increased. This facilitates the interaction of platelets and the vessel wall and promotes platelet deposition on the exposed surface.

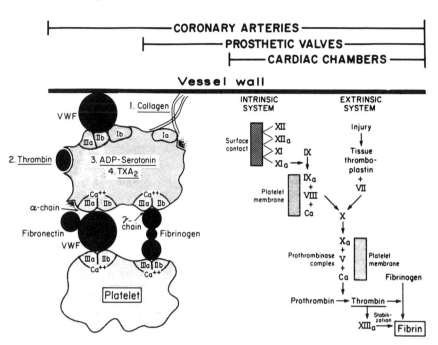

Figure 1   The mechanisms of platelet and coagulation system activation.

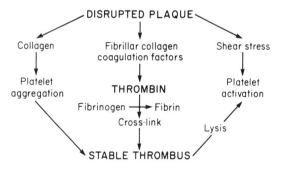

Figure 2   Proposed mechanisms of rethrombosis following thrombolysis.

The clinical importance of residual stenosis after thrombolysis has been demonstrated by a number of clinical studies (11–13). A residual stenosis > 75% luminal diameter was associated with an increased risk of early rethrombosis. Furthermore, Badger et al. (14) showed that a residual luminal diameter < 0.6 mm or Thrombolysis in Myocardial Infarction (TIMI) perfusion protocol grade 1 or 2 (partial perfusion) was associated with higher angiographic reocclusion at 5 weeks and a higher 1-year mortality rate. These clinical observations are supported by data from our laboratory, which showed that higher degrees of luminal stenosis and higher shear rates are both associated with increased platelet deposition and thrombus formation (10). However, a recent large clinical study (15) of 192 patients reported that residual stenosis following thrombolysis did not predict recurrent ischemia. This discrepancy from the previous smaller studies may be explained by the differences in methodologies and the thrombolytic agents used. In addition, this may simply indicate the complexity of the pathophysiological process of rethrombosis following thrombolysis.

Thrombogenicity of Residual Thrombus

Not only can residual thrombus following thrombolysis produce a high shear stress condition and promote thrombus growth, but it can induce a high thrombogenic environment. We found that the presence of a residual thrombus, which is common after thrombolysis, is one of the most powerful thrombogenic surfaces encountered in the laboratory. In the ex vivo model using the perfusion preparation (16), we studied the degree of deposition of platelets on stripped tunica media exposed to different degrees of stenosis. When the stenosis was severe, platelet deposition increased with time as a result of the increased shear rate. After 30 min of perfusion, platelet deposition and associated fibrin formation abruptly decreased, probably because of spontaneous thrombolysis or platelet disaggregation. This was followed immediately by a rapid increase in platelet deposition in the affected area, which suggests that the thrombus that remained after spontaneous lysis or platelet disaggregation was markedly thrombogenic and stimulated the massive deposition of platelets on its surface. With continued perfusion, a recurrent cycle of platelet deposition was observed. This finding is supported by clinical studies that have shown an increased risk of rethrombosis when a residual thrombus is seen angiographically after thrombolysis compared with cases without evidence of a residual thrombus (11,17).

Thrombin Generation and Platelet Activation

Accumulating evidence suggests that increases in platelet activation and thrombin generation occur during thrombolysis. For example, Fitzgerald et al. (18) observed a marked elevation in plasma and urinary metabolites of thromboxane A2 following the administration of streptokinase in patients with acute myocardial infarction. In another study, Eisenberg et al. (19) showed an increase in fibrino-peptide A (which is released by the action of thrombin on fibrinogen) immediately after thrombolytic therapy with streptokinase in patients with acute myocardial infarction. Similarly, Androitte and co-workers (20) recently demonstrated a substantial increase in thrombin generation in patients with acute myocardial infarction receiving intravenous infusions of rt-PA. The mechanisms for this increase in platelet and thrombin activity are unclear, but it may be due to a direct effect of plasmin on platelets and activation of the coagulation system.

The dominant pathophysiological role of thrombin in rethrombosis following thrombolysis is exemplified by the multiple important hematological roles it plays in the coagulation system. For example, thrombin is one of the most potent stimulators of platelet activation by a mechanism that is independent of ADP, thromboxane A2, and fibrin generation. In fact, there is a putative receptor for thrombin on the platelet surface, and continuous occupancy of this "receptor" is required for phosphatate synthesis and alpha-granule and acid hydrolase secretion; thus, in various experimental models, thrombin has been demonstrated to be an important mediator in platelet-dependent arterial thrombus formation irrespective of whether the thrombogenic stimuli was a foreign surface (21), mural thrombi (22), damaged vessel wall (23), or adventitial tissue (24). In addition, thrombin converts fibrinogen into fibrin and facilitates cross-linking of fibrin by factor XIII. Thus, intracoronary rethrombosis following thrombolytic therapy is a complex process occurring within a thrombogenic milieu created by shear stress, residual thrombus, and increased thrombin and platelet activation. One emerging approach to the problem of reocclusion is the use of specific antithrombin agents. The list of antithrombin agents has grown over the past few years as accumulating experimental evidence suggests a potential application for these compounds as adjuvant therapeutic agents in patients with acute myocardial infarction. In the following sections, we will discuss in detail the pharmacological action of these agents as well as their potential therapeutic roles.

ANTITHROMBIN AGENTS

Pharmacological agents that inhibit thrombin can be divided into two classes based on their mechanisms of action: (a) antithrombin III–dependent agents, such as heparin, (b) antithrombin III–independent agents, such as hirudin, activated protein C, and the synthetic antithrombins such as Argatroban (Table 2).

Antithrombin III–Dependent Agents

Heparin is the agent with which most clinical experience is available in this class. Heparin is an anticoagulant that acts as a cofactor for the protease inhibitor antithrombin III. Antithrombin III inhibits the enzymatic activities of thrombin and

Table 2   Antithrombin Agents

	Mechanism
1. Antithrombin III dependent	
Heparin	Cofactor of antithrombin III
2. Antithrombin III independent	
Hirudin	Direct inhibitor of thrombin
Activated protein C	Inactivates factor Va/VIIIa
Synthetic peptides	Direct inhibitor of thrombin

factors IXa, Xa, XIa, and XIIa. In vitro heparin enhances the rate of formation of irreversible complexes of antithrombin III with thrombin by a factor of 2000. Heparin is not only a thrombin inhibitor, but also a modulator of the coagulation cascade and the thrombin generation rate, owing to its inhibitory role on enzymatic activities of factors that lead to thrombin formation (factors Xa, IXa, XIa, and XIIa) (25) (Fig. 1).

Various experimental models simulating the anatomical and pathophysiological environment of coronary thrombosis leading to acute myocardial infarction in humans have studied the effectiveness of heparin in preventing reocclusion following thrombolysis. Experimental studies (23,26) in a porcine model of deep arterial injury by balloon dilatation have shown that heparin produces a dose-dependent reduction in both platelet and fibrinogen deposition and a reduction in the incidence of mural thrombosis at dose of 35–250 U/kg. However, at dosages that can be practically used in humans, heparin does not significantly reduce arterial platelet thrombosis (Fig. 3). In a canine model of copper coil–induced arterial thrombosis, Cereck and others (27) demonstrated that pretreatment with heparin (200–300 U/kg) potentiated the thrombolytic effects of rt-PA or scu-PA and reduced the time to perfusion. In one of our studies (16), thrombus actually accumulated during the rt-PA infusion when the concurrent heparin infusion was stopped. More recently, in a canine model of coronary artery thrombosis with superimposed high-grade stenosis, heparin in the dosage of 150 U/kg did not significantly decrease the rate of reocclusion (28). Similar findings were reported in a canine model with copper coil–induced coronary artery thrombosis or with local thrombosis with endothelial damage by external trauma (29). In a rabbit femoral artery eversion graft model, Jang et al. (24) demonstrated that the use of high-dose heparin failed to prevent arterial occlusion. The reason for this apparent ineffectiveness of heparin in preventing rethrombosis is unclear, but it has been suggested recently that clot-bound thrombin is relatively inaccessible to the large heparin–antithrombin III complex (30).

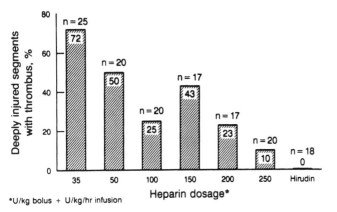

Figure 3   Number of arterial segments with deep vascular injury that had mural thrombosis. n = number of segments with deep injury. Height of the bar represents the percentage with thrombus. There was a reduction from 72% in the lowest heparin group to 10% in the highest heparin group. No thrombus was found in the hirudin group. [Reprinted with permission from Heras et al. (23).]

The clinical experience, so far, with heparin in preventing reocclusion following thrombolysis has been mixed and controversial (31). The Thrombolysis and Angioplasty in Myocardial Infarction Group (TAMI-3) trial (4) evaluated 134 patients receiving intravenous t-PA for acute myocardial infarction; half the patients were given a single bolus of 10,000 U heparin, and half the patients received placebo. The major endpoint, infarct-related patency at 90 min, was 79% in both treatment and control groups. However, this trial cannot be regarded as conclusive because of the limited number of patients, and the single injection of heparin may have been insufficient. Two recent randomized trials, however, reported beneficial effects of heparin on later patency rates. Hsia et al. (7) randomized 205 patients with acute myocardial infarction who received rt-PA to either aspirin (80 mg/day) or early intravenous heparin (5000 U bolus with 1000 U/hr infusion titrated to $2 \times$ PTT control). Patency at 18 hr in the aspirin group was 52% versus 82% in the heparin group ($p < 0.001$). Similarly, Bleich et al. (8) randomized 83 patients to receive either rt-PA alone or rt-PA with heparin therapy (5000 U bolus with 1000 U/hr infusion titrated to $2 \times$ PTT control). Patency rates at 48–72 hr were 44% in the control group and 71% in the heparin group. In addition, the SCATI trial (32) also reported significant differences in hospital mortality and reinfarction rates in patients receiving streptokinase and heparin (intravenous bolus early and subcutaneously late) compared to patients receiving streptokinase alone. However, the recently completed GISSI-2 trial (5), involving more than 12,000 patients receiving either rt-PA or streptokinase, demonstrated no significant improvement in the rate of reinfarction, postinfarction angina, and overall ischemic events in patients starting 12,500 U heparin subcutaneously 12 hr after thrombolytic therapy compared with placebo. The International Study Group (6) evaluated more than 20,000 patients using a similar design and also reported the lack of beneficial effects of subcutaneous heparin in preventing the clinical sequelae of rethrombosis. However, delaying subcutaneous heparin for 4–12 hr may be inferior to immediate intravenous therapy for preventing reocclusion.

Thus, the role of heparin as adjunctive therapy to accelerate thrombolysis and prevent reocclusion is controversial. Further clinical trials are needed to define the usefulness of heparin as an adjuvant therapy in patients with acute myocardial infarction.

Antithrombin III–Independent Agents

This class of antithrombins inhibit thrombin either by directly binding to thrombin (e.g., hirudin) or by inhibiting a cofactor that is essential for thrombin formation (e.g., activated protein C). Experiences with these agents are predominantly experimental, although preclinical dose response studies are ongoing in both American and European institutions.

Hirudin

Hirudin is a protein of low molecular weight [7.5 kilodalton (kDa), or about one-tenth the size of the heparin–antithrombin III complex] and a very potent, specific, noncovalent, irreversible inhibitor of thrombin (33). Hirudin occurs naturally in the salivary secretions of medicinal leeches, and recombinant hirudin, produced through advanced DNA technology, is available and generally used in experimental studies.

Hirudin interacts directly with thrombin and induces significant conformational changes in the thrombin molecule, which cause the loss of its coagulant activity (34). Thrombin activates platelets in part by binding to glycoprotein Ib on the platelet membrane and by producing a proteolytic degradation of glycoprotein V (35). The site where hirudin binds thrombin appears important for the reaction between thrombin and platelet. Hirudin has a high affinity for thrombin (Ki = 10–15 m) and the platelet-thrombin receptor (approximately 10–100 times higher than the Ki for thrombin). Hirudin can displace thrombin from its binding sites on platelets and thus might cause disaggregation (36). There are no circulatory inhibitors to hirudin. In contrast, platelet factor 4 from alpha granules is the natural inhibitor for heparin. Because no naturally occurring inhibitor has been described, the dosage of hirudin administered is the only limiting factor in blocking thrombin. In addition to its inhibitory effect on thrombin, hirudin also prevents the activation of factors V, VIII, and XIII and thus can markedly suppress thrombin generation and the powerful coagulation and positive feedback effects of thrombin on the activation of coagulation factors and platelets.

The effects of hirudin on thrombosis have been extensively studied in various animal models. Using deep arterial balloon injury in a pig model, our laboratory compared the efficacy of heparin and recombinant hirudin in the prevention of platelet aggregation, fibrinogen deposition, and thrombus formation (23). We showed that heparin, at a dose that prolonged the aPTT to twice the control time, did not prevent mural thrombosis or significantly reduce platelet deposition compared with placebo but did reduce fibrinogen deposition. Recombinant hirudin markedly reduced platelet and fibrinogen deposition in a dose-related manner and totally eliminated mural thrombosis at an aPTT of 2–3 × that of control (Figs. 3,4). Platelet deposition was restricted to only a single layer in animals pretreated with recombinant hirudin. Furthermore, we found that the aPTT is a valuable index of plasma hirudin concentration and correlated inversely with quantitative platelet and fibrinogen deposition (Fig. 5). Using a similar deep arterial injury model preparation (37), we recently compared the lytic effect of rt-PA plus recombinant hirudin with rt-PA alone. Intravenous rt-PA was administered at 30 min and continued for 210 min after the creation of occlusive platelet-rich thrombi in the left carotid artery by balloon dilatation. rt-PA was administered as 0.3 mg/kg bolus, 3 mg/kg over 90 min, then 1 mg/kg over 120 min; the hirudin dosage was 1 mg/kg bolus, then 0.7 mg/kg/hr. Only one of six pigs given rt-PA alone reperfused at 120 min by angiography, while all pigs treated with rt-PA plus hirudin reperfused at 90 min. The aPTT was prolonged 2.4 × control in pigs given the combination therapy. Residual platelet deposition was also markedly reduced in pigs given hirudin and rt-PA. Garratt et al. (38), using an arterial stent vascular injury model in the pig, demonstrated that hirudin (1 mg/kg bolus with infusion of 1 mg/kg/hr) significantly reduced platelet deposition, in response to stenting and balloon angioplasty, compared with the use of aspirin and dipyridamole. Hirudin was also tested in an open-chest dog model (39). Intimal injury to the coronary arteries was produced with direct current. Hirudin was administered at a dose sufficient to increase the aPTT to 2–3 × control. Platelet deposition and thrombus formation were markedly decreased compared with placebo. Similarly, in a femoral arteriovenous shunt model in baboons (40), recombinant hirudin profoundly inhibited the deposition of platelets and thrombus formation in a dose-dependent manner.

Intrinsic pharmacological properties of hirudin may explain its superiority to heparin as an antithrombotic agent. First, residual thrombus contains active thrombin bound to fibrin, which is poorly accessible to the large heparin–antithrombin III complex. Second, a platelet-rich arterial thrombus releases large amounts of platelet factor 4, which inhibits heparin. Third, fibrin II monomer, formed by the action of thrombin on fibrinogen, also inhibits heparin. Finally, hirudin is at least 10 times smaller than the heparin–antithrombin III complex, has

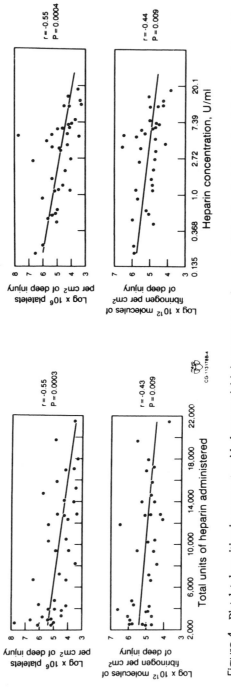

Figure 4 Platelet deposition in segments with deep arterial injury versus total amount of hirudin administered and the relationship with the aPTT. (Reprinted with permission from Heras et al. Circulation 1990; 82:1476–84.)

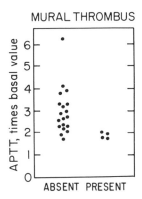

Figure 5 Activated partial thromboplastin time (aPTT) prolongation measured in each hirudin treated pig. Note the total absence of mural thrombosis when the aPTT prolongation is 2× basal value. (Reprinted from Heras et al. Circulation 1990; 82:1476-84.)

no natural inhibitors, and, therefore, has greater accessibility to thrombin bound to fibrin.

Preclinical studies of recombinant hirudin in humans have already begun. Verstraete et al. (41) demonstrated a dose-dependent antithrombotic effect in volunteers with intravenous recombinant hirudin. Further studies of the duration of therapy for both prevention of thrombosis and arrest of the growth of preexisting thrombus are required before clinical trials on this promising agent are initiated.

Activated Protein C

Activated protein C (APC) is an antithrombotic serine protease (42). It is generated from vitamin K–dependent plasma protein C by the catalytic complex of thrombin and thrombomodulin. APC functions as a potent inhibitor of thrombin by inactivating coagulation cofactors V and VIII, which are essential for the generation of thrombin. The rate of inactivation of these cofactors (especially in their activated forms) in plasma is rapid, since greater than 80% of their activity is destroyed in 3 min by 3 μg/ml of APC (43). Human protein C must be proteolytically activated to function as an anticoagulant. APC loses its anticoagulant properties upon incubation with the serine protease inhibitor, implying that protein C functions enzymatically by proteolytic inactivation. The potent inactivation of factors V and VIII in plasma is entirely sufficient to explain the prolongation of the aPTT. Human factor VIIIa, an activated form of factor VIII generated by thrombin, is inactivated very rapidly by APC but not by the inactivated form of protein C. Human protein C can be activated in vivo by several proteolytic enzymes, such as thrombin. These pharmacological features enable APC to provide a very responsive mechanism for antithrombotic regulation. Thus, when APC is available

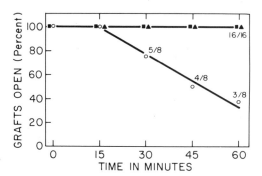

Figure 6   Plot of patency of arteriovenous Dacron vascular graft of control primates (o-o) and during infusion of activated protein C 0.25 mg/kg (▲-▲) and 1.0 mg/kg (■-■). [Reprinted with permission from Gruber et al. (47).]

on the cell surface, it effectively shuts down the generation of clotting factor Xa and the generation of thrombin (43). Since thrombin is essential for the conversion of V to Va and VIII to VIIIa, APC will essentially exert its effect only where thrombin is generated. This is in contrast to heparin, which blocks all the activated serine proteases in the system at all times. Thus, these features may render APC less likely to cause substantial bleeding complications.

The physiological significance of protein C is shown by the clinical observation that the incidence of heterozygous protein C deficiency is higher in patients with thrombophilia than in healthy individuals (44); in addition, there is a positive correlation between thrombotic events and heterozygous protein C deficiency (45).

Experimental results obtained in various animal models indicate that APC is a potent antithrombotic agent without significant impairment of primary hemostasis. Using a stenotic venous model in dogs and Rhesus monkies, Emerick et al. (43) demonstrated that the use of APC significantly decreased the rate of fibrin acretion onto thrombi compared with controls. APC infusions resulted in a 3–6 sec prolongation in aPTT with no changes in PT, and bleeding was minimal in the animals studied. In a primate model of arterial graft thrombosis, Gruber and co-workers (46) demonstrated a marked reduction in platelet deposition as measured by the real-time scintillation camera imaging of indium-labeled platelet deposition. In addition, all the grafts of the treated animals were patent, compared to none of the control grafts. More recently, the same group of investigators confirmed the remarkable efficacy of APC in a chronic arteriovenous shunt thrombosis model in primates (47) (Fig. 6). Infusion of APC at doses of 0.25 and 1.0 mg/kg/hr significantly reduced the extent of platelets and fibrinogen deposition on the shunt in a dose-dependent manner. All the shunts in the treated animals remained patent, while five of eight control shunts were occluded within 60 min. Circulating plasma markers of thrombus formation and of fibrinolysis did not increase significantly during the infusion, and measurements of bleeding time were within normal limits despite the profound effects on the coagulation time in vitro.

Finally, the additive beneficial effect of APC during thrombolysis was demonstrated in a recent study using a primate arterial graft model. Griffin et al. (48) showed that the use of urokinase and APC (0.25 mg/kg) in combination markedly interrupted platelet-dependent thrombus formation compared with the use of urokinase monotherapy. This antithrombotic effect was seen without the impairment of the normal hemostatic mechanism. These observations suggest that the administration of APC in a clinical setting may be less likely to cause bleeding then the administration of other available platelet antagonists and thrombin inhibitors.

Synthetic Antithrombins

Over the past few years, the list of new synthetic antithrombin peptides being investigated in experimental models has grown. All of these synthetic peptides inhibit thrombin by antithrombin III–independent mechanisms and prevent platelet aggregation and thrombin formation in animal models. Although there is some variation among these different agents, the administration of effective antithrombotic doses of each results in impairment of normal hemostasis and prolongation of bleeding time. Two of the typical synthetic antithrombin peptides will be discussed below.

Argatroban (Argipidine). Argatroban [(2R,4R)-4-methyl-1-[N2-(3- methy-1,2,3-4-tetrahydro-8-quinolinesulfonyl)-2-arginyl]-2 piperidinecarboxylic acid monohydrate] is a substituted arginine derivative with three binding regimens that correspond to (a) a positively charged guaninide group, (b) an aromatic N2 substituent, and (c) a hydrophobic carboxamide portion. The specificity of this agent has been shown to be dependent in stereospecific interactions between the carboxyamide substituent and a hydrophobic binding pocket of the thrombin. Its antithrombin action is independent of antithrombin III.

This arginyl peptide has been tested in various animal models of thrombosis. Eidt and co-workers (50) studied the effects of heparin and intra-arterial argatroban on the cyclical variation of coronary blood flow (CFV) in dogs with experimental coronary artery stenosis and endothelial injury. The CFVs result primarily from the aggregation of platelets and thrombin formation at the site of the stenosis followed by dislodgment and distal embolization. Using this canine model, argatroban abolished CFVs in a dose-dependent manner. At the same time, the bleeding time and aPTT were also prolonged. Heparin also appears to be effective in a short period of time but not for prolonged periods of CFVs. In a rabbit femoral arterial eversion graft model, Jang et al. (24) evaluated the efficacy of

heparin and argatroban in the prevention of arterial platelet-rich thrombus formation. High-dose intravenous heparin (200 U/kg) failed to prevent occlusion in 60
min whereas intravenous argatroban infusion at a rate of 100 or 200 μg/kg/min for
60 min, which prolonged thrombin time more than fourfold, prevented thrombosis in 70% of the rabbits studied. Patency of femoral arterial segments was maintained after the end of intraarterial argatroban infusion for 3 hr despite
normalization of the thrombin time and aPTT. Pathological examination of the
graft in the treated animals revealed that the adventitial surfaces were covered by
layers of platelets without platelet aggregation or fibrin deposition. A potential
significant drawback of this peptide is the marked prolongation of both thrombin
time and the aPTT in the pharmacological dose used. More recently, Yasuda et al.
(51) provided additional information concerning acceleration of thrombolysis and
reduction of early reocclusion during the first 2 hr after the start of rt-PA administration with a simultaneous infusion of argatroban or aspirin or the combination
of both. With a dose successful in prolonging the mean aPTT to more than sixfold,
argatrobin significantly decreased the time to reperfusion by 50% compared with
groups receiving aspirin alone. The groups receiving the combination of aspirin
and argatroban had the lowest incidence of reocclusion compared with groups
treated with either agent alone. However, the antithrombotic effect of the peptide
is associated with a concomitant significant impairment of normal hemostasis.

Arginine Chloromethyl Ketone. Phenylalanine-L-propyl L-arginine chloromethyl ketone (PPACK) is a synthetic, selective, irreversible thrombin inhibitor
(52). The process of the covalent inactivation of thrombin probably occurs in two
processes: (a) reversible active-site complex formation followed by (b) rapid irreversible alkylation of the active center histidine by the agent. In a vascular graft
thrombosis model in primates (21), Hanson and Harker demonstrated that the use
of PPACK abolished vascular graft platelet deposition, aggregation, thrombus
formation, and the associated in vivo release of platelet-specific proteins and
fibrinopeptides. In addition, all the grafts were patent at the end of the study. The
effects of PPACK largely disappeared within 15 min after the infusion was
stopped. In contrast, sustained comparable anticoagulation levels with heparin
had no effect on platelet deposition, aggregation, thrombus formation, or graft
patency. Similarly, Collen et al. (53) eliminated intravascular thrombosis in a rabbit model with the use of PPACK. Concomitant marked elevation of thrombin
time and aPTT was observed.

SUMMARY

We have discussed the pathophysiological process of coronary reocclusion following thrombolysis and highlighted the central role of thrombin in the patho-
genic process. In addition to heparin, new thrombin inhibitors are emerging as

promising agents in the prevention of the rethrombotic process. Although investigations of these agents are still in the experimental stage and several major issues remain unresolved (the dosage, duration of therapy, and potential bleeding complications), they hold considerable promise as future adjunctive agents in the treatment of acute myocardial infarction.

REFERENCES

1. Fuster V, Stein B, Badimon L, Chesebro J. Antithrombotic therapy after myocardial reperfusion in acute myocardial infarction. J Am Coll Cardiol 1988; 12(Suppl A):78A-84A.
2. Heras M, Chesebro JH, Thompson PL, Fuster V. Prevention of early and late rethrombosis and future strategies after coronary reprefusion. In Julian D, et al., eds. Thrombolysis in cardiovascular disease. New York: Marcel Dekker, 1990:203-31.
3. Collen D. Synergism of thrombolytic agents: investigational procedures and clinical potential. Circulation 1988; 77:731-5.
4. Topol EJ, George BS, Kereiakes DJ, et al. A randomized clinical trial of intravenous tissue type plasminogen activator and early intravenous heparin in acute myocardial infarction. Circulation 1989; 79:281-6.
5. GISSI 2: a factorial randomization trial of alteplase versus streptokinase and heparin versus no heparin among 12,490 patients in acute myocardial infarction. Lancet 1990; 336:65-70.
6. The International Study Group. In hospital mortality and clinical course of 20,381 patients in suspected acute myocardial infarction randomized between alteplase and streptokinase with or without heparin. Lancet 1990; 336:71-5.
7. Hsia J, Hamilton N, Kleiman N, Roberts R, Chaitmen BR, Prss AM. A comparison between heparin and low dose aspirin as adjunctive therapy with tissue plasminogen activator for acute myocardial infarction. N Engl J Med 1990; 323:1433-8.
8. Bleich SD, Nichols T, Schumacher H, Looke DH, Tate DA, Teichman SL. Effect of heparin on coronary arterial patency after thrombolysis with tissue plasminogen activator in acute myocardial infarction. Am J Cardiol 1990; 66:1412-7.
9. Runge MS. Prevention of thrombosis and rethrombosis: new approaches. Circulation 1990; 82:655-8.
10. Lassila R, Badimon JJ, Vallabhajosula S, Badimon L. Dynamic monitoring of platelet deposition on severely damaged vessel wall in flowing blood. Effects of different stenosis on thrombus formation. Arteriosclerosis 1990; 10:306-15.
11. Gash AK, Spain JF, Sherry F, et al. Factors influencing reocclusion after coronary thrombolysis for acute myocardial infarction. Am J Cardiol 1986; 57:175-7.
12. Harrison DG, Ferguson DW, Collins SW, et al. Rethrombosis after reperfusion with streptokinase: importance of geometry of residual lesion. Circulation 1984; 69:991-9.
13. Schaer DH, Leiboff RH, Katz RJ, et al. Recurrent early ischemic events after thrombolysis for acute myocardial infarction. Am J Cardiol 1987; 59:788-92.
14. Badger RS, Brown BG, Kennedy JW, et al. Usefulness of recanalization of luminal diameter of 0.6 mm or more with intracoronary streptokinase during acute myocardial

infarction in predicting normal perfusion status, continued arterial patency and survival at one year. Am J Cardiol 1987; 59:519-22.

15. Ellis SG, Topol EJ, George BJ, et al. Recurrent ischemia without warning. Analysis of risk factors for in hospital ischemic events following successful thrombolysis with intravenous tissue plasminogen activator. Circulation 1989; 80:1159-65.

16. Badimon L, Badimon JJ. Mechanism of arterial thrombosis in nonparallel streamlines: platelet thrombi grow at the apex of stenotic injured vessel wall. Experimental study in the pig model. J Clin Invest 1989; 84:1134-44.

17. De Guise P, Theroux P, Bonan R, et al. Rethrombosis after successful thrombolysis and angioplasty in acute myocardial infarction. J Am Coll Cardiol 1988; 1:192A (abstract).

18. Fitzgerald DJ, Catella F, Roy L, Fitzgerald GA. Marked platelet activation in vivo after intravenous streptokinase in patients with acute myocardial infarction. Circulation 1988; 77:142-54.

19. Eisenberg PR, Sherman LA, Jaffe AS. Paradoxical elevation of fibrinopeptide A after streptokinase: evidence for continued thrombosis despite intense fibrinolysis. J Am Coll Cardiol 1987; 10:527-9.

20. Androitte F, Klutt C, Hackett D, et al. High dose infusion of t-PA is associated with enhanced thrombin generation in acute myocardial infarction. Circulation 1990; 82(Suppl II):II-771.

21. Hanson SR, Harker LA. Interruption of acute platelet-dependent thrombosis by the synthetic antithrombin PPACK. Proc Natl Acad Sci USA 1988; 85:3184-8.

22. Badimon L, Lassila R, Badimon J, et al. Thrombin is more thrombogenic than the severely damaged vessel wall. Circulation 1988; 78(Suppl II):II-119.

23. Heras M, Chesebro JH, Penny WJ, et al. Effects of thrombin inhibitor on the development of platelet-thrombosis deposite during angioplasty in pigs. Heparin versus hirudin, a synthetic thrombin inhibitor. Circulation 1989; 79:657-65.

24. Jang IK, Gold HK, Ziskind AA, et al. Prevention of platelet-rich arterial thrombosis by selective thrombin inhibitor. Circulation 1990; 81:219-25.

25. Wessler S, Gitel SN. Pharmacology of heparin and warfarin. J Am Coll Cardiol 1986; 8:10-20.

26. Heras M, Chesebro JH, Penny WJ, et al. Importance of adequate heparin dosage in arterial angioplasty in the porcine model. Circulation 1988; 78:654-60.

27. Cereck B, Lewis AS, Hold H, et al. Enhancement of thrombolysis with t-PA with pretreatment with heparin. Circulation 1986; 74:583-7.

28. Yasuda T, Gold HK, Fallon TY, et al. A canine model of coronary artery thrombosis with superimposed high grade stenosis from the investigation of rethrombosis after thrombolysis. J Am Coll Cardiol 1989; 13:1409-14.

29. Bergmann SR, Fox KAA, Ter-Pogossian MM, et al. Clot-selective coronary thrombolysis with t-PA. Science 1987; 220:1181-3.

30. Massel DR, Hadoba M, Weitz JI. Clot-bound thrombosis is protected from heparin inhibition. A potential mechanism for rethrombosis after lytic therapy. Circulation 1989; 80(Suppl II):II-420 (abstract).

31. White DH. GISSI-2 and the heparin controversy. Lancet 1990; 336:297-301.

32. The SCATI Group. Randomized controlled trial of subcutaneous calcium-heparin in acute myocardial infarction. Lancet 1989; 2:182-6.

33. Markwardt F, Nowick G, Sturzebecker J, et al. Pharmacokinetics of anticoagulant effects of hirudin in man. Thromb Haemost 1984; 52:160-3.

34. Mao STJ, Yates MJ, Owen TY, et al. Interaction of Hirudin with thrombin: identification of a minimal binding domain of hirudin that inhibits clotting activity. Biochemistry 1988; 27:8170-3.

35. Siess W. Molecular mechanisms of platelet activation. Physiology 1989; 69:58-178.

36. Tam SW, Fenmton JW, Detwiler TC. Dissociation of thrombin from platelet by hirudin. J Biol Chem 1979; 254:8723-5.

37. Mruk TS, Chesbro JH, Webster MWI, et al. Hirudin markedly enhanced thrombolysis with rt-PA. Circulation 1990; 82(Suppl III):III-135 (abstract).

38. Garratt KN, Heras M, Holmes DR Jr, et al. Platelet deposition and thrombosis in arterial stents: effects of hirudin compared with heparin plus antiplatelet therapy. J Am Coll Cardiol 1990; 15(Suppl A):209A (abstract).

39. Homeister JW, Mickelson JK, Hoff PT, Luchessi BR. Recombinant hirudin prevents thrombosis in the canine coronary artery. Circulation 1989; 80(Suppl II):II-421 (abstract).

40. Kelly AB, Hanson SR, Marzec M, Harker LA. Recombinant hirudin interruption of platelet-dependent thrombus formation. Circulation 1989; 80(Suppl II):II-211 (abstract).

41. Verstraete M, Hoet B, Tormia I, et al. Hirudin, a specific thrombin inhibitor: pharmacological and hemostatic effect in man. Circulation 1989; 80(Suppl II):II-421 (abstract).

42. Marler RA, Kleiss AJ, Griffin JH. Mechanism of action of human APC, a thrombin dependent anticoagulant enzyme. Blood 1982; 59:1067-72.

43. Emerick SC, Murayama H, Yan SB, et al. Preclinical pharmacology of activated protein C. In Holdenberg JC, ed. The pharmacology and toxicity of proteins. New York: Alan R Liss, 1989:356-7.

44. Gladson CL, Scharrer I, Hack KH, Griffin JH. The frequency of type I heterozygous protein S and protein C deficiency in 141 unrelated young patients with venous thrombosis. Thromb Haemost 1988; 59:18-22.

45. Bovill EG, Bauer KA, Dickerman JD, et al. The clinical spectrum of heterozygous protein C deficiency in a large New England kindred. Blood 1989; 73:712-7.

46. Gruber A, Griffin JH, Harker LA, Hanson SR. Inhibition of platelet-dependent thrombus formation by human activated protein C in a primate model. Blood 1989; 73:639-42.

47. Gruber A, Hanson SR, Kelly A, et al. Inhibition of thrombin formation by activated recombinant protein C in a primate model of arterial thrombosis. Circulation 1990; 82:578-85.

48. Griffin JH, Hanson SR, Gruber A, et al. Antithrombotic effect of combining activated protein C with urokinase in a primate model of arterial thrombosis. Thromb Heamost 1989; 62:482 (abstract).

49. Kikomoto R, Tamao Y, Tejuka T, et al. Selective inhibitor of thrombin by argatroban. Biochemistry 1984; 23:85-90.

50. Eidt JF, Allison P, Noble S, et al. Thrombin is an important mediator of platelet aggregation in stenosed canine coronary arteries with endothelial injury. J Clin Invest 1989; 84:18-27.

51. Yasuda T, Gold HK, Yaoita H, et al. Comparative effects of aspirin, a synthetic thrombin inhibitor and a monoclonal antibody glycoprotein IIb/IIIa antibody on coronary artery reperfusion, reocclusion and bleeding with rt-PA in a canine preparation. J Am Coll Cardiol 1990; 16:714-22.

52. Kettner C, Shaw E. D-Phe-Pro-ArgCH2-Cl-A. Selective affinity label for thrombin. Thromb Res 1979; 14:969-73.

53. Collen D, Marsuo D, Stasseu JM, et al. In vivo studies of a synthetic inhibitor of thrombin. J Lab Clin Med 1982; 99:76-83.

12

Warfarin

Samuel Z. Goldhaber
*Harvard Medical School and Brigham and
Women's Hospital, Boston, Massachusetts*

INTRODUCTION

Research supported by the Wisconsin Alumni Research Foundation in the 1930s led to the recognition that a bleeding disease in cattle ("sweet clover disease") was due to spoiled sweet clover. Bishydroxycoumarin was identified as the culprit, and over the next few years, multiple congeners were synthesized. Warfarin has very favorable biological properties and has become the most widely used coumarin compound in North America (1,2).

PHARMACOLOGY

The coumarin compounds are similar structurally to vitamin K and inhibit competitively the enzyme vitamin K_1 epoxide reductase, which is crucial for vitamin K metabolism. This prevents regeneration of the active reduced form—vitamin K_1H_2—so that carboxylation of the vitamin K-dependent clotting factors—factors II, VII, IX, and X—is inhibited (Fig. 1A). Therefore, the unmodified clotting factors (known by hematologists as PIVKAs—proteins induced in vitamin K absence) are released into the plasma but are functionally inactive because they have not undergone a vitamin K-dependent addition of carboxyl groups onto glutamic acid residues (3). These glutamic acid residues bind calcium cation (Fig. 1B); this

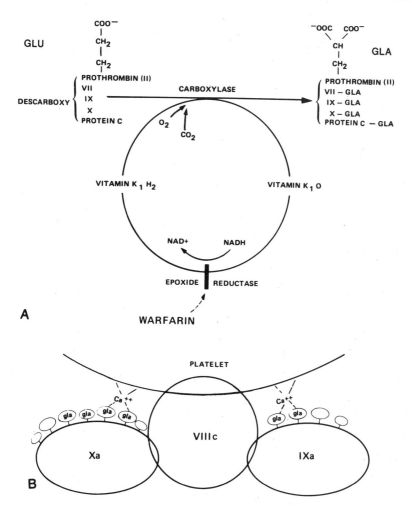

Figure 1   (A) Mechanism of action of warfarin. Warfarin inhibits an important step in vitamin K metabolism, decreasing vitamin K_1H_2-dependent carboxylation of factors II, VII, IX, X, and protein C. (B) The gamma-carboxyglutamic acid (GLA) residues on the vitamin K–dependent factors are essential for participation of these factors in coagulation reactions. glu = glutamic acid. (Reprinted from Ref. 2 with permission from W. B. Saunders Co.)

permits the coagulation protein to bind to phospholipids on activated platelets or endothelial cells.

As the biological activity of the vitamin K-dependent procoagulants decreases, the anticoagulant effects of the coumarin derivatives are realized. Factor VII, with a half-life of approximately 6 hr, is the first vitamin K-dependent factor to decrease. This leads to a prolongation of the prothrombin time (PT), which is utilized to monitor the activity of the extrinsic coagulation pathway (Fig. 2). However, prolongation of the PT is not equivalent to antithrombotic effect because the other vitamin K-dependent clotting factors have longer half-lives. Factor II, for example, has a half-life of 60–100 hr (2,3). This is why we usually heparinize patients during the first 4–5 days of warfarin therapy, even if the PT appears to be prolonged to the therapeutic target range. In addition, coumarin derivatives ultimately prolong the partial thromboplastin time (PTT) as well as the PT because they inhibit vitamin K_1H_2-dependent carboxylation of factor IX, which affects the intrinsic pathway, monitored by the PTT, as well as the extrinsic pathway, monitored by the PT (Fig. 2).

Coumarin derivatives also rapidly depress protein C anticoagulant activity. Protein C circulates as an inactive molecule that is activated by thrombin in the presence of a cofactor, thrombomodulin, on the endothelial surface (4). Activated protein C limits coagulation by inactivating factors V_a and VIII_c, which, in turn, decreases thrombin production (Fig. 2). Decreased protein C activity may produce paradoxically a hypercoagulable state and can lead to the development of skin necrosis associated with coumarin anticoagulation. Therefore, large loading doses (more than 10 mg) should not be administered because of the possibility of rapidly depressing the protein C level.

Certain drugs potentiate coumarin derivatives whereas others have inhibitory action (Table 1). Although bleeding is the most common side effect, other less common adverse effects may occur (Table 2).

Bleeding from warfarin tends to be correlated with the intensity of anticoagulation. A study at Brigham and Women's Hospital demonstrated that the risk of bleeding increases as the PT increases. Of 130 cases of bleeding, 38% were due to remediable lesions, half of which were occult prior to warfarin administration (5). Therefore, if bleeding occurs when the PT is within the therapeutic range, occult malignancy should be investigated. Minor bleeding with a prolonged PT may merely require interruption of warfarin therapy, without administration of fresh frozen plasma, until the PT has returned to the therapeutic range. Extensive investigation of patients with minor bleeding and a PT above the therapeutic range is usually not productive.

A study at Boston City Hospital showed that switching from Coumadin to generic warfarin was associated with increased morbidity and increased expense due to widely fluctuating PT levels (6). This finding probably reflects the more erratic bioavailability of generic warfarin.

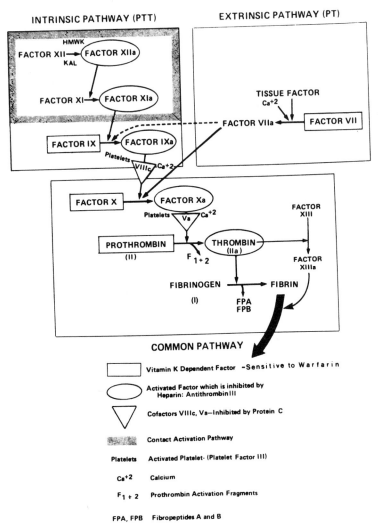

Figure 2   Important features of the coagulation pathways include the vitamin K–dependent factors affected by warfarin, the activated serine proteases inhibited by heparin: antithrombin III, and the role of platelets and calcium. The nonenzymatic cofactors VIII$_c$ and V$_a$ are inactivated by protein C. The prothrombin time (PT) measures the function of the extrinsic and common pathways; the partial thromboplastin time (PTT) measures the function of the intrinsic and common pathways. HMWK = high-molecular-weight kininogen; KAL = kallikrein. (Reprinted from Ref. 4 with permission from W. B. Saunders Co.)

Table 1   Examples of Drugs that Affect Coumarin Derivatives

Increase PT Response	Decrease PT Response
Cephalosporins	Antacids
Cimetidine	Antihistamines
Narcotics	Barbiturates
NSAIDs	Cholestyramine
Quinidine	Oral contraceptives
Sulfonamides	Rifampin
Sulfonylurea hypoglycemic	Vitamin C
agents	

SECONDARY PREVENTION OF MYOCARDIAL INFARCTION

The Warfarin Re-Infarction Study (WARIS) was initiated in Oslo, Norway, to assess the effect of long-term treatment with warfarin after myocardial infarction (7). Eligible patients had to be 75 years of age or younger and could not have standard contraindications to warfarin therapy. Importantly, patients were not allowed to use antiplatelet drugs such as aspirin. Those who enrolled were randomized to warfarin or to placebo. Treatment began, on average, 27 days after myocardial infarction. The PT target range was approximately equivalent to a prothrombin time ratio of 1.5-2.0 using a typical North American thromboplastin.

From 1983-1986, 1214 patients were enrolled. Using an intention-to-treat analysis, 20% in the placebo group and 15% in the warfarin group died—a significant reduction in risk of 24% (p = 0.027) (Fig. 3). When only patients who were actually receiving study medication or who were within 1 month of discontinuing it were analyzed, the risk reduction was 35%.

Table 2   Side Effects of Coumadin Derivatives

Bleeding
Alopecia
Purple toe syndrome
Dermatitis
Embryopathy, especially during the 6th-12th week of gestation
Skin necrosis
Diarrhea

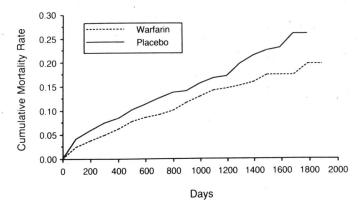

Figure 3 Cumulative rates of death from all causes, according to original treatment assignment, in the WARIS trial. (Reprinted from Ref. 7 with permission.)

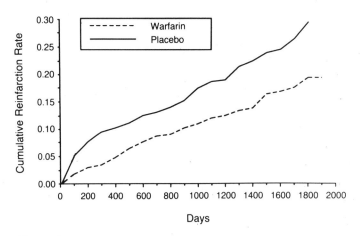

Figure 4 Cumulative rates of reinfarction, according to original treatment assignment, in the WARIS trial. (Reprinted from Ref. 7 with permission.)

With regard to recurrent myocardial infarction, the risk reduction with warfarin was 34% (Fig. 4). For patients actually continuing on study treatment, the reduction in risk was 43%.

There were 55% fewer strokes in the warfarin group. Overall, 14 strokes were fatal: four hemorrhagic strokes in the warfarin group and 10 nonhemorrhagic strokes in the placebo group.

During the trial, eight warfarin-treated patients had major extracranial bleeding events, of which five were gastrointestinal. All five of the latter patients had subsequently identified pathological lesions in the gastrointestinal tract.

Thus, WARIS provides a rationale for prescribing warfarin for secondary prevention of myocardial infarction. It would have been interesting to examine whether less intensive anticoagulation would have produced as beneficial an effect or to compare warfarin to an aspirin control. Also, the combination of warfarin plus aspirin might have provided even superior results, but this was not tested in WARIS, which specifically proscribed the use of aspirin or other antiplatelet agents.

PRIMARY PREVENTION OF CORONARY ARTERY DISEASE

The Northwick Park Heart Study (NPHS) recruited 1511 white men, aged 40–64 years, from northwest London (8). The NPHS evaluated prospectively the relationships between entry levels of factor VII, fibrinogen, and cholesterol and subsequent coronary heart disease incidence. High levels of factor VII coagulant activity and of plasma fibrinogen were associated with increased risk, especially for events occurring within 5 years of recruitment. These associations appeared to be stronger than for cholesterol (9). Elevations of one standard deviation in factor VII activity, fibrinogen, and cholesterol were associated with increases in the risk of an episode of coronary heart disease within 5 years of 62%, 84%, and 43%, respectively (Fig. 5).

The NPHS demonstrates that a hypercoagulable state increases the risk of coronary heart disease. Restriction of dietary fat can reduce factor VII levels. However, factor VII is also the procoagulatory vitamin K–dependent protein that is most rapidly inhibited by warfarin.

Factor VII coagulant activity probably increases the rate of thrombin production (10). In addition, factor VII concentrates can successfully treat factor VIII–resistant hemophiliacs, probably because of enhanced extrinsic pathway activity on thrombin production (Fig. 6).

Would warfarin and aspirin together reduce the incidence of coronary heart disease more than either agent alone? This question is addressed in the ongoing Thrombosis Prevention Trial (TPT) (10). Men aged 45–69 years, without contraindications to warfarin or aspirin, are recruited if they have elevated factor VII

IHD within 5 years of examination

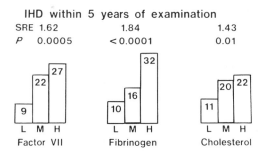

Figure 5   The Northwick Park Heart Study evaluated prospectively the relationships between entry levels of factor VII, fibrinogen, cholesterol, and coronary heart disease incidence. The number of coronary heart disease events that occurred within 5 years of examination correspond to the low (L), middle (M), and high (H) thirds of the distribution at entry of factor VII, fibrinogen, and cholesterol. The standardized regression effect (SRE) is the increase in risk of an event per one standard deviation increase. Increased levels of factor VII coagulant activity, fibrinogen, and cholesterol were associated with an increased coronary heart disease incidence. For example, a one standard deviation increase in factor VII activity corresponded to an increased risk of 62% of having an ischemic event within 5 years. (Reprinted from Ref. 9 with permission.)

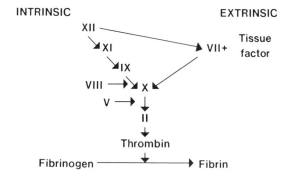

Figure 6   A summary of the coagulation cascade.

coagulant activity levels. The aim of the warfarin is to reduce factor VII coagulant activity from a level of about 120% of normal to approximately 70%. (Full anticoagulation reduces factor VII coagulant activity to approximately 30% of normal.)

Warfarin (or placebo) is initiated with 2.5 mg daily and is increased by 0.5 or 1.0 mg/day at monthly intervals until the desired effect on factor VII coagulant activity (among those patients receiving active warfarin) is achieved. The average warfarin dose is 4.6 mg/day. The aspirin component is a 75-mg, controlled-release preparation (10). The trial will continue until 1996.

LEFT VENTRICULAR THROMBUS AFTER ANTERIOR MYOCARDIAL INFARCTION

One-third of anterior myocardial infarctions are complicated by left ventricular thrombus formation. This frequency can be halved by anticoagulation. Echocardiography should be undertaken about 1 week after anterior myocardial infarction because more than 90% of thrombi will be evident at this stage. Resolution of the thrombus can then be monitored with serial echocardiograms. This type of echocardiographically guided anticoagulation might prevent three strokes, with one major bleeding complication, for every 100 patients with anterior myocardial infarction (11). Alternatively, all patients with anterior myocardial infarction could be anticoagulated with warfarin. However, formal decision analysis shows that this latter strategy will lead to more frequent bleeding events (12).

NONVALVULAR ATRIAL FIBRILLATION

Atrial fibrillation (AF) not related to valvular heart disease is associated with nearly half the arterial emboli presumed to be of cardiac origin. It starts at an average age of 64 years and affects 2–5% of the U.S. population over 60 years of age. AF is associated with a fivefold increase in risk of ischemic stroke, which eventually occurs in as many as 35% of patients with nonvalvular AF (13).

Since 1989, four prospective trials (14–16) of primary stroke prevention in nonvalvular atrial fibrillation have been terminated early, at the recommendation of the respective data-monitoring committees (Table 3). All have demonstrated an advantage for warfarin-treated patients compared with those who received placebo. One trial (14) showed that warfarin was effective but that aspirin in a dose of 75 mg/day was not more effective than placebo.

Table 3   Trials of Warfarin in Nonvalvular Atrial Fibrillation

Trial name (Ref. #)	Protocol	Results
The Copenhagen AFASAK Study (14)	Warfarin vs. low-dose aspirin (75 mg/day) vs. placebo; principal endpoint was thromboembolism; secondary endpoint was vascular death.	4 times as many thromboemboli and 4–5 times as many death in the aspirin and in the placebo groups compared with warfarin.
SPAF: Stroke Prevention in Atrial Fibrillation (15)	Warfarin vs. aspirin (325 mg/day) vs. placebo; endpoint is prevention of ischemic stroke and systemic thromboembolism.	Risk reduction of 81% among patients who are eligible to receive warfarin and who receive active therapy with warfarin or aspirin.
BAATAF: Boston Area Anticoagulation Trial for Atrial Fibrillation (16)	Unblinded, randomized, controlled trial of low-dose warfarin; the control group was not given but could choose to take aspirin.	Warfarin causes an 86% reduction in stroke; 62% reduction in death; one fatal hemorrhage in each group.
VA Cooperative Study #308: SPINAF: Stroke Prevention in Nonvalvular Atrial Fibrillation (unpublished)	Principal endpoint is cerebral infarction; randomized, double-blind, placebo-controlled trial of low-dose warfarin therapy.	Warfarin causes a reduction in stroke, myocardial infarction, and cardiovascular mortality.

PREVENTION OF RESTENOSIS AFTER ANGIOPLASTY

Warfarin (high dose) was compared with aspirin (325 mg/day) in a randomized trial of 248 patients who had undergone successful coronary angioplasty. The objective was to prevent restenosis, and patients had repeat coronary angiograms 3–6 months after the initial angioplasty. Overall, 36% randomized to warfarin had restenosis compared with 27% allocated to aspirin. Among patients with at least a 6-month history of angina prior to angioplasty, the restenosis rates were twice as high among the warfarin patients (44%) compared with the aspirin patients (21%). Thus, aspirin was superior to warfarin among patients with a longer history of angina.

UNPROVEN BUT COMMONLY PRESCRIBED ADJUNCTIVE USES IN CORONARY ARTERY DISEASE

Warfarin is frequently used for coronary arterial disease indications which seem logical but which have not yet been proven to be effective in randomized controlled trials. Among patients heparinized for an acute ischemic syndrome, angiographically visualized coronary arterial thrombus, or a complicated angioplasty, the cardiologist is understandably reluctant to stop heparin and withdraw abruptly systemic anticoagulation. Therefore, these patients (Table 4) are frequently switched to warfarin and overlapped on heparin and warfarin for 4–5 days, before the heparin is discontinued.

REGULATION OF THE PROTHROMBIN TIME

Thromboplastin reagents prepared from human brain are more responsive to the reduction in vitamin K–dependent coagulation factors than are thromboplastins prepared from rabbit brain. Therefore, the dose of warfarin required to prolong the PT using a human brain thromboplastin is less than for a similar prolongation using rabbit brain thromboplastin. In North America, more than 90% of all PT reagents are provided by three manufacturers of relatively unresponsive rabbit brain thromboplastins. In contrast, most laboratories in the United Kingdom use a more responsive human brain thromboplastin (19).

To standardize reporting of PT results, a common thromboplastin reagent could be used worldwide, but this is not feasible. A practical alternative is to relate the PT result to the common standard of the international normalized ratio (INR). The INR is the PT ratio that would be observed if the thromboplastin were international reference material derived from a standard brain preparation. For example, to prevent systemic embolism in atrial fibrillation, the recommended ratio of 1.3–1.6 for rabbit brain thromboplastin is approximately equivalent to an INR of 2.0–3.0 (20).

Table 4   Unproven, Commonly Prescribed Indications for Adjunctive Use of Warfarin

1. Following PTCA for unstable angina with residual thrombus or stenosis.
2. Following PTCA for an acute ischemic syndrome if the patient has just recovered from an acute coronary occlusion.
3. Following PTCA if a stent has been used.
4. Following acute MI with catheterization revealing a high-grade residual lesion; such patients may be treated with warfarin for 3–6 months plus aspirin (low dose) indefinitely (18).
5. Following CABG among patients with grafts at high risk of occlusion (e.g., after right coronary artery endarterectomy).

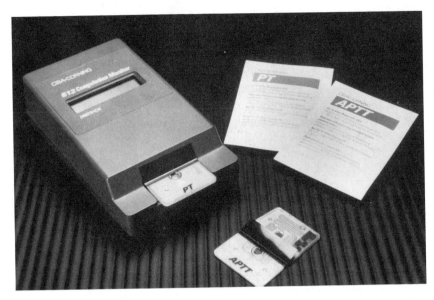

Figure 7   The Biotrack laser optical system. In the Biotrack prothrombin time test, the monitor detects the time from application of blood to the cartridge to cessation of flow and converts it into a prothrombin time.

OUTPATIENT REGULATION OF WARFARIN

Most warfarin is administered in the outpatient setting. Until recently, we adjusted the dose of warfarin based on the plasma PT. After the laboratory telephoned us with PT results, we used to contact our patients either to reassure them that their dosing regimen was appropriate or to make dosage adjustments. Unfortunately, it can be quite difficult to explain changes in anticoagulation dosing by telephone. Therefore, we now utilize the Biotrack (Fig. 7) to make in-office assessments of warfarin dosing regimens. The Biotrack provides the PT result in 2 min by analyzing a drop of whole blood obtained from a fingertip puncture. It has been demonstrated that devices of this type (21) can be given to patients who can then monitor their PT at home (22,23).

THE FUTURE

Multiple mechanisms appear to contribute to the increased procoagulant activity during thrombolysis. The consequences of increased procoagulant activity include delay or failure of clot lysis and rethrombosis. Although warfarin has never been shown to be an effective adjunctive therapy for thrombolysis, new strategies are emerging. These adjunctive therapies include more potent thrombin inhibition and inhibition of factors that initiate thrombosis (24). In the meantime, warfarin will assume an increasingly prominent role in the secondary and primary prevention of myocardial infarction and in the treatment of chronic atrial fibrillation regardless of its etiology.

REFERENCES

1. Wessler S, Gitel SN. Warfarin. From bedside to bench. N Engl J Med 1984; 311:645-52.
2. Stead RB. Clinical pharmacology. In Goldhaber SZ, ed., Pulmonary embolism and deep venous thrombosis. Philadelphia: Saunders, 1985, 99-119.
3. Kessler CM. The pharmacology of aspirin, heparin, coumarin, and thrombolytic agents. Implications for therapeutic use in cardiopulmonary disease. Chest 1991; 99:97S-112S.
4. Stead RB. Regulation of hemostasis. In Goldhaber SZ, ed., Pulmonary embolism and deep venous thrombosis. Philadelphia: Saunders, 1985, 27-40.
5. Landefeld CS, Rosenblatt MW, Goldman L. Bleeding in outpatients treated with warfarin: relation to the prothrombin time and important remediable lesions. Am J Med 1989; 87:153-9.
6. Richton-Hewett S, Foster E, Apstein CS. Medical and economic consequences of a blinded oral anticoagulant brand change at a municipal hospital. Arch Intern Med 1988; 148:806-8.
7. Smith P, Arnesen H, Holme I. The effect of warfarin on mortality and reinfarction after myocardial infarction. N Engl J Med 1990; 323:147-52.
8. Meade TW, North WRS, Chakrabarti R, Stirling Y, Haines AP, Thompson SG. Haemostatic function and cardiovascular death: early results of a prospective study. Lancet 1980; 1:1050-3.
9. Meade TW, Mellows S, Brozovic M, Miller GJ, Chakrabarti RR, North WRS, Haines AP, Stirling Y, Imeson JD, Thompson SG. Haemostatic function and ischaemic heart disease: principal results of the Northwick Park Heart Study. Lancet 1986; 2:533-7.
10. Meade TW. Low-dose warfarin and low-dose aspirin in the primary prevention of ischemic heart disease. Am J Cardiol 1990; 65:7C-11C.
11. Left ventricular thrombosis and stroke following myocardial infarction. Lancet 1990; 1:759-60.
12. Weintraub WS, Ba'albaki HA. Decision analysis concerning the application of echocardiography to the diagnosis and treatment of mural thrombi after anterior wall acute myocardial infarction. Am J Cardiol 1989; 64:708-16.
13. Chesebro JH, Fuster V, Halperin JL. Atrial fibrillation—risk marker for stroke. N Engl J Med 1990; 323:1556-8.
14. Petersen P, Boysen G, Godfredsen J, Andersen ED, Andersen B. Placebo-controlled, randomized trial of warfarin and aspirin for prevention of thromboembolic complica-

tions in chronic atrial fibrillation. The Copenhagen AFASAK Study. Lancet 1989; 1:175-9.

15. Stroke Prevention In Atrial Fibrillation Study Group Investigators. Preliminary report of the stroke prevention in atrial fibrillation study. N Engl J Med 1990; 322:863-8.

16. The Boston Area Anticoagulation Trial for Atrial Fibrillation Investigators. The effect of low-dose warfarin on the risk of stroke in patients with nonrheumatic atrial fibrillation. N Engl J Med 1990; 323:1505-11.

17. Thornton MA, Gruentzig AR, Hollman J, King SB III, Douglas JS. Coumadin and aspirin in prevention of recurrence after transluminal coronary angioplasty: a randomized study. Circulation 1984; 69:721-7.

18. Chesebro JH, Mruk JS, Webster MWI, Fuster V. Antithrombotic therapy with coronary angioplasty, thrombolysis, and bypass graft surgery. Primary Cardiol 1991; 17:19-39.

19. Hirsh J. Is the dose of warfarin prescribed by American physicians unnecessarily high? Arch Intern Med 1987; 147:769-71.

20. Hirsh J, Levine MN. The optimal intensity of oral anticoagulant therapy. JAMA 1987; 258:2723-6.

21. Lucas FV, Duncan A, Jay R, Coleman R, Craft P, Chan B, Winfrey L, Mungall DR. A novel whole blood capillary technique for measuring the prothrombin time. Am J Clin Pathol 1987; 88:442-6.

22. White RH, McCurdy SA, von Marensdorff H, Woodruff DE Jr, Leftgoff L. Home prothrombin time monitoring after the initiation of warfarin therapy. A randomized, prospective study. Ann Intern Med 1989; 111:730-7.

23. Ansell J, Holden A, Knapic N. Patient self-management of oral anticoagulation guided by capillary (fingerstick) whole blood prothrombin times. Arch Intern Med 1989; 149:2509-11.

24. Eisenberg PR. Role of new anticoagulants as adjunctive therapy during thrombolysis. Am J Cardiol 1991; 67:19A-24A.

13

The Emerging Role of Combination Thrombolytic Therapy in Acute Myocardial Infarction

Cindy Grines and William O'Neill
William Beaumont Hospital, Royal Oak, Michigan

Eric Topol
The Cleveland Clinic Foundation, Cleveland, Ohio

INTRODUCTION

The objectives of thrombolytic therapy are to rapidly restore coronary patency, prevent reocclusion, salvage myocardium, and enhance survival. Although thrombolytic therapy for acute myocardial infarction is now widely accepted, each of the thrombolytic agents currently available has intrinsic advantages and limitations when utilized as monotherapy (Table 1). Irrespective of the dose of thrombolytic drug, it has been difficult to consistently achieve an acute patency rate greater than 75–80% (1–5). Furthermore, the time to recanalization may be protracted, with the median time being 45 min, regardless of which thrombolytic drug is utilized (6,7). In addition, recurrent ischemia and reocclusion occur frequently and unpredictably after thrombolytic therapy (8). Although left ventricular function is an important prognostic indicator, serial left ventriculograms have demonstrated minimal improvement in function after thrombolytic therapy (9). Serious bleeding complications, although rare, remain the primary concern of physicians when considering the risk/benefit ratio of thrombolytic therapy for any given patient. Finally, given the concern over cost containment in medicine, the expense of the pharmaceutical agents is an important issue. For example, the administration of the newer-generation thrombolytic drugs could consume one-half

Table 1   Current Limitations of Thrombolytic
Monotherapy

Patency plateau of approximately 75-80%
Protracted time to recanalization
Recurrent ischemia/reocclusion
Modest improvement in ventricular function
Serious bleeding complications
Cost

or more of the Medicare reimbursement for the diagnosis-related groups (DRG) category of uncomplicated myocardial infarction (10).

Because of their deficiencies, combinations of various thrombolytic agents have recently received a great deal of attention. There are many potential benefits of combining thrombolytic drugs. It was initially hoped that by administering two very potent thrombolytic agents, a reperfusion rate approaching 100% might be achieved. This phenomenon was referred to as "super efficacy." Second, by utilizing an agent that depletes serum fibrinogen levels and has a very long half-life, the rate of infarct vessel reocclusion might be reduced. Addition of an agent that reduces serum viscosity and left ventricular afterload (streptokinase, anistreplase) might further improve left ventricular function. Other studies have utilized drugs thought to have synergistic relationships, thereby allowing a lower dose of each thrombolytic agent and potentially reducing the risk of bleeding complications, as well as the cost of very expensive second-generation thrombolytic drugs.

EARLY EXPERIMENTAL COMBINATION THROMBOLYTIC DRUGS

Tissue plasminogen activator (t-PA) and single-chain urokinase type plasminogen activator (scu-PA, prourokinase) are fibrin-specific thrombolytic agents. However, when these agents are used alone, high doses are required to achieve thrombolysis in humans. These high doses result in a significant depletion of serum fibrinogen (11-13). Therefore, in an attempt to reduce the dose requirement using monotherapy, investigations have been undertaken to determine synergistic effects between various agents. "Synergism" of thrombolytic agents is thought to occur when the combined effect of the agents is greater than the expected additive effect of the individual agents based on a dose/effect relationship (14). For instance, initial in vitro studies performed by Gurewich and Pannell demonstrated synergism between t-PA and scu-PA (15). However, Collen et al. reported that there was no evidence of synergism between urokinase and scu-PA, and that the effects seen between these agents merely represented an additive effect (16). Both authors noted a "threshold phenomenon" and a "lag phase" with scu-PA–induced thrombolysis.

In a jugular vein thrombosis model, Collen et al. demonstrated that synergistic effects did exist between t-PA and urokinase, as well as between t-PA and scu-PA (16). They could not demonstrate any definitive interaction, however, between scu-PA and urokinase. In a canine model of coronary artery thrombosis, Ziskind et al. found synergism between t-PA and prourokinase within a narrow dose range (17). However, reocclusion was a frequent occurrence despite the very high rate of reperfusion observed.

Two small pilot studies suggested that recombinant t-PA and scu-PA might act synergistically in fibrinolysis (18,19). In addition, small doses of t-PA with urokinase were found to result in successful reperfusion in three of four treated patients (18). As a result of these very early studies, several recent clinical investigations have centered on the evaluation of combinations of various thrombolytic drugs.

COMBINATION PROUROKINASE WITH t-PA OR UROKINASE

Some investigators believe that the use of nonspecific plasminogen activators that induce systemic fibrinolysis and plasmin generation may be undesirable. The reason for this is that plasminemia causes a hemostatic defect with subsequent activation of the complement system, which may lead to platelet hyperaggregability (20,21). Although controversial, some physicians also believe that depletion of serum fibrinogen may increase the risk of bleeding complications.

t-PA and scu-PA induce selective fibrinolysis. However, when they are used alone, high doses are required to reperfuse an occluded coronary artery. These high doses produce a significant reduction in serum fibrinogen levels (11). Studies utilizing combinations of t-PA with scu-PA attempt to achieve more effective thrombolysis without compromising fibrin specificity. A demonstration of a synergistic effect between these two agents may allow a lower dose of both t-PA and scu-PA, which may potentially lower the cost, as well as reducing the lag time required for thrombolysis with scu-PA. As demonstrated in Table 2, three small clinical trials have been performed addressing the relationship between scu-PA and t-PA. Collen and van de Werf studied nine patients who received a dose of 10 mg t-PA, as well as 10 mg of scu-PA. Patency was achieved in seven of nine patients (78%) by 90 min (19). Of the 38 patients who received 12 mg of t-PA and 48 mg of scu-PA in the study by Bode and colleagues, patency was achieved in 82% (22). Kirshenbaum and co-workers studied 23 patients who received combination t-PA (20 mg) and scu-PA (16.3 mg) and achieved a 70% early recanalization rate (23). These studies demonstrated a minimal reduction in serum fibrinogen and plasminogen levels as well as a paucity of bleeding complications. Therefore, it

Table 2   Combination Prourokinase with UK or t-PA

Study	N	scu-PA dose	UK dose	t-PA dose	Acute patency (%)
Gulba	15	4.5 MU	0.25 MU		33
	16	6.5 MU	0.25 MU		75
Kasper	35	4.5 MU	0.2 MU		66
Collen	9	10 mg		10 mg	78
Bode	38	48 mg		12 mg	82
Kirshenbaum	23	16.3 mg		20 mg	70

UK = urokinase; t-PA = tissue plasminogen activator; scu-PA = prourokinase.

appears that combined intravenous infusion of t-PA and scu-PA at appropriate doses induces coronary thrombolysis equal to the results achieved with either t-PA or scu-PA monotherapy. This high rate of coronary thrombolysis is coupled with very high fibrin specificity. Although these data initially appear to be favorable, the incidence of reocclusion has not been adequately addressed. Furthermore, there has been recent concern that agents that do not deplete circulating fibrinogen may have a higher rate of rethrombosis.

Other investigators have sought to study combinations of scu-PA with urokinase. As demonstrated in Table 2, Gulba and co-workers studied two groups of patients utilizing different doses of prourokinase (24). The first group of patients received 4.5 mega units of scu-PA, as well as 250,000 units of urokinase. Acute patency was only 33%, and 60% of these vessels subsequently reoccluded. The second series of patients received 6.5 mega units of scu-PA, as well as 250,000 units of urokinase. Patency improved to 75%, and the reocclusion rate was only 8% in this group. Although fibrinogen decreased only 13% from baseline, minor bleeding occurred in 37% of patients. Kasper et al. reported 35 patients who received combination scu-PA and urokinase (25). Acute patency was 66% in their series, with a reocclusion rate of 10%. Therefore, it appears that low-dose urokinase may reduce by 50% the dose of prourokinase required for effective thrombolysis.

COMBINATIONS OF t-PA AND UROKINASE

Since animal studies suggested a synergistic relationship between t-PA and urokinase (16,17), we conducted a dose-ranging study utilizing different combinations of t-PA and urokinase (26). The rationale for conducting the study was to test whether a synergistic relationship existed between the two drugs at very low doses and to determine whether superior infarct artery patency might occur by combining very high doses of each drug. Incremental doses of both t-PA and urokinase were infused over 60 min in 146 consecutive patients treated a mean of 3 hr from symptom onset. Coronary arteriography was performed 90 min after initiation of the infusion and 7 days later. Five different dosing regimens were utilized. Groups 1 and 2 received 25 mg of t-PA combined with either 500,000 units or 1 million units of urokinase, respectively. These drug combinations were used to test the hypothesis of low-dose synergism. Groups 3, 4 and 5 all received 1 mg/kg of t-PA with doses of urokinase ranging from 500,000 units to 2 million units. These relatively high dose combinations of thrombolytic drugs were used to determine whether a higher rate of infarct vessel patency might be achieved.

In groups 1 and 2, patency at 90 min was only 36% and 42%, respectively. With 1 mg/kg of t-PA and increasing doses of urokinase (groups 3–5), patency ranged from 72% to 75% (overall 73%). Repeat catheterization at day 7 demonstrated a reocclusion rate of 9%, which tended to be lower than our earlier experience with t-PA monotherapy. This reduction in reocclusion was particularly apparent in patients who failed thrombolysis and required angioplasty. These patients had a substantially higher patency rate at hospital discharge compared with patients treated with t-PA monotherapy and rescue PTCA in TAMI-1 (96% versus 69%, $p = 0.01$). In addition, inhospital mortality (0% versus 10.4%, $p = 0.08$) appeared to be improved.

This pilot study was unable to demonstrate a synergistic relationship between t-PA and urokinase in humans. Furthermore, a plateau of 75% infarct artery patency at 90 min existed regardless of the dose of thrombolytic drug administered. However, with the combined infusion of these agents, there appeared to be a favorable reduction in the rate of reocclusion, particularly in patients who failed thrombolysis and required rescue angioplasty, and there appeared to be no additional risk of bleeding.

In the recently completed Thrombolysis and Angioplasty in Myocardial Infarction (TAMI-5) study, patients with acute myocardial infarction were randomized to receive either t-PA alone, (100 mg administered over 3 hr), urokinase alone (3 million units over 1 hr), or the combination of t-PA (1 mg/kg) with urokinase (1.5 million units) over 1 hr (27). Patients then underwent a second randomization to emergency cardiac catheterization versus no catheterization. Patients who underwent catheterization demonstrated an early patency rate of 71% for t-PA alone, 62% for urokinase, and 78% for the combination regimen ($p = $ NS). Interestingly, reocclusion was reduced after combination therapy (2%), compared with 12% after t-PA monotherapy and 7% after urokinase monotherapy ($p = 0.004$).

The incidence of an adverse inhospital event (defined as death, stroke, reinfarction, heart failure, or recurrent ischemia) was lower after combination therapy (32%) compared with t-PA (40%) or urokinase (45%, $p = 0.04$) monotherapy. In-

Table 3   Combination t-PA with Urokinase

Study	N	t-PA dose	UK dose	90-min patency (%)	Reocc (%)
TAMI-2	112	1 mg/kg/60 min	0.5–2 MU	76	9
TAMI-5	191	1 mg/kg/60 min	1.5 MU	78	2
TAMI-7	44	1 mg/kg/30 min	1.5 MU	74	5
URALMI	129	1 mg/kg/60 min	1–2 MU	81	9
Pooled	476			78	5

UK = urokinase; t-PA = tissue plasminogen activator; Reocc = reocclusion.

terestingly, the bleeding complications after combination t-PA and urokinase did not appear to be increased. Specifically, there were no intracranial bleeds after combination therapy compared to four intracranial bleeds in the t-PA monotherapy group. Furthermore, the nadir hematocrit, number of patients who required a blood transfusion, as well as the average number of units transfused were identical in the two groups.

As demonstrated in Table 3, subsequent studies have also been performed using combinations of t-PA with urokinase (28,29). Consistently, this regimen results in a high early patency rate with a very favorable reocclusion rate compared to t-PA monotherapy.

COMBINATION t-PA WITH STREPTOKINASE

Since the above studies have suggested that substituting the longer-acting, systemic fibrinolytic agent urokinase for a t-PA maintenance infusion might reduce the rate of reocclusion with no additional risk of bleeding, subsequent investigations were centered on defining a regimen that was less costly than t-PA/urokinase. In a 40-patient pilot study, we demonstrated that the combination of half-dose t-PA with full-dose streptokinase offered high infarct artery patency and a low rate of reocclusion (30) (Table 4). Bonnet and colleagues treated 50 consecutive patients with a regimen consisting of 50 mg t-PA (administered as a 20-mg bolus followed by 30 mg over 30 min), followed by 1 million units of streptokinase over the next 30 min (31). Ninety-minute patency after combination t-PA/streptokinase in this series was 84%, and reocclusion occurred in 7% of patients. Transfusions were required in only 2%, and there were no strokes.

To determine the comparability of combination therapy to t-PA alone, we designed a prospective trial in which 216 patients were randomized within 6 hr of

Table 4   Outcome After Combined t-PA/Streptokinase

Study	N	Patency 90-min	Reocclusion Overall	Salvage PTCA	Intracranial Bleed	# Deaths
KAMIT pilot	40	30/40	3/37	1/8	0	1
KAMIT	109	80/102	3/89	1/12	1	7
Bonnet	50	42/50	3/45	0/8	0	1
Pooled	199	79%	5.2%	7.1%	0.5%	4.5%

t-PA = tissue plasminogen activator; PTCA = percutaneous transluminal coronary angioplasty.

myocardial infarction to the combination of half-dose (50 mg) t-PA with strep-tokinase (SK) (1.5 million units) over 1 hr or to the conventional dose of t-PA (100 mg/3hr) (32). Acute patency was determined by angiography at 90 min and an-gioplasty was reserved for failed thrombolysis. Intravenous heparin and oral aspi-rin were maintained until follow-up catheterization at day 7. Acute patency was significantly greater after t-PA/SK (79%) compared with t-PA alone (64%, $p <$ 0.05). After angioplasty for failed thrombolysis, acute patency increased to 96% in both groups. Marked depletion of serum fibrinogen occurred after t-PA/SK compared with t-PA alone at 4 hr (37 ± 36 versus 199 ± 66 mg/dl, $p < 0.0001$) and persisted 24 hr after therapy. Reocclusion (3% versus 10%, $p = 0.06$), reinfarction (0 versus 4%, $p < 0.05$), and the need for emergency bypass surgery (1% versus 6%, $p = 0.05$) tended to be less with the t-PA/SK group. Greater myocardial sal-vage was apparent after t-PA/SK as assessed by infarct zone function at day 7. Inhospital mortality (6% versus 4%) and serious bleeding complications (12% versus 11%) were similar in the two groups. These results suggest that a less ex-pensive regimen of half-dose t-PA with SK yields superior 90-min patency and 7-day left ventricular function and a trend toward reduced reocclusion compared with conventional monotherapy t-PA.

The low rate of reocclusion after combination of t-PA with either SK or urokinase may be due to the interference of fibrin polymerization, to the an-tiplatelet effects of fibrin degradation products, or to prolonged depletion of circu-lating fibrinogen, which may allow time for healing of injured endothelium (33–35). Although preservation of circulating fibrinogen was thought to be a po-tential advantage in reducing bleeding complications (36), laboratory measures of the "lytic state" may not correlate well with bleeding complications. Current data suggest that prolonged depletion of serum fibrinogen may be advantageous in re-ducing reocclusion. Interestingly, despite marked differences in serum fibrinogen levels, bleeding complications were similar in groups that received combination thrombolytic agents or t-PA alone. Lack of increased bleeding in these trials utilizing t-PA combined with SK or urokinase may be related to the lower dose and shorter infusion duration of t-PA.

FUTURE RESEARCH DIRECTIONS

There continue to be many new developments in the field of thromboblytic therapy. In recent years, intense interest has been apparent in combination thrombolytic therapy, the interaction between intravenous heparin and thrombolytic agents, and the use of accelerated dosing regimens of t-PA (37,38). To address these issues, a new large-scale mortality trial entitled "Global Utilization of Streptokinase and t-PA for Occluded Coronary Arteries (GUSTO)" has recently been undertaken (39). The principal objective of this trial is to test whether aggressive pharmacological regimens that quickly achieve and maintain coronary patency will translate into improved clinical outcome. As demonstrated in Figure 1, the reference standard will be intravenous streptokinase with two other randomization arms, including accelerated t-PA monotherapy, as well as combination t-PA with streptokinase. All patients will receive heparin and oral aspirin therapy. Primary endpoints include 30-day mortality, with secondary endpoints being inhospital clinical events.

The Thrombolysis in Myocardial Infarction (TIMI) phase 4 trial is currently evaluating combined therapy with anistreplase and t-PA, as shown in Figure 2. Trials such as GUSTO and TIMI-4 will help to define the potential advantage of combined thrombolytic therapy and greatly extend our perspective of safety with

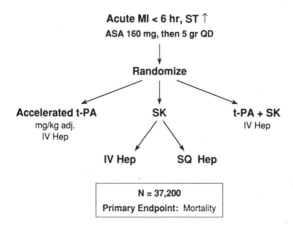

Figure 1   Study design for the ongoing Global Utilization of Streptokinase and t-PA for Occluded Coronary Arteries. (GUSTO).

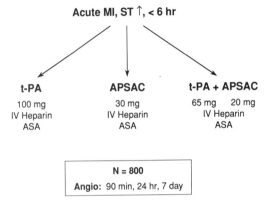

Figure 2   Proposed study design for the Thrombolysis in Myocardial Infarction (TIMI) phase 4 trial.

use of more than one plasminogen activator. While ultimately combined thrombolytics may be supplanted by specific adjunctive therapies, the current use of both a relatively fibrin specific and nonspecific activator holds considerable promise for improvement in clinical outcome after myocardial infarction.

ACKNOWLEDGMENT

The authors acknowledge Phyllis McKinney for manuscript preparation.

REFERENCES

1. The TIMI Study Group. The Thrombolysis in Myocardial Infarction (TIMI) trial. N Engl J Med 1985; 312:932–6.
2. Verstraete M, Bory M, Collen D, Erbel R, Lennane RJ, Mathey D, Michels HR, Schartel M, Uebis R, Bernard R, Brower RW, DeBono DP, Huhmann W, Lubsen J, Meyer J, Rutsch W, Schmidt W, von Essen R. Randomized trial of intravenous recombinant tissue-type plasminogen activator versus intravenous streptokinase in acute myocardial infarction. Lancet 1985; 1:842–7.
3. Topol EJ, Califf RM, George BS, Kereiakes DJ, Abbottsmith CW, Candela RJ, Lee KL, Pitt B, Stack RS, O'Neill WW, and the Thrombolysis and Angioplasty in Myocardial Infarction Study Group. A randomized trial of immediate versus delayed elective angioplasty after intravenous tissue plasminogen activator in acute myocardial infarction. N Engl J Med 1987; 317:581–8.
4. Neuhaus KL, Tebbe U, Gottwik M, Weber MAJ, Feuerer W, Niederer W, Haerer W, Praetorius F, Grosser KD, Huhmann W, Hoepp HW, Alber G, Sheikhzadeh A, Schneider B. Intravenous recombinant tissue plasminogen activator (rt-PA) and

urokinase in acute myocardial infarction: results of the German Activator Urokinase Study (GAUS). J Am Coll Cardiol 1988; 12:581-7.

5. Guerci AD, Gerstenblith G, Brinker JA, Chandra NC, Gottlieb SO, Bahr RD, Weiss JL, Shapiro EP, Flaherty JT, Bush De, Chew PH, Gottlieb SH, Halperin HR, Ouyang P, Walford GD, Bell WR, Fatterpaker AK, Llewellyn M, Topol EJ, Healy V, Siu CO, Becker LC, Weisfeldt ML. A randomized trial of intravenous tissue plasminogen activator for acute myocardial infarction with subsequent randomization to elective coronary angioplasty. N Engl J Med 1987; 317:1613-8.

6. Chesebro HK, Knatterud G, Roberts R, Borer J, Cohen LS, Dalen J, Dodge HT, Francis DK, Hillis D, Ludbrook P, Markis JE, Mueller H, Passamani ER, Powers ER, Rao AK, Robertson T, Ross A, Ryan TJ, Sobel BE, Willerson J, William SO, Zaret BL, Braunwald E. Thrombolysis in Myocardial Infarction (TIMI) Trial, Phase 1: comparison between intravenous tissue plasminogen activator and intravenous streptokinase. Clinical findings through hospital discharge. Circulation 1987; 76:142-54.

7. Anderson JL, Rothbard RL, Hackworthy RA, et al. Multicenter reperfusion trial of intravenous anisoylated plasminogen streptokinase activator complex (APSAC) in acute myocardial infarction: controlled comparison with intracoronary streptokinase. J Am Coll Cardiol 1988; 11:1153-63.

8. Ellis SG, Topol EJ, George BS, Kereiakes DJ, Debowey D, Sigmon KN, Pickel A, Lee KL, Califf RM. Recurrent ischemia without warning. Analysis of risk factors for in-hospital ischemic events following successful thrombolysis with intravenous tissue plasminogen activator. Circulation 1989; 80:1159-65.

9. The TIMI Study Group. Comparisonof invasive and conservative strategies after treatment with intravenous tissue plasminogen activator in acute myocardial infarction: results of the Thrombolysis in Myocardial Infarction (TIMI) Phase II Trial. N Engl J Med 1989; 320:618-27.

10. Vogel JHK. Management of acute myocardial infarction 1990: a perspective. Clin Cardiol 1991; 14:5-9.

11. Rao AK, Pratt C, Berke A, Jaffe A, Ockene I, Schreiber TL, Bell WR, Knatterud G, Robertson RL, Terrin ML, for the TIMI Investigators. Thrombolysis in Myocardial Infarction (TIMI) Trial—Phase I: hemorrhagic manifestations and changes in plasma fibrinogen and the fibrinolytic system in patients treated with recombinant tissue plasminogen activator and streptokinase. J Am Coll Cardiol 1988; 11:1-11.

12. Bode C, Schoner MS, Schules G, Zimmermann R, Schwarz F, Kubler W. Efficacy of intravenous pro-urokinase and a combination of pro-urokinase and urokinase in acute myocardial infarction. Am J Cardiol 1988; 61:971-4.

13. Meyer J, Bar F, Barth H, Charbonnier B, El Deeb MF, Flohe EL, Heikklia GJ, Massberg I, Mathey D, Monassier JP, Probst P, Schmitz-Hubner U, Seabra-Gomes R, Strupp G, Uebis R, Vermeer F, van der Werf T, Westerhof P, Windeler J. Randomized double-blind trial of recombinant prourokinase against streptokinase in acute myocardial infarction. Lancet 1989; 1:863-8.

14. Collen D. Synergism of thrombolytic agents: investigational procedures and clinical potential. Circulation 1988; 77:731-5.

15. Gurewich V. Pannell R. A comparative study of the efficacy and specificity of tissue

plasminogen activator and prourokinase. Demonstration of synergism and of different thresholds of non-selectivity. Thrombosis Res 1986; 44:217–28.

16. Collen D, Stassen J, Stump D, Verstraete M. Synergism of thrombolytic agents in vivo. Circulation 1986; 74:838–42.

17. Ziskind AA, Gold HK, Yasuda T, Kanke M, Guerrero JL, Fallon T, Saito T, Collen D. Synergistic combinations of recombinant human tissue-type plasminogen activator and human single-chain urokinase-type plasminogen activator. Effect on thrombolysis and reocclusion in a canine coronary artery thrombosis model with high grade stenosis. Circulation 1989; 79:393–9.

18. Collen D, Stump DC, Van de Werf F. Coronary thrombolysis in patients with acute myocardial infaction by intravenous infusion of synergic thrombolytic agents. Am Heart J 1986; 1083–4.

19. Collen D, van de Werf F. Coronary arterial thrombolysis with low-dose synergistic combinations of recombinant tissue-type plasminogen activator (rt-PA) and recombinant single-chain urokinase-type plasminogen activator (rscu-PA) for acute myocardial infarction. Am J Cardiol 1987; 60:431–4.

20. Ohlstein EH, Storer B, Fujita T, Shebinski RJ. Tissue plasminogen activator and streptokinase induce platelet hyperaggregability in the rabbit. Thrombosis Res 1987; 46:575–85.

21. Niewiarowski S, Sonyl AF, Gillies P. Plasmin-induced platelet aggregation and platelet release reaction. Effects on hemostasis. J Clin Invest 1973; 52:1647–59.

22. Bode C, Schuler G, Nordt T, Schonermark S, Baumann H, Richardt G, Dietz R, Gurewich V, Kubler W. Intravenous thrombolytic therapy with a combination of single-chain urokinase-type plasminogen activator and recombinant tissue-type plasminogen activator in acute myocardial infarction. Circulation 1990; 81:907–13.

23. Kirshenbaum JM, Flaherty JT, Bahr RD, Levine HJ, Loscalzo J, Schumacher R, Wahr D, Braunwald E. Coronary thrombolysis with low-dose synergistic combinations of pro-urokinase and recombinant tissue plasminogen activator. Circulation; 1990 (Suppl III):III-537 (abstract).

24. Gulba DCL, Fischer K, Barthels M, Polensky U, Reii G-H, Daniel WG, Weizel D, Lichtlen PR. Low dose urokinase preactivated natural pro-urokinase for thrombolysis in acute myocardial infarction. Am J Cardiol 1989; 63:1025–31.

25. Kasper W, Hohnloser SH, Engler H, Meinertz T, Wilkens J, Roth E, Lang K, Limbourg P, Just H. Coronary reperfusion studies with pro-urokinase in acute myocardial infarction: evidence for synergism of low dose urokinase. J Am Coll Cardiol 1990; 16:733–8.

26. Topol EJ, Califf RM, George BS, Kereiakes DJ, Rothbaum D, Candela RJ, Abbottsmith CW, Pinkerton CA, Stump DC, Collen D, Lee KL, Pitt B, Line E, Boswick JM, O'Neill WW, Stack RS, and the TAMI Study Group. Coronary arterial thrombolysis with combined infusion of recombinant tissue-type plasminogen activator and urokinase in patients with acute myocardial infarction. Circulation 1988; 77:1100–7.

27. Califf RM, Topol EJ, Stack RS, Ellis SG, George BS, Kereiakes DJ, Samaha JK, Worley SJ, Anderson JL, Harrelson-Woodlief L, Wall TC, Phillips HR, Abbottsmith CW, Candela RJ, Flanagan WH, Sasahara AA, Mantell SJ, Lee KL, for the TAMI Study Group. Evaluation of combination thrombolytic therapy and timing of cardiac

catheterization in acute myocardial infarction. Results of thrombolysis and angioplasty in myocrdial infarction—phase 5 randomized trial. Circulation 1991; 83:1543-56.

28. Wall TC, Topol EJ, George BS, Ellis SG, Samaha J, Kereiakes DJ, Worley SJ, Sigmon K, Califf RM, Duke University. The TAMI-7 trial of accelerated plasminogen activator dose regimens for coronary thrombolysis. Circulation 1990; (Suppl III):III-538 (abstract).

29. Verstraete M, and the Urokinase and Alteplase in Myocardial Infarction Collaborative Group. Combination of urokinase and alteplase in the treatment of myocardial infarction. Coronary Artery Dis 1991; 2:225-35.

30. Grines CL, Nissen SE, Booth DC, Branco MN, Gurley JC, Bennett KA, DeMaria AN, and the KAMIT Study Group. A new thrombolytic regimen for acute myocardial infarction using combination half dose tissue-type plasminogen activator with full dose streptokinase: a pilot study. J Am Coll Cardiol 1989; 14:573-80.

31. Bonnet JL, Bory M, D'Houdain F, Joly P, Juhan I, Djiane P, Habib G, Dubouloz F, Timone CHU. Association of tissue plasminogen activator and streptokinase in acute myocardial infarction: preliminary data. Circulation 1989; 80 (Suppl II):II-343 (abstract).

32. Grines CL, Nissen SE, Booth DC, Gurley JC, Chelliah N, Wolf R, Blankenship J, Branco MC, Bennett K, DeMaria AN, and the Kentucky Acute Myocardial Infarction Trial (KAMIT) Group. A prospective, randomized trial comparing combination half dose tissue plasminogen activator with streptokinase to full dose tissue plasminogen activator. Circulation 1991; 84:540-549.

33. Larrieu MJ. Comparative effects of fibrinogen degradation products D and E on coagulation. Br J Haematol 1973; 72:719.

34. Thorsen LI, Brosstad F, Gogstad G, Sletten K, Solum NO. Competitions between fibrinogen with its degradation products for interactions with the platelet-fibrinogen receptor. Thrombosis Res 1986; 44:611-23.

35. Wilson PA, McNicol GP, Douglas AS. Effect of fibrinogen degradation products on platelet aggregation. J Clin Pathol 1968; 21:141-53.

36. Marder VJ. Relevance of changes in blood fibrinolytic and coagulation parameters during thrombolytic therapy. Am J Med 1987; 83 (Suppl 2A):15-9.

37. White HD. GISSI-2 and the heparin controversy. Lancet 1990; 336:297-8.

38. Topol EJ, Califf RM. Intravenous heparin, thrombolytics, and medical marketing. J Intervent Cardiol 1991; 4:1-4.

39. Global Utilization of Streptokinase and tPA for Occluded Coronary Arteries (GUSTO). Study protocol, January 1, 1991, and protocol amendment, March 21, 1991.

14

The Role of Converting Enzyme Inhibitors After Myocardial Infarction

Bertram Pitt and Eric R. Bates
University of Michigan Medical Center, Ann Arbor, Michigan

INTRODUCTION

Although angiotensin-converting enzyme (ACE) inhibitors have found wide application in the therapy of patients with hypertension and congestive heart failure, their use in patients post myocardial infarction has been limited. Increasing evidence, however, suggests that ACE inhibitors may play a major role in the therapy of the post–myocardial infarction patient.

VENTRICULAR DILATION

Ventricular dilation has been recognized as an important postinfarction pathophysiological mechanism. Serial echocardiographic studies by Eaton and colleagues (1) brought to attention the fact that patients with acute anterior myocardial infarction tend to have an increase in ventricular volume over the first few weeks postinfarction due to thinning and lengthening of the infarct segment. This process appears to be correlated negatively with the degree of left ventricular hypertrophy and directly with the size and transmurality of the infarct zone (2). Additionally, a persistently occluded infarct artery contributes importantly to the process (3,4). The importance of this phenomenon has been elucidated by studies correlating infarct expansion with an increase in mortality (1,4), hemodynamic deterioration (1), left ventricular rupture (5), and left ventricular aneurysm formation (6,7). While Eaton and colleagues (1) emphasized that the left ventricle enlarged over the first few weeks postinfarction, subsequent studies have demonstrated that there may be progressive ventricular enlargement over the first year postinfarction (3). Lengthening or hypertrophy of the infarct zone contributes to this process. Dilation of the ventricle leads to progressive loss of the normal ellipsoidal shape, with a more spherical shape adding to ventricular volumes. While most attention has focused on ventricular enlargement in the patient with acute anterior myocardial infarction, the studies of Jeremy et al. (8) have pointed out that it is not the location of the infarction that is of importance, but rather the extent of the infarction. In a study of 50 patients followed over 6 months postinfarction, they noted that 21 patients demonstrated an increase in ventricular volume (12 anterior and nine inferior), 21 had a stable course (12 anterior and nine inferior), and eight showed a decrease in ventricular volume (five anterior and three inferior). Those who showed infarct expansion had a larger infarct size with peak creatinine kinase levels of 2539 ± 1468 units/liter, compared with 1741 ± 983 in those who remained stable and 1418 ± 921 in those who showed a decrease in ventricular volume during the 6-month follow-up. The importance of the extent of ventricular damage in determining infarct expansion was further emphasized by studies of Picard et al. (9), who showed that patients with a normal endocardial surface area index of ventricular damage as determined by echocardiography tended to remain stable over a 3 month follow-up period postinfarction, whereas those with an enlarged endocardial surface area index dilated. The patients with a normal endocardial surface area index had an approximate 5% mortality compared with those with enlarged endocardial surface area index and ventricular dilation, who had approximately a 20% mortality over the 3-month follow-up period.

Although it has been recognized that left ventricular ejection fraction postinfarction is an excellent predictor of survival in the first 6–12 months (10,11), White et al. (12) have recently shown that end-systolic volume is an even better predictor of survival. In patients with a left ventricular ejection fraction greater than 50%, there was relatively little discrimination in regard to prognosis by determining end-systolic volume, whereas in patients with left ventricular ejection fractions of 40–49% and in those with fractions below 40% there was a significant increase in mortality in those with the largest end-systolic volumes. Our understanding of the way in which ventricular dilation and increased end-systolic volume increase mortality postinfarction has recently been expanded by animal studies performed by Karam et al (13). These investigations also showed that in animals with extensive left ventricular infarction, there was an increase in left ventricular volume postinfarction. This increase in ventricular volume was associated with an increase in myocyte cross-sectional area and left ventricular mass in the noninfarcted areas of the left ventricle. Of particular interest was the finding that not only the left ventricle, the site of the infarction, showed hypertrophy of the noninfarcted segments, but so did the right ventricle. These investigators were also able to show that the increase in left ventricular and right ventricular hypertrophy was associated with a decrease in coronary flow reserve as evidenced by a significant reduction in coronary blood flow after the administration of the arteriolar dilator carbochrome. This decrease in coronary flow reserve could be an important pathophysiological mechanism explaining the development of progressive heart failure and death postinfarction, which, in the face of increased myocardial wall tension and hence oxygen demand resulting from ventricular dilation, might predispose to relative myocardial ischemia and progressive myocardial dysfunction. Efforts to limit infarct size and/or to prevent infarct expansion in the presence of a significant infarct should, therefore, have therapeutic value.

THE EFFECT OF REPERFUSION ON VENTRICULAR DILATION

One important approach to preventing infarct expansion is to limit infarct size by myocardial reperfusion. Experimental and clinical studies have shown that early reperfusion can limit infarct size and maintain ventricular volume and ejection fraction.

Hochman and Choo (14) subjected 68 rats to left coronary ligation and randomized them to 30-min reperfusion, 2-hr reperfusion, or permanent coronary artery ligation. The animals were euthanized and their hearts examined at 2 weeks. Thirty-minute reperfusion, as expected, reduced infarct size, extent of transmurality, and degree of infarct expansion. More significantly, the 2-hr reperfused rat hearts had infarct size and extent of transmurality similar to the permanently ligated hearts, but had less severe infarct expansion. This study suggested that shape salvage from delayed reperfusion strategies initiated after myocyte salvage might be expected could have a favorable impact on left ventricular function.

Siu and co-workers (15) performed echocardiography 2 days and 3 months after myocardial infarction in 20 patients with early infarct artery patency and in 10 patients with occluded infarct arteries. The endocardial surface area index was unchanged in patients with patent infarct arteries (60 ± 15 versus 62 ± 13), but increased in patients with occluded infarct arteries (52 ± 7 versus 62 ± 10; $p = 0.02$). Meanwhile, the extent of abnormal wall motion improved with arterial patency (28 ± 15 versus $18 \pm 16\%$; $p = 0.005$), but was unchanged with arterial occlusion (21 ± 11 versus $24 \pm 17\%$).

A retrospective review of patients with multivessel disease and first myocardial infarction by Lange et al. (16) demonstrated that spontaneous infarct artery patency improved left ventricular end-systolic volume index (65 ± 15 versus 75 ± 25 ml; $p = 0.28$), left ventricular end-systolic volume index (28 ± 15 versus 43 ± 23 ml; $p = 0.002$), and left ventricular ejection fraction (57 ± 16 versus $47 \pm 15\%$; $p = 0.002$) compared with persistent infarct artery occlusion.

An echocardiographic substudy performed on 331 patients in the GISSI-1 trial (17) demonstrated the effect of early reperfusion with streptokinase on left ventricular volumes. Evaluation at the time of hospital discharge in treated patients versus control patients showed a reduction in both left ventricular end-diastolic volume (119 ± 50 versus 135 ± 58 cc; p = 0.01) and end-systolic volume (65 ± 36 versus 75 ± 46 cc; p = 0.04). At 6 months, the benefit persisted: left ventricular end-diastolic volume, 111 ± 48 versus 128 ± 54 cc (p = 0.001); end-systolic volume 56 ± 34 versus 69 ± 42 cc (p = 0.001).

Four other trials assessing the impact of thrombolytic therapy on ventricular volumes are summarized in Chapter 2, Table 6. While thrombolysis and prevention of extensive infarction and subsequent ventricular dilation are desirable, this is often not achievable because of contraindications to therapy, delays in instituting therapy, or reocclusion after successful reperfusion. In patients who fail to undergo successful reperfusion and in those with extensive infarction despite reperfusion, other strategies seem appropriate.

ACE INHIBITORS AND VENTRICULAR DILATION

One of the most promising strategies to prevent postinfarction ventricular dilation and thereby alter prognosis is the use of ACE inhibitors. These agents lower left ventricular filling and systemic arterial pressure and decrease systemic vascular resistance while maintaining or increasing forward cardiac output.

Animal Studies

Pfeffer et al. have shown in several animal studies that ventricular dilation postinfarction can be prevented by the use of ACE inhibitors (18–22). In their rat model of myocardial infarction produced by coronary ligation, a wide range of left ventricular dysfunction results within 3 weeks related to infarct size and ventricular volume (18). Captopril therapy for 3 months prevented the increase in left ventricular end-diastolic pressure seen in controls in all but those with extensive infarct size (19). Peak stroke volume index was also maintained in those without extensive infarction, while increases in ventricular volume and decreases in left ventricular chamber stiffness were attenuated. Subsequently, 302 rats were randomized to either placebo or captopril therapy 14 days after coronary artery ligation and followed for 1 year (20). Median survival in captopril-treated animals was 260 days, compared with 197 days in the untreated group. The best survival results (21 versus 48%) were found in rats with moderate infarct size (20–40% of left ventricular surface area occupied by fibrous scar tissue). Rats with large infarct size had no significant benefit (Fig. 1).

Further evidence for a beneficial effect of ACE inhibitors postinfarction has been presented by McDonald et al. (23), who found that both ventricular enlarge-

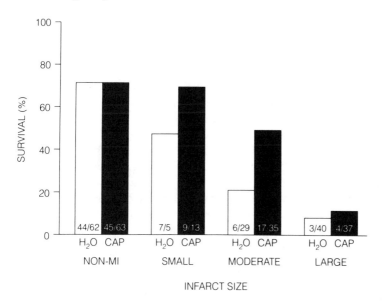

Figure 1   One-year survival after inferior infarction in rat. [CAP, captopril (solid bars)]; [H_2O, placebo (open bars)]. (Reproduced with permission from Ref. 22.)

ment and the increase in left ventricular mass in the noninfarcted left ventricular myocardium could be prevented. In view of the effects of left ventricular hypertrophy and the decrease of coronary flow reserve accompanying hypertrophy, this effect of ACE inhibitors in preventing ventricular hypertrophy might be of importance in the development of subsequent heart failure and sudden cardiac death.

Clinical Studies

Sharpe and colleagues in New Zealand (24) were the first to demonstrate the importance of ACE inhibitors in preventing infarct expansion after myocardial infarction in humans. In a randomized, double-blind study of 60 patients with left ventricular dysfunction (ejection fraction < 45%), but no evidence of heart failure 1 week after Q-wave anterior or inferior myocardial infarction, treatment was instituted with either captopril, 25 mg three times/day, furosemide, 40 mg once/day, or placebo. Cross sectional echocardiography was used to measure left ventricular volumes at baseline and at 1, 3, 6, 9, and 12 months. Although the captopril group showed only an insignificant improvement in left ventricular end-diastolic volume index, significant improvement was demonstrated for left ventricular end-systolic volume index, stroke volume index, and ejection fraction from 1 month on. In contrast, ventricular volumes significantly increased in the furosemide and placebo groups. The authors suggested that reversing the increase in afterload after myocardial infarction with captopril had a beneficial impact on progressive cardiac dilation and dysfunction compared with the lack of effect for preload reduction with diuretic treatment.

Pfeffer and colleagues (25) conducted a small randomized double-blind, placebo-controlled trial in 59 patients with first anterior myocardial infarction and ejection fraction $\leq 45\%$. Cardiac catheterization was performed 11–31 days after infarction, and patients were then assigned to placebo or captopril (target dose 50 mg tid) and followed for 1 year. Fifty-two patients had repeat catheterization, resulting in paired studies for 25 patients given placebo and 27 given captopril. Significant, but small, decreases in left ventricular end-diastolic, pulmonary capillary wedge and mean pulmonary artery pressures were noted. Neither group experienced a change in end-systolic volume. A significant increase in end-diastolic volume (21 ± 8 ml) in the placebo group was attenuated (10 + 6 ml) in the captopril group. In the placebo group, volumes increased by 31 ± 11 ml in 15 patients with occluded infarct arteries versus 5 ± 7 ml in 10 patients with patent arteries ($p < 0.02$). No difference was seen in treated patients with occluded (7 ± 6 ml, $n = 21$) or patent (19 ± 17 ml, $n = 6$) left anterior descending coronary arteries. Captopril also increased exercise capacity ($p < 0.05$).

Although the studies by Sharpe et al. (24) and Pfeffer et al. (25) demonstrated the feasibility and beneficial effects of administering an ACE inhibitor in the first few weeks postinfarction, there is increasing evidence that the addition of a converting enzyme inhibitor during the early hours of infarction might also be beneficial. McAlpine et al. (26) have shown that the renin-angiotensin system is activated in the first few days after infarction, especially in patients with evidence of heart failure. Early administration of an ACE inhibitor postinfarction could have several desirable effects. Activation of the renin-angiotensin system predisposes to an increase in systemic and coronary vascular resistance, as well as acting as a stimulus for myocardial hypertrophy. ACE inhibitors administered during the early hours postinfarction could, therefore, block these adverse effects and cause peripheral and coronary vasodilation as well as prevent subsequent left ventricular enlargement and hypertrophy with its deleterious consequences. In addition, Westlin and Mullane (27) suggested that sulfhydryl-containing ACE inhibitors such as captopril might prevent reperfusion injury by blocking free-radical generation. Sulfhydryl-containing ACE inhibitors have been shown to prevent oxidation of catecholamines (28). The oxidation products of catecholamines, adrenochromes, have been shown to depress myocardial function, cause myocardial cell necrosis, and induce ventricular arrhythmias (29, 30).

Nabel and colleagues (31) tested the combined administration of tissue plasminogen activator and intravenous captopril followed by oral captopril in 20 patients compared with 18 patients receiving rt-PA alone. At day 7 (Fig. 2) end-diastolic volume increased in placebo-treated patients (135 ± 10 versus 156 ± 9

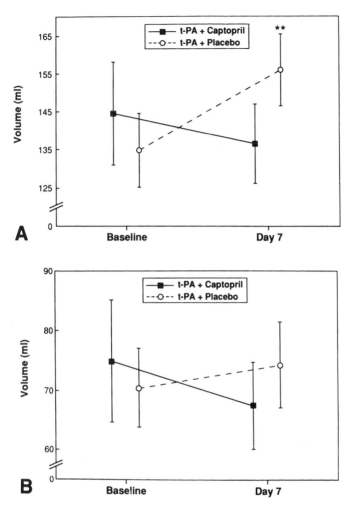

Figure 2 Left ventricular end-diastolic volume (A) and left ventricular end-systolic volume (B) measured from left ventriculography at baseline and at day 7. **p = 0.02 compared with placebo baseline. t-PA = tissue plasminogen activator. (Reproduced with permission from Ref. 31.)

ml; p = 0.02) but decreased in the captopril-treated group (145 ± 14 versus 137 ± 10 ml, p = NS). End-systolic volume increased from 70 ± 7 to 74 ± 7 cc in placebo-treated patients and decreased in captopril-treated patients from 75 ± 10 to 67 ± 7 ml, although the results were statistically insignificant. The influence of captopril in this study on the renin-angiotensin-aldosterone system in shown in Figure 3.

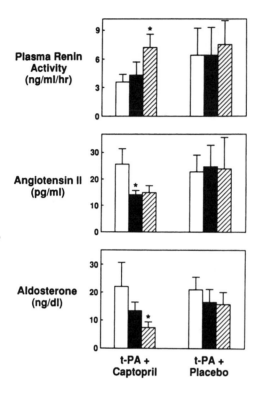

Figure 3   Measurements of plasma renin activity, angiotensin II levels, and aldosterone levels at baseline (open bars), 1 hr after intravenous therapy (closed bars), and day 7 (hatched bars). *$p < 0.05$. t-PA = tissue plasminogen activator. (Reproduced with permission from Ref. 31.)

CONCLUSION

Given the promising animal and clinical data demonstrating the effectiveness of ACE inhibitors in preventing infarct expansion and ventricular hypertrophy, it is reasonable to expect that ongoing large-scale clinical trials testing this hypothesis might be beneficial. The Survival and Ventricular Enlargement (SAVE) trial is a North American multicenter, double-blind, placebo-controlled trial of captopril in patients with left ventricular ejection fractions less than 40% after acute myocardial infarction. Eligible patients were randomized 3–16 days after infarction and will be followed for over 2 years. The acute benefit of administering ACE inhibitors is being tested in over 80,000 patients in at least five trials (Table 1). The ISIS group will be testing captopril in addition to nitroglycerin and magnesium therapy

Table 1 Mortality Trials Testing Acute ACE Inhibitor Administration

Trial	Agent	Study size	Endpoint
CONSENSUS-2	Enapril versus placebo	9,000	6-month mortality
Chinese Study	Captopril versus control	10,000	Short-term mortality
SMILE	Zofenopril versus placebo	3,000	Hospital mortality or CHF
ISIS-4	Captopril versus control	40,000	5-week mortality
GISSI-3	Lisinopril versus control	20,000	Short-term mortality

CONSENSUS: SMILE = Study of MI Late Evaluation; ISIS = International Study of Infarct Survival; GISSI = Gruppo Italiano per lo Studio della Streptochinasi nell'Infarto Miocardio.

(Fig. 4). The GISSI group will study lisinopril and nitroglycerin (Fig. 5). Until the results of these large-scale studies are available, however, it is prudent to consider the use of ACE inhibitors postinfarction as clinical investigation rather than clinical practice. It is possible that a reduction in arterial pressure during myocardial reperfusion or some other as yet unexplained effect on the renin-angiotensin system might have a deleterious effect. Further study will also be needed to determine whether there are any specific advantages of ACE inhibitors over other vasodila-

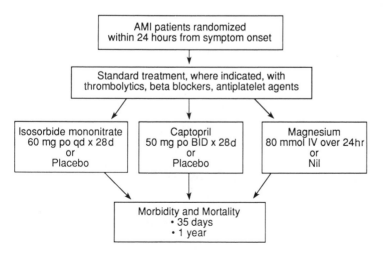

Figure 4   ISIS-4 protocol algorithm.

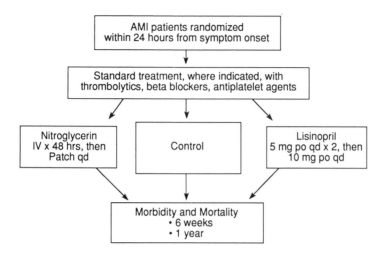

Figure 5   GISSI-3 protocol algorithm.

tors, such as nitroglycerin, which also prevent infarct expansion (32). Finally, it will be important to determine whether the benefit of vasodilator therapy is limited to patients with occluded infarct arteries or whether there is additional benefit in patients who achieve successful reperfusion.

REFERENCES

1. Eaton LW, Weiss JL, Bulkley BH, Garrison JB, Weisfeldt ML. Regional cardiac dilation after acute myocardial infarction. Recognition by two-dimensional echocardiography. N Engl J Med 1979; 300:57-62.
2. Pirolo JS, Hutchins GM, Moore GW. Infarct expansion: pathologic analysis of 204 patients with a single myocardial infarction. J Am Coll Cardiol 1986; 7:349-54.
3. Warren SE, Royal HD, Markis JE, Grossman W, McKay RG. Time course of left ventricular dilation after myocardial infarction: influence of infarct-related artery and success of coronary thrombolysis. J Am Coll Cardiol 1977; 11:12-9.
4. Force T, Kemper A, Leavitt M, Parisi AF. Acute reduction in functional infarct expansion with late coronary reperfusion: assessment with quantitative two-dimensional echocardiography. J Am Coll Cardiol 1988; 11:192-200.
5. Schuster EG, Bulkley BH. Expansion of transmural myocardial infarction: a pathophysiologic factor in cardiac rupture. Circulation 1979; 60:1532-8.
6. Hochman JS, Bulkley, BH. The pathogenesis of left ventricular aneurysms: an experimental study in the rat model. Am J Cardiol 1982; 50:83-8.
7. Merzlish JL., Berger HJ, Plankey M, Errico D, Levy W, Zarat BL. Functional left ventricular aneurysm formation after acute anterior transmural myocardial infarction:

incidence, natural history and prognostic implications. N Engl J Med 1984; 311: 1001-6.

8. Jeremy RW, Allman KC, Bautovich G, Harris PJ. Patterns of left ventricular dilation during the six months after myocardial infarction. J Am Coll Cardiol 1989; 13: 304-10.

9. Picard MH, Wilkins GT, Roy PA, Weyman AZ. Natural history of left ventricular size and function after acute myocardial infarction: assessment and prediction by echocardiographic surface mapping. Circulation 1990; 82:484-90.

10. Schulze RA, Strauss HW, Pitt B. Sudden death in the year following myocardial infarction. Am J Med 1977; 62:192-9.

11. The Multicenter Post-Infarction Research Group: Risk stratification and survival after myocardial infarction. N Engl J Med 1983; 209:331-6.

12. White HD, Norris RM, Brown MA., Brandt PWT, Whitlock RML, Wild CJ, Left ventricular end-systolic volumes as the major determinant of survival after recovery from myocardial infarction. Circulation 1987; 76:44-51.

13. Karam R, Healy BP, Wicker P. Coronary reserve is depressed in post myocardial infarction reactive cardiac hypertrophy. Circulation 1990; 81:238-46.

14. Hochman JS, Choo H. Limitation of myocardial infarct expansion by reperfusion independent of myocardial salvage. Circulation 1987; 75:299-306.

15. Siu SC, Picard MH, Ray PA., Weymen AE. Effects of a patent infarct-related coronary artery on left ventricular morphology and regional function. J Am Coll Cardiol 1991; 17:314A (abstract).

16. Lange RA., Cigarroa RC, Hillis LD. Influence of residual antegrade coronary blood flow on survival after myocardial infarction in patients with multivessel coronary artery disease. Cor Artery Dis 1990; 1:59-63.

17. Marino P, Zanolla L, Zardini P. Effect of streptokinase on left ventricular modeling and function after myocardial infarction: the GISSI (Gruppo Italiano per lo Studio della Streptochinasi nell'Infarto Miocardico) Trial. J Am Coll Cardiol 1989; 14: 1149-58.

18. Pfeffer MA, Pfeffer JM, Fishbein MC. Myocardial infarct size and ventricular function in rats. Circ Res 1979; 44:503-12.

19. Pfeffer JM, Pfeffer MA, Braunwald E. Influence of chronic captopril therapy on the infarcted left ventricle of the rat. Circ Res 1985; 57:84-95.

20. Pfeffer MA, Pfeffer JM, Steinberg C, Finn P. Survival after an experimental myocardial infarction: beneficial effects of long-term therapy with captopril. Circulation 1985; 72:406-12.

21. Pfeffer MA, Pfeffer JM. Ventricular enlargement and reduced survival after myocardial infarction. Circulation 1987; 75(Suppl IV):IV-93–IV-97.

22. Lamas GA, Pfeffer MA. Left ventricular remodeling after acute myocardial infarction: clinical course and beneficial effects of angiotensin-converting enzyme inhibition. Am Heart J 1991; 121:1194-1202.

23. McDonald K, Carlyle P, Hauer K, Elbers T, Hunter D, Cohn JN. Early ventricular remodeling after myocardial damage in the dog and its prevention by converting enzyme inhibitions. Clin Res 1990; 38:414A (abstract).

24. Sharpe N, Murphy J, Smith H, Hannan S. Treatment of patients with symptomless left ventricular dysfunction after myocardial infarction. Lancet 1988; 1:255-9.

25. Pfeffer MA, Lamas GA, Vaughan DE. Effect of captopril on progressive ventricular dilation after anterior myocardial infarction. N Engl J Med 1988; 319:80-6.

26. McAlpine HM, Morton JJ, Leckie B, Rumley A, Gillen G, Dargie HJ. Neuroendocrine activation after acute myocardial infarction. Brit Heart J 1988; 60:117-24.

27. Westlin W, Mullane K. Does captopril attenuate reperfusion-induced myocardial dysfunction by scavenging free radicals? Circulation 1988; 77(Suppl I)I-3-I-9.

28. Kukreya RC, Kontos HA. Hess ML. Captopril and enalaprilat do not scavenge the superoxide anion. Am J Cardiol 1990; 65:241-71.

29. Yates JC, Beamish RE, Dhalla NS. Ventricular dysfunction and necrosis produced by adrenochrome metabolite of epinephrine: relation to pathogenesis of catecholamine cardiomyopathy. Am Heart J 1981; 102:210-21.

30. Beamish RE, Dhillon KS, Singal PK., Shalla NS. Protective effect of sulfinpyrazone against catecholamine metabolite adrenodrone-induced arrhythmias. Am Heart J 1981; 102:149-56.

31. Nabel EG, Topol EJ, Galeana A, Ellis SG, Bates ER, Werns WS, Walton JA, Muller DW, Schwaiger M, Pitt B. A randomized placebo-controlled trial of combined early intravenous captopril and recombinant tissue-type plasminogen activator therapy in acute myocardial infarction. J Am Coll Cardiol 1991; 17:467-73.

32. Jugdutt BI, Warnica JW. Intravenous nitroglycerin therapy to limit myocardial infarct size, expansion, and complications. Circulation 1988; 78:906-19.

15

Free Radical Scavengers

Steven W. Werns
University of Michigan Medical Center, Ann Arbor, Michigan

INTRODUCTION

The fundamental assumption underlying the current therapy of acute myocardial infarction is that the early restoration of myocardial blood flow arrests the progression of myocardial cell death, permitting the ultimate functional recovery of reversibly injured myocardium. There is experimental evidence, however, that reperfusion of ischemic myocardium may simultaneously cause the extension of myocardial injury beyond that which occurs as a result of the ischemic process, a concept that has been termed "reperfusion injury." There is considerable controversy regarding the existence of reperfusion injury. The purpose of this chapter is to review critically the evidence that either supports or opposes the hypothesis that leukocytes and oxygen radicals cause postischemic tissue injury.

OXYGEN RADICALS

Sources of Free Radicals

Excellent reviews of the biochemistry of free radicals, and their role in human disease, have been published (1,2). Superoxide anion (O_2^-), hydrogen peroxide (H_2O_2), and hydroxyl radical (OH·) are formed via the sequential, univalent reduction of molecular oxygen (Fig. 1). Superoxide anions and hydroxyl radicals

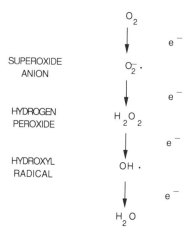

Figure 1   Univalent reduction of oxygen. The sequential addition of single electrons (e^-) results in the formation of superoxide anion, hydrogen peroxide, hydroxyl radical, and water.

are classified as free radicals because they possess unpaired electrons. H_2O_2, which is not a free radical, can be converted to hydroxyl radical by a metal ion-dependent reaction. Iron, which may be derived from ferritin when it reacts with O_2^- (3) or from hemoglobin (4) or myoglobin (5) that is degraded by H_2O_2, is the most likely promoter of hydroxyl radical formation.

Oxygen free radicals can be generated by a number of mechanisms that may be activated by ischemia and reperfusion (Table 1). Free radicals may be formed via the autooxidation of catecholamines that are released within ischemic myocardium (1). The mitochondria isolated from ischemic myocardium exhibit enhanced production of oxygen radicals (6). The release of arachidonic acid from ischemic cell membranes (7,8) may stimulate free radical production via the cyclooxygenase and lipoxygenase pathways of arachidonic acid metabolism (9). Xanthine

Table 1   Sources of Free Radicals

Autooxidation of catecholamines
Mitochondria
Cyclooxygenase and lipoxygenase
Xanthine oxidase
Neutrophils

dehydrogenase, which utilizes nicotinamide adenine dinucleotide (NAD) as an electron receptor and does not generate free radicals, may be converted to xanthine oxidase, which can reduce oxygen to superoxide anion (10). Activated neutrophils that accumulate during reperfusion of ischemic myocardium may release superoxide anion, hydrogen peroxide, and hypochlorous acid, an oxidant formed by the myeloperoxidase-catalyzed reaction of hydrogen peroxide with chloride anion (11).

Biochemical Reactivity of Free Radicals

The reaction of free radicals with intracellular or extracellular molecules can exert diverse biochemical effects. Hydrogen peroxide causes damage to DNA, which activates a repair enzyme that consumes NAD, resulting in impaired synthesis of adenosine triphosphate (ATP) (12). Hypochlorous acid, an oxidant produced by activated neutrophils, also may deplete cellular ATP (13). Hypochlorous acid also promotes destruction of tissue by activating a latent collagenase and oxidizing alpha-1-proteinase inhibitor, permitting neutrophil-derived elastase to attack sensitive substrates (11). Oxygen radicals cause peroxidation of unsaturated fatty acids and oxidation of unsaturated and sulfur-containing amino acids, disturbing the conformation of proteins by the cross-linking of amino acid residues. The peroxidation of membrane lipids may alter membrane permeability and ion transport.

Effects of Free Radicals on Cardiac Tissue

Numerous studies have demonstrated that oxygen radicals are able to injure cardiac tissue. Oxygen radicals have been shown to depress the contractile function of isolated papillary muscles (14), ventricular septae (15), and isolated hearts (16,17). Cardiac tissue exposed to free radicals developed swollen mitochondria (15,16), endothelial damage (15,16), and abnormal vascular permeability (18).

Antioxidant Mechanisms

Several defense mechanisms protect cells from oxidative damage by the free radicals that are formed during normal metabolism. The alpha-tocopherol (vitamin E) content of myocardial membranes is thought to be an important determinant of susceptibility to peroxidative damage to the membrane lipids (19). Superoxide dismutase (SOD) catalyzes the formation of hydrogen peroxide from superoxide anions (Fig. 2). The decomposition of hydrogen peroxide to water and oxygen can be catalyzed by the enzymes catalase and glutathione peroxidase (Fig. 2). The latter enzyme also catalyzes the reduction of lipid peroxides. Glutathione peroxidase utilizes glutathione as a cofactor, resulting in the formation of glutathione disulfide.

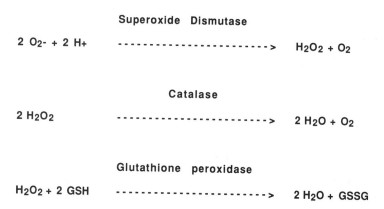

Figure 2   Reactions catalyzed by the endogenous antioxidant enzymes superoxide dismutase, catalase, and glutathione peroxidase. GSH, glutathione; GSSG, glutathione disulfide.

Glutathione and glutathione peroxidase constitute the major protection within cardiac tissue against damage by hydrogen peroxide and lipid hydroperoxides (20). Under conditions of increased production of hydrogen peroxide or lipid peroxides, regeneration of glutathione may be inadequate to prevent the peroxidation of membrane lipids (21). Ischemia may predispose the heart to damage by free radicals by reducing the myocardial concentrations of free radical scavengers, such as superoxide dismutase and glutathione (22).

The activities of SOD, catalase, and glutathione peroxidase in the plasma are negligible (23). Circulating erythrocytes, however appear to constitute a defense against hydrogen peroxide formed in the extracellular space (24–27).

DETECTION OF FREE RADICALS IN THE ISCHEMIC HEART

Electron paramagnetic resonance (EPR) spectroscopy has been employed to demonstrate that oxygen radicals are generated during reperfusion after transient regional or global myocardial ischemia (28–35). During reperfusion after either a brief (15 min) or prolonged (90 min) period of canine coronary artery occlusion, EPR signals characteristic of free radical adducts were detected in samples of both myocardium and the coronary venous blood draining from the ischemic bed (32–35). Treatment with either N-2-mercaptopropionyl glycine, a scavenger of hydroxyl radicals, or SOD plus catalase markedly suppressed the production of free radicals (29,30,32,34,35).

EXPERIMENTAL MODELS OF MYOCARDIAL INJURY

The concept of reperfusion injury, along with the advent of thrombolytic therapy and coronary angioplasty as a means of reperfusing ischemic myocardium in patients with acute myocardial infarction, have spurred attempts to identify agents that improve myocardial salvage after transient regional ischemia followed by reperfusion. A primary goal has been to determine whether administration of agents at the time of reperfusion, rather than during coronary occlusion, can limit myocardial injury, both to provide supportive evidence for the concept of reperfusion injury and to mimic clinical conditions, which usually preclude the initiation of therapy before the onset of coronary thrombosis.

Several experimental paradigms have been employed to investigate the concept of reperfusion injury. One approach has been to study the recovery of regional myocardial function after a brief coronary artery occlusion that results in "myocardial stunning" but no irreversible tissue injury, i.e., necrosis. Another approach has been to measure the extent of irreversible myocardial injury after transient coronary artery occlusion. Each of the experimental paradigms will be discussed separately because the data indicate that different mechanisms of injury may be involved.

XANTHINE OXIDASE AND EXPERIMENTAL MYOCARDIAL INFARCTION

Oxygen radicals formed by the enzyme xanthine oxidase are one of the proposed causes of cellular injury during reperfusion of ischemic tissue (10). A small clinical trial reported better postoperative cardiac performance in patients who were treated with allopurinol, a xanthine oxidase inhibitor, before coronary bypass surgery (36). The role of xanthine oxidase in the pathogenesis of ischemic myocardial injury, however, is controversial. There is evidence that myocardial xanthine dehydrogenase, which does not generate oxygen radicals, may be converted to xanthine oxidase during regional myocardial ischemia in some species (10,37). It is unclear, however, whether xanthine oxidase exists in the human heart (see below), and there have been variable effects of xanthine oxidase inhibitors on the extent of experimental myocardial infarction (MI).

Several xanthine oxidase inhibitors have been employed in studies of experimental MI: allopurinol, oxypurinol, which is a metabolite of allopurinol, and amflutizole, which is unrelated chemically to the latter compounds. Treatment with allopurinol beginning one or more days before coronary artery occlusion was shown to limit the extent of canine myocardial injury after coronary artery occlusion for 60 (37) or 90 (38) min followed by reperfusion for 4 or 6 hr, respectively. The acute administration of allopurinol beginning either 30 min before coronary artery occlusion (39) or 15 min before reperfusion (40) did not reduce canine infarct size. The inability of acute treatment with allopurinol to limit infarct size supported the idea that cardioprotection by allopurinol was dependent on the conversion of allopurinol, a competitive inhibitor of xanthine oxidase, to oxypurinol, a noncompetitive inhibitor with a longer half-life (41,42). Thus, it was hypothesized that formation of xanthine oxidase substrates within ischemic myocardium would attenuate the inhibition of xanthine oxidase by allopurinol, but not inhibition by oxypurinol (42).

Several recent studies have tested the ability of oxypurinol or amflutizole to limit reperfusion injury. Treatment with oxypurinol did not produce a sustained reduction of infarct size (43–45), although the negative results might relate to an inadequate duration of therapy. Administration of amflutizole, which is a more potent inhibitor of xanthine oxidase than either allopurinol or oxypurinol, also did not reduce canine infarct size (46).

Recent evidence indicates that the myocardial protection afforded by treatment with either allopurinol or oxypurinol may be independent of xanthine oxidase inhibition. Several laboratories have reported that rabbit and pig hearts lack xanthine oxidase activity (47–53), implying that xanthine oxidase inhibitors should not reduce ischemic myocardial injury in either species. Nevertheless, some workers have observed beneficial effects of allopurinol on ischemic rabbit and pig hearts (47,51,54), although others have reported that allopurinol did not attenuate ischemic myocardial injury in the rabbit (50,55).

The mechanism of allopurinol's cardioprotective effect is important because there are conflicting data regarding the activity of xanthine oxidase in the human heart. Biochemical assays have not detected xanthine oxidase activity in homogenates of human myocardium (52,53,56,57), while immunohistochemical techniques indicated the presence of xanthine oxidase in the capillary endothelium of the human heart (58). One group of investigators demonstrated uric acid release from the human heart during transient myocardial ischemia induced by coronary angioplasty (59). Recently, however, the same group studied the ability of perfused hearts to convert exogenous hypoxanthine to urate (53). Rabbit, pig, and human hearts exhibited negligible ability to produce uric acid, implying that extracardiac components, e.g., neutrophils, may be responsible for the apparent xanthine oxidase activity observed previously.

MYOCARDIAL ISCHEMIA AND LEUKOCYTES

Mechanisms of Neutrophil Accumulation

One postulated mechanism of reperfusion injury is the infiltration of reperfused ischemic myocardium by leukocytes. There is abundant evidence that reperfusion of ischemic myocardium is accompanied by the accumulation of neutrophils. Early histological investigations of experimental myocardial infarction revealed that neutrophils are present in the ischemic myocardium within 50 min of reperfusion after 40 min of ischemia (60). Both biochemical indices of neutrophil accumulation and radiolabeled neutrophils have been employed to confirm that neutrophils progressively invade ischemic myocardium after reperfusion. After 90 min of coronary artery occlusion, the myocardial activity of nyeloperoxidase, which correlates with the extent of neutrophils measured histologically, exhibited a 23-fold increase 5 hr after reperfusion, compared to only a sixfold increase at the end of the ischemic period (61). Go et al. (62) demonstrated that 12 min of ischemia is insufficient to stimulate neutrophil accumulation during reperfusion, but the number of neutrophils is significantly increased within 1 hr of reperfusion after a coronary artery occlusion lasting either 40 or 90 min. Subsequently, the latter investigators also observed that the presence of a critical stenosis that abolished the hyperemic blood flow after reperfusion did not alter the accumulation of neutrophils (63).

There are several possible stimuli of neutrophil accumulation within ischemic myocardium. Within 30 min of occlusion of a canine coronary artery, chemotactic activity for neutrophils is present in coronary sinus blood (64). Increased concentrations of leukotriene B_4, a neutrophil chemoattractant that is a product of the lipoxygenase pathway of arachidonic acid metabolism, have been detected within ischemic myocardium (65–67). Recent studies have described a neutrophil chemotactic factor (NCF) that is secreted by endothelial cells that have been treated with interleukin-1 or tumor necrosis factor alpha (68). NCF that is distinct from other known chemotactic factors also was detected in the effluent of isolated hearts (69).

Substantial evidence suggests that activation of the complement system is a principal stimulus for the migration of neutrophils to ischemic myocardium. C5a, for example, is a potent activator of neutrophil chemotaxis, degranulation, and superoxide anion generation (70). More than 20 years ago, a tissue protease that cleaves the third component of complement was detected within ischemic myocardium (71,72). Current data indicate that molecules derived from ischemic mitochondria may be responsible for formation of complement-derived chemoattractants during ischemic myocardial injury. Constituents of mitochondria are able to activate the complement system in vitro (73,74). Mitochondrial peptides that activate complement are present in the cardiac lymph during reperfusion after coronary artery occlusion in dogs (75,76). Further support for the importance of complement is provided by the observation that complement depletion before or after coronary artery occlusion reduced the myocardial loss of creatine kinase and the infiltration of neutrophils (77,78).

Clinical studies also indicate that the complement system and neutrophils are activated in patients with acute M.I. Mehta et al. (79) collected samples of blood from patients with acute MI within 1 hr of their chest pain. The plasma concentrations of peptide $B\beta$, a product of fibrin degradation by neutrophil elastase, were about 15-fold higher those of control patients. Examination of neutrophil morphology suggested that the neutrophils had been activated in vivo. C5b-9 complement complexes are present in the plasma of patients with acute myocardial infarction (80) and within infarcted regions of human myocardium (81), providing evidence of the generation of C5a, a chemoattractant for neutrophils. The plasma concentration of C5b-9 correlated directly with the peak plasma creatine kinase and inversely with the left ventricular ejection fraction. The data can be interpreted in two ways: greater activation of complement may cause more extensive injury, or it may be a reflection of the extent of injury.

Activation of plasmin by thrombolytic drugs, such as streptokinase and tissue plasminogen activator, also activates complement (82,83). One may speculate whether activation of complement by thrombolytic agents is beneficial or detrimental. On one hand, activation of complement may amplify the inflammatory response to ischemia and thereby exert a deleterious effect on the heart (83). Alternatively, intravascular complement activation might limit the ability of neutrophils to adhere to the damaged endothelium within ischemic myocardium because circulating granulocytes that are activated by complement exhibit down-regulation of their chemotactic response during a subsequent exposure to a chemotactic stimulus (84,85). Bell et al. (86) employed technetium 99m pyrophosphate and neutrophils labeled with indium 111 to quantitate the extent of infarction and the myocardial accumulation of neutrophils in patients with acute MI. The ratio of 111 In to 99m Tc, a measure of the inflammatory response normalized for infarct size, was 0.41 in patients treated with a thrombolytic drug, compared to 0.79 in patients not treated with a thrombolytic drug ($p < 0.05$). Thus, the activation of complement by thrombolytic agents may suppress inflammation by deactivating neutrophils.

Effects of Neutrophil Depletion

Many studies have demonstrated the limitation of experimental myocardial injury by agents that deplete circulating neutrophils, inhibit neutrophil function, or counteract the cytotoxic effects of neutrophil-derived products. Romson et al. (87) were the first investigators to show a reduction of experimental infarct size by the depletion of neutrophils. Compared to a control group of dogs, a group of dogs treated with antineutrophil antiserum exhibited a 77% reduction in the blood leukocyte count and a 43% smaller infarct size after coronary artery occlusion for 90 min followed by reperfusion. A series of studies conducted by Lucchesi and co-workers (88–90) have confirmed and extended the previous data. The paper authored by Simpson et al. (88) reported a sustained limitation of infarct size in neutropenic dogs undergoing 72 hr of reperfusion after 90 min of ischemia, supporting the argument that neutrophil depletion results in a permanent salvage of tissue rather than a mere delay of necrosis. Additional supportive data were reported by Litt et al. (91), who examined the effect of neutrophil depletion that was instituted at the time of reperfusion. After coronary artery occlusion for 90 min, the ischemic myocardium was reperfused with blood depleted of neutrophils via extracorporeal circulation through a leukocyte filter. Compared to the control group, infarct size was 40% less in the treatment group, a difference nearly identical to that observed in previous studies that employed antineutrophil antibodies (87).

The ability of neutrophil depletion to modify the extent of myocardial injury appears to depend on the duration of coronary artery occlusion. Neutrophil depletion limited the extent of myocardial injury in dogs after 2 hr of ischemia (92), but not after 3 hr (93) or 4 hr (89) of ischemia. Thus, neutrophil-mediated injury may not significantly increase the extent of myocardial injury after extensive irreversible ischemic injury caused by prolonged coronary artery occlusion.

Drugs that Inhibit Neutrophil Function

Ibuprofen

A study that employed ibuprofen, an inhibitor of cyclooxygenase, provided an important insight into the role of neutrophils in ischemic myocardial injury. Ibuprofen limited the extent of myocardial injury in dogs undergoing coronary artery occlusion for 60 or 90 min followed by reperfusion, although it did not reduce myocardial oxygen demand or increase regional myocardial blood flow (94,95). Treatment with ibuprofen suppressed the accumulation of neutrophils, but not platelets, within the ischemic myocardium (95), and depletion of platelets with antiserum did not limit infarct size in similar experiments (96,97). Thus, it was inferred that ibuprofen protected ischemic myocardium by inhibiting neutrophil function. Also, the failure of ibuprofen to reduce infarct size in dogs subjected to 3 hr of ischemia followed by reperfusion is consistent with the inability of neutrophil depletion to limit the myocardial injury after 3 hr of ischemia (93,98). Unfortunately, treatment with ibuprofen also resulted in impaired myocardial healing after myocardial infarction in dogs (99,100).

Prostaglandins

Inhibition of neutrophil function may also explain the limitation of ischemic myocardial injury by prostaglandin E_1 (PGE_1), prostacyclin (PGI_2), and iloprost, a stable analog of PGI_2 (88,101-103). Each of the agents inhibited the generation of superoxide anions by activated neutrophils in vitro and decreased the extent of canine myocardial injury caused by coronary artery occlusion and reperfusion in vivo. The compound SC39902, another stable analog of PGI_2, displayed hemodynamic effects similar to those of PGI_2, but it did not inhibit neutrophil function or reduce infarct size (102). Thus, it was concluded that PGI_2, PGE_1, and iloprost reduced ischemic myocardial injury by suppressing neutrophil-mediated tissue damage.

The effects of iloprost on canine myocardial injury illustrated the relationship between treatment duration and therapeutic efficacy. An infusion of iloprost that was terminated 2 hr after reperfusion did not alter the extent of infarction measured 72 hr after reperfusion (88). A sustained infusion of iloprost until 48 hr after reperfusion, however, significantly reduced infarct size assessed 72 hr after reperfusion (88). Thus, agents with short pharmacological half-lives, such as iloprost, may require prolonged administration to limit the ultimate extent of myocardial injury.

Adenosine

Coronary artery occlusion causes increased formation and release of adenosine from the ischemic myocardium (104–106). It has been postulated that the adenosine formed within the ischemic myocardium may act as an endogenous inhibitor of neutrophil-mediated injury to endothelial cells (107,108). Neutrophils have two distinct adenosine receptors; stimulation of one class promotes neutrophil chemotaxis, while stimulation of the other inhibits superoxide anion generation (109). Concentrations of adenosine that are present in plasma in vivo have been shown to inhibit the generation of superoxide anion by stimulated human neutrophils in vitro (110). Depletion of endogenously released adenosine by the addition of adenosine deaminase enhanced the susceptibility of endothelial cells to neutrophils, and an adenosine analog that inhibited the adherence of stimulated neutrophils to cultured endothelial cells reduced neutrophil-induced endothelial cell injury (107).

Several studies have investigated the effects of adenosine administration on experimental myocardial infarction in dogs. An intracoronary infusion of adenosine was administered over 1 hr beginning at the onset of coronary artery reperfusion (111–113). Dogs that were subjected to 90 min of coronary artery occlusion exhibited an impressive reduction of infarct size compared to control dogs (41% versus 10% of the area at risk) (111), while there was no apparent benefit in dogs that underwent 3 hr of myocardial ischemia before reperfusion (113). The inability of adenosine to limit injury caused by a 3-hr period of ischemia is consistent with the previously discussed studies that demonstrated a similar dichotomy in dogs treated with antineutrophil antibodies.

Recently, an additional study examined the effects of intravenous adenosine on experimental MI (114). Dogs underwent coronary artery occlusion for 30 min followed by reperfusion. The animals were randomly assigned to treatment with either intravenous adenosine (0.15 mg/kg/min) or Ringer's lactate during the first 150 min of reperfusion. After reperfusion for 72 hr, infarct size, expressed as a percentage of the area at risk, was 17.1% in the adenosine a group, compared to 35.3% in the control group ($p < 0.01$).

Each of the studies of adenosine's effect on MI has employed lidocaine as an antiarrhythmic agent. Homeister et al. (115) recently studied the independent effects of lidocaine and adenosine on experimental myocardial injury in dogs subjected to 90 min of coronary artery occlusion followed by reperfusion. Neither drug alone altered the extent of injury, while infarct size was 20.8% in dogs receiving the combination of adenosine and lidocaine compared to 47.8% in control dogs. The authors speculated that adenosine and lidocaine exerted a synergistic inhibition of neutrophil-mediated vascular injury. Studies that directly examined the structure and function of the vascular endothelium have demonstrated less injury in adenosine-treated dogs compared to control dogs, which is consistent with the proposal that adenosine inhibits neutrophil-mediated reperfusion injury (111,112,114). Infusion of adenosine during hypoxia reduced the posthypoxic contractile dysfunction and creatine kinase release of rabbit hearts perfused with a crystalloid solution devoid of leukocytes (116). Thus, additional actions of adenosine also may contribute to its cardioprotective effect.

Perfluorochemical

Perfluorochemicals are characterized by small particle size ($1-2 \mu M$) low viscosity, and high oxygen-carrying capacity. Fluosol-DA, an emulsion of two perfluorochemicals, a detergent, glycerol, phospholipids, and various electrolytes, has been approved by the Food and Drug Administration for intracoronary infusion during coronary angioplasty. Fluosol-DA also has been proposed as a means of preventing neutrophil-mediated reperfusion injury. Experimental data have shown that Fluosol-DA inhibits neutrophil-mediated endothelial injury in vitro by attenuating neutrophil chemotaxis, adherence, protease release, and oxygen radical formation (117,118). Several studies have examined the effect of both intracoronary and intravenous Fluosol-DA on experimental myocardial infarction (119–123). Dogs were treated with intracoronary Fluosol-DA during the initial 30 min of reperfusion after coronary artery occlusion for 90 min. After reperfusion for either 1 day or 2 weeks, the Fluosol-treated dogs had smaller infarcts and better left ventricular function than the control dogs (119,120). Subsequently, it was shown that administration of Fluosol intravenously beginning 30 min before reperfusion reduced infarct size and improved wall motion in the ischemic zone (122). The in vivo studies also demonstrated that Fluosol suppresses neutrophil infiltration and preserves endothelial cell structure and function within the ischemic myocardium (121,122). Therefore, it has been concluded that Fluosol-DA prevents experimental reperfusion injury after myocardial ischemia by attenuating neutrophil-induced endothelial injury. Current clinical trials are evaluating the ability of intravenous Fluosol to limit reperfusion injury in patients receiving thrombolytic therapy for acute MI.

Antibodies to Neutrophil Surface Glycoproteins

Adherence to leukocytes to target cells, a prerequisite for cytotoxicity, is mediated by leukocyte cell surface glycoprotein complexes, referred to as the CDw18 complex (124,125). The adherence molecules are heterodimers consisting of common beta subunits with different alpha subunits that determine the molecular specificity. CDllb/CD18, also known as Mo1, is expressed on both human and animal phagocytic cells, and mediates cellular interactions with C3bi, a complement component deposited at sites of inflammation. Neutrophil activation increases the expression of the adhesion-promoting receptors (125). During reperfusion of ischemic myocardium, the neutrophils isolated from canine cardiac lymph exhibited enhanced expression of Cdllb/CD18 (126). Also, the lymph itself stimulated the expression of CDllb/CD18 by neutrophils isolated from normal dogs. Monoclonal antibodies directed against the neutrophil surface receptors have been shown to inhibit adhesion of the neutrophils to target cells, thereby reducing cytotoxicity (124,127). Consequently, a number of the antibodies have been studied to determine whether they limit myocardial reperfusion injury.

Simpson et al. (128,129) studied an anti-Mo1 murine IgG monoclonal antibody that binds to an epitope on the CDllb alpha subunit of the Mo1 glycoprotein. Administration of the anti-Mo1 antibody, or F(ab')2 fragments of the antibody, beginning 45 min after coronary artery occlusion, significantly reduced infarct size in dogs subjected to 90 min of occlusion followed by reperfusion for up to 72 hr (128,129). The antibody had no effects on arterial blood pressure, heart rate, or collateral blood flow that could account for the observed limitation of myocardial injury.

An alternative approach to limiting neutrophil adhesion within ischemic myocardium is to inhibit activation of the complement system. Complement receptor 1 (CR-1) is a member of a family of proteins that regulate complement activation. Soluble CR1 (sCR1) is a recombinant, soluble form of CR1 that inhibits the activation of both the classical and alternative pathways in vitro (130). Treatment with SCR1 reduced myocardial infarct size by 44% in a rat model of reperfusion injury (130).

The ability of sCR1 and anti-Mo1 antibodies to limit infarct size implies that complement activation and neutrophil adhesion are potential therapeutic targets to prevent neutrophil-mediated myocardial injury and to optimize the benefits of myocardial reperfusion.

MEDIATORS OF LEUKOCYTE-INDUCED INJURY

Neutrophils are capable of causing myocardial injury via several different mechanisms (Table 2). One is mechanical obstruction of the microcirculation because of

Table 2   Mediators of Neutrophil-Induced Injury

Enzymes
    Proteinases—collagenase and gelatinase degrade collagen
    Myeloperoxidase—catalyzes formation of hypochlorous acid
Lipid metabolites
    Leukotriene B_4—increases neutrophil chemotaxis, adhesion, and superoxide anion
      generation
    Leukotrienes C_4 and D_4—increase vascular permeability and coronary vascular
      resistance
    Platelet-activating factor—increases neutrophil activation and coronary vascular
      resistance
Oxygen metabolites
    Superoxide anion
    Hydrogen peroxide
    Hypochlorous acid

---

the poor deformability of neutrophils (131). Sixty percent of the capillaries within the ischemic bed were obstructed by leukocytes and displayed evidence of the "no reflow" phenomenon after regional ischemia and reperfusion of the canine heart (132). Progressive obstruction of the capillary bed may exacerbate ischemic injury by impeding reflow to the previously ischemic myocardial region.

Proteinases

The destruction of tissue by neutrophils may represent a cooperative interaction of hydrogen peroxide, myeloperoxidase, and proteinases. Release of hydrogen peroxide and myeloperoxidase by activated neutrophils results in the formation of hypochlorous acid, which reacts with amines to produce highly reactive chlorinated oxidants. Collagenase and gelatinase, two metalloproteinases contained within the neutrophil granules, are released as inactive proenzymes which are activated by the hypochlorous acid generated by activated neutrophils (11). Activated collagenase and gelatinase appear to have a dual function, having the ability to degrade collagen and inactivate alpha-1-proteinase inhibitor, an antiproteinase located in plasma and interstitial fluid. Hypochlorous acid or its derivatives also are able to inactivate the alpha-1-proteinase inhibitor by oxidizing a methionine that is critical to the ability of the protein to inhibit elastase.

    The role of neutrophil-derived proteinases in the pathogenesis of ischemic myocardial injury has not been studied extensively. A combination of three protease inhibitors did not reduce ischemic myocardial injury in rats, but the experimental protocol entailed 6 hr of ischemia without reperfusion, which probably minimizes leukocyte-mediated injury (133). Although aprotinin, a nonspecific inhibitor of proteolysis, reduced the severity of ischemic myocardial injury in dogs (64), the mechanism of aprotinin's cardioprotective effect is unclear because it also inhibited the generation of superoxide anions by neutrophils in vitro (134).

Eicosanoids

Activated neutrophils synthesize and release leukotrienes and other products of the lipoxygenase pathway of arachidonic acid metabolism (65,135,136). Leukotriene B4, a potent chemotactic factor, may amplify the inflammatory response to ischemia (65,136). Leukotrienes C4 and D4 increase vascular permeability and coronary vascular resistance, which may exacerbate ischemic myocardial injury (136). Although several drugs that inhibit the lipoxygenase pathway have been shown to reduce the extent of neutrophil infiltration and myocardial injury caused by regional ischemia, the multiple pharmacological effects of each agent confound interpretation of the results (137,138). One drug that is believed to be a selective 5-lipoxygenase inhibitor, REV-5901, also was reported to limit canine infarct size (139). A compound that antagonizes leukotriene B4 receptors, however, did not alter neutrophil infiltration or the extent of canine ischemic injury (140). Thus, it is unclear whether leukotrienes are important mediators of the inflammatory events associated with myocardial ischemia and reperfusion.

Platelet-Activating factor

Platelet-activating factor (PAF), a phospholipid that is synthesized by neutrophils, macrophages, platelets, and endothelial cells, exerts several actions that may directly or indirectly exacerbate ischemic myocardial injury (141). The cardiac effects of PAF are coronary vasoconstriction that is mediated by the endogenous production of leukotrienes, and a direct negative inotropic effect (142-144). PAF may enhance neutrophil-mediated injury via its capacity to stimulate neutrophil chemotaxis, adherence, granule secretion, and oxygen radical release, both independently and by priming the neutrophil responses to other agonists (145,146). Montrucchio et al. (147,148) reported that PAF is released from the rabbit heart during reperfusion after global ischemia and from the human heart during pacing-induced ischemia in patients with coronary artery disease. Treatment with either of two structurally unrelated PAF antagonists reduced myocardial injury in dogs subjected to coronary artery occlusion for 90 min followed by reperfusion (149).

EFFECTS OF FREE RADICAL SCAVENGERS

Superoxide Dismutase

The effects of oxygen radical scavengers on experimental myocardial infarction have been studied widely, and a satisfactory explanation for the conflicting results has not arisen despite extensive review and discussion (150–153). The controversy is focused primarily on whether treatment with superoxide dismustase (SOD), which metabolizes superoxide anions, is able to limit reperfusion injury. Several studies performed at the University of Michigan (154–157) and at Johns Hopkins University (158) have concluded that treatment with SOD does reduce canine myocardial reperfusion injury. Treatment with SOD reduced infarct size in dogs subjected to coronary artery occlusion for 90 min followed by reperfusion for 1 or 2 days (156,158). The administration of PEG-SOD, which has a prolonged plasma half-life due to the polyethylene glycol conjugate, limited the extent of infarction after coronary artery occlusion for 90 min followed by reperfusion for 4 days (157). Infarct size, expressed as a percent of the area at risk, was 29% in the PEG-SOD group, compared to 44% in the control group ($p < 0.005$).

Prolonged coronary artery occlusion is associated with vascular injury that is characterized by impaired vasodilation (159,160) and increased vascular permeability (161). Mehta et al. (159,160) demonstrated that treatment with SOD attenuates the loss of vascular relaxation in dogs subjected to 1 hr of coronary artery occlusion followed by reperfusion. Also, the increased microvascular permeability observed after 1 hr of ischemia was significantly blunted by infusion of SOD (161). Thus, a number of laboratories have reported that SOD exerts beneficial effects on ischemic myocardium.

Other laboratories, however, have consistently produced negative results with SOD. Two independent studies have concluded that treatment with "native" SOD did not limit canine infarct size after coronary artery occlusion for 90 min followed by reperfusion for 4 days (45) or 1 week (162). Additional groups have reported that "native" SOD did not alter the extent of canine myocardial injury after occlusion of a coronary artery for 2, 3, or 6 hr followed by reperfusion (163–166). Tanaka et al. (167) studied the effects of PEG-SOD plus catalase in dogs that underwent 90 min of regional myocardial ischemia followed by 4 days of reperfusion. Infarct size, expressed as a percent of the area at risk, was 37% in the treated group compared to 45% in the controls (p = NS). The dose of PEG-SOD in the latter study was 10,000 units/kg, while the previously described study by Tamura et al. (157) employed a dose of 1000 units/kg. Preliminary data have suggested that SOD may be deleterious at excessive doses (168), which may explain the apparent discrepancy between the studies by Tamura (157) and Tanaka (167).

Shirato and colleagues (169) proposed that the positive results observed with SOD treatment reflect an artifact of SOD's effect on the histochemical method used to measure infarct size. Their contention is that SOD causes dead tissue to retain the ability to reduce the tetrazolium salts that some laboratories have employed to measure infarct size. Lucchesi and co-workers (personal communication), however, found that SOD did not interfere with the tetrazolium method of assessing infarct size. Thus, further study will be necessary to reconcile the discordant data regarding SOD's ability to limit reperfusion injury.

Sulfhydryl Compounds

An important intracellular defense against oxidative injury is the enzyme glutathione peroxidase, which catalyzes the reduction of hydrogen peroxide or lipid peroxides by transferring electrons from glutathione, a cysteine-containing tripeptide. Both experimental and clinical studies indicate that myocardial glutathione stores may be inadequate to prevent oxidative injury during postischemic reperfusion (22,170–172). Glutathione and other low-molecular-weight sulfhydryl compounds, such as N-2-mercaptopropionyl glycine (MPG), have been shown to inhibit the peroxidation of lipids by oxygen free radicals in vitro (173).

Several studies have examined the ability of sulfhydryl compounds to limit myocardial reperfusion injury in vivo. The administration of MPG either before coronary artery occlusion or before coronary reflow, but not 40 min after reflow, significantly reduced the extent of injury after 90 min of ischemia followed by reperfusion (90,174). Administration of N-acetylcysteine, another sulfhydryl compound, did not limit the extent of myocardial injury in dogs subjected to 90 min of ischemia followed by reperfusion (175). Treatment was terminated 3 hr after reperfusion, however, while infarct size was determined 24 hr after reperfusion. As noted earlier, studies utilizing iloprost and "native" SOD suggest that free radical–mediated injury may not be confined to the initial hours of reperfusion. Thus, the inefficacy of N-acetylcysteine may relate to the short duration of therapy.

Some investigators have proposed that captopril, an inhibitor of angiotensin converting enzyme (ACE), acts as a free radical scavenger because of its sulfhydryl group (176,177), while more recent studies concluded that captopril is not an effective scavenger of free radicals (178,179).

FREE RADICALS AND MYOCARDIAL "STUNNING"

The term "stunned myocardium" has been adopted to denote the delayed recovery of contractile function by viable myocardium after ischemia and reperfusion (180, 181). The experimental protocol usually used to investigate the pathogenesis of stunned myocardium involves the measurement of regional systolic wall thickening or segment shortening before and after occlusion of a canine coronary artery for 15 min, a period of ischemia insufficient to cause tissue necrosis. Considerable evidence supports the theory that oxygen radicals formed during reperfusion play a pathogenetic role in myocardial stunning after reversible injury (180,181).

Effects of Free Radical "Scavengers"

Numerous free radical "scavengers" have been reported to enhance the recovery of myocardial function in dogs subjected to coronary artery occlusion for 15 min. Three independent laboratories reported that the combination of SOD and catalase improved the return of wall thickening or segment shortening after 15 min of ischemia followed by reperfusion for 2 or 3 hr (182–184). Neither SOD alone nor catalase alone, however, exerted independent protection against myocardial stunning (185).

Dimethylthiourea (DMTU), a putative scavenger of hydroxyl radicals, and MPG, the low-molecular-weight sulfhydryl compound referred to above, also have been shown to limit myocardial stunning (186,187). The beneficial effect of DMTU has been attributed to scavenging of hydroxyl radicals, but the compound may not be a specific "scavenger" of hydroxyl radicals because it also reacts with hypochlorous acid, which is formed via the release of hydrogen peroxide and myeloperoxidase by activated neutrophils (188). Strong evidence for the importance of hydroxyl radicals in the pathogenesis of myocardial stunning is the reduction of myocardial stunning by deferoxamine, which chelates the iron that is believed to catalyze the formation of hydroxyl radical from superoxide anion and hydrogen peroxide (189–191).

Administration of the free radical scavengers commenced before coronary artery occlusion in each of the studies described above, precluding any conclusion regarding the relative importance of ischemia and reperfusion in the development of myocardial stunning. Recently, however, Bolli and colleagues (34,191) demonstrated that antioxidant therapy begun at the time of reperfusion markedly reduces both contractile dysfunction and free radical generation. Infusion of MPG beginning 1 min before reperfusion was associated with improved recovery of wall thickening, while there was no improvement in dogs that received MPG starting 1 min after reperfusion (34). Similarly, the production of free radicals was markedly reduced only if MPG treatment was begun before reperfusion. Subsequently, analogous experiments were performed with deferoxamine (191). Administration of deferoxamine beginning 2 min before reperfusion limited both stunning and free radical formation, but treatment with deferoxamine 1 min after reperfusion did not prevent stunning.

Effects of Neutrophil Inhibition or Depletion

The role of neutrophils in the pathogenesis of myocardial stunning is unclear. Occlusion of a canine coronary artery for 12 min did not stimulate the accumulation of neutrophils during reperfusion of the myocardium (62), but there are conflicting data regarding the effect of neutrophil depletion on myocardial stunning. Three laboratories have studied the role of neutrophils in myocardial stunning by using extracorporeal circulation through filters to reperfuse ischemic myocardium with agranulocytic blood (192–194). Engler and Covell (192) observed nearly complete prevention of myocardial stunning. Westlin and Mullane (193) reported that myocardial segment shortening after 15 min of ischemia followed by 3 hr of reperfusion recovered to 55% of baseline in the neutropenic group compared to 6% of baseline in the control group ($p < 0.05$). Jeremy and Becker (194), however, found no difference between the functional recovery of control and neutropenic dogs.

Myocardial stunning was not altered by a 90% reduction of the peripheral neutrophil count in dogs treated with an antibody that previously had been shown to limit myocardial injury after 90 min of ischemia (195,196). Postischemic contractile function was not alleviated by administration of the anti-Mo1 antibody that reduced canine infarct size after 90 min of ischemia (197). Thus, two laboratories have reported favorable effects of neutrophil depletion by filters, but the contribution that neutrophils make to the dysfunction of reversibly injured myocardium does not appear to be blocked by a clinically feasible approach, such as the injection of antibodies directed against neutrophils.

Effects of Xanthine Oxidase Inhibitors

Unlike the human heart, the canine heart does have significant xanthine oxidase activity (37). Nevertheless, xanthine oxidase inhibitors have had variable effects on myocardial stunning in dogs. Treatment with either allopurinol or oxypurinol has been reported to improve systolic wall thickening after 15 min of regional ischemia (198,199). Amflutizole, a potent inhibitor of xanthine oxidase, did not attenuate myocardial myocardial stunning in dogs (200).

Other Sources of Free Radicals

The conflicting data regarding the role of neutrophils and xanthine oxidase in the pathogenesis of myocardial stunning suggest that the burst of free radical production at the time of reperfusion may emanate from other sources. Mitochondria constitute one potential source of free radicals within the ischemic heart. Vandeplassche et al. (201) provided cytochemical evidence for the generation of hydrogen peroxide by a mitochondrial NADH-oxidase within viable myocardial tissue after 45 min of regional myocardial ischemia followed by reperfusion. Ueta et al. (202) measured free radical production by submitochondrial particles isolated from ischemic and nonischemic canine myocardium. Free radical production was significantly increased in the mitochondria harvested after 60 min of coronary artery occlusion compared to mitochondria prepared from nonischemic myocardium. Other investigators have reported that addition of SOD and catalase suppressed the formation of hydroxyl radicals and facilitated the production of ATP by mitochondria harvested from rabbit hearts subjected to global ischemia (6).

Recently, a number of investigators have hypothesized that myoglobin, an abundant protein in the heart, may promote free radical-induced injury to membrane transport systems (5,173,203-205). For example, peroxidation of arachidonic acid (173,203) and inhibition of the sarcoplasmic reticulum calcium ATPase (205) occur after incubation with myoglobin plus hydrogen peroxide, but not after incubation with either myoglobin or hydrogen peroxide alone. One possible mechanism of myoglobin-dependent injury is degradation of the heme by hydrogen peroxide, releasing free iron that catalzyes the formation of hydroxyl radicals from hydrogen peroxide (5). An alternative mechanism is conversion of myoglobin to a ferriperoxide derivative that can initiate lipid peroxidation (173,203). The "myoglobin" hypothesis is supported by biochemical studies that have shown that myoglobin-mediated oxidant injury is inhibited by free radical scavengers, which reduce myocardial stunning such as mercaptopropionyl glycine (173).

CURRENT CLINICAL INVESTIGATION

The cardiology division of the University of Michigan has been involved in multicenter clinical trials of several agents that have limited reperfusion injury in experimental animals: iloprost, SOD, and DA-Fluosol. The final report of the iloprost study has been published (206), and a preliminary analysis of the SOD trial has been presented at the 1989 Scientific Session of the American Heart Association (207). Patient enrollment in the Fluosol study was scheduled for completion in mid-1991.

Iloprost

Simpson and colleagues (88,101,102) proposed that limitation of reperfusion injury by iloprost, a stable analog of PGI_2, is due to inhibition of neutrophil function. A pilot trial of iloprost therapy in patients with acute MI was conducted at the University of Michigan. Combined therapy with iloprost and tissue plasminogen activator (100 mg over 3 hr) was administered to 25 patients with acute myocardial infarction presenting within 6 hr of symptom onset. Iloprost was started at a dose of 0.5 ng/kg/min IV, with increases at 5-min intervals to 1 and then 2 ng/kg/min. The latter dose was maintained for 48 hr unless a reduction was required for hypotension or serious side effects.

After initiation of therapy, the patients underwent left ventriculography, coronary angiography, and angioplasty of the infarct vessel if it was occluded at 90 min after therapy; i.e., flow was TIMI grade 0 or 1. The patients underwent fol-

Table 3   Clinical and Angiographic Effects of Iloprost and t-PA

	t-PA and iloprost	t-PA	p
Number of patients	25	25	
Patency at 90 min	11 (44%)	15 (60%)	0.26
Patency at end of cath[a]	21 (84%)	23 (92%)	
Reocclusion[b]	3 (14%)	6 (26%)	0.46
Baseline ejection fraction[c]	51.3 ± 10.1%	47.3 ± 11.5%	
7-day ejection fraction	49.0 ± 9.4%	50.4 ± 9.8%	
Change in wall motion of infarct zone (SD/chord)	0.21 ± 0.90	0.76 ± 0.89	0.05

[a]Acute patency (TIMI 2 or 3) on discharge from the catheterization laboratory (i.e., after diagnostic angiography or rescue PTCA if performed).
[b]Angiographic reocclusion after discharge from the catheterization laboratory.
[c]All data are mean ± SD.

low-up ventriculography and angiography 7 days after admission, or earlier if indicated for treatment of recurrent ischemia.

The 25 patients treated with iloprost and t-PA were compared to a subsequent series of 25 patients treated with t-PA alone with respect to angiographic, ventriculographic, hematological, and clinical outcomes. The rates of infarct vessel patency for the iloprost plus t-PA and t-PA alone groups were not significantly different at 90 min, 44% versus 60% (p = 0.26), or at the end of procedure, 84% versus 92% (Table 3). The rates of reocclusion at 1 week were 14% in the iloprost group and 26% in the t-PA alone group (p = 0.46). Neither regional nor global left ventricular function was improved by the combination of t-PA and iloprost compared to t-PA alone (Table 3).

Administration of iloprost was associated with a smaller decrease in serum fibrinogen and a smaller increase in fibrinogen degradation products (Table 4). There were no differences in the frequency of bleeding complications or need for transfusion. Hypotension required termination of the iloprost infusion in three patients, and a reduction of the dose in five additional patients. Vomiting was a prominent side effect of iloprost, occurring in 16 of 25 patients treated with iloprost compared to 7 of 25 patients treated with t-PA alone (p = 0.02).

Although this was a relatively small pilot study, the results are disappointing from several perspectives. First, there was no apparent benefit with respect to initial patency or reocclusion of the infarct vessel, or recovery of left ventricular function, despite experimental evidence that iloprost or prostacyclin should augment thrombolysis (208), reduce infarct size (88,101), and alleviate myocardial

Table 4   Hematological Effects of Iloprost and t-PA

	t-PA and iloprost	t-PA
Number of patients	25	19[a]
Baseline fibrinogen (mg/dl)	2.70 ± 0.52	3.45 ± 1.07
4-hr fibrinogen (mg/dl)	1.80 ± 0.66	1.65 ± 0.89
% change	33%	52%

[a]Six patients in the t-PA group who subsequently received urokinase were deleted from the analysis.

stunning (209). Second, an iloprost dose of 2 ng/kg/min was poorly tolerated owing to gastrointestinal side effects, which would preclude increasing the dose to the range of 50–100 ng/kg/min employed in experimental studies (88,209). Finally, there was less degradation of fibrinogen in the patients treated with iloprost, which may reflect an accelerated clearance of t-PA via an increase in hepatic blood flow by iloprost. Thus, it is possible that iloprost, and perhaps other vasodilators, may actually reduce the thrombolytic efficacy of t-PA.

Superoxide Dismutase

The cardiology divisions of Johns Hopkins University and the University of Michigan have coordinated a randomized, double-blind Multicenter clinical trial of recombinant human SOD in patients who underwent coronary angioplasty for acute MI. Patients were eligible for inclusion if coronary angiography within 6 hr of symptom onset demonstrated an occluded (TIMI grade 0 or 1) infarct vessel that was suitable for angioplasty (Fig. 3). Eligible patients were randomized to administration of either placebo or SOD, which was administered as a 10 mg/kg bolus and an infusion of 0.2 mg/kg/min for 1 hr beginning at the time of angioplasty. The primary endpoints were regional and global left ventricular function assessed by contrast ventriculography 7 days after therapy. Left ventricular function also was evaluated by radionuclide ventriculography 4–6 weeks after infarction. The baseline patient characteristics, patency of the infarct vessel, and recovery of regional and global left ventricular function were similar for the placebo and SOD groups (Tables 5, 6, and 7; Figure 4). There are several possible reasons for the negative result. First, the study was terminated before achieving the sample size of 170 patients that was required to have a power of 90% assuming that the true effect of SOD on the change in ejection fraction is an increase of 5 absolute percent. Second, the mean time to reperfusion was 4 hr after the onset of chest pain, and most experimental studies have not demonstrated a reduction of infarct size by SOD when the duration of ischemia was 2 hr or greater. Finally, recent experimental studies suggest that 1 hr of SOD therapy is inadequate to achieve sus-

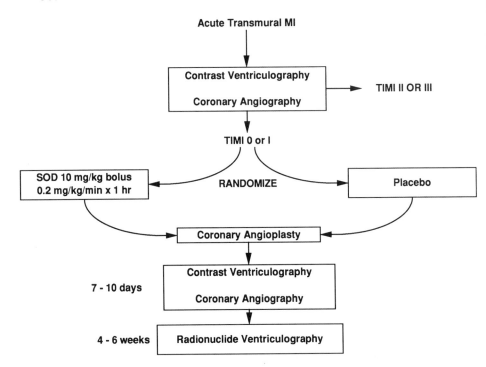

Figure 3   Superoxide dismutase protocol.

Table 5   Patient Population Enrolled in SOD Trial

	SOD	Placebo
n	59	55
Age (years)	58.8	57.7
% Male	75%	84%
Infarct vessel		
LAD	46%	47%
LCX	17%	6%
RCA	37%	47%
Baseline EF	50.9 ± 14.0%	50.1 ± 16.7%
Time to reperfusion	4.1 ± 1.4 hr	4.1 ± 1.5 hr
Thrombolytics	26%	18%

EF = ejection fraction.

Table 6   Early Recovery of Left Ventricular Function in SOD Trial

| | | Contrast ventriculography | | | |
| | | LV ejection fraction (%) | | Wall motion (SD/chord) | |
	n	Acute	7-10 days	Acute	7-10 days
SOD	36	52.1 ± 13.7	52.4 ± 13.7	-2.95 ± 0.85	-2.56 ± 1.19
Control	35	51.8 ± 14.7	55.6 ± 12.6	-3.03 ± 0.83	-2.30 ± 1.39
p		NS	NS	NS	NS

All data are mean ± SD.

tained limitation of myocardial injury (157). Thus, future clinical trials of SOD should be designed to achieve a larger sample size, earlier reperfusion, and a longer duration of therapy, e.g., by using PEG-SOD.

Fluosol

Several experimental studies have demonstrated the ability of Fluosol to limit reperfusion injury in canine models of myocardial infarction (119–123). Forman et al. (210) reported the results of a pilot trial of Fluosol in patients with acute anterior MI who underwent emergency PTCA of the left anterior descending coronary artery (LAD). The Fluosol group (*n* = 5) received oxygenated Fluosol via the proximal LAD at a rate of 40 ml/min for 30 min beginning immediately after restoration of coronary flow, while the control group underwent conventional PTCA (*n* = 6). Contrast left ventriculography was performed at the time of

Table 7   Late Recovery of Left Ventricular Function in SOD Trial

| | | Radionuclide ventriculography | | | |
| | | LV EF (%) | | Regional EF (%) | |
	n	Acute	4-6 weeks	Acute	4-6 weeks
SOD	31	44.8 ± 14.6	45.5 ± 14.2	24.0 ± 15.4	28.9 ± 15.1
Control	25	44.9 ± 14.9	48.2 ± 13.7	24.0 ± 17.1	33.1 ± 17.5
p		NS	NS	NS	NS

All data are mean ± SD.
EF = ejection fraction.

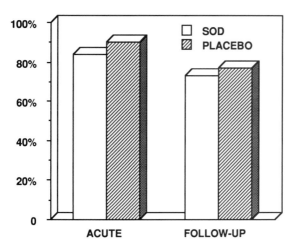

Figure 4   Infarct artery patency of SOD and placebo patients.

PTCA and an average of 12 days later. There was significantly greater recovery of regional wall motion in the ischemic zone in the Fluosol group compared to the control group.

The TAMI-9 study is a large, multicenter, randomized trial designed to evaluate the effects of intravenous Fluosol in patients treated with t-PA within 6 hr of onset of acute MI. The patients will be randomly assigned to either a control group (standard thrombolytic therapy) or a treatment group (standard thrombolytic therapy with intravenous Fluosol). The Fluosol group will be administered 100% oxygen via a nonrebreathing mask and 15 ml/kg of Fluosol intravenously at a rate of ≤20 ml/min over 12 hr. All patients will receive aspirin 325 mg daily, intravenous heparin for 1 week, intravenous lidocaine, and both metoprolol (5 mg IV × 3, then 50–100 mg twice daily) and a calcium antagonist unless contraindicated. The primary physiological endpoint is the left ventricular ejection fraction measured by contrast ventriculography 7–10 days posttreatment. The primary clinical endpoint is a combined endpoint of the following clinical events: death, recurrent angina or MI, congestive heart failure, and PTCA or bypass surgery before the predischarge cardiac catheterization. The projected sample size is 400 subjects.

FUTURE PROSPECTS

Experimental models of myocardial stunning after brief periods of ischemia have provided convincing evidence of the role of free radicals in the pathogenesis of reperfusion injury. The stunning model may be relevant to patients with exertional angina, transient coronary artery spasm, or unstable angina, but transient left ventricular dysfunction is seldom clinically important under those circumstances. Left ventricular dysfunction is a major determinant of clinical outcome in patients with acute MI. Unfortunately, the experimental studies of MI have produced conflicting data regarding the ability of free radical scavengers to limit myocardial injury. A recent study has claimed to disprove the existence of reperfusion injury. Ganz et al. (211) performed a study that compared the extent of necrosis in the reperfused and nonreperfused halves of a single ischemic territory. The authors concluded that reperfusion did not extend the boundary of necrosis, but the duration of reperfusion was limited to 5 min, which is probably insufficient to exclude the existence of neutrophil-mediated injury after reperfusion.

Undoubtedly, reperfusion injury will be the subject of continued basic investigation. Meanwhile, the results of the TAMI trial of Fluosol are eagerly awaited. If Fluosol fails to improve left ventricular function, it is likely that there will be diminished enthusiasm for further clinical trials. A positive result, however, should provide impetus for further basic and clinical studies of myocardial reperfusion injury.

REFERENCES

1. Southorn PA, Powis G. Free radicals in medicine. I. Chemical nature and biologic reactions. Mayo Clin Proc 1988; 63:381-9.
2. Southern PA. Powis G. Free radicals in medicine. II. Involvement in human disease. Mayo Clin Proc 1988; 63:390-408.
3. Biemond P, Van Eijk HG, Swaak AJG, Koster JF. Iron mobilization from ferritin by 02- derived from stimulated polymorphonuclear leukocytes. Possible mechanism in inflammation disease. J Clin Invest 1984; 73:1576-9.
4. Puppo A, Halliwell B. Formation of hydroxyl radicals from hydrogen peroxide in the presence of iron. Is haemoglobin a biological Fenton reagent? Biochem J 1988; 249: 185-90.
5. Puppo A, Halliwell B. Formation of hydroxyl radicals in biological systems. Does myoglobin stimulate hydroxyl radical formation from hydrogen peroxide? Free Rad Res Commun 1988; 4:415-22.
6. Otani H, Tanaka H, Inoue T, Umemoto M, Omoto K,Tanaka K, Sato T, Osako T, Masuda A, Nonoyama A, Kagawa T. In vitro study on contribution of oxidative metabolism of isolated rabbit heart mitochondria to myocardial reperfusion injury. Circ Res 1984; 55:168-75.
7. Chien KR, Han A, Sen A, Buja LM, Willerson JT. Accumulation of unesterified arachidonic acid in ischemic canine myocardium. Circ Res 1984; 54:313-22.
8. Chien KR, Sen A, Reynolds R, Chang A, Kim Y, Gunn MD, Buja LM, Willerson JT. Release of arachidonate from membrane phospholipids in cultured neonatal rat myocardial cells during adenosine triphosphate depletion. J Clin Invest 1985; 75:1770-80.

9. Kukreja RC, Kontos HA, Hess ML, Ellis EF. PGH synthase and lipoxygenase generate superoxide in the presence of NADH or NADPH. Circ Res 1986; 59:612-9.

10. McCord JM. Oxygen-derived free radicals in post ischemic tissue injury. N Engl J Med 1985; 312:159-63.

11. Weiss SJ. Tissue destruction by neutrophils. N Engl J Med 1989; 320:365-75.

12. Schraufstatter IU, Hinshaw DB, Hyslop PA, Spragg RG, Cochrane CG. Oxidant injury of cells. J Clin Invest 1986; 77:1312-20.

13. Dallegri F, Goretti R, Ballestrero, Ottonello L, Patrone F. Neutrophil induced depletion of adenosine triphosphate in target cells: evidence for a hypochlorous acid-mediated process. J Lab Clin Med 1988; 112:765-72.

14. Blaustein AS, Schine L, Brooks WW, Fanburg BL, Bing OHL. Influene of exogenously generated oxidant species on myocardial function. Am J Physiol 1986; 250: H595-9.

15. Burton KP, McCord JM, Ghai G. Myocardial alterations due to free-radical generation. Am J Physiol 1984; 246:H776-83.

16. Ytrehus K, Muyklebust R, Mjos R. Influence of oxygen radicals generated by xanthine oxidase in the isolated perfused rat heart Cardiovasc Res 1986; 20:597-603.

17. Gillespie MN, Kojima S, Kunitomo M, Jay J. Coronary and myocardial effects of activated neutrophils in perfused rabbit hearts. J Pharmacol Exp Ther 1986; 239:836-40.

18. Jackson CV, Mickelson JK, Pope TK, Rao PS, Lucchesi BR. O_2 free radical-mediated myocardial and vascular dysfunction. Am J Physiol 1986; 25:H1225-H1231.

19. Janero DR, Burghardt B. Oxidative injury to myocardial membrane: direct modulation by endogenous alpha-tocopherol. J Mol Cell Cardiol 1989; 21:1111-24.

20. Tribble DL, Kennedy FG, Jones DP: Contrasting features of peroxide metabolism in heart and liver. In: Singal PK (ed). Oxygen radicals in the pathophysiology of heart disease. Boston: Kluwer, 1988: 25-40.

21. Noronha-Dutra AA, Steen EM. Lipid peroxidation as a mechanism of injury in cardiac myocytes. Lab Invest 1982; 47:346-53.

22. Roth E, Torok B, Zsoldos T, Matkovics B. Lipid peroxidation and scavenger mechanism in experimentally induced heart infarcts. Basic Res Cardiol 1985; 80:530-6.

23. Halliwell B, Gutteridge JMC. Oxygen free radicals and iron in relation to biology and medicine: some problems and concepts. Arch Biochem Biophys 1986; 246:501-4.

24. Toth KM, Clifford DP, Berger EM, White CW, Repine JE. Intact human erythrocytes prevent hydrogen peroxide-mediated damage to isolated perfused rat lungs and cultured bovine pulmonary artery endothelial cells. J Clin Invest 1984; 74:292-5.

25. Agar NS, Sadrzadeh SMH, Hallaway EP, Eaton JW. Erythrocyte catalase: a somatic oxidant defense. J Clin Invest 1986; 77:319-21.

26. Winterbourn CC, Stern A. Human red cells scavenge extracellular hydrogen peroxide and inhibit formation of hypochlorous acid and hydroxyl radical. J Clin Invest 1987; 80:1486-91.

27. Brown JM, Grosso MA, Terada LS, Beehler CJ, Toth KM, Whitman GJ, Harken AH, Repine JE. Erythrocytes decrease myocardial hydrogen peroxide levels and reperfusion injury. Am J Physiol 1989; 256:H584-H588.

28. Zweier JL, Flaherty JT, Weisfeldt ML. Direct measurement of free radical generation

following reperfusion of ischemic myocardium Proc Natl Acad Sci USA 1987; 84: 1404-7.

29. Zweier JL, Rayburn BK, Flaherty JT, Weisfeldt ML. Recombinant superoxide dismutase reduces oxygen free radical concentrations in reperfused myocardium. J Clin Invest 1987; 80:1728-34.

30. Zweier JL. Measurement of superoxide-derived free radicals in the reperfused heart. J Biol Chem 1988; 263:1353-7.

31. Garlick PB, Davies MJ, Hearse DJ, Slater TF. Direct detection of free radicals in the reperfused rat heart using electron spin resonance spectroscopy. Circ Res 1987; 61: 757-60.

32. Kuzuya T, Hoshida S, Kim Y, Nishida M, Fuji H, Kitabatake A, Tada M, Kamada T. Detection of oxygen-derived free radical generation in the canine postischemic heart during late phase of reperfusion. Circ Res 1990; 66:1160-5.

33. Bolli R, Patel BS, Jeroudi MO, Lau EK, McCay PB. Demonstration of free radical generation in "stunned" myocardium of intact dogs with the use of the spin trap alphaphenyl N-tert-butyl nitrone. J Clin Invest 1988; 82:476-85.

34. Bolli R, Jeroudi MO, Patel BS, Aruoma OI, Halliwell B, Lau EK, McCay PB. Marked reduction of free radical generation and contactile dysfunction by antioxidant therapy begun at the time of reperfusion. Circ Res 1989; 65:607-22.

35. Bolli R, Jeroudi MO, Patel BS, DuBose CM, Lai EK, Roberts R, McCay PB. Direct evidence that oxygen-derived free radicals contribute to postischemic myocardial dysfunction in the intact dog. Proc Natl Acad Sci USA 1989; 86:4695-9.

36. Johnson WD, Kayser KL, Brenowitz JB, Saedi SF. A randomized controlled trial of allopurinol in coronary bypass surgery. Am Heart J 1991; 121:20-4.

37. Chambers DE, Parts DA, Patterson G, Roy R, McCord JM, Yoshida S, Parmley LF, Downey JM. Xanthine oxidase as a source of free radical damage in myocardial ischemia. J Mol Cell Cardiol 1985: 17:145-52.

38. Werns SW, Shea MJ, Mitsos SE, Dysko RD, Fantone JC, Schork MA, Abrams GD, Pitt B, Lucchesi BR. Reduction of the size of infarction by allopurinol in the ischemic-reperfused canine heart. Circulation 1986; 73:518-24.

39. Reimer KA, Jennings RB. Failure of the xanthine oxidase inhibitor allopurinol to limit infarct size after ischemia and reperfusion in dogs. Circulation 1985: 71:1069-75.

40. Werns SW, Grum CM, Ventura A, Lucchesi BR. Effects of allopurinol or oxypurinol on myocardial reperfusion injury. Circulation 1987; 76:IV-97 (abstract).

41. Spector T. Inhibition of urate production by allopurinol, Biochem Pharmacol 1977: 26:355-8.

42. Spector T. Oxypurinol as an inhibitor of xanthine oxidase-catalyzed production of superoxide radical. Biochem Pharmacol 1988; 37:349-52.

43. Kinsman JM, Murry CE, Richard VJ, Jennings RB, Reimer KA. The xanthine oxidase inhibitor oxypurinol does not limit infarct size in a canine model of 40 minutes of ischemia with reperfusion. J Am Coll Cardiol 1988; 12:209-17.

44. Puett DW, Forman MB, Cates CU, Wilson BH, Hande KR, Friesinger GC, Virmani R. Oxypurinol limits myocardial stunning but does not reduce infarct size after reperfusion. Circulation 1987; 76:678-86.

45. Richard VJ, Murry CE, Jennings RB, Reimer KA. Therapy to reduce free radicals during early reperfusion does not limit the size of myocardial infarcts caused by 90 minutes of ischemia in dogs. Circulation 1988; 78:473-80.

46. Werns SW, Grum CM, Ventura A, Hahn RA, Ho PPK, Towner RD, Fantone JC, Schork MA, Lucchesi BR. Xanthine oxidase inhibition does not limit canine infarct size. Circulation 1991; 83:995-1005.

47. Godin DV, Bhimji S. Effects of allopurinol on myocardial ischemic injury induced by coronary artery ligation and reperfusion. Biochem Pharmacol 1987; 36:2101-7.

48. Godin DV, Bhimji S, McNeill JH. Effects of allopurinol pretreatment on myocardial ultrastructure and arrhythmias following coronary artery occlusion and reperfusion. Cell Pathol 1986; 52:327-41.

49. Grum CM, Ragsdale RA, Ketai LH, Shlafer M. Absence of xanthine oxidase or xanthine dehydrogenase in the rabbit myocardium. Biochem Biophys Res Commun 1986; 141:1104-8.

50. Grum CM, Ketai LH, Myers CL, Shlafer M. Purine efflux after cardiac ischemia: relevance to allopurinol cardioprotection. Am J Physiol 1987; 252:H368-73.

51. Das DK, Engelman RM, Clement R, Otani H, Prasad MR, Rao PS. Role of xanthine oxidase inhibitor as free radical scavenger: a novel mechanism of action of allopurinol and oxypurinol in myocardial salvage. Biochem Biophys Res Commun 1987; 148: 314-9.

52. Muxfeldt M, Schaper W. The activity of xanthine oxidase in heart of pigs, guinea pigs, rabbits, rats, and humans. Basic Res Cardiol 1987; 82:486-92.

53. deJong JW, van der Meer P, Nieukoop AS, Huizer T, Stroeve RJ, Bos E. Xanthine oxidoreductase activity in perfused hearts of various species, including humans. Circ Res 1990; 67:770-3.

54. Terada LS, Rubinstein JD, Lesnefsky EJ, Horwitz LD, Leff JA, Repine JE. Existence and participation of xanthine oxidase in reperfusion injury of ischemic rabbit myocardium. Am J Physiol 1991; 260:H805-H810.

55. Downey JM, Miura T, Eddy LJ, Chambers DE, Mellert T, Hearse DJ, Yellon DM. Xanthine oxidase is not a source of free radicals in the ischemic rabbit heart. J Mol Cell Cardiol 1987; 19:1053-60.

56. Eddy LJ, Stewart JR, Jones HP, Engerson TD, McCord JM, Downey JM. The free radical producing enzyme, xanthine oxidase, is undetectable in human hearts. Am J Physiol 1987; 253:H709-H711.

57. Grum CM, Gallagher KP, Kirsh MM, Shlafer M. Absence of detectable xanthine oxidase in human myocardium. J Mol Cell Cardiol 1989; 21:263-7.

58. Jarasch E-D, Bruder G, Heid HW. Significance of xanthine oxidase in capillary endothelial cells. Acta Physiol Scand 1986; 548:39-46.

59. Huizer T, DeJong JW, Nelson JA, Czarnecki W, Serruys PW, Bonnier JJRM, Troquay R. Urate production by human heart. J Mol Cell Cardiol 1989; 21:691-5.

60. Sommers HM, Jennings RB. Experimental acute myocardial infarction: histologic and histochemical studies of early myocardial infarcts induced by temporary or permanent occlusion of a coronary artery. Lab Invest 1964; 13:1491-1503.

61. Mullane KM, Kraemer R, Smith B. Myeloperoxidase activity as a quantitative assess-

ment of nuetrophil infiltration into ischemic myocardium. J Pharmacol Methods 1985; 14:157-67.

62. Go LO, Murry CE, Richard VJ, Weischedel GR, Jennings RB, Reimer KA. Myocardial neutrophil accumulation during reperfusion after reversible or irreversible ischemic injury. Am J Physiol 1988; 255:H1188-H1198.

63. Richard VJ, Brooks SE, Jennings RB, Reimer KA. Effect of a critical coronary stenosis on myocardial neutrophil accumulation during ischemia and early reperfusion in dogs. Circulation 1989; 80:1805-15.

64. Hartmann JR, Robinson JA, Gunnar RM. Chemotactic activity in the coronary sinus after experimental myocardial infarction. Effects of pharmacologic interventions on ischemic injury. Am J Cardiol 1977; 40:550-5.

65. Mullane KM, Salmon JA, Kraemer R. Leukocyte-derived metabolites of arachidonic acid in ischemia-induced myocardial injury. Fed Proc 1987; 46:2422-33.

66. Kuzuya T, Hoshida S, Nishida M, Kim Y, Kamada T, Tada M. Increased production of arachidonate metabolites in an occlusion-reperfusion model of canine myocardial infarction. Cardiovasc Res 1987; 21:551-8.

67. Sasaki K, Ueno A, Katori M, Kikawada R. Detection of leukotriene B4 in cardiac tissue and its role in infarct extension through leucocyte migration. Cardiovasc Res 1988; 22:142-8.

68. Strieter RM, Kunkel SL, Showell HG, Marks RM. Monokine induced gene expression of a human endothelial cell-derived neutrophil chemotactic factor. Biochem Biophys Res Commun 1988; 156:1340-5.

69. Elgebaly SA, Masetti P, Allam M, Forouhar F. Cardiac derived neutrophil chemotactic factors; preliminary biochemical characterization. J Mol Cell Cardiol 1989; 21: 585-93.

70. Fernandez HN, Henson PM, Otani A, Hugli TE. Chemotactic response to human C3a and C5a anaphylatoxins. J Immunol 1978; 120:109-15.

71. Hill JH, Ward PA. C3 leukotactic factors produced by a tissue protease. J Exp Med 1969; 130:505-18.

72. Hill JH, Ward PA. The phlogistic role of C3 leukotactic fragments in myocardial infarcts of rats. J Exp Med 1971; 133:885-900.

73. Pinckard RN, Olson MS, Giclas PC, Terry R, Boyer JT, O'Rourke RA. Consumption of classical complement components by heart subcellular membranes in vitro and in patients after acute myocardial infarction. J Clin Invest 1975; 56:740-50.

74. Giclas PC, Pinckard RN, Olson MS. In vitro activation of complement by isolated human heart subcellular membranes. J Immunol 1979; 122:146-51.

75. Rossen RD, Michael LH, Kagiyama A, Savage HE, Hanson G, Reisberg MA, Moake JN, Kim SH, Self D, Weakley S, Giannini E, Entmann ML. Mechanism of complement activation after coronary artery occlusion: Evidence that myocardial ischemia in dogs causes release of constituents of myocardial subcellular origin that complex with human C1q in vivo. Circ Res 1988; 62:572-84.

76. Kagiyama A, Savage HE, Michael LH, Hanson G, Entman ML, Rossen RD. Molecular basis of complement activation in ischemic myocardium: identification of specific molecules of mitochondrial origin that bind human C1q and fix complement. Circ Res 1989; 64:607-15.

77. Pinckard RN, O'Rourke RA, Crawford MH, Grover FS, McManus LM, Ghidoni JJ, Storrs SB, Olson MS. Complement localization and mediation of ischemic injury in baboon myocardium. J Clin Invest 1980; 66:1050-6.

78. Crawford MH, Grover FL, Kolb WP McMahan CA, O'Rourke RA, McManus LM, Pinckard RN. Complement and neutrophil activation in the pathogenesis of ischemic myocardial injury. Circulation 1988; 78:1449-58.

79. Mehta J, Dinerman J, Mehta P, Saldeen TGP, Lawson D, Donnelly WH, Wallin R. Neutrophil function in ischemic heart disease. Circulation 1989; 79:549-56.

80. Yasuda M, Takeuchi K, Hiruma M, Iida H, Tahara A, Itagane H, Toda I, Akioka K, Teragaki M, Oku H, Kanayama Y, Takeda T, Kolb WP, Tamerius JD. The complement system in ischemic heart disease. Circulation 1990; 81:156-63.

81. Schafer J, Mathey D, Hugo F, Bhakdi S. Deposition of the terminal C5b-9 complement complex in infarcted areas of human myocardium. J Immunology 1986; 137: 1945-9.

82. Gewirz H, Lint TF. Alternative modes and pathways of complement activation. In Day NK, Good RA (eds). Biological amplification systems in immunology. New York: Plenum Press, 1977; 17-45.

83. Bennett WR, Yawn DH, Migliore PJ, Young JB, Pratt CM, Raizner AE, Roberts R, Bolli R. Activation of the complement system by recombinant tissue plasminogen activator. J Am Coll Cardiol 1987; 10:627-32.

84. Skubitz KM, Craddock PR. Reversal of hemodialysis granulocytopenia and pulmonary leukostasis. J Clin Invest 1981; 67:1383-91.

85. Spilberg I, Mehta J, Muniain MA, Simchowitz L, Atkinson J. Receptor blockade as a mechanism of deactivation of human neutrophils by pepstatin and formyl-met-leu-phe. Inflammation 1984; 8:73-86.

86. Bell D, Jackson M, Nicoll JJ, Millar A, Dawes J, Muir AL. Inflammatory response, neutrophil ativation, and free radical production after acute myocardial infarction; effect of thrombolytic treatment. Br Heart J 1990; 63:82-7.

87. Romson JL, Hook BG, Kunkel SL, Abrams GD, Schork MA, Lucchesi BR. Reduction of the extent of ischemic myocardial injury by neutrophil depletion in the dog. Circulation 1983; 67:1016-23.

88. Simpson PJ, Fantone JC, Mickelson JK, Gallagher KP, Lucchesi BR. Identification of a time window for therapy to reduce experimental canine myocardial injury: suppression of neutrophil activation during 72 hrs of reperfusion. Circ Res 1988; 63:1070-9.

89. Jolly SR, Kane WJ, Hook BG, Abrams GD, Kunkel SL, Lucchesi BR. Reduction of myocardial infarct size by neutrophil depletion: effect of duration of occlusion. Am. Heart J 1986; 112:682-90.

90. Mitsos SE, Askew TE, Fantone JC, Kunkel SL, Abrams GD, Schork A, Lucchesi BR. Protective effects of N-2 mercaptopropionyl glycine against myocardial reperfusion injury after neutrophil depletion in the dog: evidence for the role of intracellular-derived free radicals. Circulation 1986; 73:1077-86.

91. Litt MR, Jeremy RW, Weisman FH, Winkelstein JA, Becker LC. Neutrophil depletion limited to reperfusion reduces myocardial infarct size after 90 minutes of ischemia. Circulation 1989; 80:1816-27.

92. Carlson RE, Schott RJ, Buda AJ. Neutrophil depletion fails to modify myocardial no reflow and functional recovery after coronary reperfusion. J Am Coll Cardiol 1989; 14:1803-13.

93. Chatelain P, Latour J-G, Tran D, De Lorgeril M, Dupras G, Bourassa M. Neutrophil accumulation in experimental myocardial infarcts: relation with extent of injury and effect of reperfusion. Circulation 1987; 75:1083-90.

94. Romson JL, Bush LR, Jolly SR, Lucchesi BR. Cardioprotective effects of ibuprofen in experimental regional and global myocardial ischemia. J Cardiovasc Pharmacol 1982; 4:187-96.

95. Romson JL, Hook BG, Rigot VH, Schork MA, Swanson DP, Lucchesi BR. The effect of ibuprofen on accumulation of indium-111-labeled platelets and leukocytes in experimental myocardial infarction. Circulation 1982; 66:1002-11.

96. Jolly SR, Schumacher WA, Kunkel SL, Abrams GD, Liddicoat J, Lucchesi BR. Platelet depletion in experimental myocardial infarction. Basic Res Cardiol 1985; 80:269-79.

97. Mullane KM, McGiff JC. Platelet depletion and infarct size in an occlusion-reperfusion model of myocardial ischemia in anesthetized dogs. J Cardiovasc Pharmacol 1985; 7:733-8.

98. Reimer KA, Jennings RB, Cobb FR, Murdock RH, Greenfield JC, Becker LC, Bulkley BH, Hutchins GM, Schwartz RP, Bailey KR, Passamani ER. Animal models for protecting ischemic myocardium: results of the NHLBI Cooperative Study. Circ Res 1985; 56:651-65.

99. Brown EJ, Kloner RA, Schoen FJ, Hammerman H, Hale S, Braunwald E. Scar thinning due to ibuprofen administration after experimental myocardial infarction. Am J Cardiol 1983; 51:877-83.

100. Jugdutt BI. Delayed effects of early infarct-limiting therapies on healing after myocardial infarction. Circulation 1985; 72:907-14.

101. Simpson PJ, Mickelson JK, Fantone JC, Gallagher KP, Lucchesi BR. Iloprost inhibits neutrophil function in vitro and in vivo and limits experimental infarct size in canine heart. Circ Res 1987; 60:666-73.

102. Simpson PJ, Mitsos SE, Ventura A, Gallagher KP, Fantone JC, Abrams GD, Schork MA, Lucchesi BR. Prostacyclin protects ischemic-reperfused myocardium in the dog by inhibition of neutrophil activation. Am Heart J 1987; 113:129-37.

103. Simpson PJ, Mickelson J, Fantone JC, Gallagher KP, Lucchesi BR. Reduction of experimental canine myocardial infarct size with prostaglandin E1: Inhibition of neutrophil migration and activation. J Pharmacol Exp Ther 1988; 244:619-24.

104. Jennings RB, Steenbergen C. Nucleotide metabolism and cellular damage in myocardial ischemia. Annu Rev Physiol 1985; 47:727-49.

105. Kitakaze M, Hori M, Tamai J, Iwakura K, Koretsune Y, Kagiya T, Iwai K, Kitabatake A, Inoue M, Kamada T. Alpha-1-adrenoceptor activity regulates release of adenosine from the ischemic myocardium in dogs. Circ Res 1987; 60:631-9.

106. Deussen A, Borst M, Kroll K, Schrader J. Formation of S-adenosylhomocysteine in the heart. II. A sensitive index for regional myocardial underperfusion. Circ Res 1988; 63:250-61.

107. Cronstein BN, Levin RI, Belanoff J, Weissmann G, Hirschhorn R. Adenosine: an endogenous inhibitor of neutrophil-mediated injury to endothelial cells. J Clin Invest 1986; 78:760-70.
108. Engler R. Consequences of activation and adenosine-mediated inhibition of granulocytes during myocardial ischemia. Fed Proc 1987; 46:2407-12.
109. Cronstein BN, Daguma L, Nichold D, Hutchinson AJ, Williams M. The adenosine/neutrophil paradox resolved: human neutrophils posess both A1 and A2 receptors that promote chemotaxis and inhibit 02- generation, respectively. J Clin Invest 1990; 85:1150-7.
110. Cronstein BN, Kramer SB, Weissmann G, Hirshhorn. Adenosine: a physiological modulator of superoxide anion generation by human neutrophils. J Exp Med 1983; 158:1160-77.
111. Olafsson B, Forman MB, Puett DW, Pou A, Cates CU, Friesinger GC, Virmani R. Reduction of reperfusion injury in the canine preparation by intracoronary adenosine: importance of the endothelium and the no-flow phenomenon. Circulation 1987; 76:1135-45.
112. Babbitt DG, Virmani R, Forman MB. Intracoronary adenosine administered after reperfusion limits vascular injury after prolonged ischemia in the canine model. Circulation 1989; 80:1388-99.
113. Babbitt DG, Virmani R, Vildibill HD, Norton ED, Forman MB. Intracoronary adenosine administration during reperfusion following 3 hours of ischemia: effects on infarct size, ventricular function and regional myocardial blood flow. Am Heart J 1990; 120:808-18.
114. Pitrarys CJ, Virmani R, Vildibill HD, Jackson EK, Forman MB. Reduction of myocardial reperfusion injury by intravenous adenosine administered during the early reperfusion period. Circulation 1991; 83:237-47.
115. Homeister JW, Hoff PT, Fletcher DD, Lucchesi BR. Combined adenosine and lidocaine administration limits myocardial reperfusion injury. Circulation 1990; 82: 595-608.
116. Takeo S, Tanonaka K, Miyake K, Imago M. Adenine nucleotide metabolites are beneficial for recovery of cardiac contractile force after hypoxia. J Mol Cell Cardiol 1988; 20:187-99.
117. Virmani R, Warren D, Rees R, Fink LM, English D. Effects of perfluorochemical on phagocytic function of leukocytes. Transfusion 1983; 23:512-5.
118. Babbit DG, Forman MB, Jones R, Bajaj AK, Hoover RL. Prevention of neutrophil-mediated injury to endothelial cells by perfluorochemical. Am J Pathol 1990; 136: 451-9.
119. Forman MB, Bingham S, Kopelman HA, Wehr C, Sandler MP, Kolodgie F, Vaughn WK, Friesinger GC, Virmani R. Reduction of infarct size with intracoronary perfluorochemical in a canine preparation of reperfusion. Circulation 1985; 71:1060-8.
120. Forman MB, Puett DW, Wilson BH, Vaughn WK, Friesinger GC, Virmani R. Beneficial long-term effect of intracoronary perfluorochemical on infarct size and ventricular function in a canine reperfusion model. J Am Coll Cardiol 1987; 9:1082-90.
121. Forman MB, Puett DW, Bingham SE, Virmani R, Tantengco MV, Light TR, Bajaj A, Price R, Friesinger G. Preservation of endothelial cell structure and function by in-

tracoronary perfluorochemical in a canine preparation of reperfusion. Circulation 1987; 76:469–79.

122. Bajaj AK, Cobb MA, Virmani R, Gay JC, Light FT, Forman MB. Limitation of myocardial reperfusion injury by intraveneous perfluorochemicals. Circulation 1989; 79: 645–56.

123. Schaer GL, Karas SP, Santoian EC, Gold G, Visner MS, Virmani R. Reduction in reperfusion injury by blood-free reperfusion after experimental myocardial infarction. J Am Coll Cardiol 1990; 15:1385–93.

124. Todd RF, Simpson PJ, Lucchesi BR. The anti-inflammatory properties of monoclonal anti-mol (CD11B/CD18) antibodies in vitro and in vivo. In: Rosenthal AS, Springer, TA, Anderson DC, Rothlein R. (eds). Structure and function of molecules involved in leukocyte adhesion. New York: Springer-Verlag, 1989.

125. Berger M, O'Shea J, Cross AS. Human neutrophils increase expression of C3bi as well as C3b receptors upon activation. J Clin Invest 1984; 74:1566–71.

126. Dreyer WJ, Smith CW, Michael LH, Rossen RD, Hughes BJ, Entman ML, Anderson DC. Canine neutrophil activation by cardiac lymph obtained during reperfusion of ischemic myocardium. Circ Res 1989; 65:1751–62.

127. Simon RH, DeHart PD, Todd RF. Neutrophil-induced injury of rat pulmonary alveolar epithelial cells. J Clin Invest 1986; 78:1375–86.

128. Simpson PJ, Todd RF, Fantone JC, Mickelson JK, Griffin JD, Lucchesi BR. Reduction of experimental canine myocardial reperfusion injury by a monoclonal antibody (anti-Mo-1, anti-CD11b) that inhibits leukocyte adhesion. J Clin Invest 1988; 81: 624–9.

129. Simpson PJ, Todd RF, Mickelson JK, Fantone JC, Gallagher KP, Lee KA, Tamura Y, Cronin M, Lucchesi BR. Sustained limitation of myocardial reperfusion injury by a monoclonal antibody that alters leukocyte function. Circulation 1990; 81:226–37.

130. Weisman HF, Bartow T, Leppo MK, Marsh HC, Carson GR, Concino MF, Boyle MP, Roux KH, WeisfeldtML, Fearon DT. Soluble human complement receptor type 1: in vivo inhibitor of complement suppressing post-ischemic myocardial inflammation and necrosis. Science 1990; 249:146–51.

131. Schmid-Schonbein GW. Capillary plugging by granulocytes and the no-reflow phenomenon in the microcirculation. Fed Proc 1987; 46:2397–2401.

132. Engler RL, Schmid-Schonbein GW, Pavelec RS. Leukocyte capillary plugging in myocardial ischemia and reperfusion in the dog. Am J Pathol 1983; 111:98–111.

133. Bolli R, Cannon RO, Speir E., Goldstein RE, Epstein SE. Role of cellular proteinases in acute myocardial infarction. II. Influence of in vivo suppression of myocardial proteolysis by antipain, leupeptin and pepstatein on myocardial infarct size in the rat. J Am Coll Cardiol 1983; 2:681–8.

134. Hallett MB, Shandall A, Young HL. Mechanism of protection against 'reperfusion injury' by aprotinin: roles of polymorphonuclear leukocytes and oxygen radicals. Biochem Pharmacol 1985; 34:1757–61.

135. Henderson WR, Klebanoff SJ. Leukotriene production and inactivation by normal, chronic granulomatous disease and myeloperoxidase-deficient neutrophils. J Biol Chem 1983; 258:13522–7.

136. Lewis RA, Austen KF. The biologically active leukotrienes. J Clin Invest 1984; 73: 889-97.

137. Mullane KM, Read N, Salmon JA, Moncada S. Role for leukocytes in acute myocardial infarction in anesthetized dogs: relationship to myocardial salvage by anti-inflammatory drugs. J Pharmacol Exp Ther 1984; 228:510-52.

138. Bednar M, Smith B, Pinto A, Mullane KM. Nafazatrom-induced salvage of ischemic myocardium in anesthetized dogs is mediated through inhibition of neutrophil function. Circ Res 1985; 57:131-41.

139. Mullane K, Hatala MA, Kraemer R, Sessa W, Westlin W. Myocardial salvage induced by REV-5901: an inhibitor and antagonist of the leukotrienes. J Cardiovasc Pharmacol 1987; 10:398-406.

140. Hahn RA, MacDonald BR, Simpson PH, Potts BD, Parli CJ. Antagonism of leukotriene B4 receptors does not limit canine myocardial infarct size. J Pharmacol Exp Ther 1990; 253:58-65.

141. Hanahan DJ. Platelet activating factor: a biologically acitve phosphoglyceride. Annu Rev Biochem 1986; 55:483-509.

142. Kenzora JL, Perez JE, Bergmann SR, Lange LG. Effects of acetyl glyceryl ether of phosphorylcholine (platelet activating factor) on ventricular preload, afterload, and contractility in dogs. J Clin Invest 1984; 74:1193-1203.

143. Stahl GL, Lefer AM. Mechanisms of platelet-activating factor-induced cardiac depression in the isolated perfused rat heart. Circulatory Shock 1987; 23:165-77.

144. Robertson DA, Genovese A, Levi R. Negative intropic effect of platelet-activating factor on human myocardium: a pharmacological study. J Pharmacol Exp Ther 1987; 243:834-9.

145. Gay JC, Beckman JK, Zaboy KA, Lukens JN. Modulation of neutrophil oxidative responses to soluble stimuli by platelet-activating factor. Blood 1986; 67:931-6.

146. Vercelloti GM, Yin HQ, Gustafson KS, Nelson RD, Jacob HS. Platelet-activating factor primes neutrophil responses to agonists: role in promoting neutrophil-mediated endothelial damage. Blood 1988; 71:1100-7.

147. Montrucchio G, Alloatti G, Tetta C, De Luca R, Saunders RN, Emanuelli G, Camusi G. Release of platelet-activating factor from ischemic-reperfused rabbit heart. Am J Physiol 1989; 256:H1236-46.

148. Montrucchio G, Camussi G, Tetta C, Emanuelli G, Orzan F, Libero L, Brusca A. Intravascular release of platelet-activating factor during atrial pacing. Lancet 1986; 2:293.

149. Maruyama M, Farber NE, Vercellotti GM, Jacob HS, Gross GJ. Evidence for a role of platelet activating factor in the pathogenesis of irreversible but not reversible myocardial injury after reperfusion in dogs. Am Heart J 1990; 120:510-20.

150. Kloner RA, Przyklenk K, Whittaker P. Deleterious effects of oxygen radicals in ischemia/reperfusion. Circulation 1989; 80:1115-27.

151. Engler R, Gilpin E. Can superoxide dismutase alter myocardial infarct size? Circulation 1989; 79:1137-42.

152. Reimer KA, Murry CE, Richard VJ, The role of neutrophils and free radicals in the ischemic-reperfused heart: why the confusion and controversy? J Mol Cell Cardiol 1989; 21:1225-39.

153. Lucchesi BR, Werns SW, Fantone JC. The role of the neutrophil and free radicals in ischemic myocardial injury. J Mol Cell Cardiol 1989; 21:1241-51.

154. Jolly SR, Kane WJ, Bailie MB, Abrams GD, Lucchesi BR. Canine myocardial reperfusion injury: its reduction by the combined administration of superoxide dismutase and catalase. Circ Res 1984; 54:277-85.

155. Werns SW, Shea MJ, Driscoll DM, Cohen C, Abrams GD, Pitt B, Lucchesi BR. The independent effects of oxygen radical scavengers on canine infarct size; reduction by superoxide dismutase but not catalase. Circ Res 1985; 56:895-8.

156. Werns SW, Simpson PJ, Mickelson JK, Shea MJ, Pitt B, Lucchesi BR. Sustained limitation by superoxide dismutase of canine myocardial injury due to regional ischemia followed by reperfusion. J Cardiovasc Pharmacol 1988; 11:36-44.

157. Tamura Y, Chi L, Driscoll EM, Hoff PT, Freeman BA, Gallagher KP, Lucchesi BR. Superoxide dismutase conjugated to polyethylene glycol provides sustained protection against myocardial ischemia/reperfusion injury in canine heart. Circ Res 1988; 63:944-59.

158. Ambrosio G, Becker LC, Hutchins GM, Weisman HF, Weisfeldt ML. Reduction in experimental infarct size by recombinant human superoxide dismutase: insights into the pathophysiology of reperfusion injury. Circulation 1986; 74:1424-33.

159. Mehta JL, Nichols WW, Donnelly WH, Lawson DL, Thompson L, ter Riet M, Saldeen TGP. Protection by superoxide dismutase from myocardial dysfunction and attenuation of vasodilator reserve after coronary occlusion and reperfusion in dog. Circ Res 1989; 65:1283-95.

160. Mehta JL, Lawson DL, Nichols WW. Attenuated coronary relaxation after reperfusion: effects of superoxide dismutase and TxA2 inhibitor U 63557A. Am J Physiol 1989; 257:H1240-H1246.

161. Dauber IM, Lesnefsky EJ, VanBenthuysen KM, Weil JV, Horwitz LD. Reactive oxygen metabolite scavengers decrease functional coronary microvascular injury due to ischemia-reperfusion. Am J Physiol 1991; 260:H42-H49

162. Nejima J, Knight DR, Fallon JT, Umemura N, Manders WT, Canfield DR, Cohen MV, Vatner SF. Superoxide dismutase reduces reperfusion arrhythmias but fails to salvage regional function or myocardium at risk in conscious dogs. Circulation 1989; 79:143-53.

163. Przyklenk K, Kloner RA. "Reperfusion injury" by oxygen-derived free radicals? Circ Res 1989; 64:86-96.

164. Gallagher KP, Buda AJ, Pace D, Gerren RA, Shlafer M. Failure of superoxide dismutase and catalase to alter size of infarction in conscious dogs after 3 hours of occlusion followed by reperfusion. Circulation 1986; 73:1065-76.

165. Przyklenk K, Kloner RA. Effect of oxygen-derived free radical scavengers on infarct size following six hours of permanent coronary artery occlusion: salvage or delay of myocyte necrosis? Basic Res Cardiol 1987; 82:146-58.

166. Patel BS, Jeroudi MO, O'Neill PG, Roberts R, Bolli R. Effect of human recombinant superoxide dismutase on canine myocardial infarction. Am J Physiol 1990; 258: H369-H380.

167. Tanaka M, Stoler RC, FitzHarris GP, Jennings RB, Reimer KA. Evidence against the

"early protection-delayed death" hypothesis of superoxide dismutase therapy in experimental myocardial infarction. Circ Res 1990; 67:636-44.

168. Omar BA, Jordan MC, Downey JM, McCord JM. Protection afforded by superoxide dismutase is dose dependent in the in situ reperfused rabbit heart. Circulation 1989; 80(Suppl II):II-294 (abstract).

169. Shirato C, Miura T, Ooiwa H, Toyofuku T, Wilborn WH, Downey JM. Tetrazolium artifactually indicates superoxide dismutase-induced salvage in reperfused rabbit heart. J Mol Cell Cardiol 1989; 21:1187-93.

170. Ceconi C, Curello S, Cargnoni A, Ferrari R, Albertini A, Visioli O. The role of glutathione status in the protection against ischaemic and reperfusion damage: effects of N-acetyl cysteine. J Mol Cell Cardiol 1988; 20:5-13.

171. Ferrari R, Alfieri O, Curello S, Ceconi C, Cargnoni A, Marzollo P, Pardini A, Caradonna E, Visioli O. Occurence of oxidative stress during reperfusion of the human heart. Circulation 1990; 81:201-11.

172. Lesnefsky EJ, Dauber IM, Horowitz LD. Myocardial sulfhydryl pool alterations occur during reperfusion after brief and prolonged myocardial ischemia in vivo. Circ Res 1991; 68:605-13.

173. Mitsos SE, Kim D, Lucchesi BR, Fantone JC. Modulation of myoglobin-H_2O_2-mediated peroxidation reactions by sulfhydryl compounds. Lab Invest 1988;59:824-30.

174. Mitsos SE, Fantone JC, Gallagher KP, Walden KM, Simpson PJ, Abrams GD, Schork MA, Lucchesi BR. Canine myocardial reperfusion injury: protection by a free radical scavenger, N-2-mercaptopropionyl glycine. J Cardiovasc Pharmcol 1986; 8:978-88.

175. Forman MB, Puett DW, Cates CU, McCroskey DE, Beckman JK, Greene HL, Virmani R. Glutathione redox pathway and reperfusion injury. Effect of N-acetylcysteine on infarct size and ventricular function. Circulation 1988; 78:202-13.

176. Westlin W, Mullane K. Does captopril attenuate reperfusion-induced myocardial dysfunction by scavenging free radicals? Circulation 1988; 77(Suppl I):I-30-I-39.

177. Bagchi D, Prasad R, Das DK. Direct scavenging of free radicals by captopril, an angiotensin converting enzyme inhibitor. Biochem Biophysical Res Commun 1989; 158:52-7.

178. Kukreja RC, Kontos HA, Hess ML. Captopril and enalaprilat do not scavenge the superoxide anion. Am J Cardiol 1990; 65:241-71.

179. Mehta JL, Nicolini FA, Lawson DL. Sulfhydryl group in angiotensin converting enzyme inhibitors and superoxide radical formation. J Cardiovasc Pharmacol 1990; 16:847-9.

180. Bolli R. Oxygen-derived free radicals and postischemic myocardial dysfunction ("stunned myocardium"). J Am Coll Cardiol 1988; 12:239-49.

181. Bolli R. Mechanism of myocardial "stunning." Circulation 1990; 82:723-38.

182. Myers ML, Bolli R, Lekich RF, Hartley CJ, Roberts R. Enhancement of recovery of myocardial function by oxygen free-radical scavengers after reversible regional ischemia. Circulation 1985; 72:915-21.

183. Przyklenk K, Kloner RA. Superoxide dismutase plus catalase improve contractile function in the canine model of the "stunned myocardium." Circ Res 1986; 58:148-56.

184. Gross GJ, Farber NE, Hardman HF, Warltier DC. Beneficial actions of superoxide dismutase and catalase in stunned myocardium of dogs. Am J Physiol 1986; 250: H373-H377.

185. Jeroudi MO, Triana FJ, Patel BS, Bolli R. Effect of superoxide dismutase and catalase, given separately, on myocardial "stunning." Am J Physiol 1990; 259:H889-H901.

186. Myers ML, Bolli R, Lekich R, Hartley CJ, Roberts R. N-2 mercaptopropionylglycine improves recovery of myocardial function after reversible regional ischemia. J Am Coll Cardiol 1986; 8:1161-8.

187. Bolli R, Zhu W, Hartley CJ, Michael LH, Repine JE, Hess ML, Kukreja RC, Roberts R. Attenuation of dysfunction in the postischemic 'stunned' myocardium by dimethylthiourea. Circulation 1987; 76:458-68.

188. Wasil M, Halliwell B, Grootveld M, Moorhouse CP, Hutchinson DCS, Baum H. The specificity of thiourea, dimethylthiourea and dimethyl sulphoxide as scavengers of hydroxyl radicals. Biochem J 1987; 243:867-70.

189. Bolli R, Patel BS, Zhu W, O'Neill PG, Hartley CJ, Charlat ML, Roberts R. The iron chelator desferrioxamine attenuates postischemic ventricular dysfunction. Am J Physiol 1987; 253:H1372-H1380.

190. Farber NE, Vercellotti GM, Jacob HS, Pieper GM, Gross GJ. Evidence for a role of iron-catalyzed oxidants in functional and metabolic stunning in the canine heart. Circ Res 1988; 63:351-60.

191. Bolli R, Patel BS, Jeroudi MO, Li XY, Triana JF, Lai EK, McCay PB. Iron-mediated radical reactions upon reperfusion contribute to myocardial "stunning." Am J Physiol 1990; 259:H1901-H1911.

192. Engler R, Covell JW. Granulocytes cause reperfusion ventricular dysfunction after 15-minute ischemia in the dog. Circ Res 1987; 61:20-8.

193. Westlin W, Mullane KM. Alleviation of myocardial stunning by leukocyte and platelet depletion. Circulation 1989; 80:1828-36.

194. Jeremy RW, Becker LC. Neutrophil depletion does not prevent myocardial dysfunction after brief coronary occlusion. J Am Coll Cardiol 1989; 13:1155-63.

195. O'Neill PG, Charlat ML, Michael LH, Roberts R, Bolli R. Influence of neutrophil depletion on myocardial function and flow after reversible ischemia. Am J Physiol 1989; 256:H341-51.

196. Shea MJ, Simpson PJ, Werns SW, Buda AJ, Alborzy-Khaghany AS, Hoff PT, Pitt B, Lucchesi BR. Effect of neutrophil depletion on recovery of "stunned" myocardium. Clin Res 1987; 35:327A (abstract).

197. Schott RJ, Nao BS, McClanahan TB, Simpson PJ, Stirling MC, Todd RF, Gallagher KP. F(ab')2 fragments of anti-Mol (904) monoclonal antibodies do not prevent myocardial stunning. Circ Res 1989; 65:1112-24.

198. Charlat ML, O'Neill PG, Egan JM, Abernethy DR, Michael LH, Myers ML, Roberts R, Bolli R. Evidence for a pathogenetic role of xanthine oxidase in the "stunned" myocardium. Am J Physiol 1987; 252:H566-H577.

199. Holzgrefe HH, Gibson JK. Beneficial effects of oxypurinol pretreatment in stunned, reperfused canine myocardium. Cardiovasc Res 1989; 23:340-50.

200. Werns S, Ventura A, Li GC, Lucchesi BR. Amflutizole, a xanthine oxidase inhibitor,

does not attenuate myocardial stunning in the canine heart. Circulation 1989; 80 (Suppl II): II-295 (abstract).

201. Vandeplassche G, Hermans C, Thone F, Borgers M. Mitochondrial hydrogen peroxide generation by NADH-oxidase activity following regional myocardial ischemia in the dog. J Mol Cell Cardiol 1989; 21:383-92.

202. Ueta H, Ogura R, Sugiyama M, Kagiyama A, Shin G. O2- spin trapping on cardiac submitochondrial partaicles isolated from ischemic and non-ischemic myocardium. J Mol Cell Cardiol 1990; 22:893-9.

203. Grisham MB. Myoglobin-catalyzed hydrogen peroxide dependent arachidonic acid peroxidation. J Free Rad Biol Med 1985; 1:227-32.

204. Fantone JC, Jester S, Loomis T. Metmyoglobin promotes arachidonic acid peroxidation at acid pH. J Biol Chem 1989; 264:9408-11.

205. Buckmaster MJ, Werns SW, Shlafer M, Lucchesi BR, Fantone JC. Inhibition of sarcoplasmic reticulum Ca2+-dependent ATPase by myoglobin- hydrogen peroxide. FASEB J 1990; 4:A1217.

206. Topol EJ, Ellis SG, Califf RM, George BS, Stump DC, Bates ER, Nabel EG, Walton JA, Candela RJ, Lee KL, Bline EM, Pitt B. Combined tissue-type plasminogen activator and prostacyclin therapy for acute myocardial infarction. J Am Coll Cardiol 1989; 14:877-84.

207. Werns SW, Brinker J, Gruber J, Rothbaum D, Heuser R, George B, Burwell L, Kereiakes D, Mancini GBJ, Flaherrty J. A randomized, double-blind trial of recombinant human superoxide dismutase (SOD) in patients undergoing PTCA for acute MI. Circulation 80 (Suppl II): II-113, 1989.

208. Schumacher WA, Lee EC, Lucchesi Br. Augmentaion of streptokinase-induced thrombolysis by heparin and prostacyclin. J Cardiovasc Pharmacol 1985; 7:739-46.

209. Farber NE, Pieper GM, Thomas JP, Gross GJ. Beneficial effects of iloprost in the stunned canine myocardium. Circ Res 1988; 62:204-15.

210. Forman MB, Perry JM, Wilson BH, Verani MS, Kaplan PR, Shawl FA, Friesinger GC. Demonstration of myocardial reperfusion injury in humans: results of a pilot study utilizing coronary angioplasty with perfluorochemical in anterior myocardial infarction. J Am Coll Cardiol 1991; 18:911-8.

211. Ganz W, Watanabe I, Kanamasa K, Yano J, Han DS, Fishbein MC. Does reperfusion extend necrosis? A study in a single territory of myocardial ischemia-half reperfused and half not reperfused. Circulation 1990; 82:1020-1033.

16

Inotropic Therapy for Cardiogenic Shock Complicating Acute Myocardial Infarction

John M. Nicklas
University of Michigan Medical Center, Ann Arbor, Michigan

INTRODUCTION

Cardiogenic shock is a poorly tolerated complication of acute myocardial infarction. If a patient develops cardiogenic shock, urgent diagnostic evaluation and rapid pharmacological intervention are indicated. In patients who have received thrombolytic agents and undergone early revascularization, pharmacological support for shock may be especially beneficial. This chapter will review the principles and practical application of positive inotropic therapy for cardiogenic shock complicating acute myocardial infarction.

INCIDENCE OF CARDIOGENIC SHOCK IN ACUTE MYOCARDIAL INFARCTION

Between 20% and 30% of patients with acute myocardial infarction present with some degree of congestive heart failure (1-3). Approximately 8% develop cardiogenic shock (1-4). For patients who present with mild heart failure (Killip class II), in-hospital mortality rates are nearly 20% (1-5). However, for patients with cardiogenic shock, in-hospital mortality rates range between 65% and 90% (1-8). Even if a patient with shock survives hospitalization, there is an additional 35% 1-year mortality (1-4). Aspirin and thrombolytic therapy have improved in-hospital survival for patients with mild heart failure (Killip class II), but they have not altered the prognosis for patients with shock (1, 6).

EFFECT OF INTRAVENOUS POSITIVE INOTROPES ON IN-HOSPITAL SURVIVAL

Most patients with cardiogenic shock complicating an acute myocardial infarction currently receive intravenous positive inotropes (2). However, the effect of this pharmacological support on prognosis is uncertain. Early reports suggested that in-hospital survival was improved, but concurrently controlled, randomized trials have not been performed (7, 8). Mortality rates for patients with shock in the 1980s, when positive inotropes were widely utilized, are similar to mortality rates in the 1950s, before such pharmacological support was available (1-8). Nevertheless, significant benefit from treatment with inotropes cannot be excluded. Even if pharmacological support alone does not improve prognosis, treatment may stabilize patients long enough for other, more potent interventions to be performed.

EFFECT OF INTRAVENOUS INOTROPES ON STUNNED MYOCARDIUM

Although the primary goal of thrombolytic therapy for acute myocardial infarction is to induce early recanalization of the infarct-related coronary artery and, thereby, to salvage jeopardized myocardium, early recanalization does not restore contractility immediately. Instead, the reversibly injured myocardium exhibits a prolonged depression in contractile function, which can last for several days, a condition commonly known as "myocardial stunning" (9). In patients with cardiogenic shock and early infarct artery recanalization, pharmacological support can be critical until the contractile function of stunned myocardium returns.

Positive inotropes are effective in restoring contractile function to stunned myocardium. In animal models of stunning, brief intravenous infusions of dopamine, norepinephrine, and epinephrine augment regional contractility to nearly normal levels (10-12). Although the effects of prolonged stimulation are unknown, 2-hr infusions do not deplete high-energy phosphate stores or alter the course of contractile recovery of stunned myocardium (13).

MECHANISM OF CONTRACTION AND ACTIONS OF POSITIVE INOTROPES

Cytoplasmic Calcium

Cytoplasmic calcium is the critical mediator of the contractile process. In the resting myocyte, most intracellular calcium is stored in the sarcoplasmic reticulum and the level of free cytoplasmic calcium is low compared to the level in the extracellular space (14, 15). When an action potential depolarizes cellular membranes, some calcium enters the cytoplasm from the extracellular space and large amounts of calcium are released from the sarcoplasmic reticulum. Free cytoplasmic calcium then combines with troponin, activating the myofilaments to contract. The force of contraction is determined by the amount of calcium delivered to the troponin, the rate of delivery, and the sensitivity of the myofibrils to calcium (14-17). In stunned myocardium, decreased myofibrillar sensitivity to calcium and/or decreased delivery of free calcium to the myofibrils appears to be responsible for the impairment in contractile function (18, 19).

Actions of Positive Inotropes

Nonglycosidic positive inotropic agents improve contractile function either by increasing delivery of calcium to the contractile apparatus or by increasing myofibrillar sensitivity to calcium activation. Endogenous catecholamines and their derivatives interact with adrenoreceptors on the cell surface. Beta- adrenoreceptor agonists activate adenylate cyclase, increasing levels of cyclic adenosine 3',5' -monophosphate (cAMP), which, in turn, activates cAMP-dependent protein kinases (20-22). The kinases increase phosphorylation of membrane-bound proteins serving as calcium channels in the cell membrane and sarcoplasmic reticulum. Phosphorylation of these proteins increases the number of channels available for transmembrane calcium flux, thus augmenting the concentration of cytoplasmic calcium during the action potential. Alpha-adrenoreceptor activation appears to mediate an increase in cytoplasmic calcium influx without intermediary activation of cAMP (23). Phosphodiesterase-III enzyme inhibitors decrease cAMP breakdown and activate cAMP-dependent protein kinases, producing effects similar to beta-receptor stimulation. Some phosphodiesterase-III inhibitors also increase myofibrillar sensitivity to calcium (24, 25).

Cardiovascular Effects Induced by Activation of Adrenoreceptor Subtypes

Alpha-and beta-adrenoreceptors each have two subtypes distinguished by their location and cardiovascular effects (26, 27). Alpha$_1$ receptors are postsynaptic and are located in both vascular smooth muscle and myocardium. Alpha$_1$ receptor activation produces peripheral vasoconstriction, mild increases in myocardial contractility, and decreases in heart rate. Alpha$_2$ receptors are located in persynaptic sympathetic nerve terminals and postsynaptic vascular effector cells. Presynaptic alpha$_2$ receptor activation decreases peripheral norepinephrine release and central sympathetic nervous system outflow. Postsynaptic alpha$_2$ activation produces peripheral vasoconstriction. Beta$_1$ receptors are located in the heart. Activation of beta1 receptors produces increases in myocardial contractility, increases in heart rate, and increases in the rate of intracardiac conduction. Beta2 receptors are located in peripheral smooth muscle and the sinoatrial node. Activation of beta2 receptors produces peripheral vasodilation and increases in heart rate.

Nonadrenoreceptor Effects of Positive Inotropic Agents

Some positive inotropic agents act on nonadrenoreceptors to produce direct vasodilation. Dopaminergic receptors are located peripherally in the renal and hepatosplanchnic vascular beds (28). Activation of dopaminergic1 receptors increases intracellular cAMP. Activation of dopaminergic2 receptors inhibits peripheral sympathetic nerve transmission. Activation of both types of dopaminergic receptors produces renal and hepatosplanchnic vasodilation. Dopamine can also activate serotonin receptors to produce vasoconstriction (29).

Since phosphodiesterase-III inhibitors increase intracellular cAMP levels, they also increase transmembrane calcium flux. The increase in calcium flux increases cardiac contractility and produces peripheral arterial and venous vasodilation (30).

LIMITATIONS OF POSITIVE INOTROPIC THERAPY

Despite the positive inotropic actions of sympathomimetic amines and phosphodiesterase-III inhibitors, these agents may produce unwanted effects, including supraventricular and ventricular arrhythmias, excessive peripheral vasoconstriction or vasodilation, and increases in myocardial oxygen consumption. Chronic administration of catecholamines is at least partly limited by beta- receptor downregulation and the development of tolerance. Long-term oral administration of some positive inotropes to patients with chronic congestive heart failure has been associated with excess mortality (31, 32). Careful monitoring of the effects of positive inotropes is indicated, and intravenous administration is preferred because it permits rapid drug titration in response to changes in clinical condition.

Arrhythmias

Sympathomimetic amines induce arrhythmias directly by increasing the rate of phase 4 depolarization of automatic cells in the sinoatrial node and Purkinje system and by decreasing the refractory period in ventricular and atrial myocardium (33). In addition, these agents induce arrhythmias indirectly by reducing serum potassium levels. Thus, catecholamines can produce sinus tachycardia and activate latent pacemaker cells in the ventricular conducting system. Dopamine and dobutamine differ from other sympathomimetic amines in producing less tachycardia and ventricular ectopy (34, 35). Dopexamine appears to cause even less sinus tachycardia than either dopamine or dobutamine (36).

Excessive Vasodilation or Vasoconstriction

The majority of positive inotropic agents can induce significant peripheral vasoconstriction mediated via alpha1 adrenoreceptor stimulation. Even dopamine, which also activates beta2 adrenoreceptors, can cause peripheral gangrene (37). In patients with peripheral vascular disease, there is an increased risk of tissue necrosis with catecholamine infusions. In contrast, positive inotropes with significant beta2 activity or direct vasodilator properties can produce significant hypotension.

Myocardial Blood Flow

Sympathomimetic amines can cause both vasoconstriction and vasodilation of coronary arteries (38). In isolated vascular strips, dopamine can induce coronary vasoconstriction via alpha1 and serotonin receptor activation as well as coronary vasodilation (28). Norepinephrine and epinephrine cause beta receptor-mediated coronary vasodilation in vascular strips (39). In intact animal models, catecholamines increase myocardial oxygen consumption and induce proportionate increases in coronary blood flow (40). Although infarct extension has not been documented, catecholamines can precipitate angina pectoris (41–43).

Beta-Adrenoreceptor Down-Regulation

Prolonged administration of beta agonists produces down-regulation and tolerance to sympathomimetic stimulation (44). Down-regulation is associated with decreases in beta receptor density and, at least in animal models, desensitization of the receptors to high-affinity agonist binding (45–48). In patients with preexisting heart failure, beta1 rather than beta2 receptors are down-regulated (49). This selective down-regulation probably reflects the high circulating levels of norepinephrine in patients with heart failure and the associated selective stimulation of beta1 rather than beta2 receptors (50). Pharmacological agonist stimulation can also induce beta2 receptor down-regulation (51, 52). However, it is unclear whether agonists down-regulate the two beta receptor subtypes via the same mechanisms or to the same degree.

Tolerance to beta agonist stimulation develops rapidly. Continuous intravenous infusions of dobutamine, a beta1 agonist, can elicit significant tolerance (one-third loss of hemodynamic effect) within 72 hrs (53). In contrast, intermittent 48-hr infusions of dobutamine administered weekly are not associated with the development of tolerance (54). However, even these intermittent infusions may not produce clinical benefit (55).

Table 1   Receptor Activity of Sympathomimetic Amines

	Alpha$_1$	Beta$_1$	Beta$_2$	Dopa$_1$	Sero
Dopamine	++++	++++	++	+++	+
Dobutamine	+	++++	++	-	-
Norepinephrine	++++	++++	-	-	-
Epinephrine	++++	++++	+++	-	-
Isoproterenol	-	++++	++++	-	-
Methoxamine	++++	-	-	-	-
Dopexamine	-	+	++++	++	-

SYMPATHOMIMETIC AMINES

The adrenoreceptor activity of the commonly available sympathomimetic amines is shown in Table 1 (28). Norepinephrine, epinephrine, dopamine, and methoxamine can produce powerful vasoconstriction via their stimulation of alpha$_1$ receptors. Norepinephrine, epinephrine, dopamine, isoproterenol, and dobutamine are beta$_1$ agonists and potent cardiac stimulants. Isoproterenol and, to a lesser extent, epinephrine, dopamine, and dobutamine produce beta$_2$- mediated vasodilation. Dopamine also elicits renal and hepatosplanchnic vasodilation via dopaminergic$_1$ receptor activation. Because they produce the fewest unwanted side effects, dopamine and dobutamine are the most commonly administered positive inotropes in the early period following a myocardial infarction.

Dopamine

Dopamine is an endogenous catecholamine and the metabolic precursor of both norepinephrine and epinephrine. Dopamine is rapidly metabolized by monoamine oxidase (MAO) and catechol-O-methyltransferase (COMT) (56). The metabolites are excreted primarily in the urine.

Dopamine activates dopaminergic$_1$ and dopaminergic$_2$ receptors at low concentrations and beta$_1$ and alpha adrenoreceptors, and serotonergic receptors at high concentrations (28, 38). At low infusion rates less than 5 mg/kg/min, dopamine produces renal and hepatosplanchnic vasodilation. Cardiac output is redistributed and flow to the kidneys increases (57). At infusion rates above 2 μg/kg/min, dopamine activates beta$_1$receptors, increases stunned myocardial contractility, and augments cardiac output. At high infusion rates, greater than 5 μg/kg/min, dopamine activates alpha adrenoreceptors and serotonergic receptors, leading to significant increases in peripheral vascular resistance (29, 57).

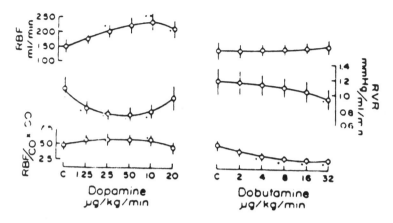

Figure 1   Renal hemodynamic responses to intravenous infusions of dopamine and dobutamine. Renal blood flow (RBF) determined by electromagnetic flowprobe. RVR, renal vascular resistance; RBF/CO × 100 percent of cardiac output perfusing renal artery. Values are mean ± 1 standard error of mean.
*Significantly different from control ($p < 0.05$).
**Significantly different from control ($p < 0.01$).
[From Ref. 57 (Fig. 3), with permission].

   Dopamine is useful therapeutically because it selectively activates receptors at in fusion rates less than 5 μg/kg/min. At low infusion rates, dopamine can redirect cardiac output to the kidneys and induce a diuresis in patients with oliguria secondary to decreased renal blood flow (59)(Fig. 1). At low infusion rates, dopamine can also augment cardiac output by increasing stroke volume without increasing vascular resistance or significantly altering automaticity (57)(Fig. 1). At high infusion rates greater than 5 μg/kg/min, dopamine can further increase cardiac output, but only by increasing heart rate and at the expense of increased renal and systemic vascular resistance. High infusion rates are usually associated with significant increases in systemic blood pressure and left ventricular filling pressure (60).
   Because dopamine is metabolized via MAO, it should not be administered to patients who have received MAO inhibitors (56). It can induce nausea and vomiting, presumably via activation of central nervous system dopaminergic receptors, but this is rare since infusions of dopamine do not usually reach these central receptors. Extreme vasoconstriction and necrosis have been reported with extravasation of large amounts of dopamine. Phentolamine, an alpha blocker, can be used to relieve the vasoconstriction.

Dobutamine

Dobutamine is a synthetic derivative of isoproterenol (61). The drug has a half-life of approximately 2 min. It is metabolized by methylation and conjugation, and the metabolites are primarily excreted in the urine (56).

Dobutamine is a racemic mixture of two enantiomers (56). The (+)-isomer of dobutamine is a potent beta$_1$ agonist and a potent alpha$_1$ antagonist. The (-)-isomer is a weak beta agonist and a potent alpha$_1$ agonist. Unlike dopamine, dobutamine does not selectively activate receptors in a dose-dependent fashion. The pharmacological effects of dobutamine represent the net activity of a complex receptor interaction.

Of the currently available sympathomimetic amines, dobutamine produces the greatest increase in myocardial contractility and cardiac output for the smallest cost in automaticity and peripheral vasoconstriction (60, 62). It induces a dose-dependent increase in stroke volume at infusion rates as high as 10 μg/kg/min (57)(Fig. 2). At higher doses, dobutamine increases cardiac output only by increasing heart rate. It produces a dose-dependent decrease in systemic vascular resistance up to infusion rates as high as 32 μg/kg/min. Dobutamine does not significantly alter left ventricular filling pressures at infusion rates below 10 μg/kg/min and tends to decrease right ventricular filling pressures (60). Unlike dopamine, dobutamine does not increase renal blood flow, but, instead, tends to redistribute cardiac output to the skeletal muscles (57)(Fig. 1).

Administration of dobutamine to patients following acute myocardial infarction appears to be relatively safe. Although dobutamine increases myocardial oxygen consumption, at least in the absence of critical epicardial coronary artery disease, it also induces a proportionate increase in coronary blood flow (42, 63). In contrast, administration of dopamine is not associated with an increase in coronary blood flow proportionate to the increment in oxygen consumption. In animal models of ischemia and reperfusion, dobutamine does not increase infarct size (41). Similarly, in small anecdotal clinical reports, dobutamine in doses up to 40 μg/kg/min did not increase plasma levels of creatine kinase in patients with evolving myocardial infarctions (64).

Administration of dobutamine is limited primarily by increases in automaticity and atrioventricular conduction. Dobutamine increases heart rate in a dose-dependent fashion. A dose of 10 μg/kg/min can induce a 25 beat/min increment in heart rate (57, 60). Dobutamine can also increase ventricular response rates to atrial fibrillation by increasing AV nodal conduction (56).

Norepinephrine

Norepinephrine is a potent endogenous catecholamine that activates alpha$_1$ and beta$_1$ receptors (Table 1). Norepinephrine is rapidly metabolized by COMT and

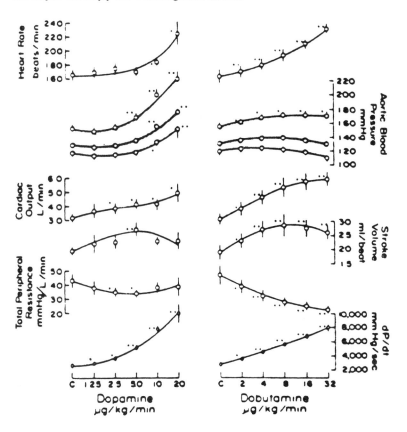

Figure 2   Systemic hemodynamic effects of dopamine and dobutamine. Values are mean ± 1 standard error of mean.
*Significantly different from control ($p < 0.05$).
**Significantly different from control ($p < 0.01$).
[From Ref. 57 (Fig. 1), with permission.]

MAO. It augments contractility in normal and stunned myocardium (11, 56). Norepinephrine is also a powerful vasoconstrictor and increases systemic blood pressure and ventricular filling pressures (65)(Fig. 3). Although norepinephrine produces relatively small changes in heart rate directly, vagal reflex responses to increases in blood pressure mediate decreases in heart rate.

Norepinephrine increases blood pressure by raising systemic vascular resistance. Although it also increases myocardial contractility, cardiac output is not usually increased because of the concomitant rise in vascular resistance. Since cerebral vessels are relatively insensitive to catecholamine-induced vasoconstric-

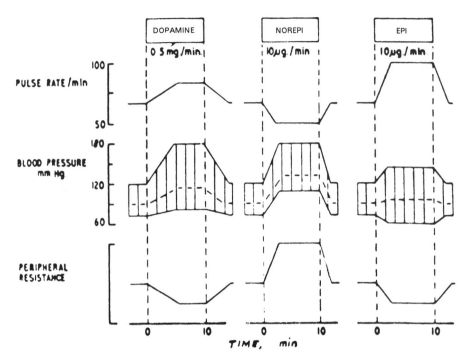

Figure 3 Comparision of some cardiovascular effects in humans of intravenous infusions of dopamine, norepinephrine (norepi), and epinephrine (epi). (From Ref. 65, with
permission.)

tion, norepinephrine can improve cerebral blood flow in severe hypotension by
raising systemic pressures (56). By elevating diastolic pressure and by direct coronary vasodilation, norepinephrine can also increase coronary perfusion. The degree of vasoconstriction induced by norepinephrine is dose-dependent and can
usually be detected at infusion rates as low as 2 μg/kg/min.

Norepinephrine should only be administered when severe systemic hypotension compromises cerebral perfusion. Norepinephrine decreases renal, hepatic,
and splanchnic blood flow (56). Extravasation of norepinephrine can cause tissue
necrosis and sloughing. It can also induce severe ventricular arrhythmias.

Epinephrine, Isoproterenol, Methoxamine

Epinephrine, isoproterenol, and methoxamine are potent sympathomimetic
amines. Their pharmacological effects reflect their activation of adrenergic receptors (Table 1). However, their value in the treatment of cardiogenic shock is limited because they produce more unwanted side effects than alternative agents. For

example, epinephrine increases cardiac output and decreases systemic vascular resistance, but also markedly increases heart rate and arrhythmias (65)(Fig. 3). Infusions of epinephrine frequently induce angina (56). Isoproterenol is also associated with significant increases in heart rate. Methoxamine increases blood pressure by raising systemic vascular resistance, but frequently causes cardiac output to fall. Infusions of epinephrine, isoproterenol, and methoxamine should not be administered to patients following acute myocardial infarction.

Dopexamine

Dopexamine is a new dopamine analog not currently approved by the Food and Drug Administration in the United States. Dopexamine is a potent beta1 and moderate dopaminergic agonist but it has no alpha1 and little beta1 activity (36, 66–68). In moderate to high doses, it may be superior to dobutamine and dopamine in increasing cardiac output while simultaneously increasing renal blood flow.

Xamoterol

Xamoterol is a synthetic sympathomimetic amine also not approved by the Food and Drug Administration in the United States. Xamoterol is a partial beta1 agonist and partial beta antagonist. In a randomized, placebo-controlled clinical trial, treatment for 3 months with oral xamoterol was associated with a nearly three fold increase in mortality (31).

PHOSPHODIESTERASE-III INHIBITORS

Both phosphodiesterase-III inhibitors and sympathomimetic amines increase intracellular cAMP levels. However, since phosphodiesterase-III inhibitors do not activate adrenergic receptors, they do not cause alpha-mediated peripheral vasoconstriction, nor do they induce beta receptor down-regulation or pharmacological tolerance. Instead, phosphodiesterase-III inhibitors cause peripheral vasodilation and deliver potent inotropic stimulation regardless of the density or sensitivity of the beta receptors. Thus, phosphodiesterase-III inhibitors have advantages over sympathomimetic amines during prolonged therapy and in patients with preexisting conditions associated with beta receptor down-regulation (69). A number of chemically divergent compounds, including amrinone, milrinone, enoximone, and pimobendan, specifically inhibit phosphodiesterase-III.

Amrinone

Amrinone is a bipyridine derivative and the only phosphodiesterase-III-specific inhibitor currently approved by the Food and Drug Administration in the United

States. Although amrinone is well absorbed from the gastrointestinal tract, it has been associated with significant thrombocytopenia, especially during chronic therapy, and it is not approved for oral administration (70, 71). Amrinone's distribution half-life after intravenous infusion is approximately 5 min and its elimination half-life varies between 3 and 10 hr (69, 72). Amrinone therapy should be initiated with an intravenous loading dose of 0.75 mg/kg and maintained with infusion rates between 5 and 10 μg/kg/min, titrated to hemodynamic effect. The native compound and its conjugated metabolites are primarily excreted in the urine.

Amrinone is a potent vasodilator with some inotropic activity. It increases cardiac output and decreases systemic vascular resistance and ventricular filling pressures (73, 74). The increase in cardiac output is dose-dependent throughout the therapeutic range. Amrinone does not increase heart rate except at high doses. Decreases in blood pressure occur at moderate to high doses and are roughly proportional to reductions in systemic vascular resistance. Increases in cardiac output are not associated with changes in myocardial oxygen consumption, presumably because the degree of inotropic stimulation is balanced by the degree of vasodilation (75, 76).

Although amrinone enhances atrioventricular conduction, it is not associated with a significant change in automaticity (77). Amrinone can increase the ventricular response rate to atrial fibrillation or flutter. The risk of thrombocytopenia is dose-dependent and is associated with decreased platelet survival times and normal bone marrow megakaryocytes (70, 71). Withdrawal of amrinone infusions can precipitate significant decreases in cardiac output, which respond to readministration of the drug (78, 79).

Milrinone

Milrinone is a derivative of amrinone with 15–20 times more potent inotropic and vasodilator properties than the parent compound (80). Milrinone is better tolerated than amrinone when administered orally. However, in randomized, placebo-controlled clinical trials, chronic treatment with oral milrinone has been associated with significant increases in mortality (32, 81). In one trial, after 6 months of therapy, patients receiving milrinone had a 28% higher mortality rate than patients receiving placebo, with the largest increases in mortality among the high risk subgroups (32).

Enoximone

Enoximone is an imidazole derivative and phosphodiesterase-III inhibitor with pharmacological effects similar to those of amrinone and milrinone. In small clinical trials, treatment with oral enoximone has also been associated with increased mortality rates (82).

Pimobendan

Pimobendan is a pyridazinone derivative and phosphodiesterase-III inhibitor. In addition, pimobendan appears to sensitize the myofibrils to calcium (24, 25). In small clinical trials, treatment with oral pimobendan has not been associated with increased mortality rates (83).

COMBINED INOTROPIC THERAPY

Dopamine/Dobutamine

Simultaneous therapy with dopamine and dobutamine can combine the beneficial effects of each agent. Dopamine, at infusion rates less than 5 μg/kg/min, improves renal and mesenteric perfusion but does not significantly increase cardiac output. Dobutamine, at infusion rates between 2 and 10 μg/kg/min, significantly increases cardiac output but does not increase renal blood flow. Together, these agents can increase cardiac output and redistribute flow to the kidneys.

Dobutamine/Amrinone

Sympathomimetic amines and phosphodiesterase inhibitors increase intracellular cAMP levels via different pharmacological mechanisms. Theoretically, adrenergic activation combined with phosphodiesterase-III inhibition could generate higher cAMP levels than either pharmacological stimulation alone. In practice, dobutamine and amrinone are synergistic. The combination of these two agents produces a greater increase in positive left ventricular dP/dt than either individual drug (84). The combination of dobutamine's inotropic effects with amrinone's vasodilation also appears to be mechanically efficient. When administered together, these drugs are well tolerated and can be infused at high rates (5–15 μg/kg/min).

COMBINED SYMPATHOMIMETIC AMINES/VASODILATOR THERAPY

The sympathomimetic amines, dopamine and dobutamine, can be combined with the vasodilators, nitroprusside and nitroglycerin, to produce unique hemodynamic effects. For example, although dopamine can increase renal perfusion at low infusion rates, it has no effect on left ventricular filling pressure but at higher infusion rates, it can increase filling pressure. When dopamine is combined with nitroglycerin, renal perfusion can be increased while left ventricular filling pressure is decreased (86). Similarly, nitroprusside can be combined with dopamine or dobutamine to produce or accentuate venous and arteriolar dilation. Nitroglycerin and nitroprusside are usually effective only when the pulmonary capillary wedge is

Table 2   Dosages of Commonly Used Inotropic Agents

	Loading dose	Maintenance
Sympathomimetic amines		
Dopamine	None	1-5 μg/kg/min
Dobutamine	None	2-10 μg/kg/min
Norepinephrine	None	2-15 μg/kg/min
Phosphodiesterase-III Inhibitors		
Amrinone	0.75 mg/kg	5-10 μg/kg/min

greater than 15 mmHg (14). The therapeutic range for intravenous nitroglycerin is 25-500 μg/min and the therapeutic range for nitropusside is 50-150 μg/min.

SUMMARY

Inotropic therapy can provide critical support for patients with cardiogenic shock complicating acute myocardial infarction. Sympathomimetic amines and phosphodiesterase-III inhibitors increase cAMP levels and transmembrane calcium flux. The doses of the most commonly administered inotropes are listed in Table 2.

REFERENCES

1. Gruppo Italiano per lo Studio della Streptochinasi nell'Infarto Miocardico (GISSI). Effectiveness of intravenous thrombolytic treatment in acute myocardial infarction. Lancet 1986; 1:397-401.
2. Hands ME, Rutherford JD, Muller JE, Davies G, Stone PH, Parker C, Braunwald E, and the MILIS Study Group. The in-hospital development of cardiogenic shock after myocardial infarction: incidence, predictors of occurrence, outcome and prognostic factors. J Am Coll Cardiol 1989; 14:40-6.
3. Gruppo Italiano per lo Studio della Sopravvivenza nell'Infarto Miocardico. GISSI-2: a factorial randomised trial of alteplase versus streptokinase and heparin versus no heparin among 12,490 patients with acute myocardial infarction. Lancet 1990; 336: 65-71.
4. Goldberg RJ, Gore JM, Alpertt JS, Osganian V, de Groot J, Bade J, Chen Z, Frid D, Dalen JE. Cardiogenic shock after acute myocardial infarction. Incidence and mortality from a community-wide perspective, 1975 to 1988. N Engl J Med 1991; 325:1117-22.
5. Killip T, Kimball JT. Treatment of myocardial infarcation in a coronary care unit: a two-year experience with 250 patients. Am J Cardiol 1967; 20:457-64.
6. Bates ER, Topol EJ. Limitations of thrombolytic therapy for acute myocardial infarction complicated by congestive heart failure and cardiogenic shock. J Am Coll Cardiol 1991; 18:1077-84.

7. Griffith GC, Wallace WB, Cochran B, Nerlich WE, Frasher WG. The treatment of shock associated with myocardial infarction. Circulation 1954; 9:527-32.

8. Gunnar RM, Cruz A, Boswell J, Co BS, Pietras RJ, Tobin JR. Myocardial infarction with shock. Hemodynamic studies and results of therapy. Circulation 1966; 33:753-62.

9. Braunwald E, Kloner RA. The stunned myocardium: prolonged, postischemic ventricular dysfunction. Circulation 1982; 66:1146-9.

10. Ellis SG, Wynne J, Braunwald E, Henschke CI, Sandor T, Kloner RA. Response of reperfusion-salvage, stunned myocardium to inotropic stimulation. Am Heart J 1984; 107:13-9.

11. Ciuffo AA, Ouyang P, Becker LC, Levin L, Weisfeldt ML. Reduction of sympathetic inotropic response after ischemia in dogs. J Clin Invest 1985; 75:1504-9.

12. Becker LC, Levine JH, DiPaula AF, Guarnieri T, Aversano T. Reversal of dysfunction in postischemic stunned myocardium by epinephrine and postextrasystolic potentiation. J Am Coll Cardiol 1986; 7:580-9.

13. Przyklenk K, Kloner RA. Is "stunned myocardium" a protective mechanism? Effect of acute recruitment and acute β-blockade on recovery of contractile function and high-energy phosphate stores at 1 day post-reperfusion. Am Heart J 1989; 118:480-9.

14. Braunwald E, Ross J, Sonnenblick EH. Mechanisms of contraction of the normal and failing heart, 2d ed. Boston:Little, Brown, 1976.

15. Wingrad S. Electromechanical coupling in heart muscle, In: Berne RM, ed. Handbook of physiology, section 2. The cardiovascular system. Vol I. The heart. Bethesda, MD: American Physiological Society, 1979, pp 393-428.

16. Scheuer J, Bhan AK. Cardiac contractile proteins. Adenosine triphosphatase activity and physiological function. Circ Res 1979; 45:1-12.

17. Fabiato A, Fabiato F. Calcium and cardiac excitation-contraction coupling. Annu Rev Physiol 1979; 41:473-84.

18. Kusuoka H, Porterfield JK, Weisman HF, Weisfeldt ML, Marban E. Pathophysiology and pathogenesis of stunned myocardium. Depressed Ca^{2+} activation of contraction as a consequence of reperfusion-induced cellular calcium overload in ferret hearts. J Clin Invest 1987; 79:950-61.

19. Kusuoka H, Koretsune Y, Chacko VP, Weisfeldt ML, Marban E. Excitation-contraction coupling in postischemic mlyocardium. Does failure of activator Ca^{2+} transients underlie stunning? Circ Res 1990; 66:1268-76.

20. Tada M, Katz A. Phosphorylation of the sarcoplasmic reticulum and sarcolemma. Annu Rev 1982; 44:401-23.

21. Winegrad S, McClellan G, Horowitz R, Tucker M, Lin LE. Regulation of cardiac contractile proteins by phosphorylation. Fed Proc 1983; 42:39-44.

22. Watanabe AM. Recent advances in knowledge about beta-adrenergic receptors: application to clinical cardiology. J Am Coll Cardiol 1983; 1:82-9.

23. Wagner J, Schumann HJ.Different mechanisms underlying the stimulation of myocardial alpha- and beta-adrenoceptors. Life Sci 1979; 24:2045-52.

24. Ruegg JL. Dffects of new inotropic agents on Ca^{++} sensitivity of contractile proteins. Circulation 1986; 73III:78-84.

25. Bohm M, Morano I, Pieske B, Ruegg JC, Wankerl M, Zimmerman R, Erdmann E.

Contribution of cAMP-phosphodiesterase inhibition and sensitization of the contractile proteins for calcium to the intropic effect of pimobendan in the failing human myocardium. Res 1991; 68:689-701.

26. Ahlquist RP. A study of the adrenotropic receptors. Am J Physiol 1948; 153:586-600.
27. Hoffman BB, Lefkowitz RJ. Alpha-adrenergic receptor subtypes. N Engl J Med 1981; 302:1390-6.
28. Goldberg LI, Rajfer SI. Dopamine receptors: application in clinical cardiology. Circulation 1985; 72:245-8.
29. Gilbert JC, Goldberg LI. Characterization by cyproheptadine of the dopamine-induced contraction in canine isolated arteries. J Pharmacol Exp Ther 1975; 193:435-42.
30. Hardman JG. Cyclic nucleotide and regulation of vascular smooth muscle. J Cardiovasc Pharmacol 1984; 6:S639-S645.
31. The Xamoterol in Severe Heart Failure Study Group. Xamoterol in severe heart failure. Lancet 1990; 2:1-6.
32. Packer M, Carver JR, Rodeheffer RJ, Ivanhoe RJ, Dibianco R, Zeldis SM, Hendrix GH, Bommer WJ, Elkayam U, Kukin ML, Mallis GI, Sollano JA, Shannon J, Tandon PK, DeMets DL for the PROMISE Study Research Group. Effect of oral milrinone on mortality in severe chronic heart failure. N Engl J Med 1991; 325:1468-75.
33. Aronson RS, Gelles JM. Electrophysiologic effects of dopamine on sheep cardiac Purkinje fibers. J Pharmacol Exp Ther 1974; 188:596-604.
34. Goldberg LI. Dopamine-clinical uses of an endogenous catecholamine. N Engl J Med 1974; 291:707-10.
35. Robie NW, Goldberg LI. Comparative systemic and regional hemodynamic effects of dopamine and dobutamine. Am Heart J 1975; 90:340-5.
36. Brown RA, Dixon J, Farmer JB, Hall JC, Humphries RG, Ince F, O'Connor SE, Simpson WT, Smith GW. Dopexamine: a novel agonist at peripheral dopamine receptors and beta$_2$ adrenoceptors. Br J Pharmacol 1985; 85:599-608.
37. Greene SI, Smith JW. Dopamine gangrene. N Engl J Med 1976; 294:114.
38. Todu N, Goldberg LI. Effects of dopamine on isolated canine coronary arteries. Cardiovasc Res 1975; 9:384-9.
39. Zuberbuhler RC, Bohr DF. Responses of coronary smooth muscle to catecholamines. Circ Res 1965; 16:431-40.
40. Brooks HL, Stein PD, Matson JL, Hyland JW. Dopamine-induced alterations in coronary hemodynamics in dogs. Circ Res 1969; 24:699-704.
41. Ooiwa H, Miura T, Downey JM, Matsuki T, Shizukukda Y, Adachi T, Tsuchida A, Iwamoto T, Ogawa T, Iimura O. The effect of inotropic dose of dobutamine during reperfusion on myocardial infarct size. Jpn Circ J 1989; 53:1511-20.
42. Fowler MB, Alderman EL, Oesterle SN, Derby G, Daughters GT, Stinson EB, Ingels NB, Mitchell S, Miller DC. Dobutamine and dopamine after cardiac surgery: greater augmentation of myocardial blood flow with dobutamine. Circulation 1984; 70:I103-I111.
43. Pozen RG, DiBianco R, Katz RJ, Bortz R, Myerburg RJ, Fletcher RD. Myocardial metabolic and hemodynamic effects of dobutamine in heart failure complicationg coronary artery disease. Circulation 1981; 63:1279-85.

44. Harden TK. Agonist-induced desensitization of the β-adrenergic receptor-linked adenylate cyclase. Pharmacol Rev 1983; 35:5–32.

45. Lefkowitz TJ, Stadel JM, Caron MG. Adenyulate cyclase-coupled beta-adrenergic receptors: structure and mechanisms of activation and desensitization. Annu Rev Biochem 1983; 52:159–86.

46. Hertel C, Perkins JP. Receptor-specific mechanisms of desensitization of β-adrenergic receptor function. Mol Cell Endocrinol 1984; 37:245–56.

47. Sibley DR, Daniel K, Strader CD, Lefkowitz RJ. Phosphorylation of the β-adrenergic receptor in intact cells: relationship to heterologous and homologous mechanisms of adenylate cyclase desensitization.Arch Biochem Biophys 1987; 258:24–32.

48. Vatner DE, Vatner SF, Nejima J, Uemura N, Susanni EE, Hintze TH, Homcy CJ. Chronic norepinephrine elicits desensitization by uncoupling the β-receptor. J Clin Invest 1989; 84:1741–8.

49. Bristow MR, Ginsburg R, Umans V, Fowler M, Minobe W, Rasmussen R, Zera P, Menlove R, Shah P, Jamieson S, Stinson EB. β_1- and β_2-adrenergic-receptor subpopulations in nonfailing and failing human ventricular myocardium: coupling of both receptor subtypes to muscle contraction and selective β_1-receptor down-regulation in heart failure. Circ Rec 1986; 59:297–309.

50. Cohn JN, Levine TB, Olivari MT, Garberg V, Lura D, Francis GS, Simon AB, Rector T. Plasma norepinephrine as a guide to prognosis in patients with chronic congestive heart failure. N Engl J Med 1984; 311:819–23.

51. Jenne JW, Chick TW, Strickland RD, Wall FJ. Subsensitivity of beta resopnses during therapy with a long-acting beta-2 preparation. J Allergy Clin Immunol 1977; 59:383–90.

52. Georgopoulos D, Wong D, Anthonisen NR. Tolerance to beta$_2$-agonists in patients with chronic obstructive pulmonary disease. Chest 1990; 97:280–4.

53. Unverferth Dv, Blanford M, Kates RE, Leier CV. Tolerance to dobutamine after a 72 hour continuous infusion. Am J Med 1980; 69:262–5.

54 Applefeld MM, Newman KA, Grove WR, Sutton FJ, Roffman DS, Reed WP, Linberg SE. Intermittent, continuous outpatient dobutamine infusion in the management of congestive heart failure. Am J Cardiol 1983; 51:455–8.

55. Krell MJ, Kline EM, Bates ER, Hodgson JM, Dilworth LR, Laufer N, Vogel Ra, Pitt B. Intermittent, ambulatory dobutamine infusions in patients with severe congestive heart failure. Am Heart J 1986; 112:787–91.

56. Hoffman BB, Lejkowitz RJ. Catecholamines and sympathomimetic drugs. In: Goodman LS, Gilman AG, eds. The pharmacological basis of therapeutics. New York: Pergamon Press, 1990, pp 187–220.

57. Robie NW, Goldberg LI. Comparative systemic and regional hemodynamic effects of dopamine and dobutamine. Am Heart J 1975; 90:340–5.

58. Beregovich J, Bianchi C, Rubler S, Lomnitz E, Cagin N, Levitt B. Dose-related hemodynamic and renal effects of dopamine in congestive heart failure. Am Heart J 1974; 87:550–7.

59. Goldberg LI, McDonald RH, Zimmerman AM. Sodium diuresis produced by dopamine in patients with congestive heart failure. N Engl J Med 1963; 269:1060–4.

60. Francis GS, Sharma B, Hodges M. Comparative hemodynamic effects of dopamine

and dobutamine in patients with acute cardiogenic circulatory collapse. Am Heart J 1982; 103:995-1000.

61. Tuttle RR, Mills. Dobutamine. Development of a new catecholamine to selectively increase cardiac contractility. Circ Res 1975; 36:185-96.

62. Loeb HS, Bredakis J, Gunnar RM. Superiority of dobutamine over dopamine for augmentation of cardiac output in patients with chronic low output cardiac failure. Circulation 1977; 55:375-81.

63. Bendersky R, Chatterjee K, Parmley WW, Brundage BH, Ports TA. Dobutamine in chronic ischemic heart failure: alterations in left ventricular function and coronary hemodynamics. Am J Cardiol 1981; 48:554-8.

64. Gillespie TA, Ambos HD, Sobel BE, Roberts R. Effects of dobutamine in patients with acute myocardial infarction. Am J Cardiol 1977; 39:588-94.

65. Allwood MJ, Ginsburg J. Peripheral Vascular and other effects of dopamine infusions in man. Clin Sci 1964; 27:271-81.

66. Baumann G, Gutting M, Pfafferot C, Ningel K, Klein G. Comparison of acute hemodynamic effects of dopexamine hydrochloride dobutamine and sodium nitroprusside in chronic heart failure. Eur Heart J 1988; 9:503-12.

67. Leier CV, Binkley PF, Carpenter J, Randolph PH, Unverferth DV. Cardiovascular pharmacology of dopexamine in low output congestive heart failure. Am J Cardiol 1988; 62:94-9.

68. Gollub SB, Elkayam U, Young JB, Miller LW, Haffey KA, for the Dopexamine Investigators and Their Associates. Efficacy and safety of a short-term (6-h) intravenous infusion of dopexamine in patients with severe congestive heart failure: a randomized, double-blind, parallel, placebo-controlled multicenter study. J Am Coll Cardiol 1991; 18:383-90.

69 Colucci WS, Wright RF, Braunwald E. New Positive inotropic agents in the treatment of congestive heart failure. Mechanisms of action and recent clinical developments. N Engl J Med 1986; 314:349-58.

70. Wynne J, Malacoff RF, Benotti JR, Curfman GD, Grossman W, Holman BL, Smith TW, Braunwald E. Oral amrinone in refractory congestive heart failure. Am J Cardiol 1980; 45:1245-9.

71. Massie B, Bourassa M, DiBianco R, Hess M, Konstam M, Likoff M, Packer M. Long-term administration of amrinone for congestive heart failure: lack of efficiacy in a multicenter controlled trial. Circulation 1985; 71:963-71.

72. Benotti JR, Lesko LJ, McCue JE. Acute pharmacodynamics and pharmacokinetics of oral amrinone. J Clin Pharmacol 1982; 22:425-32.

73. Benotti JR, Grossman W, Braunwald E, Davolos DD, Alousi AA. Hemodynamic assessment of amrinone: a new inotropic agent. N Engl J Med 1978; 299:1373-7.

74. LeJemtel TH, Keung E, Sonnenblick EH, Ribner HS, Matsumoto M, Davis R, Schwartz W, Alousi AA, Davolos D. Amrinone: a new non-glycosidic, non-glycosidic, non-adrenergic cardiotonic agent effective in the treatment of intractable myocardial failur in man. Circulation 1979; 59:1098-1104.

75. Benotti Jr, Grossman W, Braunwald E, Carabello BA. Effects of amrinone on myocardial energy metabolism and hemodynamics in patients with severe congestive heart failure due to coronary artery disease. Circulation 1980; 62:28-34.

76. Jentzer JH, LeJemtel TH, Sonnenblick EH, Kirk ES. Beneficial effect of amrinone on myocardial oxygen consumption during acute left ventricular failure in dogs. Am J Cardiol 1981; 48:75-83.

77. Naccarelli GV, Gary EL, Dougherty AH, Hanna JE, Goldstein RA. Amrinone: Acute electrophysiologic and hemodynamic effects in patients with congestive heart failure. Am J Cardiol 1984; 54:600-4.

78. Maskin CS, Forman R, Klein NA, Sonnenblick EH, LeJemtel TH. Long-term amrinone therapy in patients with severe heart failure: drug-dependent hemodynamic benefits despite progression of disease. Am J Med 1982; 72:113-8.

79. Packer M, Medina N, Yushak M. Hemodynamic and clinical limitations of long-term inotropic therapy with amrinone in patients with severe chronic heart failure. Circulation 1984; 70:1038-47.

80. Baim DS, McDowell AV, Cherniles J, Monrad ES, Parker JA, Edelson J, Braunwald E, Grossman W. Evaluation of a new bipyridine inotropic agent—milrinone—in patients with severe congestive heart failure. N Engl J Med 1983; 309:748-56.

81. DiBianco R, Shabetai R, Kostuk W, Moran J, Schlant RC, Wright R, for the Milrinone Multicenter Trial Group. A comparison of oral milrinone, digoxin, and their combination in the treatment of patients with chronic heart failure. N Engl J Med 1989; 320: 677-83.

82. Uretsky BF, Jessup M, Konstam MA, Dec GW, Leier CV, Benotti J, Murali S, Herrmann HC, Sandberg JA, for the Enoximone Multicenter Trial Group. Multicenter trial of oral enoximone in patients with moderate to moderately severe congestive heart failure. Lack of benefit compared with placebo. Circulation 1990; 82:774-80.

83. Kubo SH, Gollub S, Bourge R, Rahko P, Cobb F, Jessup M, Brozena S, Brodsky M, Kirlin P, Shanes J, Konstam M, Gradman A, Morledge J, Cinquegrani M, Singh S, LeJemtel T, Nicklas J, Troha J, Cohn JN, for the Pimobendan Multicenter Research Group. Beneficial effects of pimobendan on exercise tolerance and quality of life in patients with heart failure: results of a multicenter trial. Circulation (in press).

84. Gage J, Rutman H, Lucido D, LeJemtel TH. Additive effects of dobutamine and amrinone on myocardial contractility and ventricular performance in patients with severe heart failure. Circulation 1986; 74:367-73.

85. Sundram P, Reddy HK, McElroy PA, Janicki JS, Wever KT. Myocardial energetics and efficiency in patients with idiopathic cardiomyopathy: response to dobutamine and amrinone. Am Heart J 1990; 119:891-8.

86. Loeb HS, Ostrenga JP, Gaul W, Witt J, Freeman G, Scanlon P, Gunnar RM. Beneficial effects of dopamine combined with intravenous nitroglycerin on hemodynamics in patients with severe left ventricular failure. Circulation 1983; 68:813-20.

17

Therapy of Arrhythmias in Acute Myocardial Infarction

Steven J. Kalbfleisch and Fred Morady
University of Michigan Medical Center, Ann Arbor, Michigan

INTRODUCTION

Arrhythmias are extremely common in the setting of acute myocardial infarction (MI). Many rhythm disturbances are benign and require no specific therapy while others, such as ventricular fibrillation, require immediate treatment. The clinical significance of an arrhythmia generally relates to its potential to produce hemodynamic instability, to worsen ischemia, or to aggravate congestive heart failure. This chapter will review the various arrhythmias and summarize treatment options.

SINUS BRADYCARDIA

Sinus bradycardia is a common rhythm disturbance in the setting of acute MI, particularly inferior MI, and is observed in 25–40% of patients monitored within the first hour of symptom onset (1,2). The prevalence of sinus bradycardia decreases to less then 15% after 4 hr of symptoms. Thrombolytic therapy appears to increase the incidence of sinus bradycardia (3,4), possibly due to the reperfusion-induced Bezold-Jarish reflex in inferior MI (5).

Patients with sinus bradycardia have a lower hospital mortality rate than those without (6). However, the association of hypotension with sinus bradycardia, present in 20–30% of these patients (7,8), represents a high-risk subgroup with mortality rates as great as 75% if untreated, compared with 10% if treated successfully (9). Patients who are normotensive with sinus bradycardia have a low mortality rate whether or not they are treated with atropine (9).

Since patients without associated hypotension or electrical instability have a low mortality rate without treatment, simple observation is appropriate. In patients with hypotension, frequent ventricular ectopy, or heart failure, intravenous atropine is the mainstay of therapy. Atropine has been shown to increase heart rate and blood pressure in roughly 85–90% of patients and suppress associated ventricular ectopy in 87% (8,10). Since low-dose atropine (<0.3 mg) may cause a paradoxical slowing of the heart rate (11) and high initial doses (>1 mg) or large cumulative doses (>2 mg) are associated with increased side effects (8), the recommended dosage regimen is 0.5 mg every 5–10 min, for a total dose of 2 mg or until the desired clinical effect is achieved (Table 1). The onset of action is rapid, usually minutes, and the duration of action is approximately 30 min when atropine is given intravenously (12) (Fig. 1).

The major noncardiac side effects of atropine are urinary retention, acute-angle glaucoma, and toxic psychosis. These are due to the anticholinergic properties of atropine and are more frequent at larger cumulative doses and in the elderly. The major cardiac side effects are sinus tachycardia, which may worsen myocardial ischemia, and ventricular dysrrhythmias. A variety of reports have documented these serious cardiac complications with doses as low as 0.5 mg (13,14), emphasizing again that treatment should be reserved for bradycardia-related hypotension, electrical instability, or heart failure.

Table 1   Medications Used for the Treatment of Bradycardia and AV Block

Medication	Indications	Dosage	Side effects
Atropine	Symptomatic brady-cardia or 2°/3° AV block	0.5 mg IV every 5–10 min (maximum of 2 mg)	Delirium, urinary retention, acute angle glaucoma, ventricular fibrillation
Isoproterenol	Symptomatic brady-cardia or 2°/3° AV block	2–10 μg/min IV titrated to heart rate	Excessive tachy-cardia, hypotension, increased oxygen demand, arrhythmias
Aminophylline	Atropine-resistant heart block	300–400 mg IV over 15–30 min	Tachycardia, atrial arrhythmias, CNS toxicity

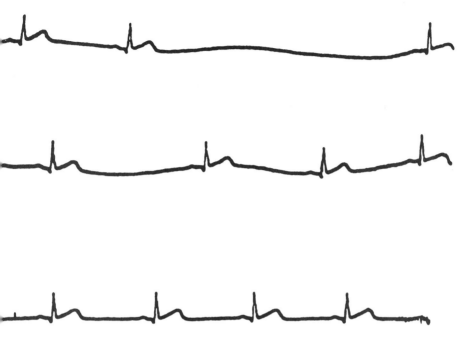

Figure 1   Sinus bradycardia. Rhythm strip demonstrating sinus bradycardia and a 3.8-sec sinus pause in a patient with an inferior infarction. The patient had associated hypotension and therefore was treated with atropine, which caused resolution of the sinus bradycardia (as seen in the last rhythm strip).

For patients refractory to atropine, the preferred second line of therapy is cardiac pacing. If the situation is acute and more immediate therapy is needed, intravenous isoproterenol at doses of 2-10 μg/min may be used as a temporizing measure (15). This is not recommended as definitive therapy because it will increase the metabolic demands of the heart, possibly increase infarct size, and is arrhythmogenic (16).

ATRIOVENTRICULAR BLOCK

First-degree atrioventricular (AV) block occurs in approximately 10% of patients with acute MI and is more frequent in inferior infarction, being present in up to 25% of patients. The major significance of first-degree AV block lies in its potential to progress to second- or third-degree block, which may occur in up to 40-60% of cases (6).

Higher-grade AV block (second or third degree) may be seen in up to 30% of acute MI patients if monitoring is begun within the first hour of symptom onset

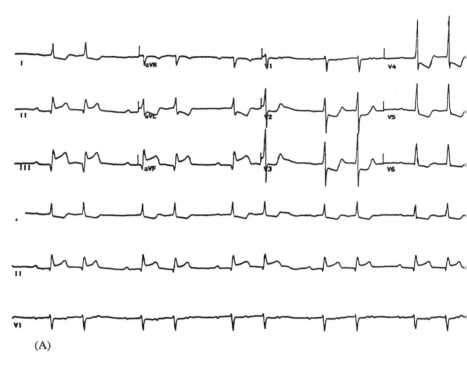

(A)

Figure 2   Second-degree AV block. (A) ECG showing a typical example of 3:2 Mobitz type I block in a patient with an acute inferior MI. Note the PR interval prolongation preceding the blocked P wave, indicative of a Mobitz type I pattern. The patient was not symptomatic and therefore no therapy was required. (B) ECG demonstrating a Mobitz type I AV block in a patient with inferior infarction. Note the PR interval following the dropped beat is shorter than the PR interval preceding the dropped beat, which is diagnostic of a Mobitz type I block.

(1). As with first-degree AV block, the incidence of second- or third-degree AV block is higher in inferior MI (27%) than anterior MI (5%) and usually appears within the first 24 hr of the MI (17) (Fig. 2). Thrombolytic therapy does not alter the frequency of high-grade AV block (3,18,19), but it does appear to decrease the duration of the block from a mean duration of 1.5–2.5 days without thrombolytics (6,17) to less than 12 hr with thrombolytics (19).

The prognosis for patients who develop high-grade AV block with an acute MI is worse than for patients without this complication. Most patients with anterior MI and high-grade AV block have either Mobitz type II block or complete AV block. These patients generally have extensive myocardial damage and extremely poor prognosis, with a 78% mortality rate even with successful treatment of the

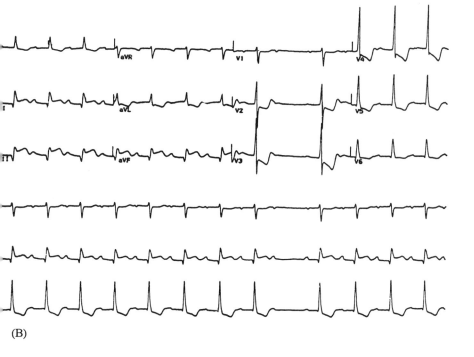

(B)

AV block (6,12). Patients with inferior MI and complete AV block also have a greater in-hospital mortality (29%) than those without complete AV block (6%), which appears primarily related to more extensive myocardial damage and worsened LV function (20). This difference in hospital mortality between those with and without complete AV block is also present with the use of thrombolytic therapy (19), although the overall mortality rates are lower (21). The long-term prognosis for patients with transient complete AV block and inferior infarction who survive the initial hospitalization does not appear to be different from the prognosis for those who did not develop this complication, indicating that the excess mortality is confined to the hospital period (22).

Patients with first-degree AV block require no specific therapy. High-grade AV block (second or third degree) complicating anterior MI is an indication for urgent temporary pacing, because these patients usually have necrosis of the infranodal conduction system and an unstable ventricular escape rhythm. If the situation is emergent, intravenous atropine in doses of 0.5 mg every 5 min for a maximum of 2 mg or isoproterenol at 2–10 μg/min titrated to heart rate may be used until pacemaker therapy is instituted.

In inferior MI, high-grade AV block is usually located in the AV node and associated with a stable junctional escape rate of 50–60 beats/min. The indications for treatment in this setting are the same as for sinus bradycardia and include hypotension, heart failure, or electrical instability as a result of the bradycardia. Stable patients do not require prophylactic pacing.

Early high-grade AV block in inferior MI, defined as occurring less than 6 hr from symptom onset, differs from late AV block in its response to therapy and probably in its etiology. Early AV block is most likely secondary to increased vagal tone and is generally responsive to standard doses of atropine (Table 1), whereas late AV block may be mediated by increased concentrations of adenosine in the AV node (20,24,25), which is released in response to the ischemic insult. Case reports indicate that this late form of atropine-resistant block is responsive to intravenous aminophylline (a competitive antagonist of adenosine) in doses of 300–500 mg given over 15–30 min (24,25) (Table 1). If initial pharmacological measures are not successful, isoproterenol at doses of 2–10 μg/min may be used until temporary pacing is instituted.

SUPRAVENTRICULAR TACHYARRHYTHMIAS

Sinus Tachycardia

Sinus tachycardia is another common rhythm disturbance in the setting of acute MI and occurs in approximately one-third of patients within the first 72 hr of symptom onset (26). This is often associated with a precipitating factor such as anxiety, continued ischemic pain, or LV dysfunction. These contributing factors should be treated in an effort to control heart rate and reduce myocardial oxygen demand before using specific drug therapy. Persistent sinus tachycardia is associated with a high hospital mortality of approximately 30% (27), probably because of an association with significant LV dysfunction, although some studies have indicated that it is an independent negative prognostic factor in patients without manifest congestive heart failure (28).

Some patients appear to have isolated tachycardia without any clear precipitating factors due to sympathetic overactivity occurring in the early stages of acute MI (29). These patients should be treated with intravenous beta blockade (Table 2) to slow the heart rate and reduce myocardial oxygen demand, especially since there is evidence in both the prethrombolytic and thrombolytic era that beta blockade, if given early in the course of the infarction, has a favorable effect on clinical outcome (30,31). When beta blockers are used, patients must be watched closely for evidence of worsening congestive heart failure, bronchospasm, hypotension, or development of heart block. If there is particular concern about possible side effects, a trial of esmolol would be advisable because of its ultrashort half-life.

Table 2 Medications Used for the Treatment of Supraventricular Tachyarrhythmias

Medication	Indications	Dosage	Side effects
Beta-blockers	Rate control of sinus tachycardia, atrial fibrillation/flutter		Congestive heart failure, bronchospasm, heart block, hypotension
Esmolol		500 μg/kg IV load over 1 min, then 50-250 μg/kg/min	Ultrashort half-life allows quick reversal of adverse effects
Metoprolol		5 mg IV over 2 min every 5 min for 3 doses	
Propranolol		1-2 mg over 2 min every 5 min (maximum 0.1 mg/kg)	
Atenolol		5 mg over 2 min, repeated 10 min later	
Digoxin	Rate control of atrial fibrillation/flutter	0.5 mg IV over 5 min, then 0.25 mg every 2-4 hr for a total of 1.5 mg	Worsening of arrhythmias (especially ventricular), development of heart block, increase in infarct size
Verapamil	Rate control of atrial fibrillation/flutter and termination of PSVT	5 mg IV over 2 min, then 1-2 mg every 1-2 min (maximum 20 mg)	Congestive heart failure, hypotension, heart block, asystole (especially if used in combination with beta-blockers)
Procainamide	Conversion of atrial fibrillation/flutter	20 mg/min IV (maximum 1 g) then 2-4 mg/min	Hypotension
Adenosine	Conversion of PSVT	6 mg IV bolus followed by 9 mg and 12 mg if not effective	Flushing, chest pain, dyspnea, sinus pauses

Atrial Fibrillation

Atrial fibrillation is the second most common supraventricular arrhythmia in the setting of acute MI, occurring in 10-20% of patients (6,32-34). Studies have shown that it is associated with a hospital mortality of up to 25-40% (33-35), probably attributable to its association with greater degrees of LV dysfunction. Ninety percent of patients who develop atrial fibrillation do so within 4 days of the onset of the MI (37), with most episodes being transient; 90% resolve within a 24-hr period (6,26). Factors associated with the development of atrial fibrillation are increased age (36), elevated intracardiac pressures (34), pericarditis (37), electrolyte disturbances, hypoxia, and atrial ischemia (38).

Precipitating factors should be sought and corrected. Treatment urgency depends on the hemodynamic and clinical status. The goals of therapy are both ventricular rate control and conversion to normal sinus rhythm (Fig. 3). If the patient is clinically unstable (i.e., has associated hypotension, chest pain, or worsening congestive heart failure), electrical cardioversion should be followed by pharmacotherapy to prevent recurrences and control the ventricular rate if atrial fibrillation does recur. Pharmacological agents useful in treating atrial fibrillation include digitalis, verapamil, beta-blockers, and procainamide.

Digitalis

For many years digitalis preparations, especially digoxin, were the mainstay of therapy for rate control in atrial fibrillation. There are disadvantages to the use of digoxin in the setting of acute MI, one being its relatively slow onset of action of up to 3-4 hr. Other drawbacks include inability to control ventricular rate during periods of enhanced sympathetic activity (39,40), a lower threshold for toxicity, and the potential to increase myocardial oxygen demand and infarct size (41). The side effect of most concern with digoxin is its potential to aggravate ventricular arrhythmias, especially in the setting of hypokalemia, which is common in acute MI. One advantage of digoxin is that it does not produce hypotension or have a negative inotropic effect as do calcium channel blockers and beta-blockers the other agents used for rate control in atrial fibrillation.

Digoxin is useful for controlling the ventricular rate during atrial fibrillation in patients with significant LV dysfunction who may not tolerate either a calcium channel blocker or beta-blocker. Often, digoxin may be used in combination with one of these other agents for enhanced rate control (40). Care must be taken when using the combination of verapamil and digoxin since this may increase digoxin levels by up to 50% by decreasing both the renal and nonrenal clearance of digoxin (39). A standard dosing regimen for digoxin is 0.5 mg given intravenously over 5-10 min (to avoid vasoconstriction) followed by 0.25 mg every 2-4 hr, for a total loading dose of 1.5 mg in a 24-hr period (Table 2). This may then be followed by daily doses of 0.25 mg to maintain serum levels of 1-1.5 μg/ml. Pa-

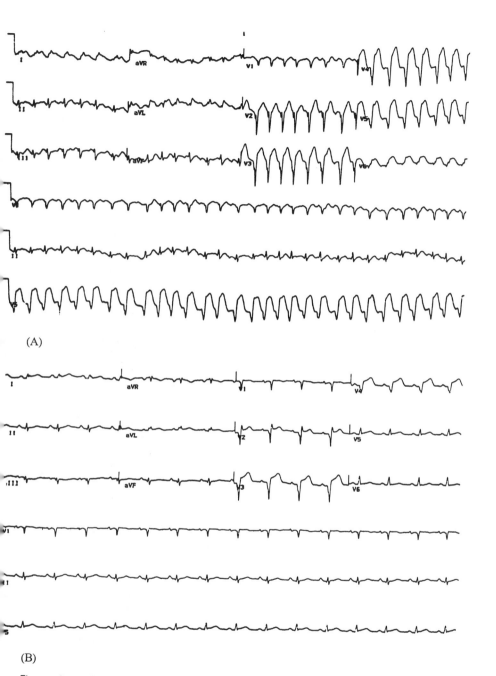

(A)

(B)

Figure 3　Atrial fibrillation. (A) ECG demonstrating atrial fibrillation with a ventricular response of 180 bpm in a patient 2 days after an anterior MI. The atrial fibrillation was associated with a worsening of congestive heart failure. (B) The patient converted to a sinus rhythm after 500 mg of procainamide and had an improvement in the heart failure symptoms. Esmolol was used for rate control prior to conversion.

tients with renal insufficiency require a downward adjustment of the maintenance dose.

Verapamil

Verapamil is the only calcium channel blocking agent commercially available in intravenous form in the United States. Verapamil controls the rate in atrial fibrillation by increasing the AV node refractory period and slowing AV node conduction. In contrast to digoxin, verapamil's effects do not rely on indirect vagal effects and, therefore, verapamil may be effective even during periods of high adrenergic tone (39). A major advantage of verapamil is its ability to control the rate quickly, with most patients showing a prompt response that lasts for at least 30 min, depending on the dose (42). The major limitation of intravenous verapamil in the setting of acute MI is its potential to aggravate heart failure, hypotension, and heart block.

Intravenous verapamil has been shown to be effective in slowing the ventricular response during atrial fibrillation in up to 80% of patients (39). A study by Hagemeijer (43) examined specifically the use of intravenous verapamil for the control of supraventricular tachyarrhythmias occurring in the first 72 hr of an MI. In this study, eight patients who had atrial fibrillation and a ventricular rate ranging from 130 to 180 bpm were treated with incremental doses of 1 mg of verapamil at 1-min intervals for a maximum dose of 20 mg. The ventricular rate decreased to less than 105 bpm in all patients with an average dose of 10 mg. Two patients developed new hypotension. Other studies have confirmed the safety and efficacy of intravenous verapamil for rapid control of atrial fibrillation (42,44). A recommended dosage regimen (Table 2) is an initial bolus of 5 mg with additional doses of 1-2 mg at intervals of 1-2 min until the desired effect is seen, or a maximum of 20 mg has been given. If the patient tolerates this with good control of the ventricular rate, a continuous infusion of 2.5-5.0 μg/kg/min may be instituted and titrated as needed. If excessive hypotension occurs with the use of verapamil, intravenous calcium should be given in an attempt to reverse this side effect. Special caution must be used if the patient is also being treated with a beta-adrenergic blocking agent, because this increases the risk for side effects such as heart failure, hypotension, and heart block.

Beta Blockade

The two intravenous beta-blockers used most commonly for control of supraventricular tachyarrhythmias are propranolol and esmolol. These differ primarily in serum half-life, beta-1 receptor selectivity, and lipid solubility, but both share the potential to precipitate heart failure, hypotension, AV block, and bronchospasm. Propranolol is a beta-1 nonselective agent with a relatively short half-life of 3-4 hr, and a high degree of lipid solubility. Esmolol is one of the newest beta-blockers available. It is a beta-1 selective agent with a low degree of lipid solubility. A major advantage of esmolol is its ultrashort half-life of approximately 10 min, which allows one to quickly discontinue therapy should adverse side effects occur. Because of the proven benefits of beta blockade in decreasing to recurrent ischemic events in acute MI (30,31), beta-blockers may be preferable to verapamil for control of atrial fibrillation unless there is a contraindication for use, such as active bronchospasm.

Propranolol is the beta-blocker that has been available for the longest period of time (45). Lemberg et al. found that 18 episodes of atrial fibrillation in 15 patients were treated effectively with intravenous propranolol, usually with a total dose of 4–5 mg. Thirteen episodes reverted to sinus rhythm and all other episodes were controlled to a rate of less than 100 bpm. Only one patient developed new hypotension and no patient had worsening of congestive heart failure. Intravenous propranolol is usually given in 1- to 2-mg boluses every 5 min until the desired effect is seen or until a total dose of 0.1 mg/kg is given (Table 2). During infusion of propranolol patients must be observed carefully for the development of adverse side effects (i.e., hypotension, heart failure, atrioventricular block, and bronchospasm).

Esmolol is the newest beta-blocker available in intravenous form for the treatment of supraventricular arrhythmias. A previous study has shown that it is as effective as propranolol for rate control in atrial fibrillation, with a success rate of approximately 75% (46). The average time for resolution of the beta-blockade effect after termination of the infusion is less than 30 min (47). The short-term use of esmolol has been shown to be safe in patients with moderate obstructive airways disease and does not cause any significant change in pulmonary function testing (48). Dosing of esmolol is somewhat complex (Table 2); it is given as a loading dose of $500 \mu g/kg$ over 1 min followed by a continuous infusion starting at $50 \mu g/kg/min$ and titrated up to a maximum of $250 \mu g/kg/min$ in $50 \mu g/kg/min$ increments. For each increase in the infusion rate, an additional bolus of $500 \mu g/kg$ is recommended. Adjustments in dosing may be made every 10 min if the patient has not had an adequate response and is free of adverse side effects. The average dose of esmolol required to control the ventricular rate during atrial fibrillation is $150 \mu g/kg/min$ (46).

Procainamide

The drugs mentioned previously for the treatment of atrial fibrillation are for rate control and are not generally effective for conversion to sinus rhythm. Chemical cardioversion is usually performed with a class 1A antiarrhythmic drug, and procainamide is the one generally used for acute intravenous therapy. Intravenous procainamide is effective in terminating recent-onset atrial fibrillation. In one study, 10 of 13 episodes of atrial fibrillation of less than 10 days' duration were terminated successfully during procainamide infusion at an average dose of 10 mg/kg (49). The usual dose of intravenous procainamide is 20 mg/min for a total of 750-1000 mg, followed by a 2-4 mg/min continuous infusion (Table 2). Procainamide's half-life is roughly 3-4 hr and is not altered in patients with acute MI or congestive heart failure (50) but is prolonged in patients with renal insufficiency, who therefore may require dosage adjustments. The most common acute side effect with intravenous procainamide is hypotension, which can be avoided by close monitoring of the blood pressure and infusion rate. The usual therapeutic range for serum procainamide levels is 4-8 μg/ml.

Atrial Flutter

Compared to atrial fibrillation, atrial flutter is a relatively uncommon arrhythmia in acute MI, being encountered in less than 5% of patients (49). It usually presents with 2:1 AV conduction and a ventricular response rate of 150 bpm. Atrial flutter more often than atrial fibrillation leads to clinical deterioration and requires emergent therapy (37). The medications used in the treatment of atrial flutter are the same as for atrial fibrillation, but it may be more resistant to pharmacotherapy (49). Unlike atrial fibrillation, atrial flutter may resolve with atrial overdrive pacing (50,51) and often can be converted electrically with shocks of 25-50 joules (52).

Paroxysmal Supraventricular Tachycardia

Paroxysmal supraventricular tachycardia (PSVT) also is uncommon in acute myocardial infarction and occurs in less than 5% of patients (51). Its deleterious effects result from the rapid ventricular rate, which increases oxygen demand and may result in hypotension. Because of its potential to worsen ischemia and extend infarct size, it generally requires aggressive management.

As with atrial fibrillation and flutter, a direct-current countershock may be used to terminate this arrhythmia if the patient is hemodynamically unstable. The two most important intravenous pharmacological agents for the acute treatment of PSVT are verapamil and adenosine, but prior to drug therapy, vagal maneuvers should be attempted to terminate the tachycardia.

Verapamil

Verapamil has been the first-line agent for termination of PSVT for a number of years. It has an 80-90% success rate with doses of 5-10 mg given intravenously and is usually effective within minutes of administration (Table 2) (55-57). It is generally a safe agent in the setting of acute MI, but one must be aware of its potential to cause LV dysfunction, hypotension, and AV block, especially if used concomitantly with beta blockade.

Adenosine

Adenosine is a new agent with some advantages for the treatment of PSVT. It is an extremely short-acting agent with a half-life of less than 20 sec (56); therefore, any adverse hemodynamic or arrhythmic effects are very transient. The most common side effects are flushing, dyspnea, chest pain, and sinus pauses upon termination of PSVT (58). Adenosine has a success rate of greater than 95% for termination of PSVT and generally is effective within 30 sec of administration (56–58). A recommended dosage regimen (Table 2) for adults is a 6-mg intravenous bolus with repeat doses of 9 mg and 12 mg given at 1-min intervals if the preceding dose is not effective. Of note is that patients taking theophylline preparations may be resistant to the effects of adenosine and require alternative therapy. Patients taking dipyridamole may be very sensitive to the effects of adenosine and should receive smaller initial doses (58).

VENTRICULAR ARRHYTHMIAS

Ventricular arrhythmias are common during the initial phases of acute MI. They range in significance from benign ventricular premature depolarizations to life-threatening ventricular tachycardia and fibrillation.

Ventricular Premature Depolarizations

The occurrence of ventricular premature depolarizations in the acute phase of MI is almost universal. The reported incidence ranges from 34% to 100%, depending on the duration and timing of electrocardiographic monitoring (6). Ventricular premature depolarizations are most prevalent within the first hour of symptom onset and decline thereafter (1). With the use of thrombolytic therapy, the incidence of both single and repetitive forms of ventricular premature depolarizations is increased after therapy, while the incidence of more malignant ventricular arrhythmias in the first few hours appears unchanged (3).

It is generally agreed that the prognostic value of ventricular premature depolarizations in predicting the occurrence of more serious arrhythmias is limited, since up to 40% of episodes of primary ventricular fibrillation are unheralded by ventricular premature depolarizations or complex ventricular ectopy, and 55% of patients without ventricular fibrillation have ventricular premature depolarizations or complex ventricular ectopy (59,60). Since premature ventricular depolarizations are nearly universal and have a limited predictive value and because the medications used in their therapy are potentially toxic, treatment is generally not necessary or advisable. There are some exceptions to this, such as patients who have a crescendo pattern of ventricular ectopy and frequent runs of nonsustained ventricular tachycardia. In these cases, antiarrhythmic therapy should be used in the hope of preventing more serious ventricular arrhythmias. The agent of first choice is lidocaine, followed by procainamide (Table 3).

Accelerated Idioventricular Rhythm

The incidence of accelerated idioventricular rhythm (AIVR) is difficult to ascertain because of the varying definitions of this rhythm disturbance in different studies. In general, it is defined as a ventricular rhythm with a rate between 60 and 120 bpm. It has an incidence reported to be between 8% and 46% in the first few days of an MI (6). With the use of thrombolytic therapy, the incidence of AIVR is increased early after drug administration compared with patients who do not receive thrombolytic therapy and may occur in up to 80% of patients who reperfuse, probably as part of the phenomenon of reperfusion arrhythmias (3,61).

The majority of episodes of AIVR are felt to be due to enhanced automaticity of ectopic ventricular sites and often are seen in the setting of bradycardia, which allows the automatic foci to become manifest. Most episodes are benign and are not felt to adversely affect prognosis. Some reports have indicated that there is an association between AIVR and more rapid forms of ventricular tachycardia (62–64). Mechanistically, this may be due to varying degrees of exit block from a single ectopic focus, with the slower rhythms being a manifestation of greater degrees of block. One report showed that the association of AIVR and the development of ventricular tachycardia was present only with rates greater than 75 bpm (64).

The need for treatment of this rhythm disturbance is controversial. Patients with slow AIVR (<75 bpm) may have hypotension due to the loss of AV synchrony. Intravenous atropine has been effective in 85% of patients for accelerating the sinus rate, suppressing the AIVR, and restoring AV synchrony (8). Because of the potential for atropine to cause serious side effects such as ventricular fibrillation (13,14), slow AIVR should be treated only if it is associated with hemodynamic instability. If atropine is not effective, atrial or AV sequential pacing may be used to restore AV synchrony. Even though patients with more rapid AIVR (>75 bpm) are at higher risk of developing life-threatening ventricular arrhythmias, there is no definitive evidence that treating this will reduce that risk or improve survival. Treatment is recommended if the episodes are frequent, have rates greater than 100 bpm, or are associated with hypotension. The treatment strategy in patients with the rapid form of AIVR is the same as for patients with ventricular tachycardia, starting first with lidocaine and progressing to procainamide and bretylium if needed.

Ventricular Tachycardia

Ventricular tachycardia may be categorized by duration (nonsustained versus sustained), morphology (polymorphic versus monomorphic), time of occurrence

Table 3   Medications Used for the Treatment of Ventricular Arrhythmias

Medication	Indications	Dosage	Side effects
Isoproterenol	Torsades de pointes	2-20 μg/min titrated to HR of >90 bpm	Worsened ischemia, increased infarct size, arrhythmias
Magnesium sulfate	Torsades de pointes	2-g IV bolus, may be repeated at 5-15-min intervals for a maximum of 6 g	Neurological depression, apnea at very high serum levels
Lidocaine	Ventricular tachycardia and fibrillation	100 mg (1.5 mg/kg) IV bolus followed by 1-4 mg/min infusion, second bolus of 0.5 mg/kg at 10-20 min. May repeat 0.5 mg/kg boluses for maximum of 200 mg	CNS hyperactivity, seizures, delirium, numbness, asystole. Increased incidence of toxicity in CHF, liver disease, and elderly
Procainamide	Ventricular tachycardia	20 mg/min IV for a maximum load of 1 g followed by 1-4 mg/min infusion	Hypotension
Bretylium	Ventricular tachycardia and fibrillation	5 mg/kg IV bolus, may repeat 5-10 mg/kg boluses every 15-30 min for a maximum of 30 mg/kg load followed by 1-2 mg/min infusion	Transient tachycardia and hypertension followed by late hypotension (primarily orthostatic)
Amiodarone	Refractory ventricular tachycardia and fibrillation	600 mg PO tid to qid for 10 days, then taper to 200-400 mg/day maintenance dose	Hypotension, myocardial depression, bradycardia, and conduction disturbances

relative to the MI (early, <48 hr, versus late, >48 hr), and relation to other clinical parameters (primary, unassociated with hemodynamic compromise, versus secondary, associated with hypotension and heart failure). In most studies that have evaluated its incidence, ventricular tachycardia has been defined as three or more consecutive ventricular beats at a rate of greater than 120 bpm. When defined in this manner, ventricular tachycardia is present in approximately 70% of patients during the first 24 hr from symptom onset (65). Episodes of ventricular tachycardia more than 10 beats in duration occur in up to 25% of patients, while sustained monomorphic ventricular tachycardia is uncommon during the first day of an MI (65). The incidence of ventricular tachycardia does not appear to be altered with the use of thrombolytic agents, at least during the first 3 hr after therapy has been given (3).

Patients who sustain a cardiac arrest due to ventricular tachycardia during the hospitalization have a higher mortality than those who do not, but almost all the excess mortality is in patients who have had ventricular tachycardia secondary to hypotension or significant heart failure. In the MILIS study, patients with cardiac arrest due to primary ventricular tachycardia within the first 72 hr of the MI had a similar hospital and long-term mortality as those who did not have a cardiac arrest (66).

Another high-risk subgroup of patients besides those with secondary ventricular tachycardia are those who develop sustained monomorphic ventricular tachycardia 2 days to 2 months after AMI. These patients have a mortality rate exceeding 50% at 1 year of follow-up, even with antiarrhythmic therapy guided by electrophysiological evaluation (67,68).

Polymorphic ventricular tachycardia in the setting of acute MI can pose a difficult diagnostic and therapeutic dilemma, especially if the patient is already receiving antiarrhythmic medications. The differential diagnosis includes ischemia-induced ventricular tachycardia versus torsades de pointes (Fig. 4). An important feature in differentiating these two conditions is the presence of a prolonged QT interval during sinus rhythm in patients who have torsades (69). Torsades de pointes also has a typical initiation sequence of a long RR interval followed by a short RR interval due to a late coupled extrasystole and is often preceded by a period of bradycardia (70).

As with other rhythm disturbances, the urgency and mode of therapy are primarily dictated by the hemodynamic consequences of the arrhythmia. If ventricular tachycardia is sustained, hemodynamically compromising, or associated with evidence of myocardial ischemia, immediate DC cardioversion is required along with concomitant pharmacotherapy to prevent recurrence. Patients who have ventricular tachycardia early in the course of an MI (<48 hr) do not necessarily require long-term therapy since, as mentioned previously, their long-term prognosis does not differ from that of patients who do not have significant ventricular arrhythmias. Patients who have sustained monomorphic ventricular tachycardia more

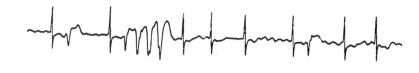

250 BPM

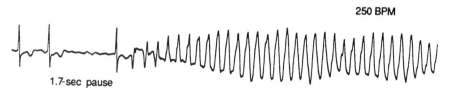

1.7-sec pause

Figure 4   Torsades de pointes. Rhythm strip demonstrating the typical initiation and morphology of torsades de pointes. Note the long RR interval (1.7-sec pause) followed by an extrasystole, which initiates the tachycardia. Note also the QT interval is greater than 50% of the RR interval in the beat preceding the pause. This patient was being treated with quinidine and had hypokalemia.

than 2 days after an MI should have long-term therapy guided by electrophysiological testing (68). Options for therapy include antiarrhythmic medications, endocardial resection, or automatic cardioverter/defibrillator implantation. For the prevention and treatment of significant ventricular arrhythmias in acute MI, the importance of potassium homeostasis cannot be overstated. A number of studies have shown a strong correlation between hypokalemia and the development of ventricular dysrhythmias (66,71). The drugs used in the acute management of ventricular tachycardia are lidocaine, procainamide, bretylium, and amiodarone, generally in this order.

In patients who have torsades de pointes, the primary therapy is elimination of the initiating and aggravating factors. In the setting of acute MI, there are usually electrolyte disturbances (hypokalemia, hypomagnesemia), medications (most commonly quinidine or procainamide), and episodes of bradycardia. While the underlying cause is being corrected, these patients may be treated with pacing or isoproterenol to increase the heart rate to 90 bpm, in order to suppress further episodes (72). Others have also reported success with magnesium sulfate using intravenous boluses of 2 g, which may be repeated at intervals of 5–15 min for a total of 6 g, if necessary (Table 3) (73). Polymorphic ventricular tachycardia not associated with a long QT interval is treated with standard antiarrhythmic medications; attempts should also be made to identify and treat underlying ischemia.

Lidocaine

Lidocaine, a class IB antiarrhythmic, is the drug of first choice when patients have significant ventricular arrhythmia in the setting of acute MI. Lidocaine has been shown to have an 80–90% success rate for the suppression of ventricular tachycardia and complex ventricular ectopy (74). The major concern with the use of lidocaine are its toxic side effects. The organ system most affected by toxicity is the central nervous system (CNS), with symptoms ranging from mild numbness and tingling to delirium and seizures. Patients who are especially prone to developing CNS toxicity are the elderly and those with underlying liver disease, congestive heart failure, or borderline mental function at the start of therapy.

Many dosing regimens for lidocaine have been developed. One method for administering lidocaine is to use an initial intravenous bolus of 100 mg or 1.5 mg/kg followed by a continuous infusion of 1–4 mg/min or 20–50 μg/kg/min. Patients should also receive a second smaller bolus of 50 mg or 0.5 mg/kg 10–20 min after the initial bolus to compensate for the predictable decline in serum levels at this time. If the initial bolus of lidocaine was ineffective, it may be followed by subsequent boluses of 50 mg at 5- to 10-min intervals, up to a maximum of 200 mg.

Since lidocaine is primarily metabolized by the liver, patients suspected of having altered hepatic metabolism or reduced hepatic blood flow should receive half the usual maintenance infusion and should undergo close monitoring of the plasma lidocaine concentrations; this includes patients with cirrhosis, congestive heart failure, and hypotension. Commonly used drugs, such as cimetidine and propranolol, decrease lidocaine clearance owing to their effects on hepatic metabolism or blood flow. In patients who are at high risk of developing toxicity, the lidocaine dose should be calculated on the basis of body weight, levels should be followed closely, and the infusion should be discontinued as soon as it is no longer needed (75). Lidocaine's half-life with normal hepatic clearance is approximately 2 hr but may increase to up to 30 hr if significant heart failure is present. The usual range of therapeutic levels is 1.5–5 μg/ml.

Procainamide

Procainamide, a class IA agent, is considered the drug of second choice for the treatment of ventricular tachycardia and frequent ventricular ectopy in acute MI. In this setting, procainamide has been shown to be up to 90% effective for the control of ventricular ectopy at serum levels of 4–10 μg/ml (76). A standard dosing regimen is to give 20 mg/min until the arrhythmia is controlled, a total of 1 g is given, or acute side effects occur. This is then followed by a continuous infusion of 2–4 mg/min (20–80 μg/kg/min) (Table 3), adjusted based on serum levels and response to therapy. In acute MI, the average serum level required for suppression of ventricular ectopy is 5.0 μg/ml, which is roughly half the level required for VPD suppression in chronic ischemic heart disease (77).

The pharmacokinetics of procainamide are not altered during acute MI or in the presence of congestive heart failure and, therefore, no dosage adjustments need to be made in these circumstances (50). The half-life of procainamide is approximately 3 hr but may be substantially increased in the presence of renal insufficiency, which may result in accumulation of serum procainamide and its active metabolite, N-acetyl-procainamide (NAPA). In the presence of renal insufficiency, the maintenance infusion should be decreased and serum levels of procainamide and NAPA should be followed closely. The major acute toxicity of intravenous procainamide is hypotension, but the incidence of this is minimal if the drug is administered using the guidelines given above (76,78). One must be cautious with the use of class IA antiarrhythmics in the setting of polymorphic ventricular tachycardia. Patients with a long QT interval and polymorphic ventricular tachycardia should not receive procainamide because this may aggravate the arrhythmia.

Bretylium

Bretylium is a class III antiarrhythmic agent used for the treatment of ventricular tachycardia refractory to lidocaine and procainamide (Fig. 5). When compared directly to lidocaine, it offers no advantage as first-line therapy, with both drugs being effective in approximately 90% of patients (79–81).

The initial dose of bretylium is 5 mg/kg, given as a rapid intravenous infusion. If this is not effective, additional doses of 5–10 mg/kg may be given at 15- to 30-min intervals for a total of 30 mg/kg loading dose, followed by a continuous infusion 1–2 mg/min (Table 3) (15). In animal studies, the peak antiarrhythmic effect occurs at 3–6 hr (82), but clinical studies have shown that a therapeutic effect may be seen within minutes after a dose is given (83). In the setting of acute MI, bretylium has been shown to cause an initial transient sinus tachycardia and hypertension, which are followed by mild hypotension (primarily orthostatic), with no significant effect on left ventricular function (84). These effects are due to bretylium's action at the sympathetic ganglia, where it initially causes a release of norepinephrine and later a postganglionic blockade (85). The dose of bretylium should be reduced in patients with renal insufficiency to avoid toxicity, because it is primarily excreted by the kidneys. The average half-life of bretylium is 8 hr.

Amiodarone

Amiodarone, also a class III antiarrhythmic agent, is the drug of last resort when a patient has ventricular dysrhythmias refractory to conventional medications. At present it is available only in oral form in the United States, but numerous studies have shown it to be highly efficacious when given intravenously for acute control of refractory ventricular arrhythmias (86–91). Collectively, these studies have shown that intravenous bolus therapy with amiodarone is greater than 50% effec-

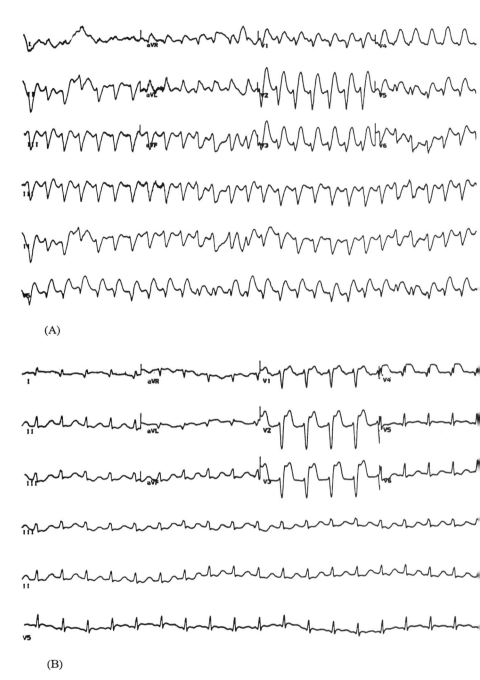

Figure 5 Sustained monomorphic ventricular tachycardia. (A) This patient developed ventricular tachycardia 4 days following an extensive anterior MI. The VT was refractory to both lidocaine and procainamide. (B) The ventricular tachycardia was finally controlled after two 350-mg (5 mg/kg) boluses of bretylium, which resulted in conversion to sinus rhythm.

tive for the control of life-threatening ventricular tachycardia and fibrillation refractory to other antiarrhythmic medications.

Since intravenous amiodarone is not currently available for general use, amiodarone must be administered orally in clinical practice. Studies have shown that very high oral doses of 2 g given 2-3 times daily may have an antiarrhythmic effect within 3-8 hr of a single dose and may be effective in completely suppressing episodes of ventricular tachycardia within 2 days of starting therapy (92,93). An appropriate dosing regimen is 600 mg 3-4 times daily for 10 days, followed by 200-400 mg/day as a maintenance dose.

Drug-Refractory Ventricular Tachycardia

Patients with drug-refractory ventricular tachycardia in the setting of acute MI generally have a poor prognosis. In the postinfarction patient, it is important to always look for ischemia as a possible trigger, especially if the patient is having polymorphic ventricular tachycardia with a normal QT interval. If ischemia is felt to be a contributing factor, the patient should receive aggressive anti-ischemic therapy, and use of intra-aortic balloon counterpulsation and/or percutaneous or surgical revascularization should be considered. Some patients may have bradycardia-dependent ventricular tachycardia, which can be effectively treated by pacing. Patients with drug-refractory ventricular tachycardia or fibrillation not secondary to ischemia may be candidates for endocardial mapping and resection. Although this carries a substantial surgical mortality of up to 30%, for those patients who survive to hospital discharge, the 1-year survival may approach 95% (94). Implantation of an automatic internal cardioverter/defibrillator may be appropriate, but not if the episodes of ventricular tachycardia are frequent.

Ventricular Fibrillation

Primary ventricular fibrillation is the most common cause of death in the early hours of acute MI. Up to 65% of deaths from infarction occur within the first hour of symptom onset and most of these deaths are due to ventricular fibrillation (95). Nearly all episodes of primary ventricular fibrillation occur within the first 6 hr from symptom onset, and it is uncommon for primary ventricular fibrillation to occur more than 8 hr after the onset of the infarction (1,2). In recent studies, the incidence of ventricular fibrillation after arrival to the coronary care unit has been less than 5% (65). There is evidence that this complication is more common in younger individuals than in patients over the age of 70 (74). With the use of thrombolytic therapy, the incidence of ventricular fibrillation less than 3 hr after drug administration does not appear to be different from placebo and is approximately 5% (3,4), while the incidence of ventricular fibrillation occurring after 3 hr may be decreased (96).

The prognosis for patients with ventricular fibrillation depends on whether the episode was primary, i.e., not associated with severe heart failure or hypotension, or secondary, i.e., occurring in the presence of severe hemodynamic compromise. The mortality rate in patients with secondary ventricular fibrillation is high, with only 20% surviving to be discharged from the hospital (6).

The prognostic importance of primary ventricular fibrillation is controversial, with two large studies showing conflicting results. The MILIS study (66) demonstrated that primary ventricular fibrillation had no effect on hospital mortality. However, the results of the GISSI trial indicated that it was associated with a higher hospital mortality (97). For patients with primary ventricular fibrillation who survive to hospital discharge there does not appear to be any additional excess long-term mortality (98,99).

The most important therapy for ventricular fibrillation is immediate electrical defibrillation. After a patient is successfully defibrillated, intravenous antiarrhythmics should be administered for 12–24 hr in an attempt to prevent a recurrence because up to 65% of patients will experience another episode, usually within 8 hr of the initial event (74). The first-line agent is lidocaine. If ventricular fibrillation is refractory to lidocaine, the second-line agent is bretylium, which has proven efficacy as an antifibrillatory drug (79–81). In patients who are refractory to these two drugs, amiodarone may be useful (Table 3).

LIDOCAINE PROPHYLAXIS

The issue of lidocaine prophylaxis in the early stages of an evolving MI is still controversial. It was once almost universally recommended after studies in the early 1970s showed a reduction in the incidence of primary ventricular fibrillation (100) and possibly in mortality (101). More recently, large-scale studies and meta-analytic reviews of the use of lidocaine in acute MI have brought this practice into question. One of the largest studies, by Koster and Dunning (102), showed that the routine use of 400 mg of intramuscular lidocaine caused a 31% decrease in the incidence of primary ventricular fibrillation but no improvement in mortality. Meta-analyses of this topic have shown that there is a trend toward higher mortality in patients who receive lidocaine, especially if it is delivered after arrival to the hospital, even though there is a 30% reduction in the incidence of ventricular fibrillation (103,104). The higher mortality rate may be attributable to a greater number of bradyarrhythmic and asystolic events.

With the advent of thrombolytic therapy, there has been renewed interest in the use of lidocaine prophylaxis because of reperfusion arrhythmias. However, studies comparing the use of thrombolytics to placebo have not shown a higher incidence of ventricular fibrillation with thrombolysis; rather, more frequent episodes of bradyarrhythmias (3,4), which could potentially be aggravated by lidocaine, have been noted. Also, experimental studies in dogs indicate that lidocaine may not be effective in preventing reperfusion ventricular fibrillation (105). Since the benefits with respect to mortality are questionable and the potential for toxicity is high, the routine use of lidocaine prophylaxis is not appropriate even when using thrombolytics.

However, in some circumstances, the prophylactic use of lidocaine may be reasonable. Patients who are at high risk for ventricular fibrillation and who have a low potential for toxicity might benefit from prophylactic lidocaine. This would include younger patients (<60 years) seen early in the course of a definite myocardial infarction (<4 hr) without heart failure, hypotension, significant liver disease, or bradyarrhythmias. If prophylaxis is used, it is recommended that a 200-mg bolus loading dose be given in 0.5–1.0 mg/kg boluses at 5-min intervals, followed by a continuous infusion of 2 mg/min (106). The lidocaine should be discontinued at 12–24 hr if no significant ventricular arrhythmias have occurred as there is a very low probability of developing ventricular fibrillation after this time.

REPERFUSION ARRHYTHMIAS

A concern over serious reperfusion arrhythmias probably arose from the known vulnerability of the heart to ventricular fibrillation in the experimental laboratory after release of a coronary ligature, an event that occurs in up to 80% of dogs in reperfusion experiments (107,108). This has not been a problem in clinical studies, probably because of the vast differences between experimentally induced reperfusion and reperfusion that is achieved clinically with thrombolytic therapy. In experimental reperfusion, an artery is often occluded and then abruptly released, allowing complete reperfusion. In the clinical setting, patients are usually seen more than 2 hr after the onset of chest pain, and if reperfusion is achieved, it is often gradual and usually associated with a significant residual stenosis. One study comparing angioplasty to thrombolytic therapy found that patients treated with angioplasty achieved more complete reperfusion with smaller residual stenoses but had a higher incidence of serious ventricular arrhythmias, lending support to the concept that the occurrence of significant arrhythmias is related to the abruptness and completeness of reperfusion (109).

Large-scale thrombolytic trials have shown that the incidence of ventricular fibrillation and ventricular tachycardia in patients treated with thrombolytics is not different from that in patients who are given placebo (3,4,97) and may actually be decreased more than 3 hr after therapy is given (96). Several other studies have shown an increase in the occurrence of bradyarrhythmias with reperfusion, especially in the setting of an inferior infarction (3,110,111), and also a higher incidence of ventricular ectopy and accelerated idioventricular rhythm, which does not appear to be of any clinical significance (3,112). Although some arrhythmias are more prevalent with thrombolysis, they have not been useful as markers of reperfusion (113). There is no clear evidence that prophylactic antiarrhythmic therapy is warranted. In patients who are undergoing angioplasty of an occluded right coronary artery in the setting of acute MI, the risk of a serious bradyarrhythmia is high, and temporary pacing capabilities should be available (114). An intravenous injection of metaraminol (2 mg) is usually sufficient in reversing the Bezold-Jarisk reflex.

PACEMAKER THERAPY IN ACUTE MYOCARDIAL INFARCTION

Temporary pacemakers may be used either therapeutically for the treatment of symptomatic bradyarrhythmias and the conversion of supraventricular or ventricular tachyarrhythmias or prophylactically in patients who are at high risk for the development of complete AV block during acute MI (Table 4). Temporary pacing should be used with caution since it is not without complications. One series showed that temporary pacing was associated with a 20% complication rate, with the most frequent complications being ventricular tachycardia during insertion, fever, and phlebitis (115). In the present era of thrombolytic therapy with the high risk of bleeding complications during the lytic state and subsequent period of anticoagulation, one must be prudent with the use of invasive procedures. If a temporary pacemaker is indicated in a patient who has recently received thrombolytics or who is fully anticoagulated, either the brachial or femoral vein approach is preferable for central venous access because bleeding can be controlled, even though there is evidence from the prethrombolytic era that the right internal jugular approach has the lowest complication rate (116). With the advent of external

Table 4   Indications for Temporary Pacing in Acute Myocardial Infarction

Therapeutic
    Asystole
    Symptomatic sinus bradycardia unresponsive to atropine
    Symptomatic bradyarrhythmias secondary to AV block unresponsive to medical
        therapy in inferior infarction
    Any bradyarrhythmia caused by AV block in anterior infarctions
    Torsades de pointes
    Conversion of atrial flutter, PSVT, and ventricular tachycardia
Prophylactic
    Mobitz type II second-degree AV block
    New- or indeterminate-onset left bundle branch block
    New- or indeterminate-onset bilateral bundle branch block (right bundle with left
        anterior or posterior hemiblock and alternating bundle branch block)

temporary pacing, there is the potential to eliminate almost all complications of transvenous pacemakers when only brief periods of pacing are required or a prophylactic pacemaker is needed (117).

The primary indication for therapeutic temporary pacing in acute MI is high-degree AV block. Patients with anterior wall myocardial infarction who develop second- or third-degree AV block should undergo temporary pacing because this type of myocardial infarction is usually associated with significant destruction of the infranodal conduction system and an unstable escape rhythm (118). Patients with inferior MI who develop second- or third-degree AV block usually have block at the level of the AV node and a stable junctional escape rate at 50 to 60 bpm. These patients often do not require therapy, but if they do, they are usually responsive to medications such as atropine or aminophylline. In symptomatic patients who do not respond to drug therapy, temporary pacing is required. Of note is that patients with an associated right ventricular infarction may benefit from AV sequential pacing to optimize hemodynamics (119).

The treatment of tachyarrhythmias in acute MI is usually best handled with medications and DC countershock, but there are some instances in which pacing may be useful. In patients with torsades de pointes, temporary pacing at rates of 90-100 bpm may prevent recurrences of the tachycardia (72). Supraventricular tachyarrhythmias which may be treated with overdrive pacing include atrial flutter and PSVT (52,53). In some instances, ventricular tachycardia may also be terminated with overdrive pacing (120), but one must be cautious because of the potential to accelerate a previously stable tachycardia and cause hemodynamic collapse.

Prophylactic temporary pacemaker insertion is indicated in patients who are at high risk for developing complete AV block. A number of studies have examined the ECG predictors of complete AV block in acute MI (121-124). These studies have shown that patients at the highest risk for complete AV block are those with the new onset of bilateral bundle branch block associated with first-degree AV block, which carries up to a 38% risk for the development of high-degree AV block (122,123) (Fig. 6). The risk for developing complete heart block with a new-onset, isolated left bundle branch block is more controversial; Hindman et al. (122) reported a risk of only 11%. The generally accepted indications for prophylactic placement of a temporary pacemaker are new- or indeterminate-onset bilaterial bundle branch block (right bundle branch block with either left anterior or left posterior hemiblock and alternating bundle branch block), new- or indeterminate-onset left bundle branch block and Mobitz type II second-degree AV block (106). In patients who develop transient complete heart block in anterior MI, a permanent pacemaker before discharge is advisable since this may improve the 1-year survival by reducing the incidence of sudden death due to complete heart block (122,125).

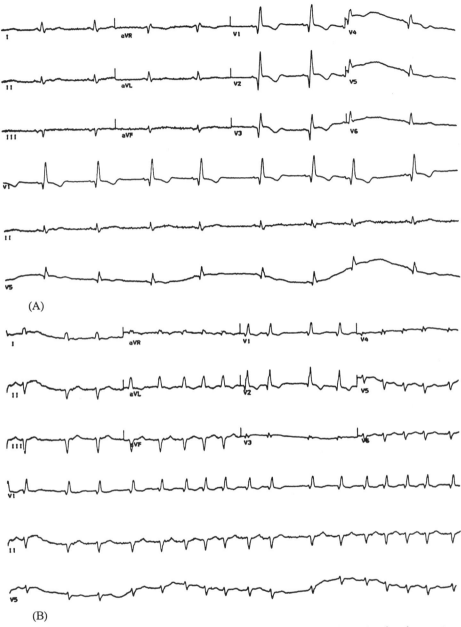

Figure 6 Bifascicular block. (A) This patient was admitted nearly 24 hr after the onset of chest pain. The initial ECG showed evidence of anterior MI and a right bundle branch block. (B) Later the patient developed atrial fibrillation and progressive left-axis deviation indicative of a left anterior hemiblock in combination with the right bundle branch block. A prophylactic temporary pacemaker was placed because of the new-onset bifascicular block, which is associated with a 30% incidence of progression to complete heart block.

ARRHYTHMIA RISK STRATIFICATION
POSTMYOCARDIAL INFARCTION

Ventricular tachyarrhythmias are the major cause of sudden cardiac death in the post-MI patient. Early studies found that both left ventricular dysfunction and complex ventricular ectopy were independent predictors for the occurrence of arrhythmic events in the first 2 years after MI (126,127). The MILIS study showed that patients with ejection fractions <40% and frequent ventricular ectopy (>10 VPDs per hour) had an 18% incidence of sudden cardiac death over a 2-year period whereas those with ejection fractions >40% and less than 10 VPDs per hour had only a 2% sudden cardiac death rate over 2 years (126). Importantly, in this study 79% of the sudden cardiac deaths occurred in the first 7 months post-MI.

Signal-averaged electrocardiograms (SAECG) have also been shown to predict arrhythmic events in the first year after MI (128,129). Patients with an abnormal SAECG have roughly a 20–30% arrhythmic event rate (VT or sudden cardiac death) compared to a <5% event rate for patients with a normal SAECG (128, 129). With the use of thrombolytic therapy, there is a four- to fivefold decrease in the incidence of abnormal SAECGs after MI (130). Using a combination of noninvasive tests (ejection fraction, SAECG, and 24-hr Holter), it is possible to identify patients at high risk of ventricular tachycardia and sudden cardiac death. Patients who have left ventricular dysfunction, ejection fraction <40%, an abnormal SAECG, and nonsustained ventricular tachycardia on a 24-hr Holter have an arrhythmic event rate of up to 50% at 1 year, whereas patients in which all these tests are normal have a very low risk (<2%) of a significant ventricular arrhythmia at 1 year post-MI (129). Although noninvasive testing may assist in risk stratification post-MI, the recent CAST study results have shown that Holter-guided arrhythmia therapy in the post-MI patient may result in increased mortality (131).

Therapy based on electrophysiological testing may reduce mortality in patients with spontaneous ventricular arrhythmias and aborted sudden cardiac death (132). However, the use of electrophysiology (EP) studies in the postinfarction period is controversial, because the incidence of inducibility of ventricular arrhythmias varies with the time from the MI, and the significance of these induced arrhythmias in patients without spontaneous arrhythmic events is not known. The incidence of inducibility during electrophysiological study increases from roughly 10% at 1 week post-MI to approximately 50% at 2–4 weeks and decreases again to about 30% at 4–5 months (133,134), showing the dynamic nature of the arrhythmic substrate during the healing phase in the post-MI period. In patients who have been successfully reperfused with thrombolytics, the incidence of inducibility at EP study is less than in patients who do not reperfuse, 12% versus 74% at 3–4 weeks post-MI in one trial (135). Another study indicated that inducible ventricular tachycardia at electrophysiological study was the best single predictor of spontaneous ventricular tachycardia or sudden cardiac death in the first year after MI when testing was done at 1–2 weeks post-MI, but this had a positive predictive value of only 30% (136).

There is mounting evidence that therapy guided by electrophysiological testing in patients with coronary artery disease, depressed LV function, and nonsustained ventricular tachycardia may reduce mortality. Wilber et al. found that in this high-risk subgroup, patients who were noninducible had a 6% 2-year cardiac arrest or sudden cardiac death rate, those who had inducible VT that was suppressed by drug therapy had roughly a 10% incidence of cardiac arrest or sudden cardiac death at 2 years, while those who had inducible VT that was not suppressible had a 50% event rate at 2 years (137). A reasonable approach to the post-MI patient is first to determine left ventricular function. If the patient has a depressed ejection fraction of <40%, a SAECG or a 24-hr Holter should be obtained. If either test is abnormal, the patient falls into a high-risk subgroup with a ventricular arrhythmic event rate of roughly 35% at 1 year (129), and electrophysiological testing is recommended. The evidence that this is an appropriate method for evaluating patients comes from nonrandomized clinical trials (137–139). Randomized clinical trials are needed to further define the role of electrophysiologically guided therapy in the post-MI patient.

REFERENCES

1. Adgey AAJ, Geddes JS, Webb SW, Allen JD, James RGG, Zaidi SA, Pantridge JF. Acute phase of myocardial infarction. Lancet 1971; 2:501–4.
2. O'Doherty M, Tayler DI, Quinn E, Vincent R, Chamberlin DA. Five hundred patients with myocardial infarction monitored within one hour of symptoms. Br Med J 1983; 286:1405–8.
3. The I.S.A.M. Study Group. A prospective trial of intravenous streptokinase in acute myocardial infarction (I.S.A.M.). N Engl J Med 1986; 314:1465–71.
4. AIMS Trial Study Group. Long term effects of intravenous anistreplase in acute myocardial infarction: final report of the AIMS study. Lancet 1990; 335:427–31.
5. Koren G, Weiss AT, Ben-David Y, Hasin Y, Luria MH, Gotsman MS. Bradycardia and hypotension following reperfusion with streptokinase (Bezold-Jarish reflex): a sign of coronary thrombolysis and myocardial salvage. Am Heart J 1986; 112:468–71.
6. Bigger JT, Dresdale RJ, Heissenbuttel RH, Weld FM, Wit AL. Ventricular arrhythmias in ischemic heart disease: mechanism, prevalence, significance, and management. Prog Cardiovasc Dis 1977; 19::255–300.
7. Grauer LE, Gershen BJ, Orlando MM, Epstein SE. Bradycardia and its complications in the prehospital phase of acute myocardial infarction. Am J Cardiol 1973; 32:607–11.
8. Scheinman MM, Thorburn D, Abbott JA. Use of atropine with acute myocardial infarction and sinus bradycardia. Circulation 1975; 52:627–33.
9. Warren JV, Lewis RP. Beneficial effects of atropine in the pre-hospital phase of coronary care. Am J Cardiol 1976; 37:69–72.

10. Chadda KD, Lichstein E, Gupta PK, Choy R. Bradycardia-hypotension syndrome acute myocardial infarction. Am J Med 1975; 59:158-64.
11. Dauchot P, Gravenstein JS. Bradycardia after myocardial ischemia and its treatment with atropine. Anesthesiology 1976; 44:501-10.
12. Rotman M, Wagner GS, Wallace AG. Bradyarrhythmias in acute myocardial infarction. Circulation 1972; 45:703-18.
13. Cooper MJ, Abinader EG. Atropine induced ventricular fibrillation: case report and review of the literature. Am Heart J 1979; 97:225-7.
14. Massumi RA, Mason DT, Amsterdam EA, DeMaria A, Miller RR, Scheinman MM, Zelis R. Ventricular fibrillation and tachycardia after intravenous atropine for the treatment of bradycardia. N Engl J Med 1972; 287:336-8.
15. Standards and guidelines for cardiopulmonary resuscitation and emergency cardiac care. JAMA 1986; 225:2841-3044.
16. Vatner SF, Baig H. Comparison of the effects of oubain and isoproterenol on ischemic myocardium of conscious dogs. Circulation 1978; 58:654-62.
17. Norris RM. Heart block in posterior and anterior myocardial infarction. Br Heart J 1969; 31:352-6.
18. Italian Group for the Study of Streptokinase in Myocardial Infarction (GISSI). Effectiveness of intravenous thrombolytic treatment in acute myocardial infarction. Lancet 1986; 1:397-407.
19. Clemmensen P, Bates ER, Califf RM, Hlatky M, Aronson L, George BS, Lee K, Kereiakas DJ, Gacioch G, Berrios E, Topol EJ, and the TAMI Study Group. Complete atrioventricular block complicating inferior wall myocardial infarction treated with reperfusion therapy. Am J Cardiol 1991; 67:225-30.
20. Berger PB, Thomas RJ. Inferior myocardial infarction high risk subgroups. Circulation 1990; 81:401-11.
21. Berger PB, Ruocco NA, Jacobs AK, Ryan TJ, and the TIMI Investigators. Increased mortality associated with heart block during inferior infarction. Results from TIMI II. Circulation 1989; 80(Suppl II):II-347 (abstract).
22. Nicod P, Gilpin E, Dittrich H, Polikar R, Henning H, Ross J. Long term outcome in patients with inferior myocardial infarction and complete atrioventricular block. J Am Coll Cardiol 1988; 12:589-94.
23. Feigl D, Ashkenazy J, Kishon Y. Early and late atrioventricular block in acute inferior myocardial infarction. J Am Coll Cardiol 1984; 4:35-8.
24. Wesley RC, Lerman BB, DiMarco JP, Berne RM, Belardinelli L. Mechanism of atropine-resistant atrioventricular block during inferior myocardial infarction: possible role of adenosine. J Am Coll Cardiol 1986; 8:1232-4.
25. Shah PK, Nalos P, Peter T. Atropine resistant post infarction complete AV block: possible role of adenosine and improvement with aminophylline. Am Heart J 1987; 113:194-5.
26. Jewitt DE, Raferty EB, Balcon R, Oram S. Incidence and management of supraventricular arrhythmias after acute myocardial infarction. Lancet 1967; 1: 724-8.
27. Hjalmarson A, Gilpin E, Kjekshus J, Schieman G, Nicod P, Henning H, Ross J. Influence of heart rate on mortality after myocardial infarction. Am J Cardiol 1990; 65: 547-53.

28. Crimm A, Severance HW, Coffey K, McKinnis R, Wagner GS, Califf RM. Prognostic significance of isolated sinus tachycardia during first three days of acute myocardial infarction. Am J Med 1984; 76:983-8.

29. Webb SW, Adgey AA, Pantridge JF. Autonomic disturbances at the onset of acute myocardial infarction. Br Med J 1972; 3:89-95.

30. The TIMI Study Group. Comparison of invasive and conservative strategies after treatment with intravenous tissue plasminogen activator in acute myocardial infarction. N Engl J Med 1989; 320:618-27.

31. Conti RC. Beta-adrenergic blockade and acute myocardial infarction. J Am Coll Cardiol 1989; 14:1824-5.

32. Hunt D, Sloman G, Penington C. Effects of atrial fibrillation on prognosis of acute myocardial infarction. Br Heart J 1978; 40:303-7.

33. Sugiura T, Iwasaka T, Ogawa A, Shiroyama Y, Tsuji H, Onoyama H, Inada M. Atrial fibrillation in acute myocardial infarction. Am J Cardiol 1985; 56:27-9.

34. Helmers C, Lundman T, Morgensen L, Orinius E, Sjogren A, Wester PO. Atrial fibrillation in acute myocardial infarction. Acta Med Scand 1973; 193:39-44.

35. Goldberg RJ, Seeley D, Becker RC, Brady P, Chen Z, Osganian V, Gore JM, Alpert JS, Dalen JE. Impact of atrial fibrillation on the in-hospital and long-term survival of patients with acute myocardial infarction: a community-wide perspective. Am Heart J 1990; 119:996-1001.

36. Cristal N, Peterburg I, Szwarberg J. Atrial fibrillation developing the acute phase of myocardial infarction, prognostic implications. Chest 1976; 70:8-11.

37. Liberthson RR, Salisbury KW, Hutter AM, Desanctis RW. Atrial tachyarrhythmias in acute myocardial infarction. Am J Med 1976; 60:956-60.

38. Hod H, Lew AS, Keltai M, Cereck B, Geft II, Shah PK, Ganz W. Early atrial fibrillation during evolving myocardial infarction: a consequence of impaired left atrial perfusion. Circulation 1987; 75:146-50.

39. Klein HO, Kaplinsky E. Verapamil and digoxin: their respective effects on atrial fibrillation and their interaction. Am J Cardiol 1982; 50:894-901.

40. David D, Segni ED, Klein HO, Kaplinsky E. Inefficacy of digitalis in the control of heart rate in patients with chronic atrial fibrillation: beneficial effect of an added beta adrenergic blocking agent. Am J Cardiol 1979; 44:1378-81.

41. Marcus FI. Use of digitalis in acute myocardial infarction. Circulation 1980; 62:17-9.

42. Rinkenberger RL, Prystowsky EN, Heger JJ, Troup PJ, Jackman WM, Zipes DP. Effects of intravenous and chronic oral verapamil administration in patients with supraventricular tachyarrhythmias. Circulation 1980; 62:996-1009.

43. Hagemeijer F. Verapamil in the management of supraventricular tachyarrhythmias occurring after a recent myocardial infarction. Circulation 1978; 57:751-5.

44. Waxman HL, Myerburg RJ, Appel R, Sung RJ. Verapamil for control of ventricular rate in paroxysmal tachycardia and atrial fibrillation. Ann Intern Med 1981; 94:1-6.

45. Lemberg L, Castellanos A, Arcebal AG. The use of propranolol in arrhythmias complicating acute myocardial infarction. Am Heart J 1970; 80:479-87.

46. Morganroth J, Horowitz LN, Anderson J, Turlapaty P, and the Esmolol Research

Group. Comparative efficacy and tolerance of esmolol to propranolol for control of supraventricular tachyarrhythmia. Am J Cardiol 1985; 56:33F-39F.

47. Kirshenbaum JM, Kloner RA, Antman EM, Braunwauld E. Use of an ultra short-acting beta-blocker in patients with acute myocardial ischemia. Circulation 1985; 72:873-80.

48. Gold MR, Dec GW, Cocca-Spofford D, Thompson T. Acute intravenous beta blockade with esmolol in cardiac patients with chronic obstructive pulmonary disease. J Am Coll Cardiol 1990; 15:24A (abstract).

49. Fenster PE, Comes KA, Marsh R, Katzenberg C, Hager D. Conversion of atrial fibrillation to sinus rhythm by acute intravenous procainamide infusion. Am Heart J 1983; 106:501-4.

50. Kessler KM, Kayden DS, Estes DM, Koslovskis PL, Sequeira R, Trohman RG, Palomo AR, Myerburg RJ. Procainamide pharmacokinetics in patients with acute myocardial infarction or congestive heart failure. J Am Coll Cardiol 1986; 7:1131-9.

51. DeSanctis RW, Block P, Hutter A. Tachyarrhythmias in myocardial infarction. Circulation 1972; 45:681-703.

52. Greenberg ML, Kelly TA, Lerman BB, DiMarco JP. Atrial pacing for conversion of atrial flutter. Am J Cardiol 1986; 58:95-9.

53. Das G, Anand GM, Ankineedu K, Chinnavaso T, Talmers FN, Weissler AM. Atrial pacing for cardioversion of atrial flutter in digitalized patients. Am J Cardiol 1978; 41:308-11.

54. Resnekov L. Present status of electroversion in the management of cardiac dysrhythmias. Circulation 1973; 47:1356-63.

55. Belhassen B, Pelleg A. Acute management of paroxysmal supraventricular tachycardia: verapamil, adenosine triphosphate or adenosine? Am J Cardiol 1984; 54:225-7.

56. Gasrratt C, Linker N, Griffith M, Ward D, Camm AJ. Comparison of adenosine and verapamil for termination of paroxysmal junctional tachycardia. Am J Cardiol 1989; 64:1310-6.

57. Viskin S, Belhassen B. Acute management of paroxysmal atrioventricular junctional reentrant supraventricular tachycardia: Pharmacologic strategies. Am Heart J 1990; 120:180-7.

58. Vidt DG, Baskt AW. Adenosine: a new drug for acute termination of supraventricular tachycardia. Cleveland Clin J Med 1990: 383-7.

59. Campbell RWF, Murray A, Julian DG. Ventricular arrhythmias in the first 12 hours of acute myocardial infarction. Br Heart J 1981; 46:351-7.

60. El-Sherif N, Myerburg RJ, Scherlag BJ, Befeler B, Aranda JM, Castellanos A, Lazzara R. Electrocardiographic antecedents of primary ventricular fibrillation, value of the R-on-T phenomenon in myocardial infarction. Br Heart J 1976; 38:415-22.

61. Miller FC, Kruchoff MW, Satler LF, Green CE, Fletcher RD, Del Negro AA, Pearle DL, Kent K, Rackey CE. Ventricular arrhythmias during reperfusion. Am Heart J 1986; 112:928-31.

62. De Soyza N, Bissett JK, Kane JJ, Murphy ML, Doherty JE. Association of accelerated idioventricular rhythm and paroxysmal ventricular tachycardia in acute myocardial infarction. Am J Cardiol 1974; 34:667-70.

63. Lichstein E, Ribas-Meneclier C, Gupta PK, Chadda KD. Incidence and description of accelerated ventricular rhythm complicating acute myocardial infarction. Am J Med 1975; 58:192-8.

64. Talbot S, Greaves M. Association of ventricular tachycardia with idioventricular rhythm. Br Heart J 1976; 38:457-64.

65. Campbell RWF. Treatment and prophylaxis of ventricular arrhythmias in acute myocardial infarction. Am J Cardiol 1983; 52:55C-59C.

66. Tofler GH, Stone PH, Muller JE, Rutherford JD, Willich SN, Gustafson NF, Poole JD, Sobel BE, Willerson JT, Robertson T, Passamani E, Braunwald E, and the MILIS Study Group. Prognosis after cardiac arrest due to ventricular tachycardia or ventricular fibrillation associated with acute myocardial infarction (the MILIS study). Am J Cardiol 1987; 60:755-61.

67. Kleiman RB, Miller JM, Buxton AE, Josephson ME, Marchlinski FE. Prognosis following sustained ventricular tachycardia occurring early after myocardial infarction. Am J Cardiol 1988; 62:528-33.

68. Marchlinski FE, Waxman HL, Buxton AE, Josephson ME. Sustained ventricular tachyarrhythmias during the early post-infarction period: electrophysiologic findings and prognosis for survival. J Am Coll Cardiol 1983; 2:240-50.

69. Tsivoni D, Keren A, Stern S. Torsades de pointes versus polymorphous ventricular tachycardia. Am J Cardiol 1983; 52:639-40.

70. Brugada, P. "Torsade de pointes." PACE 1988; 11:2246-9.

71. Nordrehaug JE, Lippe GVD. Serum potassium concentrations are inversely related to ventricular, but not to atrial, arrhythmias in acute myocardial infarction. Eur Heart J 1986; 7:204-9.

72. Keren A, Tzivoni D, Gavish D, Levi J, Gottleib S, Benhorin J, Stern S. Etiology, warning signs and therapy of torsades de pointes. Circulation 1981; 64:1167-73.

73. Tzivoni D, Banai S, Schuger C, Benhorin J, Keren A, Gottlieb S, Stern S. Treatment of torsades de pointes with magnesium sulfate. Circulation 1988; 77:392-7.

74. Ribner HS, Isaacs ES, Frishman WH. Lidocaine prophylaxis against ventricular fibrillation in acute myocardial infarction. Prog Cardiovasc Dis 1979; 21:287-310.

75. Davison R, Parker M, Atkinson AJ. Excessive serum lidocaine levels during maintenance infusions: mechanisms and prevention. Am Heart J 1982; 104:203-8.

76. Giardina ECV, Heissenbuttel RH, Bigger JT. Correlation of plasma concentration of procainamide with effect on arrhythmia, electrocardiogram, and blood pressure. Ann Intern Med 1973; 78:183-93.

77. Myerburg RJ, Kessler KM, Kiem I, Pefkaros KC, Conde CA, Cooper D, Castellanos A. Relationship between plasma levels of procainamide, suppression of premature ventricular complexes and prevention of recurrent ventricular. Circulation 1981; 64: 280-90.

78. Schienman MM, Weiss AN, Shafton E, Benowitz, N, Rowland M. Electrophysiologic effects of procainamide in patients with intraventricular conduction delay. Circulation 1974; 49:522-9.

79. Dhurandhar RW, Teasdale SJ, Mahon WA. Bretylium tosylate in the management of refractory ventricular fibrillation. Can Med Assoc J 1971; 105:161-5.

80. Holder DA, Sniderman AD, Fraser G, Fallen EL. Experience with bretylium tosylate by a hospital cardiac arrest team. Circulation 1977; 55:541-4.

81. Haynes RE, Chinn TL, Copass MK, Cobb LA. Comparison of bretylium tosylate and lidocaine in management of out of hospital ventricular fibrillation: a randomized clinical trial. Am J Cardiol 1981; 48:353-6.

82. Anderson JL, Patterson E, Conlon M, Pasyk S, Pitt B, Lucchesi BR. Kinetics of antifibrillatory effects of bretylium: correlation with myocardial drug concentrations. Am J Cardiol 1980; 46:583-91.

83. Sanna G, Arcidiacono R. Chemical ventricular defibrillation of the human heart with bretylium tosylate. Am J Cardiol 1973; 32:982-7.

84. Chatterjee K, Mandel WJ, Vyden JK, Parmley WW, Forrester JS. Cardiovascular effects of bretylium tosylate in acute myocardial infarction. JAMA 1973; 223: 757-61.

85. Koch-Wesler J. Medical intelligence: drug therapy, bretylium. N Engl J Med 1979; 300:473-7.

86. Ochi RP, Goldenberg IF, Almquist A, Pritzker M, Milstein S, Pedersen W, Gobel FL, Benditt DG. Intravenous amiodarone for the rapid treatment of life-threatening ventricular arrhythmias in critically ill patients with coronary artery disease. Am J Cardiol 1989; 64:599-603.

87. Mooss AN, Mohiuddin SM, Hee TT, Esterbrooks DJ, Hillerman DE, Rovang KS, Sketch MH. Efficacy and tolerance of high-dose intravenous amiodarone for recurrent, refractory ventricular tachycardia. Am J Cardiol 1990; 65:609-14.

88. Williams ML, Woelfel A, Cascio WE, Simpson RJ, Gettes LS, Foster JR. Intravenous amiodarone during prolonged resuscitation from cardiac arrest. Ann Intern Med 1989; 110:839-42.

89. Morady F, Scheinman MM, Shen E, Shapiro W, Sung RJ, DiCarlo L. Intravenous amiodarone in the acute treatment of recurrent symptomatic ventricular tachycardia. Am J Cardiol 1983; 51:156-9.

90. Kadish A, Morady F. The use of intravenous amiodarone in the acute therapy of life-threatening tachyarrhythmias. Prog Cardiovasc Dis 1989; 31:281-94.

91. Levine J, Massumi A, Scheinman MM, Winkle RA. The intravenous amiodarone multi-center study group: preliminary report. 1990; 15:27A (abstract).

92. Escoubet B, Coumel P, Poirier JM, Maison-Blanche P, Jaillon P, LeClerq JF, Menasche P, Cheymol G, Piwnica A, Lagier G, Slama R. Suppression of arrhythmias within hours after a single oral dose of amiodarone and relation to plasma and myocardial concentrations. Am J Cardiol 1985; 55:696-702.

93. Mostow ND, Vrobel TR, Noon D, Rakita L. Rapid suppression of complex ventricular arrhythmias with high-dose oral amiodarone. Circulation 1986; 73:1231-8.

94. Bourke JP, Hilton CJ, McComb JM, Cowan JC, Tansuphaswadikul S, Kertes PJ, Campbell RWF. Surgery for control of life-threatening ventricular tachyarrhythmias within 2 months of myocardial infarction. J Am Coll Cardiol 1990; 16:42-8.

95. Dalzell GWN, Cunningham SR, Wilson CM, Allen JD, Anderson J, Adgey AAJ. Ventricular defibrillation: the Belfast experience. Br Heart 1987; 58:441-6.

96. Schroder R. Editorial: ventricular fibrillation complicating myocardial infarction. N Engl J Med 1987; 318:381-2.

97. Volpi A, Maggioni A, Franzosi MG, Pampallona S, Mauri F, Tognoni G. In-hospital prognosis of patients with acute myocardial infarction complicated by primary ventricular fibrillation. N Engl J Med 1987; 317:257-61.

98. Nicod P, Gilpin E, Dittrich H, Wright M, Engler R, Rittlemeyer J, Henning H, Ross J. Late clinical outcome in patients with early ventricular fibrillation after myocardial infarction. J Am Coll Cardiol 1988; 11:464-70.

99. Volpi A, Cavalli A, Franzosi MG, Maggioni A, Mauri F, Santoro E, Tognoni G, and the GISSI Investigators. One-year prognosis of primary ventricular fibrillation complicating acute myocardial infarction. Am J Cardiol 1989; 63:1174-8.

100. Lie KI, Wellens HJ, Capelle FJV, Durrer D. Lidocaine in the prevention of primary ventricular fibrillation. N Engl J Med 1974; 291:1324-6.

101. Valentine PA, Frew JL, Mashford ML, Sloman JG. Lidocaine in the prevention of sudden death in the pre-hospital phase of acute infarction. N Engl J Med 1974; 291: 1327-31.

102. Koster RW, Dunning AJ. Intramuscular lidocaine for the prevention of lethal arrhythmias in the prehospitalization phase of acute myocardial infarction. N Engl J Med 1985; 313:1105-10.

103. Hine LK, Laird N, Hewitt P, Chalmers TC. Meta-analytic evidence against prophylactic use of lidocaine in acute myocardial infarction. Arch Intern Med 1989; 149: 2694-8.

104. Yusuf S, Wittes J, Friedman L. Overview of results of randomized clinical trials in heart disease. JAMA 1988; 260:2088-93.

105. Naito M, Michelson EL, Kmetzo JJ, Kaplinsky E, Dreifus LS. Failure of antiarrhythmic drugs to prevent experimental reperfusion ventricular fibrillation. Circulation 1981; 63:70-9.

106. Gunnar RM, Bourdillon PDV, Dixon DW, Fuster V, Karp RB, Kennedy JW, Klocke FJ, Passamani ER, Pitt B, Rappaport E, Reeves TJ, Russell RO, Sobel BE, Winters WL. ACC/AHA guidelines for the early management of patients with acute myocardial infarction. Circulation 1990; 82:664-707.

107. Kaplinsky E, Ogawa S, Michelson EL, Dreifus LS. Instantaneous and delayed ventricular arrhythmias after reperfusion of acutely ischemic myocardium: evidence for multiple mechanisms. Circulation 1981; 63:333-40.

108. Battle WE, Naimi S, Avitall B, Brilla AH, Banas JS, Bete JM, Levine HJ. Distinctive time course of ventricular vulnerability to fibrillation during and after release of coronary ligation. Am J Cardiol 1974; 34:42-7.

109. Timmis GC, Ramos RG, Gangadharan V, Gordon S. Determinants of reperfusion arrhythmias in a randomized trial of streptokinase vs angioplasty for acute myocardial infarction. Circulation 1985; 72:III-218 (abstract).

110. Esente P, Giambartolomei A, Gensini GG, Dator C. Coronary reperfusion and Bezold-Jarisch reflex (bradycardia and hypotension). Am J Cardiol 1983; 52:221-4.

111. Gore JM, Bull SP, Corrao JM, Goldberg RJ. Arrhythmias in the assessment of coronary artery reperfusion following thrombolytic therapy. Chest 1988; 94:727-30.

112. Cercek B, Lew AS, Laramee P, Shah PK, Peter TC, Ganz W. Time course and characteristics of ventricular arrhythmias after reperfusion in acute myocardial infarction. Am J Cardiol 1987; 60:214-8.

113. Califf RM, O'Neill W, Stack RS, Aronson L, Mark DB, Mantell S, George BS, Candella RJ, Kereiakes DJ, Abbottsmith C, Topol EJ, and the TAMI study group. Failure of simple clinical measurements to predict perfusion status after intravenous thrombolysis. Ann Intern Med 1988; 108:658-62.

114. Gacioch GM, Topol EJ. Sudden paradoxic clinical deterioration during angioplasty of the occluded right coronary artery in acute myocardial infarction. J Am Coll Cardiol 1989; 14:1202-9.

115. Austin JL, Preis LK, Crampton RS, Beller GA, Martin RP. Analysis of pacemaker malfunction and complications of temporary pacing in the coronary care unit. Am J Cardiol 1982; 49:301-6.

116. Hynes JK, Holmes DR, Harrison CE. Five year experience with temporary pacemaker therapy in the coronary care unit. Mayo Clin Proc 1983; 58:122-6.

117. Zoll PM, Zoll RH, Falk RH, Clinton JE, Eitel DR, Antman EM. External noninvasive temporary cardiac pacing: clinical trials. 1985; 71:937-44.

118. Scheinman MM, Gonzalez RP. Fascicular block and acute myocardial infarction. JAMA 1980; 244:2646-9.

119. Topol EJ, Goldschlager N, Ports TA, DiCarlo LA, Schiller NB, Botvinick EH, Chatterjee K. Hemodynamic benefit of atrial pacing in right ventricular myocardial infarction. Ann Intern Med 1982; 96:594-7.

120. Fisher JD, Mahra R, Furman S. Termination of ventricular tachycardia with bursts of rapid ventricular pacing. Am J Cardiol 1978; 41:94-102.

121. Hindman MC, Wagner GS, Jaro M, Atkins JM, Scheinman MM, DeSanctis RW, Hutter AH, Yeatmen L, Rubenfire M, Pujura C, Rubin M, Morris JJ. The clinical significance of bundle branch block complicating acute myocardial infarction: clinical characteristics, hospital mortality, and one year follow up. Circulation 1978; 58: 679-88.

122. Hindman MC, Wagner GS, Jaro M, Atkins JM, Scheinman MM, DeSanctis RW, Hutter AH, Yeatmen L, Rubenfire M, Pujura C, Rubin M, Morris JJ. The clinical significance of bundle branch block complicating acute myocardial infarction: indications for temporary and permanent pacemaker insertion. Circulation 1978; 58: 689-99.

123. Lamas GA, Muller JE, Turi ZG, Stone PH, Rutherford JD, Jaffe AS, Raabe DS, Rude RE, Mark DB, Califf RM, Gold HK, Robertson T, Passamani ER, Braunwald E, and the MILIS study group. A simplified method to predict occurrence of complete heart block during acute myocardial infarction. Am J Cardiol 1986; 57:1213-9.

124. Hollander G, Nadiminti V, Lichstein E, Greengart A, Sanders M. Bundle branch block in acute myocardial infarction. Am Heart J 1983; 105:738-43.

125. Frye RL, Collins JJ, DeSantis RW, Dodge HT, Dreifus LS, Fisch C, Gettes LS, Gillettte PC, Parsonnet V, Reeves TJ, Weinberg SL. Guidelines for permanent cardiac pacemaker implantation: a report of the joint American College of Cardiology/ American Heart Association task force on assessment of cardiovascular procedures (subcommittee on pacemaker implantation). J Am Coll Cardiol 1984; 4:434-42.

126. Mukharji J, Rude RE, Poole K, Gustafson N, Thomas LJ, Strauss W, Jaffe AS, Muller JE, Roberts R, Raabe D, Croft CH, Passamani E, Braunwald E, Willerson JT,

and the MILIS Study Group. Risk factors for sudden death after acute myocardial infarction: two-year follow-up. Am J Cardiol 1984; 54:31-6.

127. Bigger JT, Fleiss JL, Kleiger R, Miller JP, Rolnitzky LM, and The Multicenter Post-Infarction Research Group. The relationships among ventricular arrhythmias, left ventricular dysfunction, and mortality in the 2 years after myocardial infarction. Circulation 1984; 69(2):250-8.

128. Kuchar DL, Thorburn CW, Sammel NL. Late potentials detected after myocardial infarction: natural history and prognostic significance. Circulation 1986; 74(6): 1280-9.

129. Gomes JA, Winters SL, Stewart D, Horowitz S, Milner M, Barreca P. A new noninvasive index to predict sustained ventricular tachycardia and sudden death in the first year after myocardial infarction: based on signal-averaged electrocardiogram, radionuclide ejection fraction and holter monitoring. J Am Coll Cardiol 1987; 10: 349-57.

130. Gang ES, Lew AS, Hong M, Wang FZ, Siebert CA, Peter T. Decreased incidence of ventricular late potentials after successful thrombolytic therapy for acute myocardial infarction. N Engl J Med 1989; 321:712-6.

131. The Cardiac Arrhythmia Suppression Trial (CAST) Investigators: Preliminary report: effect of encainide and flecainide on mortality in a randomized trial of arrhythmia suppression after myocardial infarction. N Engl J Med 1989; 321:406-12.

132. Waller TH, Kay HR, Spielman SR, Kutalek SP, Greenspan AM, Horowitz LN. Reduction in sudden death and total mortality by antiarrhythmic therapy evaluated by electrophysiologic drug testing: criteria of efficacy in patients with sustained tachyarrhythmia. J Am Coll Cardiol 1987; 10:83-9.

133. Kuck K-H, Costard A, Schluter M, Kunze K-P. Significance of timing programmed electrical stimulation after acute myocardial infarction. J Am Coll Cardiol 1986; 8:1279-88.

134. Bhandari AK, Au PK, Rose JS, Kotlewski A, Blue S, Rahimtoola SH. Decline in inducibility of sustained ventricular tachycardia from two to twenty weeks after acute myocardial infarction. Am J Cardiol 1987; 59:284-90.

135. Kersschot IE, Brugada P, Ramentol M, Zehender M, Waldecker B, Stevenson WG, Geibel A, De Zwaan C, Wellens HJJ. Effects of early reperfusion in acute myocardial infarction on arrhythmias induced by programmed stimulation: a prospective, randomized study. J Am Coll Cardiol 1986; 7:1234-42.

136. Richards DAB, Byth K, Ross DL, Uther JB. What is the best predictor of spontaneous ventricular tachycardia and sudden death after myocardial infarction? Circulation 1991; 83:756-63.

137. Wilber DJ, Olshansky B, Moran JF, Scanlon PJ. Electrophysiological testing and nonsustained ventricular tachycardia. Use and limitations in patients with coronary artery disease and impaired ventricular function. Circulation 1990; 82:350-8.

138. Buxton AE, Marchlinski FE, Flores BT, Miller JM, Doherty JU, Josephson ME. Nonsustained ventricular tachycardia in patients with coronary artery disease: role of electrophysiologic study. Circulation 1987; 75(6):1178-87.

139. Klein RC, Machell C. Use of electrophysiologic testing in patients with nonsustained ventricular tachycardia: prognostic and therapeutic implications. J Am Coll Cardiol 1989; 14:155-61.

III

ADJUNCTIVE MECHANICAL THERAPY

18

Adjunctive Coronary Angioplasty After Thrombolytic Therapy for Acute Myocardial Infarction

Stephen G. Ellis
The Cleveland Clinic Foundation, Cleveland, Ohio

INTRODUCTION

Atherosclerotic plaque comprises on average 85% of the material obstructing coronary arteries in patients presenting with acute myocardial infarction (1). The concern that a high-grade residual stenosis after thrombolytic therapy might predispose to recurrent ischemia (2,3) or impair left ventricular functional recovery (4), as well as the failure of lytic therapy to recanalize 10-45% of coronary arteries (5-9) has stimulated tremendous interest in the potential value of percutaneous transluminal coronary angioplasty (PTCA) as an adjunct to thrombolytic therapy in the treatment of patients with acute infarction. However, it has long been recognized that the results of angioplasty are less than optimal in the presence of thrombus (10,11). The results of the recent randomized trials (12-16) have suggested that for most patients treated with intravenous thrombolytic therapy, early coronary angioplasty is not necessary and may, in fact, be harmful. This chapter will review the utility of coronary angioplasty in the several clinical settings after thrombolytic therapy in which it may be considered.

REPERFUSION THERAPY: MECHANISM OF BENEFIT

That intravenous thrombolytic therapy for acute myocardial infarction improves patient survival for those treated early after infarction by 20–25% is indisputable (17–19). However, the mechanism of benefit is controversial. The initial concept that reperfusion would salvage sufficient myocardium to improve left ventricular ejection fraction (LVEF), known from the prereperfusion era to be a strong correlate of both short- and long-term mortality after myocardial infarction (20,21), is now disputed because although many studies have demonstrated improved survival after thrombolytic therapy, few have demonstrated more than minimal improvement of left ventricular function (22–27). It has been suggested that this "function-mortality paradox" may be due to the failure to obtain left ventricular function studies in patients destined to die and thus the function measurements acquired may not be representative of the treatment groups as a whole (28). Nonetheless, the improved survival of patients leaving the hospital with a patent infarct artery, regardless of left ventricular function (29,30), as well as an apparent striking beneficial effect of reperfusion on the reduction of malignant ventricular arrhythmias (31,34), has cast doubt on the importance of salvage of large amounts of ventricular myocardium as the mechanism for improved survival with reperfusion therapy. Additional studies have suggested that even relatively late reperfusion, by means of salvaging an epicardial rim of viable myocardium or by changing the physical properties of the infarcted area, may lead to a reduction in the deleterious effects of infarct expansion (35–39). It is within this pathophysiological framework that the influence of coronary angioplasty in the setting of acute myocardial infarction must be considered.

POTENTIAL MECHANISMS OF BENEFIT BY CORONARY ANGIOPLASTY

In the many clinical settings after administration of thrombolytic therapy, coronary angioplasty might be beneficial by several mechanisms: (a) increasing infarct artery patency, (b) decreasing residual stenosis in the infarct artery, (c) reducing reocclusion compared with pharmacological treatment of the residual stenosis after thrombolytic therapy, and (d) altering the degree of potential "reperfusion injury." The importance of each of these mechanisms and the outcome after angioplasty in varied settings after thrombolytic therapy will be discussed.

THE TIMING OF CORONARY ANGIOPLASTY

The clinical setting and timing of coronary angioplasty after thrombolytic therapy are critical to its outcome. In general, coronary angioplasty can be applied in one of four settings:

1. Urgent coronary angioplasty after successful thrombolytic therapy
2. Rescue coronary angioplasty for failed thrombolytic therapy
3. "Retrieval" angioplasty for recurrent ischemia after successful thrombolytic therapy
4. Late coronary angioplasty prior to hospital discharge

URGENT CORONARY ANGIOPLASTY AFTER SUCCESSFUL THROMBOLYSIS

The rationale for the performance of urgent angioplasty after successful thrombolysis was based on the supposition that by decreasing the degree of residual stenosis, angioplasty might both decrease recurrent ischemia and improve left ventricular functional recovery. Several small-scale studies evaluating recurrent ischemia after intracoronary or intravenous streptokinase had suggested that recurrent ischemia was more common when a high-grade stenosis remained after thrombolysis (2,3,40,41). For example, in 60 patients Serruys had retrospectively noted that when a ≥58% diameter stenosis remained after thrombolysis, 63% of patients developed recurrent ischemia, whereas the risk of recurrent ischemia with a lesser stenosis was only 6%. In addition, some experimental work suggested that regional left ventricular functional recovery was superior when a vascular clamp had been removed after restoration of coronary flow compared to the effect of a partially occlusive residual stenosis (4).

This concept of enhanced ventricular recovery with lessened residual stenosis severity received initial clinical support from the work of O'Neill et al., who found in a small series of patients that recovery of LVEF was superior with coronary angioplasty compared with intracoronary streptokinase, in spite of similar patency rates (ΔLVEF: 8 ± 7 versus 1 ± 6, p = <0.001), presumably owing to the difference in residual stenosis (43 ± 31% with angioplasty versus 83 ± 17% with streptokinase) (42). These results could not be confirmed by subsequent small-scale trials of coronary angioplasty versus intravenous thrombolytic therapy, performed by DeWood (43) and Ribeiro et al. (44), although the concept has been supported by analyses performed by Sheehan et al. (45). Balanced against these potential gains are the possibility of closing an infarct artery that had been opened with thrombolytic therapy, the probability that 15% of patients with an apparent severe stenosis early after thrombolytic therapy might eventually have <50% stenosis (46), that even were the stenosis to be left alone no inducible myocardial ischemia might be demonstrated in a substantial portion of patients (47), and the cost of performing the many angioplasties that might be required. Three moderate-scale, randomized trials have been performed to assess the utility of coronary angioplasty in this setting (see Table 1) (12-14). The Thrombolysis and Angioplasty in Myocardial Infarction (TAMI) investigators screened 386 patients with emergency angiography 90 min after administration of tissue plasminogen

Table 1   Trials of Immediate Coronary Angioplasty After Thrombolysis

	TAMI (12)	TIMI-2A (13)	ECSG (14)
Patients	386	389	367
Thrombolytic agents	t-PA (100 mg)	t-PA (100–150 mg)	t-PA (100 mg)
Angiography before randomization	Yes	No	No
Patients actually having PTCA who were randomized to that group (%)	68	70	92
Immediate PTCA			
In-hospital mortality (%)	4.0	7.7	6.6
Predischarge LVEF (%)	53	50	51
Reocclusion (%)	11	NR	12
No immediate PTCA			
In-hospital mortality (%)	1.0	5.1	2.7
Predischarge LVEF (%)	56	49	51
Reocclusion (%)	13	NR	11

LVEF = left ventricular ejection fraction; PTCA = percutaneous transluminal coronary angioplasty; t-PA = recombinant tissue plasminogen activator.

activator (t-PA) and in the 197 with a patent infarct artery and anatomy suitable for PTCA, randomly allocated half the patients to immediate angioplasty and half to no further immediate mechanical intervention (12). The primary endpoint of the study, the first to report on this topic, was recovery of LVEF. There were no between-group differences in the changes in ejection fraction from baseline to follow-up (1.1 ± 8.4% for angioplasty versus 1.3 ± 8.0% for conservative therapy, p = NS). Improvements in regional infarct zone function were seen in both groups, but there was no difference in recovery between the angioplasty and conservatively managed groups (0.37 ± 0.9 versus 0.43 ± 1.0 sd/chord, p = NS). Importantly, in the two reports that followed in rapid succession, from the Thrombolysis in Myocardial Infarction (TIMI) (13) and the European Cooperative Study Group (14), despite the minor differences in study protocol the results were similar, with no improvement in left ventricular functional recovery in the angioplasty groups (Table 1). The studies also reported concordant trends toward higher mortality after coronary angioplasty (6.9% versus 3.4%, in aggregate, p = 0.027), an increase in emergency bypass surgery after angioplasty (2.3% versus 0.6%, in aggregate, p = 0.03), and no difference in the incidence of reocclusion or early reinfarction (6.7% versus 6.9%, in aggregate, p = NS). Importantly, emergency angioplasty was successful in only 86.2% of patients, compared to 94.8% of patients when later angioplasty was required in the conservatively managed patients (p = 0.01).

Widespread acceptance of these findings has occurred, but some have criticized these studies suggesting that (a) intervention was performed too late to be able to demonstrate an improvement in functional recovery even if the degree of residual stenosis had made a difference, (b) the results are not necessarily generalizable to all thrombolytic agents, and (c) subgroups of patients still might benefit from early angioplasty. In response to the first concern, most investigators feel that in each of these trials angioplasty was performed in a timely fashion and they site the inherent time delay necessary for the performance of angioplasty in this setting (48). A rational analysis of the second issue is more difficult. Both randomized (49) and nonrandomized (50) studies have shown that recurrent ischemia after angioplasty following combination of t-PA and urokinase is less frequent than when angioplasty is used after t-PA alone. The impact of recurrent ischemia in this setting may be profound (51,52), but the 3% in-hospital mortality without early angioplasty is so low that it is unlikely that even an appreciable change in the incidence of recurrent ischemia after angioplasty would change the results. Certainly in light of the cost of widespread early angioplasty and an equivalent result at best, this strategy cannot be widely advocated.

Finally, prospective and rigorous attempts to define patients at highest risk of recurrent ischemia after successful thrombolytic therapy after t-PA alone or t-PA in combination with urokinase (6,53) have been unrewarding, although trends toward a heightened risk of recurrent ischemia have been noted with delayed washout of contrast from the infarct artery and Ambrose II morphology of the infarct stenosis (53). Thus it appears that even targeted angioplasty after successful thrombolysis cannot, at this time, be defended.

RESCUE CORONARY ANGIOPLASTY AFTER FAILED THROMBOLYTIC THERAPY

The rationale for the potential benefit of rescue angioplasty is based on the above-mentioned facts that intravenous thrombolytic regimens are not always successful in achieving early infarct artery patency (5-9), that following thrombolysis, a widely patent infarct artery portends improved in-hospital (54) and long-term survival (29,30), and finally, whether achieved by thrombolysis or by rescue angioplasty, early infarct artery patency seems to convey a similar favorable short- and long-term outcome (Table 2) (55).

There are several reasons, however, why a strategy of rescue angioplasty might not prove to be beneficial. First, rapid infusion or other new regimens for administering intravenous thrombolytic and/or adjunctive therapies might improve reperfusion and infarct artery patency rates to the point that rescue angioplasty might rarely be needed (7). For instance, Neuhaus et al. recently reported a 91% patency with a front-loaded regimen of t-PA (7). Other groups have reported patency rates in excess of 80% with similar front-loaded t-PA regimens (8,9). However, given the TIMI experience with the 150-mg dose of t-PA being associ-

Table 2   Comparative In-hospital Outcome of Patients with Thrombolysis or Angioplasty-mediated Infarct Artery Patency (55)

	Thrombolysis alone	Angioplasty
No. of patients	607	169
Age (years)	56 ± 10	55 ± 9
Prior myocardial infarction (%)	13	10
Anterior Infarction (%)	40	38
Multivessel disease (%)	47	40
Baseline LVEF (%)	51 ± 11	48 ± 10*
Improvement in LVEF at hospital discharge (%EF)	1.0 ± 9	-0.1 ± 8
Reocclusion (%)	11	21**
Urgent/emergent CABG (%)	11	6*
Death (%)	4.6	5.9

$*p \leq 0.05$.
$**p \leq 0.001$.
CABG = coronary artery bypass surgery; EF = ejection fraction units; LVEF = left ventricular ejection fraction.

ated with a 1.3% incidence of intracranial hemorrhage, caution should be advocated before accepting widespread application of front-loaded t-PA regimens without demonstration of their safety in large numbers of patients. Second, it is possible that delayed thrombolytic-induced reperfusion may be sufficient to achieve nearly optimal in-hospital survival. Investigators from the PRIMI Trial (57) recently reported that while 90-min patency after the administration of intravenous streptokinase was only 64%, it increased to 85% at 24 hr. If improved patient survival requires only that an infarct artery be patent at the time of hospital discharge, then early urgent attempts to open a vessel that might otherwise open spontaneously might not be needed. Third, the potential harm from attempted, but unsuccessful rescue angioplasty might outweigh any benefit from successful rescue angioplasty. It must be noted that angioplasty performed in this setting, often with an ulcerated or fissured plaque overlaid with a large amount of thrombus and associated activated platelets, must be performed in an extremely unfavorable milieu. Several investigators have noted a lessoned primary success rate with angioplasty performed in a setting of failed versus successful thrombolysis (55,58). Particularly worrisome is that in the setting of failed rescue angioplasty, in-hospital mortalities in excess of 30% have been noted. In the summary report from the TAMI I-V series, Abbottsmith et al. reported a 39% mortality in patients with failed rescue angioplasty, considerably higher than one might expect from their baseline 48 ± 17% LVEF (55). The possibility that failed angioplasty may actually harm these patients by inducing serious arrhythmias (55,59), by further impairing left ventricular function, or by inducing recurrent ischemia cannot be dismissed. Fourth, rescue angioplasty, even when successful, may not improve survival or decrease the incidence of congestive heart failure compared to a more conservative approach. Finally, rescue angioplasty may not "be worth" the cost associated with its application in this era in which necessary limitations of resources have begun to pose constraints on the application of "high tech" medicine.

Unlike the situation with successful thrombolysis, large-scale randomized trials have not been performed to assess the utility of angioplasty performed in the "rescue" setting. In fact, only one very small study has been performed (Belenkie, personal communication). In addition, review of the published literature of nonrandomized series on rescue angioplasty finds data only from 544 patients reported in any detail (Table 3). Almost all individual series report data from fewer than 100 patients (12,60-69).

Success in establishing infarct artery patency with rescue PTCA has ranged from 71 to 92%. There has been little beneficial effect on recovery of left ventricular function demonstrated by the time of hospital discharge, although admittedly most patients were treated outside of the 1-1/2 to 2-hr window during which reperfusion apparently needs to be achieved in order to consistently see at least modest recovery of left ventricular function (70). Patients with successful rescue angioplasty have had a considerably lower mortality than their counterparts with un-

Table 3 Meta-Analysis of Rescue Coronary Angioplasty

First author	Ref.	n	Thrombolytic regimen	% success	% reocclusion	ΔEF[a]	Mortality
Topol	12	86	t-PA	73	29	-1	10.4
Califf	60	15	t-PA	87	15	+1	NR
		25	UK	84	12	+1	NR
		12	t-PA + UK	92	0	+2	NR
Fung	61	13	SK	92	16	+10	7.6
Topol	62	22	t-PA + UK	86	3	+5	0.0
Grines	63	12	t-PA + SK	100	8	NR	NR
Holmes	64	34	SK	71	NR	-11	11.0
Grines	65	10	t-PA + SK	90	12	+5	10.0
O'Connor	66	90	SK	89	14	-1	17.0
Baim	67	37	t-PA	92	26	NR	5.4
Whitlow	68	26	t-PA	81	29	-2	NR
		18	UK	89	25	+1	NR
Ellis	69	109	t-PA	79	20	+1	10.1
		5	t-PA + UK	80	20	+2	20.0
		59	SK	76	18	+4	10.2
Pooled SK, UK, or combination		292[b]		247/292 (85%)*	31/223 (14%)*	-1	11.7
Pooled t-PA only		252[c]		191/252 (76%)*	38/157 (24%)	-1	9.5
Total		544[b,c]		438/544 (80%)	69/380 (18%)	-1	10.7

[a]Change in left ventricular function from baseline to pre-hospital discharge
[b]5 patients included in both reference 17 and the current series are counted singly
[c]21 patients included in both reference 2 and the current series are counted singly
*$p = 0.01$.
NR = not reported; SK-streptokinase; t-PA-tissue plasminogen activator; UK-urokinase.

successful rescue angioplasty (55,58). Reocclusion following successful angioplasty has been reported in up to 29% of patients (12), but reocclusion rates appear
to be lower when long-acting, non-fibrin-specific agents are used (49,50).
Data from the University of Michigan Myocardial Infarct Registry support
these findings and highlight the fact that the success rate for rescue coronary angioplasty in achieving an infarct-related artery with a <70% stenosis (by com-
puter-based edge detection) and at least a TIMI grade II flow is less common than
when angioplasty is performed for a stenosis in a patent artery after thrombolysis
(77% versus 89%, p = 0.009). In the 40 cases of failed rescue angioplasty in this
registry, the cause of procedural failure was recurrent thrombosis in 31%, failure
to pass the wire through a totally occluded artery in 26%, and partial success (failure to dilate to <70% diameter stenosis) in 21%. The relation between the success
or failure of angioplasty and in-hospital survival was striking for patients with
anterior, but not inferior, infarctions. A 9.7% mortality was seen after successful
angioplasty for patients with anterior infarcts, compared with a 33% mortality for
those with failed rescue angioplasty. This difference achieved statistical significance (p = 0.017) in multivariate testing even after consideration of the effects of
LVEF and patient age, which were the other independent predictors of in-hospital
survival. However, it is not possible to say whether this difference was the result
of a benefit of successful angioplasty, harm from failed angioplasty, or both. The
success or failure of rescue angioplasty in the setting of inferior myocardial infarction appeared to be much less important, with an 8% in-hospital mortality for
both groups. There was, however, a trend toward improved survival with successful angioplasty in patients with inferior wall infarction and anterior "reciprocal"
ST-segment depression, a group generally at higher risk than the overall inferior
infarct population (21,71,72). Interestingly, the impact of successful versus failed
angioplasty in patients with anterior infarction was independent of the time after
infarction onset throughout the first 24 hr, with patients treated successfully between 6 and 24 hr after presentation having a 9% mortality and those with failed
angioplasty having a 25% mortality. Overall improvement in LVEF between hospital admission and discharge after successful angioplasty was modest (3 ±9 ejection fraction units compared with a -1 ±7 ejection fraction change in patients with
failed angioplasty), with only patients undergoing catheterization within 2 hr of
clinical presentation showing a marked improvement of ejection fraction (6 ± 7
ejection fraction units).
A further important consideration in the strategy of rescue angioplasty is the
difficulty in accurately diagnosing failed thrombolysis with current technology.
Even ST-segment improvement over the first few hours after treatment or resolution of chest pain does not assure successful thrombolysis, as emphasized by
Califf et al. from the TAMI-I experience (73). Important to the strategy of rescue
angioplasty is the difference in myoglobin and creatinine kinase (CK) isoenzyme
washout between patients with or without reperfusion (74,75), as well as real-time

digital analysis of ST-segment shifts (76,77), which may make the diagnosis of failed thrombolysis much more reliable. It appears that in the very near future bedside kits to rapidly assay myoglobin or CK isoenzymes may be available. This should improve the speed with which one can move patients eligible for rescue angioplasty to the catheterization laboratory, without requiring that all patients who have received intravenous thrombolytic therapy receive early angiography. Nonetheless, there appears to be an inherent 3 to 6-hr time delay between the onset of chest pain and possible application of rescue angioplasty (48).

What, then, is an appropriate position to take regarding rescue angioplasty? Simply stated, data are inadequate to allow scientific judgment whether or not the strategy of rescue angioplasty is justified. Based on our admittedly inadequate database, one might possibly justify application of rescue angioplasty to patients with large infarcts who present to centers with substantial experience in rescue angioplasty. Certainly, based on the apparent detrimental effect of failed rescue angioplasty, those practitioners without expertise in this area should generally refrain from its performance. Whether the strategy is beneficial or detrimental, routine application of it will be costly. The need for a randomized trial to determine the usefulness of rescue angioplasty is obvious. Hopefully, the current ongoing RESCUE trial with its expected completion in 1992 will provide some answers to this important question.

Consideration of the viability of the strategy of rescue angioplasty should also include the possibility that rapid reperfusion with whole blood may not be the most effective way of salvaging myocardium. For instance, Vinten-Johansen et al. recently demonstrated that slow reperfusion with whole blood greatly diminishes infarct size compared with abrupt reperfusion in a canine model (78), and Rosenkranz et al. found a beneficial effect of aspartate glutamate-blood cardioplegia (79). Schaer and Pitarys et al. have shown the advantageous effects of an oxygenated perfluorochemical emulsion and adenosine, respectively, in similar models (80,81). Administration of such agents via coronary catheters could easily be done. Although it must be recognized that multiple agents shown to have decreased infarct size in experimental preparations have had little or no beneficial effect in the human setting (82,83), direct coronary application of promising agents deserves to be tested.

RETRIEVAL ANGIOPLASTY FOR RECURRENT ISCHEMIA AFTER SUCCESSFUL THROMBOLYSIS

Recurrent in-hospital ischemia develops in 5–18% of patients treated with intravenous thrombolytic therapy for acute myocardial infarction, with the incidence depending on the definition and perhaps on the thrombolytic regimen utilized (12, 17,53). Furthermore, it has been associated with worsened in-hospital survival (51,52). Ohman et al. (51), reporting from the TAMI Study Group experience, found recurrent infarct-related artery ischemia in 91 of 810 consecutive patients (12.4%), and the mortality in those patients was 11.0%, compared with 4.5% in patients with sustained reperfusion (p = 0.01). Risk factors for reocclusion were right coronary artery infarction and mechanical compared with purely pharmacologically induced patency of the infarct artery. Options for treating ischemia in this setting include repeat administration of thrombolytic agents, coronary angioplasty, coronary bypass surgery, and conservative management. Currently, little is known about the comparative benefit of each of these interventions, with the exception that at least in many patients, conservative management is likely associated with a high rate of complications. Barbash et al. (84) recently reported their experience with additional thrombolytic therapy using t-PA. Forty-four of fifty-two patients (85%) had resolution of clinical signs of ischemia within 1 hr of initiation of the second t-PA infusion, but in 21 patients (48%) ischemia returned and invasive coronary intervention was required. Thirty-one patients were retreated by White et al. (85) and angiographic patency could be demonstrated in 73% of patients undergoing angiographic restudy. Importantly, four of the eight patients who had received streptokinase twice had an allergic reaction. We recently studied 75 consecutive patients with recurrent ischemia after successful reperfusion whose recurrent ischemia was treated primarily with coronary angioplasty (52). These patients had a 14.7% in-hospital mortality compared to a 2.0% mortality in patients with sustained infarct artery patency (p <0.001). Patients initially pesenting with cardiogenic shock, the elderly, and those with multivessel disease had the highest mortality with recurrent ischemia. Importantly, successful reperfusion initiated within 90 min of recurrent ischemia was associated with 100% survival in the 25 patients so treated, and this was a powerful independent predictor of improved survival even after consideration of the above-mentioned factors. Later successful reperfusion was not associated with improved hospital survival. Successful reperfusion did not appreciably improve global LVEF. Angioplasty was the primary means of achieving successful reperfusion and was successful in 39 of 52 (75%) patients in whom it was attempted. Although the importance of the timing of the successful reperfusion remains to be confirmed in larger series, it appears from these data that since repeat administration of thrombolytic agents is often at least initially successful in reestablishing coronary patency, and because this therapy can be implemented in most instances much more quickly than can coronary angioplasty, this should be the primary means of treatment in recurrent ischemia. However, many of these patients will require further mechanical coronary intervention (84).

LATE IN-HOSPITAL CORONARY ANGIOPLASTY

Late elective coronary angioplasty may be performed either after demonstration of reversible ischemia by noninvasive means or in the absence of such findings.

The distinction between these two patient subsets may be somewhat blurred, based on our recognition of the limitations of noninvasive testing in this setting. For example, Burns et al. reported that SPECT thallium stress testing performed 8 days after infarction treated with thrombolytic therapy had only a 35% sensitivity for detection of disease in the noninfarct vessel and only a 50% specificity for detection of significant disease in the infarct-related artery (86). The sensitivity for detection of disease in the infarct artery and the specificity for detection of disease in the noninfarct arteries were 95% and 84%, respectively. It must be recalled that thallium imaging is a relative flow study, and with the presence of a fixed defect due to infarction, it may be difficult to discriminate reversible changes within that area and also to detect lesser flow reductions in other coronary territories. In fact, Sutton et al. recently reported that in the presence of a significant coronary stenosis in an infarct-related artery, the primary correlate of a negative thallium stress test was the size of the infarction as estimated by the peak CK value, and not the severity of the infarct-related artery stenosis (47). That study suggests that the most common reason for inability to demonstrate reversible ischemia in this setting is a complete or nearly complete infarction. If it can be conclusively demonstrated that infarct artery patency at hospital discharge has independent predictive value above and beyond left ventricular function, and this remains somewhat controversial (28,30), then this form of screening may not be the most appropriate. The change from resting to maximum exercise-induced LVEF has somewhat similar limitations. However, even with these shortcomings, the short-term infarction-free survival in patients with negative stress tests is excellent (97% at 42 days in the TIMI-II Study (15).

The optimal timing for intervention in patients with abnormal stress tests after myocardial infarction remains to be determined. De Feyter and others (87) emphasized the relatively high complication rate after angioplasty performed in the postinfarction setting. Although a majority of patients in these studies had not been treated with thrombolytic therapy and were unstable, it must be presumed that the coronary milieu for angioplasty is still somewhat unfavorable early after infarction in patients without angina. After thrombolytic therapy, this high-risk period may possibly extend for several weeks (88). While in many patients with rest pain angioplasty cannot be deferred, in those patients in whom there is a choice, the optimal timing remains uncertain. Certainly the presence of visible thrombi on coronary angiography increases the risk of angioplasty (11), but it is possible that prolonged heparin infusion or other pharmacological means may reduce the risk of angioplasty in such patients (89).

The issue of whether or not patients should undergo routine postthrombolytic catheterization, with angioplasty as needed, compared with catheterization for ischemia has been addressed in four randomized trials (Table 4) (13,16,90,91). Importantly, in both studies large enough to adequately study the issue of survival, angioplasty was performed within 3 days of the infarction, which as previously

Table 4 Trials of Delayed Coronary Angioplasty After Thrombolysis

	Guerci (90)	TIMI-II (13)	SWIFT (16)	Barbash (91)
No. of Patients	85	3262	800	201
Allowable duration of angina before thrombolytic therapy (hr)	4	4	3	4
Thrombolytic agent	t-PA	t-PA	APSAC	t-PA
Timing of PTCA (days after MI)	3	0.75–2	2–3	3–7
PTCA attempted (% of eligible)	90	54	43	50
PTCA success (%)	84	85	87	90
Major PTCA complications (%)	3	13	13	7
F/U resting LVEF (PTCA/no PTCA)	49/51	NR	NR	51/51
F/U exercise LVEF (PTCA/no PTCA)	64/51*	NR	NR	52/53
Late mortality (%) (PTCA/no PTCA)	NR	5.2/4.7	3.3/2.7	5.1/0.0[a]

[a]mortality after randomization.

*$p \leq 0.05$.

PTCA = percutaneous transluminal coronary angioplasty; Major PTCA complications = death, infarction, emergency bypass surgery; LVEF = left ventricular ejection fraction.

noted may be too early to achieve optimal results. In the TIMI-II study, 12.8% of patients with attempted angioplasty had one or more complications within 24 hr of that procedure (15), and similarly in the SWIFT (Should We Intervene After Thrombolytic Therapy) trial (16), investigators found a rate of complications considerably higher than the generally accepted 3–5% incidence after selective coronary angioplasty (92,93). Despite their limitations, the results of each of these studies are remarkably concordant. In the TIMI-II study the risk of death or reinfarction in the group treated with routine catheterization and revascularization was 10.9% at 6 weeks compared to 9.7% in the group referred for catheterization only for demonstrable ischemia (15). No difference in resting LVEF at follow-up was noted between the two groups. From the SWIFT trial, while there was no difference in the incidence of death at 90 days (4.8% in the intervention group versus 3.2% in the conventionally treated group), there was a strong trend for a higher rate of reinfarction in the patients treated aggressively (13.6% versus 8.2%, p = 0.06). In a study that perhaps reflects more accurately the practice of many cardiologists in the United States, Barbash and colleagues randomized patients to undergo routine coronary angiography with angioplasty needed at 5 ± 2 days after thrombolytic therapy versus a group treated conservatively (91). In this study, angioplasty was successful in 90% of attempts, and 7% of patients required either emergency bypass or repeat coronary angioplasty. There was no significant difference in either 10-month mortality (8.2% in the aggressively treated group versus 3.8% in the conservatively treated group, p = 0.15) or resting LVEF at 8 weeks ($51 \pm 14\%$ in the aggressively treated group versus $51 \pm 11\%$ in the conservatively treated group, p = NS). However, if one excludes patients dying prior to catheterization (in whom the results of randomization cannot be implicated in their outcome), there was a statistically significant increase in deaths in the aggressively treated group (5.3% compared to 0.0% in the conservatively managed group, p = 0.02). In aggregate, then, these results suggest strongly that coronary angioplasty performed on the basis of the "occulostenotic reflex" is not only unnecessary, but may be harmful. Although critics of these studies point to the early timing of angioplasty and other methodological concerns, including failure in the TIMI-II study to attempt dilatation of total occlusions and the possible absence of the full antiplatelet effect of aspirin in these patients, it is unlikely, even with further delay in angioplasty or with the use of new, more powerful antiplatelet agents (94,95), that one can improve on the short-term event-free survival documented in the conservatively managed patients in all these studies. However, the results apply only to the average patient treated within these studies. In the largest study, TIMI-II, the detailed clinical characteristics of the patients treated have only been provided in abstract form (96). Furthermore, many patients (with ST-segment depression infarction, those who could not be treated within 4 hr of chest pain onset, and those with left bundle branch block) were excluded from this study and hence the patients are not entirely representative of typical infarction patients. The mean resting LVEF in these patients prior to hospital discharge was 50% and hence the majority of patients had well-preserved left ventricular function. It is uncertain how many patients had multivessel coronary disease. With these caveats, patients with prior infarction did better with catheterization 18–48 hr after infarction, whereas patients without infarction but with diabetes did worse with an invasive strategy (96).

Given these further limitations, it is perhaps noteworthy to review the long-term results in patients managed conservatively in the GISSI study (17), to ascertain which patient groups may be at particularly high mortality risk when treated without further revascularization. That study documented particularly high 1-year mortality after hospital discharge in patients with prior myocardial infarction (17% versus 6% without infarction, $p < 0.001$), in those patients ≥ 75 years old (19% versus 7% in younger patients, $p = 0.003$), in patients presenting initially with pulmonary edema or cardiogenic shock (23% versus 7%, $p = 0.01$), and also in those presenting with ST-segment depression infarction (17% versus 6%, $p = 0.01$). One can argue, therefore, that cardiac catheterization with prudent revascularization be considered in such patients, perhaps as well as in patients who require vigorous physical activity in their line of employment or in whom considerable public trust is placed (airline pilots, bus drivers, and the like).

SUMMARY

In brief, on assessment of angioplasty technology as it stands today, angioplasty can be rationally advocated for treatment of recurrent ischemia after successful thrombolytic therapy, probably for treatment of exercise-induced ischemia after successful thrombolytic therapy, and possibly for failed thrombolytic therapy in patients with large myocardial infarctions when angioplasty is performed by highly skilled practitioners. Angioplasty cannot be advocated immediately after successful thrombolytic therapy, in all patients with failed thrombolytic therapy, or in patients without evidence of overt or induced ischemia after successful thrombolytic therapy. Ongoing studies will hopefully provide important information for the circumstances under which indications are particularly speculative, for example, rescue angioplasty. Finally, although it is likely that improvements in the technique of percutaneous revascularization will be demonstrated, such as perhaps with coronary atherectomy or adjunctive use of stronger antiplatelet agents (95,97,98), it is unlikely that these improvements will reverse the results of current studies evaluating the effect of angioplasty early after successful thrombolysis and probably later after successful thrombolysis in the absence of demonstrable ischemia. One must, however, recognize that optimal medical care of patients need not be entirely dictated by the results of randomized studies, and that there is room for individualization of patient care.

ACKNOWLEDGMENT

The author would like to express his great appreciation to the secretarial assistance provided on this manuscript by Ms. Lin Nicholson.

REFERENCES

1. Brown BG, Gallery CA, Badger RS, Kennedy JW, Mathey D, Bolson,EL, Dodge HT. Incomplete lysis of thrombus in the moderate underlying atherosclerotic lesion during intracoronary infusion of streptokinase for acute myocardial infarction: quantitative angiographic observations. Circulation 1986; 73:653-61.
2. Harrison DG, Ferguson DW, Collins, SM, Skorton DJ, Ericksen EE, Kioschos JM, Marcus ML, White CS. Rethrombosis after reperfusion with streptokinase: importance of geometry of residual lesions. Circulation 1984; 69:991-9.
3. Serruys PW, Wijns W, van den Brand M, Ribeiro V, Fioretti P, Simoons ML, Kooijman CJ, Reiber JHC, Hugenholtz PG. Is transluminal coronary angioplasty mandatory after successful thrombolysis? Quantitative coronary angiographic study. Br. Heart J 1983; 50:257-65.
4. Lefkowitz CA, Pace DP, Gallagher KP, Buda AJ. The effects of a critical stenosis on myocardial blood flow, ventricular function, and infarct size after coronary reperfusion. Circulation 1988; 77:915-26.
5. TIMI. Special report: the thrombolysis in myocardial infarction (TIMI) trial. Phase I findings. N Engl J Med 1985; 312:932-6.
6. Wall T, Mark DB, Califf RM, Collins G, Burgess, R, Skelton TN, Hinohara T, Kong DF, Mantell S, Aronson L, Hlatky MA, Cusma J, Stack R, Pryor DB, Bashore TM. Prediction of early recurrent myocardial ischemia and coronary reocclusion after successful thrombolysis: a qualitative and quantitative angiographic study. Am J Cardiol 1989; 63:423-8.
7. Neuhaus KL, Feuerer W, Jeep-Tebbe S, Niederer W, Vogt A,Tebbe U. Improved thrombolysis with a modified dose regimen of recombinant tissue-type plasminogen activator. J Am Coll Cardiol 1989; 14:1566-9.
8. McKendall GR, Attubato M, Drew TM, Feit F, Sharaf B, Thomas ES, McDonald MJ, Williams DO. Improved infarct artery patency using a new modified regimen of t-PA: results of the pre-hospital administration of t-PA (PATS) pilot trial. J Am Coll Cardiol 1990; 15:3A (abstract).
9. Wall TC, Topol EJ, George BS, Ellis SG, Samaha J, Kereiakes DJ, Worlet SJ, Sigmon K, Califf RM. The TAMI -7 trial of accelerated plasminogen activator dose regimens for coronary thrombolysis. Circulation 1990; 82:III- 538 (abstract).

10. Ellis SG, Vandormael MG, Cowley MJ, DiSciascio, G, Deligonul U, Topol EJ, Bulle TM. Coronary morphologic and clinical determinants of procedural outcome with antioplasty for multivessel coronary disease. Implications for patient selection. Circulation 1990; 82:1193-1202.

11. Sugrue DD, Holmes Jr DR, Smith HC, Reeder GS, Lane GE, Vlietstra RE, Bresnahan JF, Hammes LN, Piehler JM. Coronary artery thrombus as a risk factor for acute vessel occlusion during percutaneous transluminal coronary angioplasty: improving results. Br Heart J 1986; 56:62-6.

12. Topol EJ, Califf RM, George BS, Kereiakes DJ, Abbottsmith CW, Candela RJ, Lee KL, Pitt B, Stack RS, O'Neill WW. A randomized trial of immediate versus delayed elective angioplasty after intravenous tissue plasminogen activator in myocardial infarction. N Engl J Med 1987; 317:581-8.

13. TIMI. Immediate vs. delayed catheterization and angioplasty following thrombolytic therapy for acute myocardial infarction. TIMI IIA results. JAMA 1988; 260:2849-58.

14. Simoons ML, Betriu A, Col J, Von Essen R, Lubsen J, Michel PL, Rutsch W, Schmidt W, Thery C, Vahanian A, Willems GM, Arnold AER, Debono DP, Dougherty FC, Lambertz H, Meier B, Raynaud P, Sanz GA, Uebis R, van de Werf F, Wood, D. Thrombolysis with tissue plasminogen activator in acute myocardial infarction: no additional benefit from immediate percutaneous coronary angiopasty. Lancet 1988; 2:197-202.

15. TIMI. Comparison of invasive and conservative strategies after treatment with intravenous tissue plasminogen activator in acute myocardial infarction. Results of the thrombolysis in myocardial infarction (TIMI) phase II trial. N Engl J Med 1989; 320:618-27.

16. SWIFT. SWIFT trial of delayed elective intervention vs conservative treatment after thrombolysis with anistreplase in acute myocardial infarction. Br Med J 1991; 302:555-60.

17. GISSI. Effectiveness of intravenous thrombolytic treatment in acute myocardial infarction. Lancet 1986; 1:871-4.

18. ISIS-2. Randomized trial of intravenous streptokinase, oral aspirin, both, or neither among 17 187 cases of suspected acute myocardial infarction: ISIS-2. Lancet 1988; 2:349-60.

19. Wilcox RG, Olsson CG, Skene AM, von der Lipe G, Jensen G, Hampton JR. Trial of tissue plasminogen activator for mortality reduction in acute myocardial infarction. Anglo-Scandinavian study of early thrombolysis (AS-SET). Lancet 1988; 2:525-30.

20. Kelly MJ, Thompson, Quinlan MF. Prognostic significance of left ventricular ejection fraction after acute myocardial infarction. A bedside radionuclide study. B Heart J 1985; 53: 16-24.

21. Shah PK, Pichler M. Berman DS, Singh BN, Swan HJC. Left ventricular ejection fraction determined by radionuclide ventriculography in early states of first transmural myocardial infarction. Am J Cardiol 1980; 45: 542-6.

22. ISAM. A prospective trial of intravenous streptokinase in acute myocardial infarction (I.S.A.M.). N Engl J Med 1986; 314:1465-71.

23. Kennedy JW, Martin GV, David KB, Maynard C, Stadius M, Sheehan FH, Ritchie JL. The western Washington intravenous streptokinase in acute myocardial infarction randomized trial. Circulation 1988; 77:345-52.

24. Meinertz T, Kaspter W, Schumacher M, Just H. The German multicenter trial of anisoylated plasminogen streptokinase activator complex versus heparin for acute myocardial infarction. Am J Cardiol 1988; 62:347-51.

25. Serruys PW, Simoons ML, Suryapranata H, Vermeer F, Wijns W, van den Brand M, Bar F, Zwaan C, Krauss XH, Remme WJ, Res J, Verheugt FWA, Van domburg R, Lubsen J, Hugenholtz PG. Preservation of global and regional left ventricular function after early thrombolysis in acute myocardial infarction.

26. White HD, Norris RM, Brown MA, Takayama M, Maslowski A, Bass NM, Ormiston JA, Whitlock T. Effect of intravenous streptokinase on left ventricular function and early survival after acute myocardial infarction. N Engl J Med 1987; 317:85-5.

27. Van de Werf F, Arnold AER. Intravenous tissue plasmingen activator and size of infarct, left ventricular function, and survival in acute myocardial infarction. Br Med J 1988; 297:1374-9.

28. Sheehan F H. Measurement of left ventricular function as an endpoint in trials of thrombolyic therapy. Coronary Artery Disease 1990; 1:13- 22.

29. Cigarroa RG, Lange RA, Hillis LD. Prognosis after acute myocardial infarction in patients with and without residual anterograde coronary blood flow. Am J Cardiol 1989; 64:155-60.

30. Kennedy JW, Ritchie JL, David KB, Stadius ML, Maynard C, Fritz JK. The western Washington randomized trial of intracoronary streptokinase in acute myocardial infarction. A 12-month follow-up report. N Engl J Med 1985; 312:1073-8.

31. Bourke JP, Young AA, Richards DAB, Uther JB. Reduction in incidence of inducible ventricular tachycardia after myocardial infarction by treatment with streptokinase during infarct evolution. J Am Coll Cardiol 1990; 16:1703-10.

32. Kersschot IE, Brugada P, Ramentol M, Zehender M, Waldecker B, Stevenson WG, Geibel A, de Zwaan C, Wellens HJJ. Effects of early reperfusion in acute myocardial infarction on arrhythmias induced by programmed

stimulation: a prospective, randomized study. J Am Coll Cardiol 1986; 7:1234- 42.

33. Sager PT, Perlmutter RA, Rosenfeld LE, McPherson CA, Wackers FJ, Batsford WP. Electrophysiologic effects of thrombolytic therapy in patients with a transmural anterior myocardial infarction complicated by left ventricular aneurysm formation. J Am Coll Cardiol 1988; 12:19-24.

34. Volpi A, Cavalli A, Santoro E, Tognoni G, GISSI Investigators. Incidence and prognosis of secondary ventricular fibrillation in acute myocardial infarction. Evidence for a protective effect of thrombolytic therapy. Circulation 1990; 82:1279-88.

35. Hochman JS, Choo H. Limitation of myocardial infarct expansion by reperfusion independent of myocardial salvage. Circulation 1987; 75:299-306.

36. Brown EJ, Swinford RD, Gadde P, Lillis O. Acute effects of delayed reperfusion on myocardial infarct shape and left ventricular volume: a potential mechanism of additional benefits from thrombolytic therapy. J Am Coll Cardiol 1991; 17:1641-50.

37. Jeremy RW, Hackworthy RA, Bautovich G, Hutton BF, Harris PJ. Infarct artery perfusion and changes in left ventricular volume in the month after acute myocardial infarction. J Am Coll Cardiol 1987; 9:989-95.

38. Touchstone DA, Beller GA, Nygaard TW, Tedesco C, Kaul S. Effects of successful intravenous reperfusion therapy on regional myocardial function and geometry in humans: a tomographic assessment using two-dimensional echocardiography. J Am Coll Cardiol 1989; 13:1506-13.

39. Warren SE, Royal HD, Markis JE, Grossman W, McKay RG. Time course of left ventricular dilation after myocardial infarction: influence of infarct-related artery and success of coronary thrombolysis. J Am Coll Cardiol 1988; 11:12-9.

40. Badger RS, Brown BG, Kennedy JW, Mathey D, Gallery CA, Bolson EL, Dodge HT. Usefulness of recanalization to luminal diameter of 0.6 millimeter or more with intracoronary streptokinase during acute myocardial infarction in predicting "normal" perfusion status, continued arterial patency and survival at one year. Am J Cardiol 1987; 59:519-22.

41. Gold HK, Leinbach RC, Palacios IF, Yasuda T, Block P, Buckley MJ, Akins CW, Dagget WM, Austen WG. Coronary reocclusion after selective administration of streptokinase. Circulation 1983; 68(Suppl I):I-50-I-54.

42. O'Neill W, Timmis GC, Bourdillon PD, Lai P, Ganghadarhan V, Walton J, Ramos R, Laufer N, Gordon S, Schork A, Pitt B. A prospective randomized clinical trial of intracoronary streptokinase versus coronary angioplasty for acute myocardial infarction. N Engl J Med 1986; 314:812-8.

43. DeWood MA. Direct PTCA vs intravenous t-PA in acute myocardial infarction: results from a prospective randomized trial. In Thrombolysis and

interventional therapy in acute myocardial infarction 1990, VI George Washington University Pre AHA Symposium, pp. 28-9.

44. Ribeiro EE, Silva LA, Carneiro R, D'Oliveira LG, Gasques A, Amino JG, Tavares JR, Torossian S, Buffolo E. A randomized trial of direct PTCA vs intravenous streptokinase in acute myocardial infarction. J Am Coll Cardiol 1991; 17:152A (abstract).

45. Sheenan KH, Mathey DG, Schofer J, Dodge HT, Bolson EL. Factors that determine recovery of left ventricular function after thrombolysis in patients with acute myocardial infarction. Circulation 1985; 71:1121-8.

46. Kereiakes DJ, Topol EJ, George BS, Stack RS, Abbottsmith CW, Ellis S, Candela RJ, Harrelson L, Martin LH, Califf RM. Myocardial infarction with minimal coronary atherosclerosis in the eral of thrombolytic reperfusion. J Am Coll Cardiol 1991; 17:304-12.

47. Sutton JM, Topol EJ. Significance of a negative exercise thallium test in the presence of a critical residual stenosis after thrombolysis for acute myocardial infarction. Circulation 1991; 83:1278-86.

48. Sharkey SW, Brunette DD, Ruiz E, Hession WT, Wysham DG, Goldenberg IF, Hodges M. Analysis of time delays preceding thrombolysis for myocardial infarction. Circulation 1989; 80:II-353 (abstract).

49. Califf RM, Topol EJ, Stack RS, Ellis SG, George BS, Kereiakes DJ, Samaha JK, Workey SJ, Anderson JL, Harrelson-Woodlief L, Wall TC, Phillips HR, Abbottsmith CW, Candela RJ, Flanagan WH, Sasahara AA, Mantell SJ, Lee KL. Evaluation of combination thrombolytic therapy and timing of cardiac catheterization in acute myocardial infarction. Results of Thrombolysis and Angioplasty in Myocardial Infarction—phase 5 randomized trial. Circulation 1991; 83:1543-56.

50. Topol E, Califf RM, George BS, Kereiakes DJ, Rothbaum D, Candela RJ, Abbottsmith CW, Pinkerton CA, Stump DC, Collen D, Lee KL, Pitt B, Kline EM, Boswick JM, O'Neill WW, Stack RS. Coronary arterial thrombolysis with combined infusion of recombinant tissue-type plasminogen activator and urokinase in patients with acute myocardial infarction. Circulation 1988; 77:1100-7.

51. Ohman EM, Califf RM, Topol EJ, Candela R, Abbottsmith C, Ellis S, Sigmon KN, Kereiakes D, George B, Stack R. Consequences of reocclusion after successful reperfusion therapy in acute myocardial infarction. Circulation 1990; 82:781-91.

52. Ellis SG, Debowey D, Bates ER, Topol EJ. Treatment of recurrent ischemia after thrombolysis and successful reperfusion for acute myocardial infarction: effect on in-hospital mortality and left ventricular function. J Am Coll Cardiol 1991; 17:752-7.

53. Ellis SG, Topol EJ, George BS, Kereiakes DJ, Debowey D, Sigmon KN, Pickel A, Lee KL, Califf RM. Recurrent ischemia without warning. Analysis of risk factors for in-hospital ischemic events following successful thrombolysis with intravenous tissue plasminogen activator. Circulation 1989; 80:1159–65.

54. Topol E, Califf R, George B, Kereiakes D, Lee K. Insights derived from the Thrombolysis and Angioplasty in Myocardial Infarction (TAMI) trials. J Am Coll Cardiol 1988; 12:24A–31A.

55. Abbottsmith CW, Topol EJ, George BS, Stack RJ, Kereiakes DJ, Candela RJ, Anderson LC, Harrelson-Woodlief L, Califf RM. Fate of patients with acute myocardial infarction with patency of the infarct-related vessel achieved with successful thrombolysis versus rescue angioplasty. J Am Coll Cardiol 1990; 16:770–8.

56. Carney R, Brandt T, Daley P, Pickering E, White H, McDonough T, Smith S, Smith G, Allen R, Overlie P, Vermilya S, Teichman S. Increased efficacy of rt-PA by more rapid administration: the RAAMI trial. Circulation 1990; 82:III-538 (abstract).

57. PRIMI. Randomized double-blind trial of recombinant pro-urokinase against streptokinase in acute myocardial infarction. Lancet 1989; 1:863–8.

58. Ellis SG, O'Neill WW, Bates ER, Walton JA, Nabel EG, Werns SW, Topol E. Implications for patient triage from survival and left ventricular functional recovery analyses in 500 patients treated with coronary angioplasty for acute myocardial infarction. J Am Coll Cardiol 1989; 13:1251–9.

59. Gacioch GM, Topol EJ. Sudden paradoxic clinical deterioration during angioplasty of the occluded right coronary artery in acute myocardial infarction. J Am Coll Cardiol 1989; 14:1202–9.

60. Califf RM, Topol EJ, Stack RS, Ellis SG, Kereiakes DJ, Samaha JK, Worley SJ, Anderson JL, Harrelson-Woodlief L, Wall TC, Phillips HR, Abbottsmith CW, Candela RJ, Wilson B, Sasahara AA, Mantell SJ, Lee KL. An evaluation of combination thrombolytic therapy and timing of cardiac catheterization in acute myocardial infarction: the TAMI 5 randomized trials. Circulation 1990; 83:1543–6.

61. Fung AY, Lai P, Topol EJ, Bates ER, Bourdillon DV, Walton JA, Mancini GJB, Kryski T, Pitt B, O'Neill WW. Value of percutaneous transluminal coronary angioplasty after unsuccessful intravenous streptokinase therapy in acute myocardial infarction. Am J Cardiol 1991; 58:686–89.

62. Topol EJ, Califf RM, George BS, Kereiakes DJ, Rothbaum D, Candela RJ, Abbottsmith CW, Pinkerton CA, Stump DC, Collen D, Lee KL, Pitt B, Kline EM, Boswick JM, O'Neill WW, Stack RS. Coronary arterial thrombolysis with combined infusion of recombinant tissue-type plasminogen ac-

tivator and urokinase in patients with acute myocardial infarction. Circulation 1988; 77:1100-7.

63. Grines CL, Nissen SE, Booth DC, Gurley JC, Chelliah N, Blankenship J, Branco MC, Bennett K, DeMaria AN. A prospective, randomized trial comparing combination half dose tPA with streptokinase to full dose tPA in acute myocardial infarction: preliminary report. J Am Coll Cardiol 1990; 15:4A (abstract).

64. Holmes DR, Gersh BJ, Bailey KR, Reeder GS, Bresnahan JF, Bresnahan DR, Vlietstra RE. "Rescue" percutaneous transluminal angioplasty after failed thrombolytic therapy-4 year follow-up. J Am Coll Cardiol 1989; 13:193A (abstract).

65. Grines CL, Nissen SE, Booth DC, Branco MC, Gurley JC, Bennett KA, DeMaria AN. A new thrombolytic regimen for acute myocardial infarction using combination half dose tissue-type plasminogen activator with full dose streptokinase: a pilot study. J Am Coll Cardiol 1989;14:573-80.

66. O'Connor CM, Mark DB, Hinohara T, Stack RS, Rendall D, Hlatky MA, Pryor DB, Phillips HR, Califf RM. Rescue coronary angioplasty after failure of intravenous streptokinase in acute myocardial infarction: in-hospital and long-term outcomes. J Invest Cardiol 1989; 1:85-95.

67. Baim DS, Diver DJ, Knatterud GL. PTCA "salvage" for thrombolytic failures—implications from TIMI II-A. Circulation 1988; 78:II-112 (abstract).

68. Whitlow PL. Catheterization/Rescue Angioplasty Following Thrombolysis (CRAFT) study: results of rescue angioplasty. Circulation 1990; 82:III-308 (abstract).

69. Ellis SG, Aversano T, Van de Werf F, Knudson M, Ribeiro-daSilva E, Topol EJ. Rescue coronary angioplasty: current polarization of opinion and randomized trials. J Am Coll Cardiol 1992 (in press).

70. Koren GT, Hasin Y, Appelbaum D, Welber S, Rozenman Y, Lotan C, Mosseri M, Sapoznikov D, Luria MH, Gotsman MS. Prevention of myocardial damage in acute myocardial ischemia by early treatment with intravenous streptokinase. N Engl J Med 1985; 313:1384-9.

71. Roubin GS, Shen WF, Nicholson M, Dunn RF, Kelly DT, Harris PJ. Anterolateral ST segment depression in acute inferior myocardial infarction: angiographic and clinical implications. Am Heart J 1984; 107:1177-82.

72. Berger PB, Ryan TJ. Inferior myocardial infarction. High-risk subgroups. Circulation 1990; 81:401-11.

73. Califf RM, O'Neill W, Stack RS, Aronson L, Mark DB, Mantell S, George BS, Candela RJ, Kereiakes DJ, Abbottsmith C, Topol EJ. Failure of simple clinical measurements to predict perfusion status after intravenous thrombolysis. Ann Intern Med 1988; 108:658-62.

74. Ellis AK, Little T, Masud ARZ, Liberman HA, Morris DC, Klocke FJ. Early noninvasive detection of successful reperfusion in patients with acute myocardial infarction. Circulation 1988; 78:1352-7.

75. Puelo PR, Guadagno PA, Roberts R, Scheel MV, Marian AJ, Churchill D, Perryman B. Early diagnosis of acute myocardial infarction based on assay for subforms of creatine kinase-MB. Circulation 1990; 82:759-64.

76. Clemmensen P, Ohman M, Sevilla DC, Peck S, Wagner NB, Quigley PS, Grande P, Lee KL, Wagner GS. Changes in standard electrocardiographic ST-segment elevation predictive of successful reperfusion in acute myocardial infarction. Am J Cardiol 1990; 66:1407-11.

77. Krucoff MW, Jackson YR, Burdette DL, Croll MA, Pendley LP, Aronson LG, Pope JE, Califf RM. Digital real-time 12-lead ST segment trends: a bedside noninvasive monitor of infarct vessel patency. Circulation 1989; 80:II-354 (abstract).

78. Vinten-Johansen J, Johnston WE, Lefer DJ, Smith T, Cordel AR. Controlled reperfusion attenuates no-reflow and reduces infarct size. Circulation 1990; 82:III-286 (abstract).

79. Rosenkranz E, Okamoto F, Buckberg G, Robertson J, Vinten-Johansen J, Bugyi H. Safety of prolonged aortic clamping with blood cardioplegia. III. Aspartate enrichment of glutamate-blood cardioplegia in energy-depleted hearts after ischemic and reperfusion injury. J Thorac Cardiovasc Surg 1986; 91:428-35.

80. Schaer GL, Karas SP, Santoian EC, Gold C, Visner MS, Virmani R. Reduction in reperfusion injury by blood-free reperfusion after experimental myocardial infarction. J Am Coll Cardiol 1990; 15:1385-93.

81. Pitarys CJ, Jackson EK, Virmani R, Forman MB. Permanent attenuation of myocardial reperfusion injury by intravenous adenosine. Circulation 1990; 82:III-263 (abstract).

82. Held PH, Teo KK, Yusuf S. Effects of beta-blockers, calcium channel blockers, and nitrates in acute myocardial infarction and unstable angina pectoris. In Topol EJ (ed.) Textbook of Interventional Cardiology. Philadelphia: Saunders, 1990:49-65.

83. Wilcox RG, Hampton JR, Banks DC, Birkhead JS, Brooksby IAB, Burns-Cox CJ, Hayes MJ, Joy MD, Malcolm AD, Mather HG, Rowley JM. Trial of early nifedipine in acute myocardial infarction: the TRENT study. Br Med J 1986; 293:1204-8.

84. Barbash GI, Hod H, Roth A, Faibel HE, Mandel Y, Miller HI, Rath S, Zahav YH, Rabinowitz B, Seligsohn U, Pelled B, Schlesinger Z, Motro M, Laniado S, Kaplinsky E. Repeat infusions of recombinant tissue-type plasminogen activator in patients with acute myocardial infarction and early recurrent myocardial ischemia. J Am Coll Cardiol 1990; 16:779-83.

85. White HD, Cross DB, Norris RM. Readministration of thrombolytic therapy for threatened reinfarction. Circulation 1990; 82:III-86 (abstract).

86. Burns RJ, Freeman MR, Liu P, Cox F, Morgan CD, Armstrong PW. Limitations of exercise thallium single photon tomography early after myocardial infarction. J Am Coll Cardiol 1989; 13:125A (abstract).

87. de Feyter PJ, Suryapranata H, Serruys PW, et al. Coronary angioplasty for unstable angina: immediate and late results in 200 consecutive patients with identification of risk factors of unfavorable early and late outcome. J Am Coll Cardiol 1988; 12:324-33.

88. Cleary RM, Lincoff AM, Popma JJ, Hacker JA, Ellis SG, Topol EJ, Bates ER. Increased risk for abrupt closure during elective PTCA in the post-myocardial infarction period. J Am Coll Cardiol 1991; 17:267A (abstract).

89. Douglas JS, Lutz JF, Clements SD, Robinson PH, Roubin GS, Lembo NJ, King SB. Therapy of large intracoronary thrombi in candidates for percutaneous transluminal coronary angioplasty. J Am Coll Cardiol 1988; 11:238A (abstract).

90. Guerci AD, Gerstenblith G, Brinker JA, Chandra NC, Gottlieb SO, Bahr RD, Weiss JL, Shapiro EP, Flaherty JT, Bush DE, Chew PH, Gottlieb SH, Halperin HR, Ouyang P, Walford GD, Bell WR, Fatterpaker AK, Llewellyn M, Topol EJ, Healy B, Siu CO, Becker LC, Weisfeldt ML. A randomized trial of intravenous tissue plasminogen activator for acute myocardial infarction with subsequent randomization to elective coronary angioplasty. N Engl J Med 1987; 317:1613-18.

91. Barbash GI, Roth A, Hod H, Modan M, Miller HI, Rath S, Zahav YH, Keren G, Motro M, Shachar A, Basan S, Agranat O, Rabinowitz B, Laniado S, Kaplinsky E. Randomized controlled trial of late in-hospital angiography and angioplasty versus conservative management after treatment with recombinant tissue-type plasminogen activator in acute myocardial infarction. Am J Cardiol 1990; 66:538-45.

92. Bredlau CD, Roubin GS, Leimgruber PO, Douglas JS, King SB, Gruentzig AR. In-hospital morbidity and mortality in patients undergoing elective coronary angioplasty. Circulation 1985; 72:1044-52.

93. Detre K, Holubkov R, Kelsey S, Cowley M, Kent K, Williams D, Myler R, Faxon D, Holmes D, Bourassa M, Block P, Gosselin A, Bentivoglio L, Leatherman L, Dorros G, King S, Galichia J, Al-Bassam M, Leon M, Robertson T, Passamani E. Percutaneous transluminal coronary angioplasty in 1985-1986 and 1977-1981. N Engl J Med 1988; 318:265-70.

94. Heras M, Chesebro JH, Webster MWI, Mruk JS, Grill DE, Penny WJ, Bowie EJW, Badimon L, Fuster V. Hirudin, heparin, and placebo during deep arterial injury in the pig. The in vivo role of thrombin in platelet-mediated thrombosis. Circulation 1990; 82:1476-84.

95. Ellis SG, Bates ER, Schaible T, Weisman HF, Pitt B, Topol EJ. Prospects for the use of antagonists to the platelet glycoprotein IIb/IIIa receptor to prevent postangioplasty restenosis and thrombosis. J Am Coll Cardiol 1991; 17:89B-95B.

96. Mueller H, Cohen L, Williams D, Forman S, Solomon R, Braunwald E. Subgroup analysis of the TIMI II study. J AM Coll Cardiol 1991; 17:167A (abstract).

97. Ellis SG, DeCesare NB, Pinkerton CA, Whitlow P, King SB, Ghazzal ZMB, Kereiakes DJ, Popma JJ, Menke KK, Topol EJ, Holmes DR. Relation of stenosis morphology and clinical presentation to the procedural results of directional coronary atherectomy. Circulation 1991; 84:644-53.

98. Yasuda T, Gold HK, Yaoita H, Leinbach RC, Guerrero JL, Jang I, Holt R, Fallon JT, Collen D. Comparative effects of aspirin, a synthetic thrombin inhibitor and a monoclonal antiplatelet glycoprotein IIb/IIIa antibody on coronary artery reperfusion, reocclusion and bleeding with recombinant tissue-type plasminogen activator in a canine preparation. J Am Coll Cardiol 1990; 16:714-22.

19

Support Devices

A. Michael Lincoff
The Cleveland Clinic Foundation, Cleveland, Ohio

Jeffrey J. Popma
Washington Cardiology Center, Washington, D.C.

INTRODUCTION

Over the past two decades, the early death rate associated with acute myocardial infarction has been reduced to 10–15%, principally owing to improvements in coronary care and increasing use of thrombolytic agents. Despite these encouraging results, certain subsets of patients have a less favorable prognosis; those with congestive heart failure, cardiogenic shock, or recurrent myocardial ischemia remain at particular risk for in-hospital mortality or serious morbidity. Although coronary revascularization may improve outcome in patients with cardiogenic shock (1–6) or recurrent ischemia (7) following myocardial infarction, coronary interventions in these high-risk patients are more likely to be associated with severe hemodynamic instability, end-organ injury, abrupt vessel closure, or refractory myocardial ischemia or necrosis (8–11). Some patients with circulatory compromise may not survive to reach the cardiac catheterization laboratory or surgical suite; others may develop hemodynamic collapse as a result of ischemia imparted by angioplasty balloon inflations, abrupt vessel closure, or during the hemodynamic stress associated with anesthesia induction or weaning from cardiopulmonary bypass. In patients who survive percutaneous or surgical revascularization, long-term postprocedural mortality and morbidity will be significantly greater in those with concomitant end-organ failure resulting from pre-operative hypotension and inadequate tissue perfusion. Long-term survival and functional status may be expected to be inversely related to the degree of irreversible myocardial necrosis sustained prior to revascularization.

A number of pharmacological and mechanical strategies have been advocated to support peripheral circulation, prevent irreversible end-organ injury, and limit myocardial necrosis in the settings of cardiogenic shock or recurrent myocardial ischemia following acute infarction. Whereas treatment with inotropic, vasodilator, and/or vasopressor agents may be useful in this regard, the effect of pharmacological agents on these therapeutic goals may be somewhat contradictory; improvement in systemic blood pressure using drugs such as dopamine, for example, may be achieved at the expense of increased myocardial work, wall stress, and oxygen demand. Moreover, these pharmacological approaches alone have not been shown to alter the degree of myocardial dysfunction associated with acute infarction or to limit myocardial infarct size. Pharmacological intervention in acute myocardial infarction, including thrombolytic administration, has not substantially altered the prognosis of patients presenting with clinical congestive heart failure, including those with cardiogenic shock (12-14).

Because of the limitations of pharmacological adjuncts alone, several innovative mechanical approaches have been developed for treatment of patients with profound hemodynamic instability and/or refractory ischemia associated with myocardial infarction. These techniques may be used to provide temporary hemodynamic support during coronary recanalization or revascularization or more prolonged support as a bridge to cardiac transplantation in the event of severe permanent myocardial necrosis. The current advantages, limitations, and potential applications of these devices will be described.

INTRA-AORTIC BALLOON COUNTERPULSATION

Since its clinical introduction by Kantrowitz and associates (15) in 1967, the intra-aortic balloon pump has become the most widely used circulatory support device. Operating on the principle of *counterpulsation*, the balloon pump augments arterial diastolic and coronary perfusion pressures and reduces impedance to ventricular ejection. It has been employed in the setting of myocardial infarction with or without shock, low-output heart failure following intracardiac surgery, refractory unstable angina, recurrent ventricular tachyarrhythmias, preoperative stabilization of high-risk patients, and complicated coronary angioplasty.

Principles of Operation and Hemodynamic Response

The intra-aortic counterpulsation device consists of a 30 to 40 ml catheter-mounted cylindrical balloon inserted percutaneously (or rarely by surgical arterio-

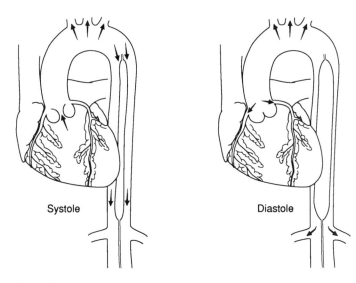

Figure 1   Mechanism of intra-aortic balloon counterpulsation. Balloon collapse during systole reduces aortic blood volume and resistance to ventricular ejection. Diastolic balloon inflation increases diastolic perfusion pressure to the coronary arteries and peripheral organs. (From Pierpont GL. Mechanical support of the failing circulation in acute coronary insufficiency and myocardial infarction. In: Francis GS and Alpert JS, eds. Modern coronary care. Boston: Little, Brown, 1990, p270. With permission.)

tomy) through a 9.5–11F femoral artery sheath into the descending aorta distal to the left subclavian artery. By electrocardiographic or hemodynamic synchronization, the balloon is cyclically inflated with helium at the onset of ventricular diastole and deflated just prior to ventricular systole. Diastolic balloon inflation rapidly forces blood from the descending aorta anterograde to peripheral organs and retrograde into the aortic root, while collapse of the balloon during systole reduces aortic blood volume and resistance to ventricular ejection (Fig. 1).

Extensive studies in humans and animal models have characterized the salutary cardiac hemodynamic effects of intra-aortic balloon counterpulsation. Reproducibly, a reduction in peak aortic systolic and left-ventricular end-diastolic pressures occurs, resulting in a decrease in the heart rate–blood pressure double product and left ventricular wall stress (16–18). Stoke work and myocardial oxygen consumption are acutely reduced by 10–20% (16,17), and cardiac output during shock states may increase by 15–30%(19,20). Peak hemodynamic improvement may be delayed until 18–24 hr after initiation of counterpulsation (21,22). Furthermore, by augmentation of mean and peak aortic diastolic pressures, coronary perfusion distal to coronary stenoses may be improved; this effect, however, has been difficult to consistently establish. Although several experimental and clinical studies have failed to demonstrate improved regional or global myocardial blood flow with intra-aortic balloon counterpulsation (18,23–25), Fuchs and co-workers (26) observed significant increases in great cardiac vein blood flow in proportion to augmented aortic diastolic pressures in patients with unstable angina using this technique. Thus, intra-aortic balloon counterpulsation ameliorates cardiac ischemia primarily by reducing myocardial work and oxygen demand; its effect on myocardial oxygen delivery appears to be variable.

Measured improvements in peripheral organ perfusion in animal models of intra-aortic balloon pump support have been somewhat inconsistent (16), and these measurements have not been made in humans. Nonetheless, improvements in mentation, diuretic responsiveness and urine output, acidosis, and peripheral vasoconstriction observed in patients treated for shock with intra-aortic balloon counterpulsation provide indirect evidence of enhanced organ perfusion.

Clinical Experience

The initial clinical experience with balloon counterpulsation was reported in 1968 (15); two patients with acute myocardial infarction and refractory cardiogenic shock were hemodynamically stabilized by insertion of the intra-aortic balloon pump. Since then, the use of balloon counterpulsation in patients with myocardial infarction (27) has been advocated to treat complications including cardiogenic shock, heart failure, recurrent ischemia, or ventricular arrhythmias, or to limit the size of uncomplicated infarction.

Cardiogenic Shock Due to Severe Left Ventricular Dysfunction

Although the clinical shock state or severe congestive heart failure can be reversed in 60–90% of patients during intra-aortic balloon pumping (21,28–31), improvement in mortality due to counterpulsation therapy alone has not been conclusively demonstrated. Scheidt and associates (30) reported an early clinical trial in which 87 patients with medically refractory postinfarction shock were treated with intra-aortic balloon counterpulsation. Normalization of hemodynamic parameters transiently occurred in up to 70% of patients, but 52/87 could not be weaned from balloon pump support. Of 35 patients in whom counterpulsation was successfully discontinued, only 15 (17% of the total group) survived to hospital discharge, and eight were alive at 1-year follow-up. Similarly, Bardet and colleagues (21) described 42 patients with cardiogenic shock secondary to myocardial infarction; of 20 patients without mechanical etiologies treated with balloon pump therapy alone, only three survived more than 1 year. Somewhat better results were obtained by Hagemeijer et al. (31), who reported a 56% rate of survival in 25 patients in cardiogenic shock or severe heart failure treated with intra-aortic balloon counterpulsation. Most studies, however, seem to corroborate the adverse outcome expected when counterpulsation therapy is used alone in patients with shock; survival rates in the Massachusetts General series (27) and other reports (22,28,29,32,33) range from 15 to 37%.

From the available data, it appears that patients with postinfarction cardiogenic shock will stratify into three groups, based on their response to balloon counterpulsation therapy. First, approximately 10–30% will not improve with placement of the intra-aortic balloon pump and will require more potent means of circulatory support. Of those patients in whom balloon therapy does produce hemodynamic stabilization, a minority (40% or less) can be weaned from the balloon pump for longer than 24 hr, though more than half of these patients may die before hospital discharge. The majority of balloon pump responders will fall into the third group and remain dependent on mechanical support or redevelop shock despite continued balloon pump therapy.

In contrast to the failure of balloon pump therapy alone to alter the overall mortality in patients with pump failure and cardiogenic shock, there is considerable uncontrolled evidence that coronary revascularization may markedly improve outcome in selected patients initially stabilized by intra-aortic counterpulsation. In an early series by Dunkman and colleagues (22), only 16% of 25 patients managed with balloon pumping for cardiogenic shock survived to hospital discharge, in contrast to the 40% survival among 15 patients who underwent emergency surgery. DeWood and associates (1) reported 75% long-term survival in 12 patients with cardiogenic shock in whom coronary artery bypass grafting was performed within 18 hr of onset of symptoms, compared to a 29% survival rate in those patients who did not undergo revascularization or in whom surgery was delayed. Alcan et. al. (28) noted that only 26% of 61 patients treated medically in their series of patients undergoing balloon pump placement for shock survived hospitalization, whereas 83% of 23 patients managed surgically survived.

In other studies, patients with shock who ultimately underwent revascularization received balloon pump support more frequently than those who were medically treated. Although the efficacy of this combined counterpulsation/revascularization therapy can be assessed from these data, the impact of either individual treatment on outcome cannot be determined. Lee and colleagues (3), for example, retrospectively analyzed survival in 87 patients with cardiogenic shock, 24 of whom were treated with coronary angioplasty (PTCA). Balloon counterpulsation was employed in 88% and 31% of patients in the PTCA and conventional therapy groups, respectively. One-month survival among patients with successful PTCA was 77%, compared to 17–18% survival among patients in whom angioplasty was unsuccessful or who were conventionally managed. Similar outcomes have been reported in two other recent series (4,34).

Mechanical Complications of Infarction

The rapid hemodynamic deterioration that almost invariably accompanies development of post infarction myocardial free-wall rupture, ventricular septal defect, or mitral valve papillary muscle rupture mandates surgical repair if the expected 50–80% 1-week mortality is to be averted (35). The timing of such operative repair was initially controversial (35–37), but most investigators now advocate early surgery before intractable hemodynamic collapse and organ failure supervene.

Intra-aortic balloon pump support, while not a curative intervention in this setting, serves as a critical adjunct for preoperative hemodynamic stabilization. Afterload reduction produced by intra-aortic counterpulsation improves forward cardiac output while reducing mitral regurgitation or left-to-right shunting across a ventricular septal defect. Clinical evidence of these effects has been provided by Gold et al. (38) and other investigators (21), who observed reductions in pulmonary-to-systemic flow ratios and pulmonary capillary wedge pressure V-wave amplitudes in patients treated with balloon therapy for ventricular septal rupture or acute mitral regurgitation, respectively. In nearly all patients with ventricular septal defect or mitral regurgitation who develop cardiogenic shock or refractory pulmonary edema, the intra-aortic balloon pump will temporarily reverse or stabilize the clinical deterioration, thus permitting emergency cardiac catheterization and providing perioperative circulatory support (21,35,36,38,39). Long-term survival following prompt operative repair has been reported to be as high as 80%. Importantly, though, hemodynamic instability usually recurs, with nearly 100% mortality in patients managed nonsurgically, despite even prolonged intra-aortic balloon pump therapy (21,36,40).

Myocardial free wall rupture, usually resulting in acute hemopericardium with immediate tamponade, cardiogenic shock, and electromechanical dissociation, accounts for nearly 10% of in-hospital deaths following myocardial infarction (41). In a minority of patients, hemodynamic decompensation may be subacute in onset or transiently improved by pericardiocentesis; prompt surgical repair in this select group of patients has resulted in survival rates of up to 65% (6). Although some authors advocate immediate surgery without cardiac catheterization (42), several groups have reported patients in whom institution of emergent intra-aortic balloon counterpulsation provided sufficient hemodynamic support for cardiac catheterization and successful operative repair to be performed (27,43,44).

Limitation of Myocardial Infarct Size

Early institution of intra-aortic counterpulsation has been investigated as a means of limiting the size and associated mortality of acute myocardial infarction. Preliminary animal experiments produced conflicting results (45,46). Leinbach and colleagues (47) initiated intra-aortic balloon therapy within 6 hr of onset of anterior infarction in 11 patients. Accelerated resolution of chest pain and ST-segment elevations with preservation of overall ventricular function and precordial R waves occurred only in the 5/11 patients who were subsequently found to have nonocclusive stenoses of their infarct-related arteries at cardiac catheterization.

Two randomized controlled trials have been performed to assess the impact of intra-aortic balloon pumping on infarction size and mortality in patients not treated with thrombolytic agents or coronary revascularization. O'Rourke et al. (48) studied 30 patients with myocardial infarction and acute heart failure, 14 of whom were assigned to counterpulsation therapy. Comparison with patients in the control group revealed no differences in peak or cumulative creatine kinase levels, hospital or long-term mortality, or follow-up functional class. Flaherty and colleagues (49) randomized 20 patients with extensive acute myocardial infarction to conventional medical therapy or intra-aortic balloon pumping with intravenous nitroglycerin initiated at a mean of 10 hr from onset of symptoms and continued for 4–5 days. No significant differences were observed in either hospital or 2-month mortality, incidence of recurrent infarction, left ventricular ejection fraction, or infarct expansion among the 10 patients in each group. Thus, the available data fail to demonstrate a reduction in mortality or improvement in ventricular function in high-risk patients with acute myocardial infarction treated with early intra-aortic balloon counterpulsation, although no trial of this type has been performed in the current era of thrombolytic therapy and acute coronary revascularization.

Postinfarction Myocardial Ischemia or Arrhythmias

Although randomized controlled trials have not been performed to assess the clinical efficacy of the intra-aortic balloon pump in stabilizing patients with refractory unstable angina, a number of retrospective analyses have demonstrated the utility of this technique (11,28,33,50–52). In the majority of postinfarction patients, recurrent myocardial ischemia is eliminated or markedly reduced by institution of intra-aortic counterpulsation, but as with cardiogenic shock, long-term survival and functional status appear to be related to successful coronary revascularization (7,33). Gold and associates (50) treated five patients with postinfarction rest angina despite maximal medical therapy with intra-aortic balloon pumping; pain did not recur in four patients and the frequency of attacks in the fifth was markedly reduced. Survival following coronary arteriography and bypass surgery in this group was 80%, with the operative death occurring in the one patient in whom initiation of balloon pump therapy had been delayed until the development of ischemia, hypotension, and ventricular arrhythmias during cardiac catheterization. Levine and colleagues (51) reported 33 patients with recurrent postinfarction ischemia managed with intra-aortic balloon counterpulsation and coronary bypass surgery. Anginal pain was abolished in 79% of patients and decreased in frequency in the others, with balloon pump support continued through weaning from cardiopulmonary bypass and the early postoperative period. Mortality in this group was 9.1%. Other investigators (11,28,33) have reported hospital mortality rates of 0–42% in patients treated with the intra-aortic balloon pump for recurrent postinfarction angina. Importantly, among 12 patients in one series (33), of whom half were managed surgically and half treated medically, mortality was 0% and 93.4% in the surgical and medical groups, respectively.

Following thrombolytic or mechanical reperfusion for acute myocardial infarction, balloon counterpulsation may be useful in *preventing* recurrent ischemic events through its augmentation of diastolic coronary perfusion pressures and improvement of blood flow across the coronary lesion. Two separate studies have reported a 0% rate of coronary reocclusion in a total of 114 patients treated with balloon therapy following myocardial infarction, in contrast to 13% and 21% rates of reocclusion in conventionally treated patients (53,54). A prospective controlled trial of the efficacy of balloon pump counterpulsation in preventing recurrent ischemia is currently underway.

The role of intra-aortic balloon counterpulsation in the management of refractory peri-infarction ventricular arrhythmias has been reported in a limited number of studies (29,55,56). Among more than 1000 patients in whom the balloon pump was placed over a 10-year period at Massachusetts General Hospital (55), the primary indication for this therapy was postinfarction ventricular arrhythmias in only 22 patients. The frequency of life-threatening recurrent arrhythmias was decreased or abolished by balloon counterpulsation in 86% of patients, with the most marked beneficial effects noted in those with associated active myocardial ischemia, heart failure, and/or hypotension. Notably, 90% of patients with myocardial ischemia survived to hospital discharge with emergency surgery, compared to only 14% survival among the seven patients whose ventricular arrhythmias were unassociated with either ischemia or hypotension. This study underscored the favorable prognosis for patients in whom ventricular arrhythmias were secondary to myocardial ischemia, whereas patients with arrhythmias unrelated to reversible causes had minimal benefit from balloon pump therapy.

Limitations and Complications

The most important limitation of intra-aortic counterpulsation in severely compromised patients is its modest augmentation of cardiac output and dependence on stable cardiac rhythm for synchronization. The balloon pump will fail to restore adequate blood pressure and systemic perfusion in up to 30% of patients with shock (19,22,29,30), and results in patients treated for cardiac arrest have been disappointing. In the series by Alcan et al. (28), for example, only one of seven patients who presented in cardiac arrest survived; Phillips (57) similarly described seven patients in cardiac arrest who failed initial attempts at resuscitation using the intra-aortic balloon pump, but were subsequently resuscitated with percutaneous cardiopulmonary bypass.

Although the speed and convenience of intra-aortic balloon pump implementation have improved with the development of the percutaneous technique, inability to insert the balloon catheter on the first attempt will occur in 11-25% of patients, with complete failure of insertion due to ileofemoral atherosclerosis in 2-14% (27,28,33,52,58-61). The incidence of complications associated with counterpulsation remains substantial (58-63). Limb ischemia resulting from thrombosis, embolization, or bleeding at the site of vascular access is by far the most common complication, occurring in up to 43% of patients despite routine anticoagulation with heparin. Nearly two-thirds of these patients may require early removal of the balloon pump and/or vascular surgical repair, although the incidence of permanent sequelae such as claudication, neurological impairment, or amputation is uncommon (approximately 5% in most series). In the recent review by Alderman and colleagues (62), for example, limb ischemia occurred in 47 of 103 patients treated with the intra-aortic balloon pump; 29 patients required premature discontinuation of counterpulsation support, 15 underwent vascular surgical repair, and nine had evidence of persistent limb ischemia (symptomatic in only two) by hospital discharge. Risk factors for development of vascular complications with intra-aortic balloon pumping include preexisting peripheral vascular occlusive disease, diabetes mellitus, and female gender (59,60,62). Several reports have noted a higher incidence of vascular complications with the percutaneous rather than the surgical arteriotomy method of balloon pump insertion (33,59,60), particularly in the presence of peripheral vascular disease; the current availability of lower-profile, wire-guided balloon catheters since these studies, however, may have improved the safety of the percutaneous technique.

Other complications of balloon counterpulsation, occurring with a cumulative incidence of approximately 10%, include aortoiliac dissection or perforation, visceral or cerebral embolization, bleeding or tamponade due to systemic anticoagulation, and fever, local infection, or bacteremia. Clinically significant thrombocytopenia occurs rarely, may be related to heparin administration,and usually resolves promptly with termination of balloon pumping and anticoagulation (61).

CORONARY SINUS RETROPERFUSION

Coronary sinus retroperfusion is a mechanical technique for providing blood flow to ischemic myocardium via the cardiac venous system, although without furnishing systemic hemodynamic support. It has been employed in patients with acute coronary ischemia and during high-risk coronary angioplasty and may have potential utility in the management of complicated myocardial infarction.

Development and Technique

Clinical use of the coronary venous system as an alternative channel for myocardial perfusion was introduced by Beck in 1948, who surgically constructed a vein graft from the aorta to the coronary sinus (64). This procedure afforded relief of

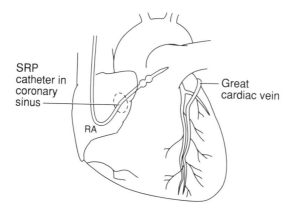

Figure 2   Positioning of synchronized retroperfusion (SRP) catheter in the coronary sinus and great cardiac vein. RA = right atrium.

angina in some patients, but led to the late development of congestive heart failure due to thrombosis of the venous drainage system and myocardial hemorrhage, edema, and fibrosis.

In 1976, Meerbaum and associates (65) renewed efforts to employ coronary sinus retroperfusion as a treatment for acute ischemic syndromes. By delivering blood in a pulsatile manner synchronized during diastole through a nonocclusive coronary sinus catheter, normal physiological coronary venous drainage resumed during systole and the adverse effects of myocardial hemorrhage and edema did not occur. Synchronized retroperfusion of arterial blood in dogs undergoing left anterior descending coronary artery ligation produced significant improvements in segmental contractile dysfunction, regional myocardial perfusion, and electro-cardiographic ST-segment elevations (64). Subsequent studies confirmed these findings and demonstrated 1.5-to sixfold reductions in infarct size with coronary sinus retroperfusion (66–68), hypothermic retroperfusion (69,70), or *retroinfusion* of prostaglandin E₁ (71). *Pressure-controlled intermittent coronary sinus occlusion* was also investigated as a means of redistributing coronary blood flow through coronary venous pressure gradients (72), but arterialization of the coronary sinus system by retroperfusion was shown to be superior in limiting infarct size (73).

The technique of synchronized retroperfusion was improved by development of an inflatable balloon-tipped coronary sinus catheter (65). Systems currently in use employ an 8F or 8.5F soft-tipped retroperfusion catheter inserted via the right or left internal jugular or left subclavian vein into the coronary sinus and advanced into the great cardiac vein (Fig. 2). Oxygenated blood is pumped from a femoral artery cannula through the coronary sinus catheter during ventricular diastole at

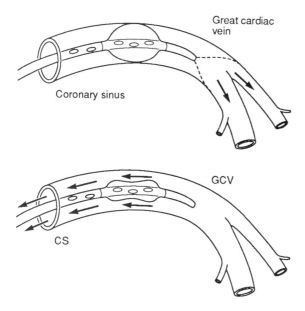

Figure 2   Operation of balloon tip catheter. During ventricular diastole (top figure), balloon inflation with blood (autoinflation) or carbon dioxide prevents efflux of blood out of the coronary sinus during retroperfusion of the great cardiac vein. Retroperfusion stops during ventricular systole, and deflation of the balloon allows systolic drainage of the coronary venous system into the right atrium. CS = coronary sinus; GCV = great cardiac vein. (From Corday E, et al. The coronary sinus: an alternate channel for administration of arterial blood and pharmacologic agents for protection and treatment of acute cardiac ischemia. J Am Coll Cardiol 1986; 7:712. With permission.)

flow rates of up to 250 cc/min (74); a 10-mm balloon located 1 cm proximal to the tip of the retroperfusion catheter inflates and deflates with blood or pressurized carbon dioxide during each cardiac cycle, preventing efflux of retroperfused blood into the right atrium.

Clinical Experience

After demonstration of the feasibility and safety of coronary sinus retroperfusion in humans (75), Gore and co-workers (76) reported its initial clinical application in five patients with refractory unstable angina and anterior myocardial ischemia. Synchronized retroperfusion, instituted within 25–60 min, completely reversed chest pain and ischemic electrocardiographic abnormalities in four patients, with relief of chest pain and partial electrocardiographic improvement in the fifth. Retroperfusion support was continued for 12–50 hr without significant hemolysis, thrombocytopenia, or changes in systemic hemodynamic parameters. Three patients treated with coronary bypass surgery survived, while two with coronary anatomy unsuitable for revascularization died.

Following this and other favorable, although uncontrolled, experience with coronary sinus retroperfusion in patients with acute ischemic syndromes (77), synchronized retroperfusion has been applied as an adjunct to coronary angioplasty (78,79). During retroperfusion, the time to onset of angina was prolonged, the frequency of angina was reduced, the magnitude of ST-segment changes was decreased, and transient regional wall motion abnormalities were ameliorated during left anterior descending coronary angioplasty. Those patients suffering abrupt vessel closure were successfully stabilized by retroperfusion support until revascularization could be accomplished. Complications, including hematoma at the venous access site, atrial fibrillation, or coronary sinus staining, have been infrequent.

The full extent to which coronary sinus retroperfusion may prove useful in the management of acute myocardial infarction remains to be defined, and experience in this patient group remains very limited. The degree of myocardial protection afforded by retroperfusion appears to be incomplete, and many patients continue to experience chest pain and exhibit significant electrocardiographic changes and regional wall motion abnormalities during supported angioplasty. Additionally, while the average time to successful coronary sinus cannulation is only 3–5 min by practiced operators, overall setup time generally exceeds 30 min and inability to cannulate the sinus will preclude use of retroperfusion in 10–15% of patients (79). Finally, this technique has been used almost exclusively for left anterior descending coronary artery occlusion, and it is unclear whether retroperfusion would protect against ischemia in other coronary distributions with substantially different patterns of venous drainage.

PERCUTANEOUS CARDIOPULMONARY BYPASS

Despite the efficacy of intra-aortic balloon counterpulsation in the hemodynamic stabilization of most patients with cardiogenic shock, this technique cannot provide total circulatory support in the event of catastrophic derangements in cardiac function or rhythm. Extracorporeal membrane oxygenation (ECMO) has been employed as a prolonged cardiopulmonary bypass support in patients with severe acute respiratory failure for nearly 20 years (80). The recent development of thin-walled, large-bore intravascular catheters and a commercially available cardiopulmonary bypass device has made rapid percutaneous initiation of cardiopulmonary support (CPS) possible, allowing application of this technique to patients with cardiogenic shock, cardiac arrest, refractory rhythm disturbances, and high-risk or complicated coronary angioplasty.

Technique and Physiological Response

Institution and maintenance of ECMO is complex and requires an experienced team. In adults, the jugular vein and axillary artery are cannulated via surgical cutdown with 36F and 22–24F tubes respectively (81). These are connected to the ECMO circuit, consisting of an occlusive roller pump servoregulated by a distensible bladder on the venous inflow line, a membrane oxygenator, and a heat exchanger. Venous blood flows by gravity siphon to the bladder and roller pump; transient decreases in venous return turn off the roller pump and prevent aspiration of air or the development of vacuum and hemolysis in the venous cannula. Blood passes from the roller pump through the membrane lung and heat exchanger and is returned to the aortic root via the arterial cannula. During long-term ECMO support, blood flow through the extracorporeal circuit is adjusted to achieve a mixed venous saturation of >70%, heparin is continuously infused to maintain the activated clotting time at 200–240 sec (82) to prevent thrombosis in the bypass circuit, and fluid balance is carefully monitored.

A percutaneous technique for institution of CPS with a commercially available cardiopulmonary support device has been described by Shawl et al. (83). Following ileofemoral arteriography to exclude significant atherosclerotic obstruction (except in those patients emergently treated for cardiac arrest), the femoral artery and vein are entered and progressively dilated to permit passage of 18F or 20F bypass sheaths; the tip of the arterial cannula is placed just below the aortic bifurcation and the long venous cannula is advanced to the right atrial-inferior vena caval junction (Fig.3). Cannulae are attached to a portable, battery-operated cardiopulmonary support system (C. R. Bard, Billerica, MA), consisting of a vortex-centrifugal Biomedicus pump in series with a membrane oxygenator. Blood is aspirated from the right atrium and returned via the oxygenator through the femoral arterial cannula; flow rates of up to 6.0 L/min may be obtained, providing nearly complete circulatory support. Fluid administration may be needed upon initiation of bypass to maintain adequate venous return and systemic arterial pressure. Activated clotting time is maintained above 400 sec by heparin infusion during short-term cardiopulmonary support, particularly if coronary revascularization is performed; a lower level of anticoagulation is adequate for prolonged bypass and may limit the incidence of bleeding complications (81). Upon discontinuation of bypass, the femoral sheaths are removed using an external compression clamp or by primary vascular surgical repair.

While ECMO and CPS operate on identical principles and consist of similar bypass circuitry, the percutaneous CPS technique differs from traditional ECMO in two respects. First, percutaneous femoral cannulation may be rapidly performed without the requirement of a surgical team, even while cardiopulmonary resuscitation is in progress. In experienced hands, emergent bypass can be instituted within 10–45 min (84). Second, by actively aspirating blood from the right

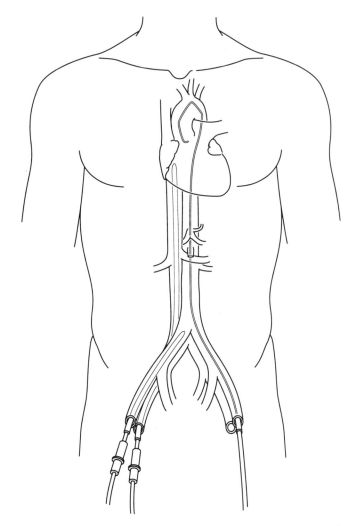

Figure 3 Diagram of the position of arterial and venous cannulae for percutaneous cardiopulmonary bypass support (either left or right femoral approaches may be used). The venous cannula is advanced to the inferior vena caval-right atrial junction. The tip of the arterial cannula is placed below the aortic bifurcation. A left Judkins coronary catheter is also present in this drawing. (From Shawl et al.[83] With permission.)

atrium using a vortex pump rather than gravity drainage, adequate flow rates are possible through the relatively small-caliber 18-20F percutaneous cannulae. Importantly, however, the percutaneous cardiopulmonary apparatus is not suitable for long-term (>6-12 hr) support, owing in part to the clinically significant hemolysis that occurs as a result of high venous flow rates through small inflow cannulae and the negative pressure produced by the unregulated centrifugal pump. Transition to the more complex ECMO apparatus should be performed if prolonged application of cardiopulmonary bypass is required.

A number of physiological changes occur during cardiopulmonary support, many of which become manifest only when bypass is maintained for more than several hours (81,85). Interaction of blood components with the surfaces of the extracorporeal circuit may cause platelet activation and aggregation, leukocyte and complement activation, and release of vasoactive substances. These, in turn, may result in transient deterioration in pulmonary function, thrombocytopenia, and capillary leakage and tissue edema. Blood pressure initially falls in many patients owing to hemodilution with the priming fluid and release of vasoactive substances. Hemolysis occurs rarely with the ECMO circuit. Finally, the impact of nonpulsatile flow in this setting is controversial. When compared to pulsatile perfusion, nonpulsatile flow may cause increased catecholamine release, impaired renal metabolism and excretion, and increased pulmonary vascular resistance, but these differences are inconsistent (86).

Clinical Experience

Initial clinical attempts at ECMO support in adults with respiratory failure met with disappointing results, primarily because of the irreversible nature of the disease in these moribund patients (81). In selected neonates with profound, but reversible pulmonary processes, however, survival rates in excess of 80% were obtained, demonstrating the efficacy and safety of prolonged cardiopulmonary support. Until recently, experience with cardiopulmonary bypass in patients with cardiac disease has been limited. Bartlett and colleagues (87) reported an early series in which one adult and three children were placed on ECMO for cardiogenic shock following intracardiac surgery; only one pediatric patient survived. Pennington and associates (88) applied cardiopulmonary support through surgical vascular cutdown to 14 patients in shock due to myocardial infarction (two patients), intracardiac surgery or postoperative complications (10 patients), or idiopathic cardiomyopathy (two patients). All patients experienced substantial hemodynamic improvement upon initiation of ECMO, although deterioration occurred in those who ultimately could not be weaned. The two patients with post infarction shock survived surgery (coronary bypass or heart transplantation), although only four patients of the entire group were long-term survivors.

With development of the percutaneous method of insertion (89), implementation of cardiopulmonary bypass became feasible on a more widespread basis. An initial favorable experience with CPS in patients undergoing high-risk coronary angioplasty led to the formation of a national registry of centers performing angioplasty under prophylactic cardiopulmonary support (90,91). Indications for support in these 363 registry patients included markedly impaired left ventricular function and/or a target vessel supplying the majority of viable myocardium. Despite the high-risk group studied, 95% of attempted vessels were successfully dilated, and overall hospital mortality was only 6%.

There has been limited experience with the emergent implementation of percutaneous cardiopulmonary bypass in patients with circulatory collapse due to myocardial infarction. Phillips et al. (92) described 11 adult patients with refractory cardiac arrest due to myocardial infarction or complicated coronary angioplasty who were successfully resuscitated by percutaneous cardiopulmonary support for up to 8 hr; five patients treated with immediate coronary revascularization survived to hospital discharge. Shawl and colleagues (93) placed eight patients with postinfarction cardiogenic shock of less than 3 hr duration on emergency cardiopulmonary bypass. All patients recovered hemodynamic stability, while two in cardiac arrest even regained consciousness while ventricular fibrillation or asystole persisted. Of seven patients in whom coronary anatomy was suitable for revascularization, long-term survival was 100%; one patient treated medically died. In another series of seven patients suffering sustained cardiac arrest during coronary angiography or angioplasty, bypass was instituted within a mean of 21 min from the onset of arrest (84). Further revascularization was attempted in five of the seven patients, and four survived.

There are several limitations of cardiopulmonary bypass support. The myocardial protective effect of this technique does not appear to be due to a significant improvement in coronary perfusion; animal experiments do not demonstrate an increase in blood flow to the distribution of an occluded coronary artery (94), and echocardiographic studies indicate that cardiopulmonary bypass does not prevent regional wall motion abnormalities or ventricular dilation induced by angioplasty balloon inflations (95). As with the intra-aortic balloon pump then, it is likely that cardiopulmonary bypass is beneficial by virtue of the hemodynamic support it provides and the consequent reduction in cardiac work and oxygen demand. During prolonged support of patients in whom the severely impaired left ventricle cannot eject against aortic root pressure, decompression of the left heart via atrial septostomy or a large catheter passed retrograde across the aortic valve must be performed in order to prevent progressive ventricular dilatation and elevation of pulmonary pressure. Percutaneous insertion of the stiff, large-bore bypass cannulae may be difficult with atherosclerotic or tortuous vessels and may require peripheral angioplasty. Finally, the attendance of a skilled perfusionist is required during all phases of cardiopulmonary support.

Complications of cardiopulmonary support occur frequently at the site of vascular cannulation. In the first year of the Supported Angioplasty Registry reported by Vogel and co-workers (90), vascular complications developed in 39% of patients and included infection at the cannula site (7.6%), thrombophlebitis (4.7%), required femoral artery repair (3.8%), femoral artery pseudoaneurysm or occlusion (3.8%), hematoma (3.8%), and transient femoral nerve injury (1.9%). Thrombocytopenia and hemolysis were rare, although transfusions were required in 43% of patients due to periprocedural blood loss. Other investigators have reported bleeding due to anticoagulation at cannulation points and other sites (pericardial tamponade, wound bleeding, and retroperitoneal, gastrointestinal, or intracranial hemorrhage) to be a major source of morbidity in patients treated with ECMO (81,87). Less frequent complications include equipment malfunction, catheter-related sepsis, and thromboembolic phenomena (81,90).

HEMOPUMP

The Hemopump, a catheter-mounted left ventricular assist device, was recently developed to overcome the limited effectiveness of the intra-aortic balloon pump and the complexities of traditional left ventricular assist devices or percutaneous cardiopulmonary bypass in the treatment of patients with profound left ventricular failure. It has been employed for periods of up to 2 weeks in patients following intracardiac surgery, cardiac allograft rejection or failure, and myocardial infarction.

Design and Hemodynamic Response

The Hemopump is a catheter-mounted axial-flow pump powered by an external drive assembly that withdraws blood directly from the left ventricular cavity and propels it into the descending aorta (Fig. 4). The 21F flexible silicone rubber inflow cannula inserted via surgical femoral arteriotomy (or rarely through the abdominal or ascending aorta) is passed retrograde across the aortic valve to rest within the left ventricular cavity; a miniature Archimedes spiral vane screw pump, housed in the distal base of the cannula, rotates at 27,000 rpm, producing nonpulsatile flow rates of up to 3.5 L/min. Power to the pump assembly is transmitted percutaneously from the external control console by a flexible drive shaft. Maximum blood flow through the Hemopump is dependent only on the resistance to flow (systemic afterload) and adequate preload and positioning of the inflow cannula within the left ventricular cavity. Hemopump output is thus independent of intrinsic left ventricular function or underlying cardiac rhythm, and the device is effective for limited periods even during ventricular fibrillation.

Animal studies have demonstrated that the Hemopump may be placed for up to 2 weeks with full-dose heparinization without the development of significant hemolysis, thrombocytopenia, hypofibrinogenemia, thromboembolic phenom-

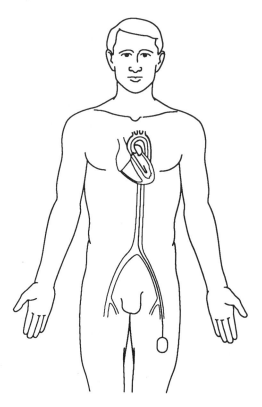

Figure 4   (A) Schematic of the placement of the Hemopump via surgical femoral arteriotomy retrograde across the aortic valve into the left ventricle. Power is transmitted through the flexible drive shaft from an external console to the pump. (From Merhige et al.[97] With permission).

ena, aortic valve or intracardiac injury, or renal or hepatic dysfunction (96). In animals undergoing experimental coronary occlusion, immediate institution of Hemo-pump circulatory support markedly reduced left ventricular end-diastolic pressure and systolic workload (97), increased collateral myocardial perfusion to the ischemic region (97), and produced modest reductions in infarct size (98). Comparison of the hemodynamic benefit afforded by the Hemopump to that of the intra-aortic balloon pump in dogs with coronary ligation demonstrated superiority of the Hemopump in reducing left ventricular workload, chamber size, and dyskinesis of the ischemic region (99).

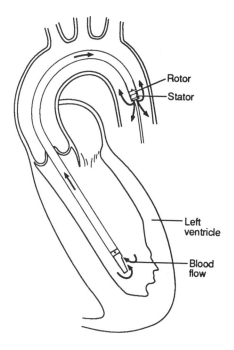

Figure 4   (B) Detail of the inflow cannula and pump housing: blood is withdrawn from the left ventricle by the Archimedes spiral vane screw pump in the base of the cannula and ejected into the aortic arch and descending aorta (From Wampler.[96] With permission.)

Clinical Experience

The reported clinical experience with the Hemopump has thus far been confined to a limited number of patients for cardiogenic shock (100-103) or during high-risk or complicated coronary angioplasty (104-107). The hemodynamic effects of Hemopump support in humans have been similar to those observed in animal models. In four patients treated with the Hemopump for cardiogenic shock following acute myocardial infarction (100), average cardiac index increased from 1.2 to 2.6 L/m^2/min, mean arterial pressure improved from 60 to 80 mm Hg, and pulmonary capillary wedge pressure declined from 27 to 17 mmHg over 48 hr. Transient increases in coronary blood flow due to left ventricular unloading have been measured in patients treated with the Hemopump for high-risk angioplasty (107).

Improvement in survival with Hemopump support among patients with cardiogenic shock has not yet been clearly demonstrated. In an uncontrolled series of

28 patients in whom insertion of the Hemopump was attempted for cardiogenic shock following myocardial infarction or cardiac surgery (103), placement failure via the femoral route occurred in six. Thirty-day survival among patients following 1 hr to 8 days of Hemopump support was 41%, while none of the six patients in whom placement failed survived. In a report in which a patient suffered acute myocardial infarction and cardiac arrest due to left main coronary artery dissection during coronary angioplasty, survival with preserved left ventricular function was aided by prompt Hemopump placement prior to coronary bypass surgery (106).

Limitations of the current Hemopump design include its relatively large profile and the substantial proportion of failed attempts at placement via the femoral artery. The inflow cannula in the left ventricular cavity may mechanically induce ventricular arrhythmias, dislodge mural thrombi, or prolapse into the aorta, causing cessation of effective support. Clinically important hemolysis, infection, or valvular damage due to the Hemopump has not been reported, although one patient suffered hemorrhagic embolic stroke in the setting of acute anterior myocardial infarction and shock (105). Finally, cardiac output through the Hemopump is limited to 3.5 L/min and is dependent on left ventricular filling and may thus be inadequate in patients with severe biventricular failure.

VENTRICULAR ASSIST DEVICE AND TOTAL ARTIFICIAL HEART

The "ultimate" mechanical support for failing circulation is the ventricular assist device (VAD) or the total artificial heart (TAH). Although several different designs have been studied as a bridge to cardiac transplantation or for the management of profound cardiac failure following heart surgery or myocardial infarction, substantial clinical experience has been reported by only a few investigators.

Design

Developed to temporarily or permanently replace the function of one or both ventricles, these devices may be broadly classified as pulsatile (valved chamber) or nonpulsatile (centrifugal) blood pumps. Despite theoretical advantages of pulsatile flow, both designs have been demonstrated to provide adequate prolonged circulatory support in humans and animal models. All require surgical placement of cannulae via median sternotomy for blood flow to and from the central circulation; heterotopic univentricular or biventricular prostheses are connected in parallel to the native heart and positioned externally or internally, while the total artificial heart replaces the patient's heart in the chest cavity.

An example of a widely used pulsatile VAD, the Pierce-Donachy prosthesis (108), consists of a valved polyurethane sac within a rigid housing, cyclically

A   B   C

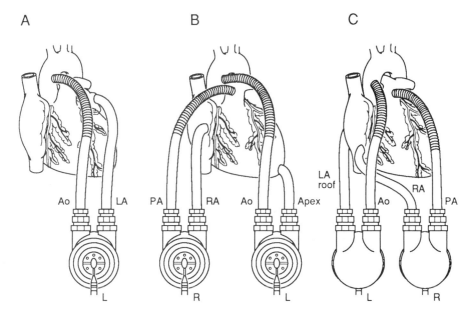

Figure 5   Cannulation alternatives for connection of the ventricular assist device. Univentricular support is provided in A; B and C depict biventricular support. Right ventricular support is accomplished by aspiration of blood from the right atrium and return to the pulmonary artery (B and C). The left ventricular assist device drains blood from the left atrial appendage (A), the left ventricular apex (B), or the roof of the left atrium (C) and returns blood to the ascending aorta. The ventricular assist devices shown in C are turned over. A₀ = ascending aorta; L = left; LA = left atrium; PA = pulmonary artery; R = right; PA = right atrium. (From Farrar et al.[112] With permission.)

compressed by a pneumatically driven diaphragm (Fig. 5). Blood pump ejection can be synchronized to the cardiac cycle or set to run independently. In calves with experimental heart failure, the Pierce-Donachy VAD restored normal systemic and left atrial pressures and provided complete left ventricular decompression; this device has been implanted for up to 110 days without development of significant hemolysis, thrombocytopenia, or embolic phenomena.

The TAH under clinical investigation is the Symbion (Jarvick-7) Total Artificial Heart. Similar to the Pierce-Donachy VAD, the Symbion TAH is a valved, pneumatically driven pulsatile pump with a smooth polyurethane sac blood surface within a rigid polycarbonate housing. The device obeys the Starling length-tension relationship, and cardiac outputs of up to 13 L/min may be obtained (109). The Symbion TAH has been implanted in growing calves for up to 9 months (110).

Clinical Experience

Ventricular Assist Device

Early trials of prosthetic left ventricular support in patients with postcardiotomy shock demonstrated that the assist device was effective in restoring systemic perfusion, relieving pulmonary edema, and decreasing myocardial oxygen demand (108,111). In a multicenter study of 29 patients receiving heterotopic ventricular assist devices as a bridge to transplantation, hospital survival among the 21 patients who underwent transplantation was 95% (112). Of patients not receiving transplants, most died of multiorgan failure or bleeding. In another series of 14 patients with cardiogenic shock receiving VADs prior to transplantation (113), seven survived to hospital discharge.

There is experimental evidence that left ventricular assist may limit infarction size and allow recovery of ventricular function after acute cardiogenic shock (108,114). Clinical experience in this setting has been limited. Noda and associates implanted a left VAD in 10 patients with cardiogenic shock following acute myocardial infarction (115). Although seven patients were successfully weaned after 6-15 days of circulatory support, only three survived to hospital discharge; five patients died of multiple organ failure felt to be due to prolonged periods of inadequate systemic perfusion prior to placement of the assist device.

A percutaneous partial left heart bypass system has recently been employed for circulatory support in two patients with cardiogenic shock (116). Using a transseptal approach, a 14 or 16.5F catheter is placed into the left atrium via the femoral vein. Oxygenated left atrial blood is returned to the circulation through a femoral artery cannula, and circulatory support has been employed for up to 10 days. While this system offers an advantage over traditional ventricular assist in that surgical implantation is not required, experience thus far is too limited to assess the incidence of significant atrial septal defect or other complications.

Total Artificial Heart

The multicenter experience of the first 100 patients to receive the Symbion TAH while awaiting cardiac transplantation has been reported (117). Duration of TAH support ranged from 1 to 243 days, with a 69% 30-day survival rate among the 68 patients who received transplants. Importantly, 32 patients died during TAH support, the majority due to multiple organ failure with or without sepsis. A trend toward improved outcome in young male patients without preexisting infection or respiratory disease was identified. Subsequent analysis demonstrated that body surface area > 1.8 m^2 is a strong correlate of systemic organ recovery and eligibility for transplantation in patients supported by the TAH, most likely owing to restricted fit of the device in the thoracic cavity and resultant impairment in ventricular filling in smaller patients (118). A heterotopic ventricular assist device may be more suitable than current designs of the TAH for bridge support in small patients.

Complications of support with both the TAH and the VAD are frequent and may cause substantial morbidity and mortality (112,117). Infection (including cannulae site or sternal wound infection and mediastinitis) and/or bleeding occurs in up to 30% of patients; less common complications include diaphragmatic paralysis and thromboembolic neurological events. The frequent development of multiple organ failure probably reflects the clinical deterioration that occurs in many of these patients before they are referred for institution of ventricular assist.

RECOMMENDATIONS

A wide array of potent mechanical support techniques are available for the management of patients with acute myocardial infarction complicated by cardiogenic shock and/or refractory myocardial ischemia (Table 1). Substantial clinical data support the use of these devices in patients with some degree of reversible underlying pathology amenable to coronary revascularization or surgical repair. Thus, urgent cardiac catheterization should be performed in most patients presenting with severe congestive heart failure, ischemia, or cardiogenic shock complicating acute myocardial infarction. Intra-aortic balloon counterpulsation will stabilize systemic hemodynamics and relieve myocardial ischemia prior to diagnostic angiography in the majority of these patients and may also be of benefit in stable patients with "high-risk" coronary lesions prior to anticipated revascularization. If refractory rhythm instability or profound left ventricular dysfunction with hemodynamic collapse supervenes, more aggressive circulatory support with percutaneous cardiopulmonary bypass, the Hemopump, or a VAD may be required. As none of these devices clearly improves myocardial oxygen supply, the addition of a perfusion technique such as coronary sinus retroperfusion may be of added benefit in limiting myocardial necrosis in patients with ongoing coronary ischemia or in improving patient tolerance of balloon inflations during coronary angioplasty.

In patients who present with cardiogenic shock due to irreversible myocardial necrosis late in the course of acute myocardial infarction, mechanical support may be appropriate as a bridge to cardiac transplantation. While prolonged circulatory assistance has been accomplished using percutaneous cardiopulmonary bypass, the Hemopump, VAD, or TAH may be more suitable means of long-term hemodynamic support.

Application of mechanical support techniques is associated with a substantial risk of vascular or infectious complications, particularly with devices requiring large-bore arterial and venous cannulation. Furthermore, the potential for dependence must be considered before mechanical circulatory assistance is instituted in patients with severely compromised ventricular function who may not be candi-

Table 1 Current Support Devices for Myocardial Infarction

Device	Advantages	Disadvantages	Applications
Intra-aortic balloon counterpulsation	↓ Myocardial oxygen demand; Ease of placement in 90% of patients; Prolonged treatment duration possible	Requires a stable cardiac rhythm; Modest augmentation of cardiac output (15–30%); 9–43% incidence of vascular complications	Prior to coronary arteriography, revascularization, or surgical repair in settings of: Cardiogenic shock due to LV dysfunction or mechanical complications; Refractory myocardial ischemia; Adjunctive therapy during high-risk coronary angioplasty
Coronary sinus retroperfusion	Improves myocardial oxygen supply; Prolonged use possible	Efficacy documented only in LAD distribution; Incomplete protection from ischemia	Therapy for refractory ischemia prior to revascularization; Possible efficacy in infarct size reduction
Percutaneous cardiopulmonary bypass	↓Myocardial oxygen demand; Independent of LV function or rhythm	No improvement in coronary perfusion; 40% incidence of vascular complications; Complex equipment requiring skilled perfusionist	Circulatory collapse or refractory arrhythmia prior to revascularization or surgical repair
Hemopump	Direct LV decompression; ↓Myocardial oxygen demand; Improves coronary perfusion; Independent of LV function or rhythm; Prolonged use possible	Requires arteriotomy and adequate femoral artery size for placement; Arrhythmogenic LV cannula; Potential for dislodgement from LV	Circulatory collapse or refractory arrhythmia prior to revascularization or surgical repair; Bridge to cardiac transplantation
Ventricular assist device; Total artificial heart	Independent of LV function or rhythm; Prolonged use possible	Requires thoracotomy for placement; 30% incidence of serious infectious or bleeding complications	Bridge to cardiac transplantation; Possible efficacy in infarct size reduction (ventricular assist device)

dates for cardiac transplantation. Judicious patient selection is required if these devices are to prove effective in improving outcome following complicated myocardial infarction.

REFERENCES

1. DeWood MA, Notske RN, Hensley GR, Shields JP, O'Grady WP, Spores J, Goldman M, Ganji JH. Intra-aortic balloon counterpulsation with and without reperfusion for mypcardial infarction shock. Circulation 1980; 61:1105-12.
2. Guyton RA, Arcidi JM, Langford DA, Morris DC, Liberman HA, Hatcher CR. Emergency coronary bypass surgery for cardiogenic shock. Circulation 1987; 76:V-22-V-27.
3. Lee L, Bates ER, Pitt B, Walton JA, Laufer N, O'Neill WW. Percutaneous transluminal coronary angioplasty improves survival in acute myocardial infarction complicated by cardiogenic shock. Circulation 1988; 78:1345-51.
4. Hibbard MD, Holmes DR, Gersh BJ, Reeder GS. Coronary angioplasty for acute myocardial infarction complicated by cardiogenic shock. Circulation 1990; 82:III-511 (abstract).
5. Kaplan AJ, Bengston JR, Aronson LG, et al. Reperfusion improves survival in patients with cardiogenic shock after acute myocardial infarction. J Am Coll Cardiol 1990; 15:155A (abstract).
6. Bolooki H. Emergency cardiac procedures in patients in cardiogenic shock due to complications of coronary artery disease. Circulation 1989; 79:I-137-I-148.
7. Ellis S. Debowey D, Bates ER, Topol EJ. Treatment of recurrent ischemia after thrombolysis and successful reperfusion for acute myocardial infarction—effect on in-hospital mortality and left ventricular function. J Am Coll Cardiol 1991; 17:752-7.
8. Ohman EM, Califf RM, Topol EJ, Candela R, Abbottsmith C, Ellis SG, Sigmon KN, Kereiakes D, George B, Stack R. Consequences of reocclusion after successful reperfusion therapy in acute myocardial infarction. Circulation 1990; 82:781-91.
9. deFeyter PJ. Coronary angioplasty for unstable angina. Am Heart J 1989; 118:860-8.
10. Hochberg MS, Parsonnet V, Gielchinsky I, Hussain SM, Fisch DA, Norman JC. Timing of coronary revascularization after acute myocardial infarction. Early and late results in patients revascularized within seven weeks. J Thorac Cardiovasc Surg 1984; 88:914-21.
11. Naunheim KS, Kesler KA, Kanter KR, Fiore AC, McBride LR, Pennington DG, Barner HB, Kaiser GC, Willman VL. Coronary artery bypass for recent infarction: predictors of mortality. Circulation 1988; 78:I-122-I-128.
12. Gruppo Italiano per lo Studio della Streptochinasi nell'Infarto Miocardico (GISSI). Effectiveness of intravenous thrombolytic treatment in acute myocardial infarction. Lancet 1986; 1:397-401.
13. The International Study Group. In-hospital mortality and clinical course of 20,891 patients with suspected acute myocardial infarction randomised between alteplase and streptokinase with or without heparin. Lancet 1990; 336:71-5.

14. Bates ER, Topol EJ. Limitations of reperfusion therapy for acute myocardial infarction complicated by congestive heart failure and cardiogenic shock. J Am Coll Cardiol 1991; 184:1077–84.

15. Kantrowitz A, Tjonneland S, Freed PS, Phillips SJ, Butner AN, Sherman JL. Initial clinical experience with intra-aortic balloon pumping in cardiogenic shock. JAMA 1968: 203:135–40.

16. Weber KT, Janicki JS. Intra-aortic balloon counterpulsation: a review of physiological principles, clinical results, and device safety. Ann Thorac Surg 1974:17:602–36.

17. Spotnitz HM, Covell JW, Ross J, Braunwald E. Left ventricular mechanics and oxygen consumption during arterial counterpulsation. Am J Physiol 1969; 217:1352–8.

18. Williams DO, Korr KS, Gerwitz H, Most AS. The effect of intra-aortic balloon counterpulsation on regional myocardial blood flow and oxygen consumption in the presence of coronary artery stenosis in patients with unstable angina. Circulation 1982; 66:593–7.

19. Ehrich DA, Biddle TL, Kronenberg MW, Yu PN. The hemodynamic response to intra-aortic balloon counterpulsation in patients with cardiogenic shock complicating acute myocardial infarction. Am Heart J 1977; 93:274–9.

20. Urschel CW, Eber L, Forrester J, Matloff J, Carpenter R, Sonnenblick E. Alteration in mechanical performance of the ventricle by intra-aortic balloon counterpulsation. Am J Cardiol 1970; 25:646–51.

21. Bardet J, Masquet C, Kahn JC, Gourgon R, Bourdarias JP, Mathivat A, Bouvrain Y. Clinical and hemodynamic results of intra-aortic balloon counterpulsation and surgery for cardiogenic shock. Am Heart J 1977; 93:280–8.

22. Dunkman WB, Leinbach RC, Buckley MJ, Mundth ED, Kantrowitz AR, Austen WG, Sanders CA. Clinical and hemodynamic results of intra-aortic balloon pumping and surgery for cardiogenic shock. Circulation 1972; 46:465–77.

23. Gerwitz H, Ohley W, Williams DO, Sun Y, Most AS. Effect of intra-aortic balloon counterpulsation on regional myocardial blood flow and oxygen consumption in the presence of coronary artery stenosis: observations in an awake animal model. Am J Cardiol 1982; 50:829–37.

24. Port SC, Patel, Schmidt DH. Effects of intra-aortic balloon counterpulsation on myocardial blood flow in patients with severe coronary artery disease. J Am Coll Cardiol 1984; 3:1367–74.

25. MacDonald RG, Hill JA, Feldman RL. Failure of intra-aortic balloon counterpulsation to augment distal coronary perfusion presure during percutaneous transluminal coronary angioplasty. Am J Cardiol 1987; 59:359–61.

26. Fuchs RM, Brin KP, Brinker JA, Guzman PA, Heuser RR, Yin FCP. Augmentation of regional coronary blood flow by intra-aortic balloon counterpulsation. Am J Cardiol 1970; 25:546–51.

27. McEnany MT, Kay JR, Buckley MJ, Daggett WM, Erdmann AJ, Mundth ED, Rao RS, DeToeuf J, Austen WG. Clinical experience with intra-aortic balloon pump support in 728 patients. Circulation 1978; 58:I-124–I-132.

28. Alcan KE, Stertzer SH, Wallsh E, Bruno MS, DePasquale NP. Current status of intra-aortic balloon counterpulsation in critical care cardiology. Crit Care Med 1984; 12: 489–95.

29. Willerson JT, Curry GC, Watson JT, Leshin SJ, Ecker RR, Mullins CB, Platt MR, Sugg WL. Intra-aortic balloon counterpulsation in patients in cardiogenic shock, medically refractory left ventricular failure, and/or recurrent ventricular tachycardia. Am J Med 1975; 58:183–91.

30. Scheidt S, Wilner G, Mueller H, Summers D, Lesch M, Wolff G, Krakauer J, Rubenfire M, Fleming P, Noon G, Oldham N, Killip T, Kantrowitz A. Intra-aortic balloon counterpulsation in cardiogenic shock. N Engl J Med 1983; 288:979–84.

31. Hagemeijer F, Laird JD, Haalebos MM, Hugenholtz PG. Effectiveness of intra-aortic balloon pumping without cardiac surgery for patients with severe heart failure secondary to recent myocardial infarction. Am J Cardiol 1977; 40:951–6.

32. O'Rourke MF, Sammel N, Chang VP. Arterial counterpulsation in severe refractory heart failure complicating acute myocardial infarction. Br Heart J 1979; 41:308–16.

33. Goldberger M, Tabak SW, Shah PK. Clinical experience with intra-aortic balloon counterpulsation in 112 consecutive patients. Am Heart J 1986; 111:497–502.

34. Waksman R, Hasin Y, Weiss TA, Gotsman MS. Intro-aortic balloon counterpulsation (IABC) improves survival of patients with acute myocardial infarction (AMI) complicated by cardiogenic shock (CS). Circulation 1990; 82:III-309 (abstract).

35. Nishimura RA, Schaff HV, Gersh BJ, Holmes DR, Tajik AJ. Early repair of mechanical complications after acute myocardial infarction. JAMA 1986; 256:47–50.

36. Daggett WM, Guyton RA, Mundth ED, Buckley MJ, McEnany T, Gold HK, Leinbach RC, Austen WG. Surgery for post-myocardial infarct ventricular septal defect. Ann Surg 1977; 186:260–71.

37. Jones MT, Schofield PM, Dark JF, Moussalli H, Deiraniya AK, Lawson RAM, Ward C, Bray CL. Surgical repair of acquired ventricular septal defect. Determinants of early and late outcome. J Thorac Cardiovasc Surg 1987; 83:680–6.

38. Gold HK, Leinbach RC, Sanders CA, Buckley MJ, Mundth ED, Austen WG. Intra-aortic balloon pumping for ventricular septal defect or mitral regurgitation complicating acute myocardial infarction. Circulation 1973; 47:1191–6.

39. Tepe NA, Edmunds LH Jr. Operation for acute postinfarction mitral insufficiency and cardiogenic shock. J Thorac Cardiovasc Surg 1985; 89:525–30.

40. Feneley MP, Chang VP, O'Rourke MF. Myocardial rupture after acute myocardial infarction. Ten year review. Br Heart J 1983; 49:550–6.

41. Bates RJ, Bentler S, Resnekov L, Anagnostopoulous CE. Cardiac rupture. Challenge in diagnosis and management. Am J Cardiol 1977; 40:429–37.

42. McMullan MH, Kilgore TL Jr, Dear HD Jr, Hindman SH. Sudden blowout rupture of the myocardium after infarction: urgent management. Report of four cases. J Thorac Cardiovasc Surg 1985; 89:259–63.

43. Hochreiter C, Goldstein J, Borer JS, Tyberg T, Goldberg HL, Subramanian V, Rosenfeld I. Myocardial free-wall rupture after acute infarction: survival aided by percutaneous intraaortic balloon counterpulsation. Circulation 1982; 65:1279–82.

44. Pifarre R, Sillivan HJ, Grieco J, Montoya A, Bakhos M, Scanlon PJ, Gunnar RM. Management of left ventricular rupture complicating myocardial infarction. J Thorac Cardiovasc Surg 1983; 86:441–3.

45. Roberts AJ, Alonso DR, Combes JR, Jacobstein JG, Post MR, Cahill PT, Ho SLT,

Abel RM, Subraanian VA, Gay WA. Role of delayed intra-aortic balloon pumping in treatment of experimental myocardial infarction. Am J Cardiol 1978; 41:1202-8.

46. Haston HH, McNamara JJ. The effects of intra-aortic balloon counterpulsation on myocardial infarct size. Ann Thoracic Surg 1979; 28:335-41.

47. Leinbach RC, Gold HK, Harper RW, Buckley MJ, Austen WG. Early intra-aortic balloon pumping for anterior myocardial infarction without shock. Circulation 1978; 58: 204-10.

48. O'Rourke MF, Norris RM, Campbell RJ, Chang VP, Sammel NL. Randomized controlled trial of intra-aortic balloon counterpulsation in early myocardial infarction with acute heart failure. Am J Cardiol 1981; 47:815-20.

49. Flaherty JT, Becker LC, Weiss JL, Brinker JA, Bulkley BH, Gerstenblith G, Kallman CH, Weisfeldt ML. Results of a randomized prospective trial of intra-aortic balloon counterpulsation and intravenous nitroglycerin in patients with acute myocardial infarction. J Am Coll Cardiol 1985; 6:434-46.

50. Gold HK, Leinbach RC, Sanders CA, Buckley MJ, Mindth ED, Austen WG. Intra-aortic balloon pumping for control of recurrent myocardial ischemia. Circulation 1973; 47:1197-1203.

51. Levine FH, Gold HK, Leinbach RC, Daggett WM, Austen WG, Buckley MJ. Management of acute myocardial ischemia with intra-aortic balloon pumping and coronary bypass surgery. Circulation 1977; 58:I-69-I-72.

52. Weintraub RM, Aroesty JM, Paulin S, Levine FH, Markis JE, LaRaia PJ, Cohen S, Kurland GF. Medically refractory unstable angina pectoris. I. Long-term follow-up of patients undergoing intra-aortic balloon counterpulsation and operation. Am J Cardiol 1979; 43:877-81.

53. Ishihara M, Sato H, Tateishi H, Uchida T, Dote K. Prevention of reocclusion after emergency coronary angioplasty for acute myocardial infarction; usefulness of intra-aortic balloon pumping. Eur Heart J 1990; 11:23 (abstract).

54. Ohman EM, Califf RM, George BS, Quigley PJ, Kereiakes DJ, Harrelson-Woodlief L, Candela RJ, Flanagan C, Stack RS, Topol EJ. The use of intraaortic balloon pumping as an adjunct to reperfusion therapy in acute myocardial infarction. Am Heart J 1991; 121:895-901.

55. Hanson EC, Levine FH, Kay HR, Leinbach RC, Gold HK, Daggett WM, Austen WG, Buckley MJ. Control of postinfarction ventricular irritability with the intra-aortic balloon pump. Circulation 62; 1980:I-130-I-137.

56. Culliford AT, Madden MR, Isom OW, Glassman E. Intra-aortic balloon counterpulsation: refractory ventricular tachycardia. JAMA 1978; 239:431-4.

57. Phillips, SJ. Percutaneous cardiopulmonary bypass and innovations in clinical counterpulsation. Crit Care Clin 1986; 2:297-318.

58. Harvey JC, Goldstein JE, McCabe JC, Hoover EL, Gay WA, Subramanian VA. Complications of percutaneous intra-aortic balloon pumping. Circulation 64; 1981:II-114-II-117.

59. Kantrowitz A, Wasfie T, Freed PS, Rubenfire M, Wajszczuk W, Schork MA. Intra-aortic balloon pumping between 1967 and 1982: analysis of complications in 733 patients. Am J Cardiol 1986; 57:976-83.

60. Gottlieb SO, Brinker JA, Borkon AM, Kallman CH, Potter A, Gott VL, Baughman KL. Identification of patients at high risk for complications of intra-aortic balloon counterpulsation: a multivariate risk factor analysis. Am J Cardiol 1984; 53:1135-9.

61. McCabe JC, Abel RM, Subramanian VA, Gay WA. Complications of intra-aortic balloon insertion and counterpulsation. Circulation 1978; 57:769-73.

62. Alderman JD, Gabliani GI, McCabe CH, Brewer CC, Lorell BH, Pasternak RC, Skillman JJ, Steer ML, Baim DS. Incidence and management of limb ischemia with percutaneous wire-guided intra-aortic balloon catheters. J Am Coll Cardiol 1987; 9: 524-30.

63. Todd GJ, Bregman D, Voorhees AB, Reemtsma K. Vascular complications associated with percutaneous intra-aortic balloon pumping. Arch Surg 1983; 118:963-4.

64. Beck CS. Revascularization of the heart. Ann Surg 1948; 128:854-64.

65. Meerbaum S, Lang T, Osher JV, Hashimoto K, Lewis GW, Feldstein C, Corday E. Diastolic retroperfusion of acute ischemic myocardium Am J Cardiol 1976; 37: 588-98.

66. Farcot JC, Meerbaum S, Lang TW, Kaplan L, Corday E. Synchronized retroperfusion of coronary veins for circulatory support of jeopardized ischemic myocardium. Am J Cardiol 1978; 41:1191-1201.

67. Geary GG, Smith GT, Suehiro GT, Zeman C, Siu B, McNamara JJ. Quantitative assessment of infarct size reduction by coronary venous retroperfusion in baboons. Am J Cardiol 1982; 50:1424-30.

68. Drury JK, Yamazaki S, Fishbein MC, Meerbaum S, Corday E. Synchronized diastolic coronary venous retroperfusion: results of a preclinical safety and efficacy study. J Am Coll Cardiol 1985; 6:328-35.

69. Meerbaum S, Haendchen RV, Corday E, Povzhitkov M, Fishbein MC, Y-Rit J, Lang TW, Uchiyama T, Aosaki N, Broffman J. Hypothermic coronary venous phased retroperfusion: a closed chest treatment of acute regional myocardial ischemia. Circulation 1982; 65:1435-45.

70. Haendchen RV, Corday E, Meerbaum S, Povzhitkov M, Rit J, Fishbein MC. Prevention of ischemic injury and early reperfusion derangements by hypothermic retroperfusion. J Am Coll Cardiol 1983; 14:1067-80.

71. Povzhitkov M, Haendchen RV, Meerbaum S, Fishbein MC, Shell W, Corday E. Prostaglandin E$_1$ coronary venous retroperfusion in acute myocardial ischemia: effects on regional left ventricular function and infarct size J Am Coll Cardiol 1984; 3:939-47.

72. Mohl W, Glogar DH, Mayr H, Losert U, Sochor H, Pachinger O, Kaindl F, Wolner E. Reduction of infarct size induced by pressure-controlled intermittent coronary sinus occlusion. Am J Cardiol 1984; 53:923-8.

73. Zalewski A, Goldberg S, Slysh S, Maroko PR. Myocardial protection via coronary sinus interventions: superior effects of arterialization compared with intermittent occlusion. Circulation 1985; 71:1215-23.

74. Hajduzki I, Kar S, Areeda J, Ryden L, Corday S, Haendchen R, Corday E. Reversal of chronic regional myocardial dysfunction (hibernating myocardium) by synchronized diastolic coronary venous retroperfusion during coronary angioplasty. J Am Coll Cardiol 1990; 15:238-42.

75. Berland J, Farcot JC, Cribier A, Bourdarias JP, Letac B. Clinical evaluation of safety and hemodynamic effects of diastolic coronary venous retroperfusion. In: Mohl W, Faxon D, Wolner E, eds. Clinics of CSI. New York: Springer-Verlag, 1986:281-7.

76. Gore JM, Weiner BH, Benotti JR, Sloan KM, Okike ON, Cuenoud HF, Faca JMJ, Alpert J, Dalen JE. Preliminary experience with synchronized coronary sinus retroperfusion in humans. Circulation 1986; 74:381-8.

77. Barnett JC,Touchon RC. Use of coronary venous retroperfusion in acute myocardial ischemia. Cardiovasc Rev Rep 1989; 10:64-5.

78. Kar S. Reduction of PTCA induced ischemia by synchronized coronary venous retroperfusion: results of multicenter clinical trial. J Am Coll Cardiol 1990; 15:250A (abstract).

79. Jacobs AK, Faxon DP. Retroperfusion and PTCA. In: Topol EJ, ed. Textbook of interventional cardiology. Philadelphia: Saunders, 1990:477-95.

80. Hill JD, O'Brien TG, Murray JJ, Dontigny L, Bramson ML, Osborn JJ, Gerbode F. Prolonged extracorporeal oxygenation for acute post-traumatic respiratory failure (shock-lung syndrome): use of a Bramson Membrane Lung. N Engl J Med 1972; 286: 629-34.

81. Hirschl RB, Bartlett RH. Extracorporeal membrane oxygenation support in cardioirespiratory failure. Adv Surg 1987; 21:189-212.

82. Sinard JM, Bartlett RH. Extracorporeal membrane oxygenation (ECMO): prolonged bedside cardiopulmonary bypass. Perfusion 1990; 5:239-49.

83. Shawl FA, Domanski MJ, Wish MH, Davis M. Percutaneous cardiopulmonary bypass support in the catheterization laboratory: technique and complications. Am Heart J 1990; 120:195-203.

84. Shawl FA, Domanski MJ, Wish M, Punja S, Hernandez TJ. Emergency percutaneous cardiopulmonary bypass in patients with cardiac arrest. Circulation 1989; 90:II-271 (abstract).

85. Bartlett RH. Physiology of extracorporeal circulation. In: D'Alessandro LC, ed. Heart Surgery 1987. Proceedings of 2nd International Symposium on Cardiac Surgery. Casa Editrichi Scientifica Internazionale, Rome, 1988:55-62.

86. Hickey PR, Buckley MJ, Philbin DM. Pulsatile and nonpulsatile cardiopulmonary bypass: review of a counteproductive controversy. Ann Thorac Surg 1983; 6:720-37.

87. Bartlett RH, Gazzaniga AB, Fong SW, Jeffries MR, Roohk HV, Haiduc N. Extracorporeal membrane oxygenator support for cardiiopulmonary failure. Experience in 28 cases. J Thorac Cardiovasc Surg 1977; 73:375-86.

88. Pennington DG, Merjavy JP, Codd JE, Swartz MT, Miller LL, Williams GA. Extracorporeal membrane oxygenation for patients with cardiogenic shock. Circulation 1984; 70:I-130-I-137.

89. Phillips SJ, Ballentine B, Slonine D, Hall J, Vandehaar J, Kongtahworn C, Zeff RH, Skinner JR, Reckmo K, Gray D. Percutaneous initiation of cardiopulmonary bypass. Ann Thorac Surg 1983; 36:223-5.

90. Vogel RA, Shawl F, Tommaso C, O'Neill W, Overlie P, O'Toole J, Vandormael M, Topol E, Tabari KK, Vogel J, Smith S, Freedmann R, White C, George B, Teirstein P. Initial report of the National Registry of Elective Cardiopulmonary Bypass Supported Coronary Angioplasty. J Am Coll Cardiol 1990; 15:23-9.

91. Vogel RA, Shawl FA. Report of the National Registry of Elective Supported Angioplasty: comparison of the 1988 and 1989 results. Circulation 1990; 82:111-653 (abstract).

92. Phillips SJ, Zeff RH, Kongtahworn C, Skinner JR, Toon RS, Grignon A, Kennerly RM, Wickemeyer W, Iannone LA. Percutaneous cardiopulmonary bypass: application and indication for use. Ann Thorac Surg 1989; 47:121-3.

93. Shawl FA, Domanski MJ, Hernandez TJ, Punja S. Emergency percutaneous cardiopulmonary bypass support in cardiogenic shock from acute myocardial infarction. Am J Cardiol 1989; 64:967-70.

94. Ward HB, Nemzek TG, McFalls EO, Gornick CC. Emergent cardiopulmonary bypass for acute myocardial ischemia in dogs. Circulation 1990; 82:III-681 (abstract).

95. Pavlides GS, Stack RK, Dudlets PI, Hauser AM, O'Neill WW. Echocardiographic assessment of global and regional myocardial function during supported angioplasty. Circulation 1989; 80:II-271 (abstract).

96. Wampler RK, Moise JC, Frazier OH, Olsen DB. In vivo evaluation of a peripheral vascular access axial flow blood pump. Trans Am Soc Artif Intern Organs 1988; 34: 450-4.

97. Merhige ME, Smalling RW, Cassidy D, Barrett R, Wise G, Short J, Wampler RK. Effect of the Hemopump left ventricular assist device on regional myocardial perfusion and function. Reduction of ischemia during coronary occlusion. Circulation 1989; 80:III-158-III-166.

98. Feindel CM, Sandhu R, Cruz J, Wilson GJ. Reduction of infarct size using the Hemopump left ventricular assist device. Circulation 1990; 82:III-589 (abstract).

99. Smalling RW, Cassidy DB, Merhige M, Felli PR, Wise GM, Barrett RL, Wampler RD. Improved hemodynamic and left ventricular unloading during acute ischemia using the Hemopump left ventricular assist device compared to intra-aortic balloon counterpulsation. J Am Coll Cardiol 1989; 130:160A (abstract).

100. Smalling RW, Sweeney MJ, Cassidy DB, Barrett RL, Morris RE, Lammermeier DE, Key PG, Haynie MP, Vrazier OH, Wampler R. Hemodynamics in cardiogenic shock after acute myocardial infarction with the Hemopump assist device. Circulation 1989; 80:II-624 (abstract).

101. Frazier OH, Nakatani T, Duncan JM, Parnis SM, Fuqua JM. Clinical experience with the Hemopump. Trans Am Soc Artif Intern Organs 1989; 35:604-6.

102. Frazier OH, Wampler RK, Duncan JM, Dear WE, Macris MP, Parnis SM, Fuqua JM. First human use of the Hemopump, a cather-mounted ventricular assist device. Ann Thorac Surg 1990; 49:299-304.

103. Wampler RK, Johnson DV, Rutan PM, Riehle RA. Multicenter clinical study of the Hemopump in the treatment of cardiogenic shock. Circulation 1989; 80:II-670 (abstract).

104. Loisance D, Dubois-Rande JL, Deleuze P, Okude J, Rosenval O, Geschwind H. Prophylactic intraventicular pumping in high risk coronary angioplasty. Lancet 1990; 335:438-40.

105. Lincoff AM, Popma JJ, Bates ER, Deeb M, Bolling SF, Meagher JS, Kelly AM, Wampler RK, Nicklas JM. Successful coronary angipolasty in two patients with car-

diogenic shock using the Nimbus Hemopump support device. Am Heart J 1990; 120: 970-2.

106. Jegaden O, Bastien O, Girard C. Temporary left ventricular assistance with a Hemopump assist device during acute myocardial infarction. J Thorac Cardiovasc Surg 1990; 1000:311-3.

107. Dubois-Rande JL, Zelinsky R, Deleuze P, Geschwind H, Loisance D. Coronary hemodynamics during Hemopump left intraventricular assistance. Circulation 1990; 82:III-680 (abstract).

108. Pierce WS, Donachy JH, Landis DL, Brighton JA, Rosenberg G, Migliore JJ, Prophet GA, White WJ, Waldhausen JA. Prolonged mechanical support of the left ventricle. Circulation 1978; 58:I-133-I-146.

109. DeVries WC, Anderson JL, Joyce LD, Anderson FL, Hammond EH, Jarvik RK, Kolff WJ. Clinical use of the total artificial heart. N Engl J Med 1984; 310:273-8.

110. Vasku J, Vasku J, Dostal M, Guba P, Gregor Z, Vasku A, Urbanek P, Necas J, Dolezel S, Cidl K. Evaluation study of calves with total artificial heart (TAH) surviving for 218-293 days of pumping. Int J Artif Organs 1990; 13:830-6.

111. Norman JC, Fuqua JM, Hibbs CW, Edmonds CH, Igo SR, Cooley DA. An intracorporeal (abdominal) left ventricular assist device. Arch Surg 1977; 112:1442-51.

112. Farrar DJ, Hill JD, Gray LA, Pennington DG, McBride LR, Pierce WS, Pae WE, Glenville B, Ross D, Galbraith TA, Zumbra GL. Heterotopic prosthetic ventricles as a bridge to cardiac transplantation. N Engl J Med 1988; 318:333-40.

113. Pennington DG, McBride LR, Kanter KR, Miller LW, Ruzevich SA, Naunheim K, Swartz MT, Termuhlen D. Bridging to heart transplantation with circulatory support devices. J Heart Transplant 1989; 8:116-23.

114. Laschinger JC, Cunningham JN, Catinella FP, Knopp EA, Glassman E, Spencer FC. "Pulsatile" left atrial-femoral artery bypass. A new method of preventing extension of myocardial infarction. Arch Surg 1983; 118:965-9.

115. Noda H, Takano H, Taenaka Y, Nakatani T, Umeau M, Kinoshita M, Tatsumi E, Yagura A, Sekii H, Kito Y, Ohara K, Tanaka K, Kumon K, Hiramori K, Yutani C, Beppu S, Fujita T, Akutsu T, Manabe H. Treatment of acute myocardial infarction with cardiogenic shock using left ventricular assist device. Int J Artif Organs 1989; 12:175-9.

116. Babic UU, Grujicic S, Djurisic Z, Vicinic M. Percutaneous left atrial-aortic bypass with a roller pump. Circulation 1989; 80:II-272.

117. Joyce LD, Johnson KE, Toninato CJ, Cabrol C, Griffity B, Copeland JG, Keon WJ, Tector A, Pifarre R, Semb B, Dembitsky W, Loisance D, Frazier OH, Noon G, Herbert Y, Halbrook H, DeVries WC, Akalin H, Aris A, Phillips SJ, Peterson A, English T, Pennington G, Carmichael MJ. Results of the first 100 patients who received Symbion total artificial hearts as a bridge to cardiac transplantation. Circulation 1989; 80:III-192-III-201.

118. Kawaguchi AT, Gandjbakhch I, Pavie A, Muneretto C, Solis E, Bors V, Leger P, Vaissier E, Levasseur JP, Szefner J, Sasako Y, Cabrol A, Cabrol C. Factors affecting survival in total artificial heart recipients before transplantation. Circulation 1990; 82: IV-322-IV-327.

20

The Evolving Role of Coronary Bypass Surgery in the Treatment of Acute Myocardial Infarction

Dean J. Kereiakes

The Christ Hospital Cardiovascular Research Center, Cincinnati, Ohio

INTRODUCTION

Surgical coronary revascularization has played both primary and adjunctive roles in strategies directed toward achieving myocardial reperfusion in evolving acute myocardial infarction (1-5). The objective benefit to be gained from emergent coronary bypass surgery and other primary reperfusion modalities is critically dependent on the early establishment of coronary reperfusion, with consequent limitation of infarct size and preservation of global and regional (infarct zone) left ventricular function (6-9). Although the immediate and long-term results of emergent coronary bypass surgery for acute myocardial infarction are promising (1-5), logistic, practical, and financial considerations have limited widespread application of this technique. Ease and rapidity of administration as well as generalized availability have made intravenous thrombolytic therapy a logical first step in a strategy aimed toward achieving timely myocardial reperfusion. However, intravenous thrombolysis fails to achieve successful coronary recanalization in 25% or more of treated patients (10-12), and coronary reocclusion in 10-20% of patients following successful thrombolysis may also limit the potential benefits of this therapy (13-15). Coronary bypass surgery may play a valuable role in maintaining coronary reperfusion that cannot be sustained by pharmacological and/or percutaneous catheter techniques. Surgery may thus be more selectively applied as a logical extension of percutaneous techniques.

In light of recent data, it is appropriate at this time to reassess the role of coronary bypass surgery in the treatment of acute myocardial infarction.

PRIMARY SURGICAL REPERFUSION

Emergent surgical revascularization during evolving acute myocardial infarction can be accomplished with a remarkably low morbidity and mortality in selected patients. Published reports suggest an overall hospital mortality of less than 5%, with surgical reexploration for postoperative hemorrhage required in less than 3% of patients not receiving thrombolytic therapy preoperatively (1-4, 16-20). Early experimental data suggested the importance of timing in surgical reperfusion of acute myocardial infarction (21,22). Left ventricular functional recovery has, however, been observed following controlled surgical reperfusion after 6-8 hr of coronary occlusion (23,24). Clinically, emergent bypass surgery performed within 6 hr of infarct symptom onset has been associated with significantly greater preservation of left ventricular function and improved hospital and long-term survival than surgery performed beyond 6 hr of chest pain onset (1,2). Interestingly, in the large series of patients studied by DeWood et al., surgical revascularization did not reduce the incidence of recurrent myocardial infarction in long-term follow-up compared with patients receiving medical therapy alone (1). However, the mortality of recurrent infarction was significantly less in surgically versus medically treated patients. The long-term survival of surgically treated patients was also influenced by the number of diseased coronary vessels in addition to the timing (less than versus greater than 6 hr) between infarct symptom onset and surgery (2).

Experimental and clinical experience with emergency reperfusion of ischemic myocardium has demonstrated the importance of a low-calcium, normothermic, amino-acid-enriched, controlled rate of reperfusion during surgery to avoid reperfusion injury and enhance myocardial functional recovery (25-28). In particular, a more gradual rate of reperfusion with lower reperfusion pressures and reperfusate that is buffered, high in Krebs cycle intermediates, and hyperosmotic may limit adverse metabolic and/or structural consequences of reperfusion. Surgical venting with decompression of the left ventricle during regional reperfusion may minimize left ventricular oxygen demand, limit histochemical damage, and further enhance immediate functional recovery (29). The saphenous vein graft conduit has been recommended in preference to the internal mammary artery for emergency primary surgical reperfusion therapy because of the potential for greater reperfusion injury if initial perfusion is established with unmodified blood and because of technical time constraints in graft harvesting (4,24). Despite concerns that the "no reflow" phenomenon secondary to myocyte swelling and capillary obliteration would limit infarct artery outflow and thus result in higher rates of early vein graft closure for grafted infarct vessels (30), graft patency rates of

90% or more have been observed in patients restudied angiographically (18,31) and appear similar to patency rates observed in noninfarct arteries following elective coronary bypass operations.

Although lacking an appropriately randomized controlled group for comparison, the cumulative primary surgical reperfusion experience demonstrates an overall in-hospital mortality of <5%, which compares favorably with an 11-24% hospital mortality reported in unselected patients treated medically (no reperfusion strategy) (32-34) with acute myocardial infarction. Importantly, mortality remains low in long-term follow-up of surgically treated patients (2-3% per year) (1,2,20,32,35) and appears less than has been reported for medically treated patients (8-15% first year; 5% per year thereafter) (36-39). The favorable outcome following surgery must be viewed in the context of potential bias in patient selection for surgical treatment.

Despite these promising reports from a small number of experienced centers, a major deterrent to the more widespread use of primary surgical reperfusion for myocardial infarction has been the fact that only 12% of the hospitals in the United States are equipped with cardiac catheterization laboratories and cardiothoracic surgical backup (40,41). The high rates of successful early infarct-related artery recanalization reported following intravenous tissue plasminogen activator (t-PA)(10) or combination t-PA and urokinase therapy (12) would make emergent surgery unnecessary in the majority of infarct victims receiving these therapies. In addition, the application of percutaneous (rescue) angioplasty to patients who fail intravenous thrombolysis has achieved successful infarct vessel recanalization in up to 96% of patients (12). These observations suggest that coronary bypass surgery will most likely serve and adjunctive rather than primary role in strategies for infarct reperfusion and will likely be of greatest benefit to a smaller subgroup of patients in whom pharmacological or catheter techniques have already been applied. In addition, concerns regarding the use of the internal mammary artery conduit during emergent primary surgical reperfusion, due to the potential for reperfusion injury discussed previously, may be less applicable when myocardial reperfusion is achieved using a sequential pharmacological-mechanical strategy. Internal mammary artery grafts may enhance long-term survival rates following coronary bypass surgery (42) and are more likely to be performed using adjunctive and particularly deferred coronary bypass surgery following pharmacological and /or catheter intervention (see below).

Although surgery may offer a more definitive treatment than thrombolysis or even PTCA for patients with multiple-vessel coronary artery disease since obstructions in noninfarct vessels can be addressed as well, logistic and economic obstacles will continue to impede the use of bypass surgery as primary therapy for myocardial infarction. In addition, recent data have suggested that bypass surgery can be deferred and safely performed in the majority of patients with multivessel coronary artery disease prior to hospital discharge (43). Still another disincentive to the use of primary catheter or surgical reperfusion therapy has been the observation that approximately 10% of patients with acute myocardial infarction will have no significant fixed coronary obstruction following intravenous thrombolytic therapy and subsequent heparin treatment (44).

One group of patients with acute myocardial infarction that may particularly benefit from emergency coronary bypass surgery are those patients who develop cardiogenic shock early during the evolution of myocardial infarction. This group of patients has previously been noted to have an especially poor prognosis (mortality exceeding 80%) (38) with conservative medical therapy and even intra-aortic balloon pump counterpulsation if revascularization (PTCA or bypass surgery)is not performed. The cumulative experience from several centers where primary surgical revascularization has been performed in patients with early cardiogenic shock complicating acute myocardial infarction has demonstrated a hospital mortality of 31% (65 of 211 patients) (3,45–48) and compares very favorably with prior reported series of medically treated patients with shock complicating myocardial infarction. Other groups of patients for whom emergency coronary bypass surgery may be beneficial are discussed later.

CORONARY BYPASS SURGERY FOLLOWING INTRAVENOUS THROMBOLYTIC THERAPY

As noted above, successful coronary thrombolysis can preserve myocardial function and reduce the early and late mortality of acute myocardial infarction. The vast majority of patients in whom thrombolysis is successful will be left with a significant fixed residual coronary stenosis in the infarct-related vessel, thus setting the stage for potential coronary reocclusion and reinfarction. Coronary reocclusion has been observed in 11–21% of patients following successful thrombolytic therapy despite concomitant treatment with intravenous heparin and antiplatelet agents (13,14,49–54). Although conflicting data have been presented (55), the risk of reocclusion may be greatest (<50%) in patients with a residual stenotic cross-sectional area of ≤ 0.4 mm^2 ($\geq 90\%$ luminal diameter stenosis) (13,51). Once myocardial reperfusion is achieved, it must be maintained before long-term salutary effects on left ventricular function and survival can be realized.

Cardiothoracic Surgical Support for Rescue Angioplasty

The capability for emergency coronary bypass surgery should be available in all centers practicing rescue PTCA for patients who fail to recanalize the infarct vessel with intravenous thrombolytic therapy alone (56). The failure rate of PTCA in

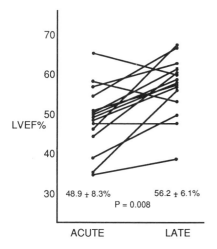

Figure 1   Left ventricular function as assessed by acute (90 min following initiation of thrombolytic therapy) and predischarge contrast left ventriculograms from patients undergoing emergency coronary artery bypass surgery following intravenous thrombolytic therapy. Significant improvement in global left ventricular ejection fraction is demonstrated. (Reprinted with permission from the American College of Cardiology (5).)

this acute situation appears to exceed the failure rate of angioplasty observed in elective cases. The success of attempted rescue PTCA may be significantly influenced by the thrombolytic regimen used, and technical success of the procedure may significantly influence the likelihood of survival (12,57,58). Coronary reocclusion following rescue PTCA is observed more frequently after t-PA monotherapy (58) or following mechanical recanalization of the right coronary artery (59). Significantly lower rates of coronary reocclusion have been observed following rescue PTCA in patients treated with t-PA/urokinase combination or urokinase monotherapy alone (57,58). We previously demonstrated significant improvement of left ventricular function in patients who have a failed attempt at rescue PTCA who have emergency surgical revascularization performed (Fig. 1). (5). For patients in whom mechanical recanalization is initially successful but coronary patency cannot be maintained (occlusive coronary dissection; rethrombosis), we have recommended placement of a perfusion balloon or perfusion catheter system to maintain coronary flow en route to surgery (60,61). Patients in whom pharmacological or mechanical recanalization cannot be achieved may also benefit from emergent coronary bypass surgery if surgery can be performed within 6–8 hr of infarct symptom onset.

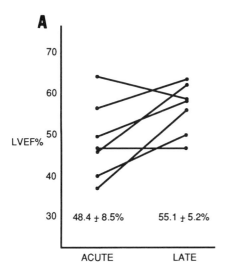

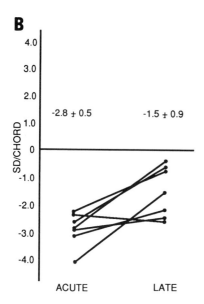

Figure 2   Analysis of left ventricular ejection fraction (LVEF) and regional infarct zone (SD/Chord) function from acute (90 min) and predischarge contrast left ventriculograms in patients undergoing emergency coronary bypass surgery following intravenous thrombolytic therapy. Changes in left ventricular ejection fraction (A)   and regional infarct zone function (B) for patients operated on less than 6 hr following infarct symptom onset.

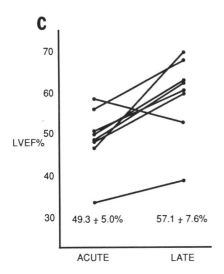

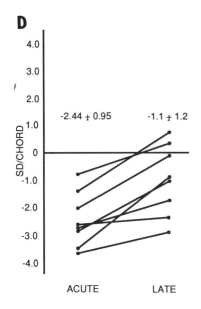

Figure 2 (continued)   Changes in left ventricular ejection fraction (C) and regional infarct zone function (D) for patients operated on >6 hr following infarct symptom onset. No
differences were apparent with respect to magnitude of change in global left ventricular
ejection fraction or regional infarct zone function based on whether patients were operated
less than versus more than 6 hr following infarct symptom onset. (Reprinted with permission from the American College of Cardiology (5).)

Emergency Coronary Bypass Surgery Following Thrombolytic Therapy

When coronary patency can be achieved at least temporarily by pharmacological means or catheter techniques preoperatively, the timing of coronary bypass surgery (less than versus greater than 6 hr after infarct symptom onset) does not appear to influence the degree of recovery in left ventricular function (Fig. 2)(5). Factors other than coronary anatomy alone may also influence the decision to proceed with emergency bypass surgery. Hemodynamic instability, the presence of cardiogenic shock, and ischemic dysfunction of noninfarct zones in patients with multivessel coronary artery disease may suggest the need for emergency surgical revascularization. We previously reported no hospital mortality in 16 patients undergoing emergency coronary bypass surgery with stable preoperative hemodynamics and three hospital deaths (38%) among eight patients with preoperative cardiogenic shock operated emergently from the cardiac catheterization laboratory following intravenous thrombolysis with or without PTCA (5). Three of these emergently operated patients (12.5%) required surgical reexploration for postoperative hemorrhage, which was found to be secondary to a generalized hemostasis abnormality in two patients and a surgically correctable cause (vein graft branch) in one patient. The overall hospital mortality in this series of patients operated emergently from the catheterization laboratory was 12.5% despite the fact that eight patients (33%) had cardiogenic shock hemodynamics preoperatively (5).

We also evaluated the immediate and long-term outcome and left ventricular function in 36 patients who had emergency coronary bypass surgery <24 hr following intravenous thrombolytic therapy from the 1387 total patients enrolled in the TAMI-1, -2, -2A, -3, and -5 trials (61). These results were compared to those in 267 patients from the same trials who had coronary bypass surgery performed more than 24 hr following thrombolytic therapy during the initial hospitalization for acute myocardial infarction. The most frequent indications for coronary bypass surgery to be performed within 24 hr of receiving intravenous thrombolytic therapy for myocardial infarction were failure of immediate or rescue PTCA (39%); left main or equivalent coronary artery disease (19%); and complex or "high risk" coronary anatomy (31%) not amenable to PTCA (Fig. 3). Failure of immediate or rescue PTCA and left main equivalent coronary disease were more frequent in patients referred to emergency compared to those who had deferred coronary bypass surgery ($p < 0.0001$ and $p = 0.032$, respectively). Complex or multivessel coronary anatomy not amenable to PTCA was a more frequent ($p = 0.01$) indication in the deferred group. Emergency coronary bypass surgery was more frequently performed in trials using t-PA monotherapy than in trials using t-PA plus urokinase combination or urokinase monotherapy (Table 1). Emergency surgery was required in 5% (29/561 patients) of all patients enrolled into

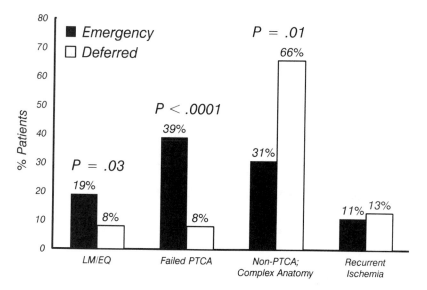

Figure 3   Relative clinical indications for emergency (n = 36) and deferred (n = 267) coronary bypass surgery following intravenous thrombolytic therapy for acute myocardial infarction. LM = left main; EQ = left main equivalent; PTCA = percutaneous transluminal coronary angioplasty.

Table 1   Relative Contribution of Each TAMI Protocol to Surgical and Nonsurgical Groups

TAMI protocol	Thrombolytic agent (s)	Type of surgery		
		Emergency [no. (%)]	Deferred [no. (%)]	None [no. (%)]
TAMI 1	t-PA	23 (64)	62 (23)	302 (28)
2	t-PA/UK	4 (11)	16 (6)	126 (12)
2A	t-PA/UK	1 (3)	32 (12)	69 (6)
3	t-PA	6 (17)	32 (12)	136 (13)
5	t-PA/UK/both	2 (6)	125 (47)	451 (42)
Total		36 (100)	267 (100)	1084 (100)

TAMI-1 and -3 versus only 0.8% (7/826 patients) of patients enrolled in TAMI-2, -2A, and -5 trials, respectively (62). The more frequent need for emergency surgery in trials using t-PA monotherapy may be explained at least in part by the more frequent occurrence of coronary reocclusion following attempted rescue PTCA in t-PA-treated patients than in patients receiving combination or urokinase monotherapy (12,57,58). Preoperative cardiogenic shock was more frequently noted in emergency versus deferred coronary bypass surgery (9/36 versus 16/267; p = 0.002), as was anterior myocardial infarction location (22/36 versus 120/267; p = 0.07).

It is important to note that although left main or equivalent coronary disease was more frequent in patients with emergency surgery (p = 0.032), it was possible to defer surgery in 21 of 28 total (75%) patients with this anatomy. Therefore, clinical factors in addition to coronary anatomical findings influenced the decision to proceed with emergency bypass surgery. The presence of hemodynamic compromise, complex ventricular ectopy, and recurrent episodes of ischemic chest pain prompted referral for emergency surgery in the vast majority of these cases. As the decision to proceed with emergency versus deferred surgery was not made in a randomized fashion, it cannot be determined whether at least some of the patients undergoing emergency surgery might have become stabilized with pharmacological or intra-aortic balloon pump support and, thus, might have had surgery safely deferred. Other perioperative complications (prolonged ventilatory assistance greater than 3 days and renal insufficiency) were more frequently observed after emergency surgery, most likely reflecting the more frequent presence of hemodynamic compromise, cardiogenic shock, and need for intra-aortic balloon pump support in emergency patients.

Death in-hospital occurred in 17% (n = 6) of emergency and 5% (n = 13) of deferred surgical patients. The hospital death rate of 17% in emergently operated patients must be viewed in the context that 24% (n = 9) of these patients had preoperative cardiogenic shock hemodynamics and 22% (n = 8) required perioperative intra-aortic balloon pump support. Conversely, the 5% hospital mortality in deferred surgical patients must be viewed from the perspective that surgery was performed for ischemic pump dysfunction in five patients and for papillary muscle dysfunction or rupture in three patients and ventricular septal rupture in three patients. These 11 patients with mechanical complications of infarction or severe left ventricular dysfunction would be expected to have a higher operative and hospital mortality rate.

Deferred (>24 Hr) Surgery Following Thrombolytic Therapy

Following successful coronary thrombolysis, the most common indications for late (>24 hr) in-hospital coronary bypass surgery are multivessel coronary artery disease (66%) and recurrent angina pectoris (13%) with coronary anatomy poorly suited for PTCA (Fig. 3) (62). A potentially important observation made by comparing the emergency and deferred surgical groups was that the timing of surgery (less than versus greater than 24 hr following thrombolysis) significantly influenced the type of bypass conduit used. Patients in whom surgery was deferred were more likely to receive an internal mammary artery conduit as part of the revascularization procedure. Recent data have supported use of the internal mammary artery conduit by demonstrating higher long-term patency rates and improved long-term survival in patients with at least one mammary artery graft compared with patients in whom only saphenous vein graft segments are used (42,63,64). Greater technical demand, constraints of time and concerns regarding the potential for sternal wound or mammary artery hemorrhage no doubt discouraged the surgeon from utilizing the internal mammary artery graft in the majority of emergency surgical procedures.

Another important observation was the significantly greater need for red blood cell transfusion in patients operated emergently. Patients undergoing emergency bypass surgery received more units of packed red blood cells within 24 hr of surgery (6.7 ± 4.5 versus 2.6 ± 2.8 units, p = 0.001) and more than 24 hr after surgery (2.9 ± 2.0 versus 1.0 ± 2.5 units, p = 0.0001) than did patients having deferred surgery. Thus, deferred surgery appears to offer potential advantages with respect to both the type of bypass conduit used and the lesser necessity for blood transfusion.

IMPACT OF SURGERY ON LEFT VENTRICULAR FUNCTION

Analysis of left ventricular function by comparison of immediate (90 min following intravenous thrombolytic therapy) and predischarge contrast left ventriculograms demonstrated remarkable preservation of left ventricular global ejection fraction and regional (infarct zone) function in 15 patients who had emergency coronary bypass surgery following intravenous thrombolytic therapy with or without attempted PTCA (Fig. 1) (5). No significant differences were apparent in the degree of global or infarct zone functional recovery when surgery was performed less than versus greater than 6 hr from infarct symptom onset (Fig. 2) (5). However, the majority of these patients had infarct artery patency achieved pharmacologically or mechanically prior to emergency surgical revascularization. Perfusion catheter systems were placed in 11 of 13 (85%) patients in whom attempted PTCA could not maintain coronary patency preoperatively. Although remarkable improvement in infarct zone function was noted for both patients with single-vessel and multivessel coronary artery disease, late improvement in non-infarct-zone function appeared to contribute to the overall greater increase in left ventricular ejection fraction observed in patients with multivessel coronary artery disease who underwent emergency coronary bypass surgery. This observation suggested that in patients with multivessel coronary disease, ischemic dysfunction of noninfarct zones may contribute to the global left ventricular compromise noted in these patients and that surgical revascularization results in substantial recovery of function in both infarct and noninfarct zones.

Significant preservation of global left ventricular ejection fraction and regional infarct zone function have also been observed in 177 patients having deferred coronary bypass surgery following intravenous thrombolytic therapy (Fig. 4). Interestingly, the degree of recovery in left ventricular ejection fraction and infarct zone function in 194 patients who have undergone bypass surgery (emergency or deferred) has exceeded the degree of functional recovery noted in nonsurgical patients following intravenous thrombolysis with or without coronary angioplasty (Fig. 5) (62). although some degree of enhancement of left ventricular function could be attributable to an increase in circulating catecholamines and other factors following major cardiac surgery (65,66), the magnitude of such changes appears small in comparison to the degree of improvement noted in the present series. Any improvement in left ventricular function attributable to surgically induced hormonal changes alone would be at least in part counterbalanced by similar hormonal changes secondary to the stress of myocardial infarction in nonsurgical patients (67,68).

LONG-TERM OUTLOOK FOLLOWING SURGERY

As a group, patients having coronary bypass surgery following intravenous thrombolysis in the TAMI trials were older, had more extensive coronary artery disease, and had more depressed left ventricular function than did patients not having surgery (43,62). Despite these adverse clinical predictors, in-hospital mortality (7% versus 6%) and post-hospital-discharge mortality (3% each) was low and was not different between surgical and nonsurgical groups, respectively (Fig. 6) (62). In addition, the need for revascularization procedures (PTCA and bypass surgery) during follow-up was more frequent in patients who did not have coronary bypass surgery during their first hospitalization for myocardial infarction. When surgical and nonsurgical patients were asked to assess their general health status at 1 year of follow-up, the majority of patients in both groups (74% surgical, 80% nonsurgical) considered themselves to be in excellent or good condition (Table 2) (43). Work status at 1 year of follow-up is shown in Table 3. A similar percentage of patients in both groups were unemployed or disabled (43). More patients in the surgical group were retired, which may reflect the significantly greater mean age of this group of patients.

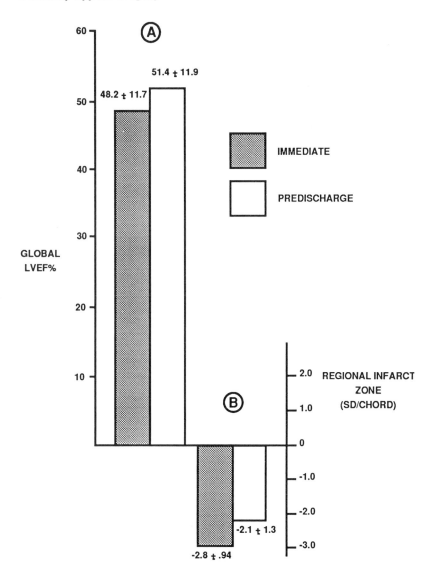

Figure 4 Changes in global left ventricular ejection fraction (LVEF) and regional infarct zone function (SD/Chord) based on preoperative (*n* = 168) and postoperative (*n* = 177) contrast left ventriculograms in patients who had deferred coronary bypass surgery following intravenous thrombolytic therapy for acute myocardial infarction.

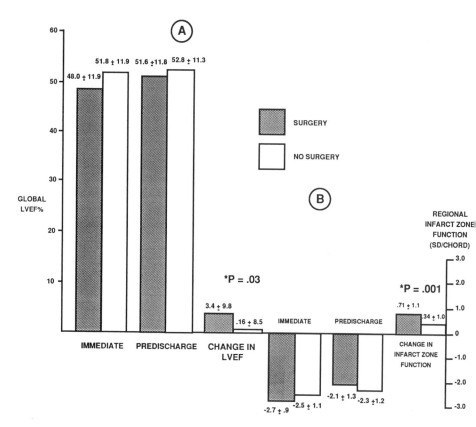

Figure 5   (A)   Preoperative and postoperative left ventricular ejection fraction (LVEF) and change in left ventricular ejection fraction for surgical patients (193 preoperative studies, 194 postoperative studies) and for nonsurgical patients (720 preoperative studies, 840 postoperative studies) treated with thrombolytic therapy with or without percutaneous transluminal coronary angioplasty.   (B)   Immediate and predischarge regional infarct zone function and change in infarct zone function for surgical patients and nonsurgical patients treated with intravenous thrombolytic therapy with or without coronary angioplasty. Greater preservation in global left ventricular ejection fraction and regional infarct zone function was observed in patients who underwent coronary bypass surgery.

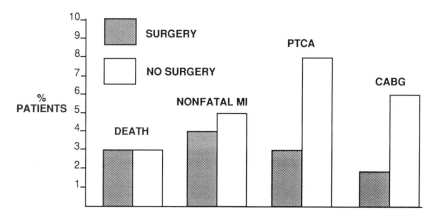

Figure 6   Incidence of posthospital discharge mortality, nonfatal myocardial infarction (MI), percutaneous transluminal coronary angioplasty (PTCA), and coronary bypass grafting (CABG) in surgical patients (n = 303) versus nonsurgical patients treated with intravenous thrombolytic therapy with or without coronary angioplasty (n = 1084). No difference in the incidence of death and nonfatal myocardial infarction was noted between groups. Revascularization procedures (PTCA, CABG) were more frequent in patients who did not undergo bypass surgery during the initial hospitalization. Average follow-up was 177.4 ± 208.6 days in surgical patients and 201.2 ± 225.8 days in nonsurgical patients.

Table 2   General Health Status at 1 Year[a]

	Surgery	No Surgery
Excellent	21/74 (28%)	52/238 (22%)
Good	34/74 (46%)	138/238 (58%)
Fair	14/74 (19%)	39/238 (16%)
Poor	5/74 (7%)	9/238 (4%)

[a]Data from 312 of 359 (87%) survivors discharged from hospital.
Source: Reproduced with permission from the *American Heart Journal* (43).

Table 3   Work Status at 1 Year

Work Status	Surgery	No surgery
Full time	28%	48%
Part time	10%	6%
Homemaker	2%	4%
Retired	46%	30%
Disabled	10%	8%
Unemployed	3%	1%
Temporarily laid off	0%	2%
Other	2%	1%

Source: Reproduced with permission from the *American Heart Journal* (43).

Table 4   Potential Indications for Emergency Bypass Surgery

1.   After successful coronary thrombolysis

   a.   >50% left main coronary artery stenosis with left anterior descending or circumflex infarct-related vessel and hemodynamic instability

   b.   >75% left main coronary artery stenosis and right coronary infarct-related vessel

   c.   Left main equivalent disease[a] with hemodynamic instability

   d.   Multivessel disease with anatomy unsuitable for coronary angioplasty and ischemic dysfunction of noninfarct zones

2.   Unsuccessful angioplasty as a result of coronary dissection/rethrombosis with a large jeopardized myocardial region

3.   Failure of or contraindications for thrombolytic or angioplasty infarct artery recanalization with infarct duration <6 hr and a large jeopardized myocardial region

4.   Cardiogenic shock in patients with multivessel disease unsuitable for coronary angioplasty

[a]≥90% stenosis of dominant circumflex coronary artery and left anterior descending infarct-related vessel or ≥90% anterior descending coronary artery stenosis with dominant circumflex infarct-related vessel.

RECOMMENDATIONS FOR USE OF CORONARY BYPASS SURGERY IN THE TREATMENT OF ACUTE MYOCARDIAL INFARCTION

Based on our experience in 303 patients, we have attempted to establish indications for emergency coronary bypass surgery following acute myocardial infarction (Table 4). Following successful coronary thrombolysis, the decision to proceed with emergency coronary bypass surgery should involve not only coronary anatomical considerations, but also hemodynamic and physiological considerations pertaining to the patients' stability. Emergency surgery should be offered to patients with severe ($\geq 75\%$) left main coronary stenosis following intravenous thrombolysis and should be considered in those patients with a significant (>50 $<75\%$) left main stenosis and a left anterior descending or circumflex infarct vessel. If hemodynamically stable, this latter group can be offered deferred (>24 hr) surgery. Likewise, in hemodynamically stable patients with left main equivalent coronary disease or multivessel disease and coronary anatomy unsuitable for PTCA, surgery can be deferred. However, if hemodynamic instability unresponsive to pharmacological or intra-aortic balloon pump support exists, bypass surgery should not be delayed but should be performed emergently. Following an unsuccessful attempt at rescue PTCA, a perfusion catheter should be placed to maintain coronary flow in surgical candidates en route to surgery. In addition, failure to recanalize the infarct artery following thrombolysis or direct angioplasty within 6 hr of infarct symptom onset or contraindications for thrombolysis or angioplasty may be considered an indication for emergency surgery in selected patients based on studies cited previously. Finally, patients in cardiogenic shock with coronary anatomy unsuitable for angioplasty should strongly be considered for surgery.

Deferred in-hospital coronary bypass surgery should be offered to selected patients with multivessel coronary artery disease and/or complex coronary anatomy not amenable to PTCA based on standard clinical criteria. These patients can be safely offered surgical revascularization prior to hospital discharge with a very low morbidity and mortality.

REFERENCES

1. DeWood MA, Notske RN, Berg R, Ganji JH, Simpson CS, Hinnen ML, Selinger SL, Fisher LD. Medical and surgical management of early Q-wave myocardial infarction. I. Effects of surgical reperfusion on survival, recurrent myocardial infarction, sudden death in functional class at 10 or more years of follow up. J Am Coll Cardiol 1989; 14:65-77.
2. DeWood MA, Leonard J, Grunwald RP, Hensley GR, Mouser LT, Burroughs RW, Berg R, Fisher LD. Medical and surgical management of early Q-wave myocardial

infarction. II. Effects on mortality and global and regional left ventricular function at 10 or more years of follow up. J Am Coll Cardiol 1989; 14:78-90.

3. Phillips S, Zeff R, Skinner J. Reperfusion protocol and results in 738 patients with evolving myocardial infarction. Ann Thorac Surg 1986; 41:119-25.

4. Phillips S. Surgery in evolving acute myocardial infarction. In Roberts A, Conti CR, eds Current Surgery of the heart. Philadelphia: Lippincott, 1987:247-56.

5. Kereiakes DJ, Topol EJ, George BS, Abbottsmith CW, Stack RS, Candela RJ, O'Neill WW, Martin LH, Califf RM. Emergency coronary bypass surgery preserves global and regional left ventricular function after intravenous tissue plasminogen activator therapy for acute myocardial infarction. J Am Coll Cardiol 1988; 11:899-907.

6. GISSI. Long term effects of intravenous thrombolysis in acute myocardial infarction: final report of the GISSI study. Lancet 1987; 1:871-4.

7. ISIS-2. A multicenter, randomized trial of intravenous streptokinase and aspirin in acute myocardial infarction. Lancet 1988; 2:349-60.

8. Simoons M, Serruys P, Brand M. Early thrombolysis in acute myocardial infarction: limitation of infarct size improves survival. J Am Coll Cardiol 1986; 7:717-28.

9. Van der Werf, Arnold S. Tissue plasminogen activator and size of infarct, left ventricular function, and survival in acute myocardial infarction. Br Med J 1988; 297:374-9.

10. Topol EJ, Califf RM, Kereiakes DJ, George BS. Thrombolysis and Angioplasty in Myocardial Infarction (TAMI) trial. J Am Coll Cardiol 1987; 10:65B-74B.

11. Califf RM, Topol EJ, George BS, Boswik JM, Lee KL, Stump D, Dillon J, Abbottsmith CW, Candela RJ, Kereiakes DJ, O'Neill WW, Stack RS. Characteristics and outcome of patients in whom reperfusion with intra-venous tissue type plasminogen activator fails: results of the Thrombolysis and Angioplasty in Myocardial Infarction (TAMI) 1 trial. Circulation 1988; 77:1090-9.

12. Califf RM, Topol EJ, Stack RS, Ellis SG, George BS, Kereiakes DJ, Samaha JK, Worley SJ, Anderson JL, Harrelson-Woodlief L, Wall TC, Phillips HR, Abbottsmith CW, Candela RJ, Flanagan WH, Sasahara AA, Mantell S, Lee KL. An evaluation of combination thrombolytic therapy and timing of cardiac catheterization in acute myocardial infarction: results of the TAMI 5 randomized trial. Circulation (in press).

13. Harrison DG, Ferguson DW, Collins SH, Skorton DJ, Erickson EE, Kioschos JM, Marcus ML, White CW. Rethrombosis after reperfusion with streptokinase: importance of geometry in residual lesions. Circulation 1984; 69:991-8.

14. Gold HK, Leinbach RC, Garabedian H, Yasuda T, Johns JA, Grossbard ED, Palacios I, Collen D. Acute coronary reocclusion after thrombolysis with recombinant human tissue-type plasminogen acitvator: prevention by a maintenance infusion. Circulation 1986; 73:347-52.

15. Fung AY, Lai P, Topol EJ, Bates ER, Bourdillon PDY Walton J, Mancini GBJ, Kryski T, Pitt B, O'Neill WW. Value of percutaneous transluminal coronary angioplasty after unsuccessful intravenous streptokinase therapy in acute myocardial infarction. Am J Cardiiol 1986; 58:686-91.

16. Van Hecke J, Flameng W, Sergent P. Emergency bypass surgery: late effects on size of infarction and ventricular function. Circulation 1985; 72 (Suppl II):II-179-II-184.

17. Berg R, Selinger S, Leonard J. Immediate coronary bypass surgery for acute myocardial infarction. J Cardiovasc Surg 1981; 81:483-7.

18. Berg R, Selinger S, Leonard J, Grunwald RP, O'Grady WP. Surgical management of acute myocardial infarction. In McGoon DC, ed. Cardiac Surgery. Philadelphia: FA Davis, 1982:61-74.

19. Katz N, Wallace R. Emergency coronary bypass surgery: indications and results. In Rackley CE, ed. Advances in critical care cardiology. Philadelphia: FA Davis, 1986: 67-72.

20. Athanasuleas CL, Geer DA, Araciniega JG, Cooper TB, Hess RG, MacLean WAH, Papapietro SE, Stanley AWH, McEachern M. A reappraisal of surgical intervention for acute myocardial. J Thorac Cardiovasc Surg 1987; 93:405-14.

21. Maroko P, Libby P, Ginks W, Bloer CM, Shell WE, Sobel BE, Ross J Jr. Coronary artery reperfusion. I. Early effects on local myocardial function in the extent of myocardial necrosis. J Clin Invest 1972; 51:2710-8.

22. Constantini C, Corday E, Lang T, Meerbaum S, Brasch J, Kaplan L, Rubins S, Gold H, Osher J. Revascularization after three hours of coronary arterial occlusion: effects on regional cardiac metabolic function in infarct size. Am J Cardiol 1975; 36:368-84.

23. Allen BS, Okamoto F, Buckberg GD, Bugyi H, Young H, Leaf J, Beyersdorf F, Sjostrand F, Maloney JV. Studies of controlled reperfusion after ischemia. XV. Immediate functional recovery after six hours of regional ischemia by careful control of conditions of reperfusion and composition of reperfusate. J Thorac Cardiovasc Surg 1986; 82:621-35.

24. Allen BS, Buckberg GD, Schwaiger M, Yeatman L, Tillisch J, Kawata N, Messenger J, Lee C. Studies of controlled reperfusion after ischemia. XVI. Early recovery of regional wall motion in patients following surgical revascularization after eight hours of acute coronary occlusion. J Thorac Cardiovasc Surg 1986; 92:636-48.

25. Vinten-Johansen J, Buckberg GD, Okamoto F, Rosenkranz E, Bugyi H, Leaf J. Studies of controlled reperfusion after ischemia. V. Superiority of surgical versus medical reperfusion after regional ischemia. J Thorac Cardiovasc Surg 1986; 92:525-34.

26. Buckberg GD. Thoracic and cardiovascular surgery. J Thorac Cardiovasc Surg 1986; 92:43-7.

27. Vinten-Johansen J, Rosenkranz E, Buckberg GD, Leaf J, Bugyi H. Studies of controlled reperfusion after ischemia. VI. Metabolic and histochemical benefits of regional blood cardioplegic reperfusion without cardiopulmonary bypass. J Thorac Cardiovasc Surg 1986; 92:535-42.

28. Allen BS, Okomoto F, Buckberg GD, Bugyi H, Leaf J. Studies of controlled reperfusion after ischemia. IX. Reperfusate composition. Benefits of marked hypocalcemia in diltiazem on regional recovery. J Thorac Cardiovasc Surg 1986; 92:564-72.

29. Allen BS, Okomoto F, Buckberg GD, Bugyi H, Leaf J. Studies in controlled reperfusion after ischemia. XIII. Reperfusion conditions: critical importance of total ventricular decompression during regional reperfusion. J Thorac Cardiovasc Surg 1986; 92:605-12.

30. Mathey D, Rodewald G, Rentrop P, Leitz K, Merx W, Messmer BJ, Rutsch W, Bucherl ES. Intracoronary streptokinase thrombolytic recanalization and subsequent surgical bypass of remaining atherosclerotic stenosis in acute myocardial infarction: complementary combined approach effecting reduced infarct size, preventing

reinfarction and improving left ventricular function. Am Heart J 1981; 102:1194-1201.

31. Phillips S, Kongthaworn C, Zeff R, Iannone L, Brown T, Gordon DF. Emergency artery revascularization: a possible therapy for acute myocardial infarction. Circulation 1979; 60:241-6.

32. DeWood M, Selinger S, Coleman W, Leonard JJ, Berg R. Surgical coronary reperfusion during acute myocardial infarction. In McGoon DC, ed. Cardiac Surgery, 2nd ed. Philadelphia: FA Davis, 1987:91-103.

33. DeWood M, Spores J, Notske R. Medical and surgical management of myocardial infarction. Am J Cardiol 1979; 44:1356-64.

34. Kennedy H, Goldberg R, Szkol M. The prognosis of anterior myocardial infarction revisited: a community wide study. Clin Cardiol 1979; 2:455-64.

35. Brower R, Fioretti P, Simoons M, Haalebos M, Rulf ENR, Hugenholtz PG. Surgical versus nonsurgical management of patients soon after myocardial infarction. Br Heart J 1985; 54:460-5.

36. Henning H, Gilpen E, Covell J. Prognosis after acute myocardial infarction: a multivaried analysis of mortality and survival. Circulation 1979; 59:1124-31.

37. Bonow K, Alpert J. The natural history and treatment of coronary artery disease. Cardiovasc Med 1978; 4:87-99.

38. Killip T, Kimball J. Treatment of myocardial infarction in a coronary care unit: a two year experience with 250 patients. Am J Cardiol 1967; 20:457-63.

39. Timmis G. Cardiovascular review 1980. Baltimore: Williams & Wilkins, 1980:53 pp.

40. Braunwald E. The aggressive treatment of acute myocardial infarction. Circulation 1985; 71:1087-92.

41. Topol EJ, Bates ER, Walton JA, Baumann G, Wolfe S, Maino J, Bayer L, Gorman L, Kline EM, O'Neill WW, Pitt B. Community hospital administration of intravenous tissue plasminogen activator in acute myocardial infarction: improved timing, thrombolytic efficacy and ventricular function. J Am Coll Cardiol 1987; 10:1173-7.

42. Loop FL, Lytle PW, Cosgrove DM. Influence of the internal mammary artery graft on 10 year survival and other cardiac events. N Engl J Med 1986; 314:1-9.

43. Kereiakes DJ, Topol EJ, Goerge BS, Abbottsmith CW, Stack RS, Candela RJ, O'Neill WW, Anderson LC, Califf RM. Favorable early and long-term prognosis following coronary bypass surgery therapy for myocardial infarction: results of a multicenter trial. Am Heart J 1989; 118:199-207.

44. Kereiakes DJ, Topol EJ, George BS, Stack RS, Abbottsmith CW, Ellis S, Candela RJ, Harrelson L, Martin LH, Califf RM. Myocardial infarction with minimal coronary atherosclerosis in the era of thrombolytic reperfusion. J Am Coll Cardiol 1991; 17:304-312.

45. DeWood M, Spores J, Berg R. Acute myocardial infarction: a decade of experience with surgical reperfusion in 701 patients. Circulation 1983; 68:118-26.

46. Kirklin JK, Blackstone EH, Zorn GL, Pacifico AD, Kirklin JW, Karp RB, Rogers WJ. Intermediate term results of coronary artery bypass grafting for acute myocardial infarction. Circulation 1985; 72(Suppl II): II-175-II-178.

47. Nunley DL, Grunkemeier GL, Teply JF, Abbruzzese PA, Davis JS, Khonsari S, Starr

A. Coronary bypass operation following acute complicated myocardial infarction. J Thorac Cardiovasc Surg 1983; 85:485-91.

48. Laks H, Rosenkranz E, Buckberg G. Surgical treatment of cardiogenic shock after myocardial infarction. Circulation 1986; 74:11-6.

49. Merx W, Dorr R, Rentrop P, Blanke H, Karsch KR, Mathey DG, Kremer P, Rutsch W, Schmutzler H. Evaluation of the effectiveness of intracoronary streptokinase infusion in acute myocardial infarction: post procedural management and hospital course in 204 patients. Am Heart J 1981; 102:1181-7.

50. Ferguson DW, White CW, Schwartz JL, Brayden GP, Kelly KJ, Kioschos JM, Kirchner PT, Marus ML. Influence of baseline ejection fraction and success of thrombolysis on mortality and ventricular function after acute myocardial infarction. Am J Cardiol 1984; 54:705-10.

51. Dodge H, Sheehan F, Mathey D, Brown BG, Kennedy JW. Usefulness of coronary artery bypass graft surgery or percutaneous transluminal coronary angioplasty after thrombolytic therapy. Circulation 1985; 72 (Suppl V):V-39-V-45.

52. Meyer J, Merx W, Dorr R. Sequential intervention procedures after intracoronary thrombolysis: balloon dilation, bypass surgery and medical treatment. Int J Cardiol 1985; 7:281-93.

53. Ban T. Emergency aortic coronary bypass surgery after percutaneous transluminal coronary recanalization: its indications and results. Jpn Circ J 1985; 49:643-8.

54. Lolley D, Emerson D, Rams J. Should coronary artery bypass be delayed following successful direct coronary artery streptokinase thrombolysis during evolving myocardial infarction? J Vasc Surg 1986; 3:330-7.

55. Ellis SG, Topol EJ, George BS, Kereiakes DJ, DeBowey D, Sigmon K, Pickel A, Lee KL, Califf RM. Recurrent ischemia without warning: analysis of risk factors for in-hospital ischemic events following successful thrombolysis with intravenous tissue plasminogen activator. Circulation 1989; 80:1159-65.

56. O'Neill WW, Kereiakes DJ, Stack RS, George BS, Califf RM, Candela RJ, Abbottsmith CW, Topol EJ. Cardiothoracic surgical support is required during interventional therapy of myocardial infarction: results from the TAMI Study Group. J Am Coll Cardiol 1987; 9:124A (abstract).

57. Abbottsmith CW, Topol EJ, George BS, Stack RS, Kereiakes DJ, Candela RJ, Anderson LC, Harrelson-Woodlief SL, Califf RM. Fate of patients with acute myocardial infarction with patency of the infarct related vessel achieved with successful thrombolysis versus rescue angioplasty. J Am Coll Cardiol 1990; 16:770-8.

58. Topol EJ, Califf RM, George BS, Kereiakes DJ, Rothbaum D, Candela RJ, Abbottsmith CW, Pinkerton C, Stump DC, Collen D, Lee KL, Ptt B, Kline EM, Boswick J, O'Neill WW, Stack RS. Coronary arterial thrombolysis with combined infusion of recombinant tissue plasminogen activator and urokinase in patients with acute myocardial infarction. Circulation 1988; 5:1100-7.

59. Gacioch GM, Topol EJ. Sudden paradoxic clinical deterioration during angioplasty of the occluded right coronary artery in acute myocardial infarction. J Am Coll Cardiol 1989; 14:1202-9.

60. Kereiakes DJ, Abbottsmith CW, Callard GM, Flege JB Jr. Emergent internal mam-

mary artery grafting following failed percutaneous transluminal coronary angioplasty: use of transluminal catheter reperfusion. Am Heart J 1987; 113:1018-20.

61. Hinohara T, Simpson JB, Phillips HR, Behar VS, Peter RH, Kong Y, Carlson EB, Stack RS. Transluminal catheter reperfusion: a new technique to reestablish blood flow after coronary occlusion during percutaneous transluminal coronary angioplasty. Am J Cardiol 1986; 57:684-8.

62. Kereiakes DJ, Califf RM, George BS, Samaha J, Anderson L, Young S, Topol EJ. Coronary bypass surgery improves global and regional left-ventricular function following thrombolytic therapy for acute myocardial infarction. Am Heart J. 1991; 122: 390-399.

63. Okies JE, Bag US, Biglow JC, Krause AH, Salomon NW. The internal mammary artery: the graft of choice. Circulation 1984; 70(Suppl):I-213-I-217.

64. Tector AJ, Schmahl TM, Canino VR. The internal mammary artery graft: the best choice for bypass of the diseased left anterior descending coronary artery. Circulation 1983; 68 (Suppl II):II-214-II-219.

65. Austin EH, Oldham HN, Sabastin DC, Jones RH. Early assessment of rest and exercise on left ventricular function following coronary artery surgery. Ann Thorac Surg 1983; 35:159-69.

66. Floyd RD, Sabastin DC, Leekel R, Jones RH. The effect of duration of hyperthermic cardioplegia on ventricular function. J Cardiovasc Surg 1983; 85:606-11.

67. Ceremuzynski L. Hormonal and metabolic reactions evoked by acute myocardial infarction. Circ Res 1981; 48:767-76.

68. Karlsberg RP, Cryer PE, Roberts R. Serial plasma catecholamine respond early in the course of clinical acute myocardial infarction: relationship to infarct extent and mortality. Am Heart J 1981; 102:24-31.

IV

ECONOMIC CONSIDERATIONS AND TREATMENT RECOMMENDATIONS

21

Economic Aspects of Therapy for Acute Myocardial Infarction

Daniel B. Mark and James G. Jollis

Duke University Medical Center, Durham, North Carolina

INTRODUCTION

Over the last decade, discussions about medical costs have moved from the eso-teric domain of the economist and health service researcher to the center stage of public attention. Medical costs now receive more attention in the national lay press than they do in the major medical journals, and much of this coverage is negative. The prevailing message is that the United States is spending too much for health care and getting too little in return. According to government figures, health spending in 1989 equaled 11.6% of the gross national product (GNP), which can be thought of as the "national pocketbook." This is about twice the rate of health spending of most other industrialized countries. Furthermore, the rate of increase in United States health spending from 1988 to 1989 was almost twice that of the increase of the overall GNP, a figure that the Secretary of Health and Hu-man Services has called "alarming" (1). Health service researchers point to unex-plained geographical variations in the frequency with which medical procedures are performed in apparently similar populations to support the contention that physicians in this country are performing too many expensive procedures (2). For example, in 1982 New Haven had a per capita rate of coronary bypass operations (CABG) that was twice that of Boston's, although the demographic characteristics of these two areas are quite similar (3). In addition, comparisons of procedure rates in the United States and Canada show substantially greater rates in the United States but no apparent associated health benefits (4).

Of all the medical specialties, cardiology has the largest share of medical expenditures (5,6). The annual total economic costs (both direct and indirect) for coronary heart disease currently exceed $80 billion (7). The cost to Medicare for the hospital care of patients age ≥ 65 with confirmed acute myocardial infarction (MI) (55% of hospitalized MI patients) is approaching $2 billion per year. Current projections are that over the next 20 years, medical spending on coronary heart disease (particularly acute MI) will rise by 25% (after adjusting for inflation) over 1990 levels (8).

Aside from occasional exhortations to each other to be more "cost effective," clinicians have generally avoided involvement in the area of medical economics, both because they are not eager to learn the unfamiliar language of the economist and because of the general feeling that such matters are not relevant to the practice of medicine. It seems to us, however, that the increasingly strong resolve of the payors in this country (i.e., primarily the federal government, private insurance companies, and the employers that pay for much of this insurance) to reduce the amount being spent on health care is on a collision course with the dramatic technological advances of modern medicine, many of which are described in this book. That "new medicine" usually costs more than "old medicine" is clearly illustrated by the over $2000 cost differential between the "high-tech" recombinant DNA product tissue plasminogen activator (t-PA) and the "low-tech" bacterial extract streptokinase (SK).

We believe that clinicians must become more involved in discussions and research on medical costs so that when cost-based decisions are required, we can be active participants in the process rather than passive bystanders. The purpose of this chapter is to introduce clinicians to some of the major concepts of medical economics, with emphasis on what is currently known about the cost of treatment of acute MI patients in the era of reperfusion therapy.

MAJOR COST CONCEPTS

In this section we shall examine some concepts that are basic to a discussion of medical costs and cost-effectiveness. In the traditional view of an economist, a "cost" is the consumption of a resource that could have been used for another purpose (9). Because our resources are ultimately limited, society is forced to make choices among alternative uses of its resources (10). Resources are usually classified in subcategories, such as labor and capital equipment. Since enumeration of all the labor and capital resources that go into production of a particular item of medical care is tedious and difficult to analyze, a useful surrogate measure of resource consumption under certain conditions is the price (more specifically the market price) that is assigned to that particular medical item or service. Thus, our first estimate of the cost of a particular medical therapy is the price of that therapy. In this sense, medical prices are entirely analogous to the price of a television or a washing machine at the local department store. When an acute MI patient receives his hospital bill after returning home, he will see on it the dollar prices (or charges) for the resources consumed during the hospital stay.

Unfortunately, medical prices or charges are a relatively inaccurate measure of medical resource consumption. The economic notion of a fair market price presumes informed consumers (patients) making rational choices, paying for these choices themselves, and producers (hospitals, doctors) competing on price. In the medical marketplace, there is little evidence that hospitals and doctors compete on prices (11). In fact, hospitals and doctors in a given area more often compete with each other to have the largest, most modern facility equipped with the newest high-technology drugs and devices regardless of the price. The major reason excessively high prices do not force these providers out of business (as would happen in a truly competitive market) is that their patients are insulated from the economic consequences of consuming too much medical care by the third-party payors (the federal government and the insurance companies). If patients had to pay completely out of pocket for thrombolytic therapy or coronary bypass surgery, there would likely be either a dramatic reduction in the price (charge) for these items or a substantial reduction in use (12). Of course, the need to preserve one's health will force patients to seek certain kinds of medical care even if they have to pay completely out-of-pocket.

In the medical market, there is another important distortion of prices at work. Many hospitals take care of patients who cannot pay their bills and who have no health insurance, or they give free services to their employees. In addition, some departments or laboratories may not have enough patient volume to cover operating expenses while other areas of the hospital are strong revenue generators. Hospital administrators, primarily concerned with keeping the hospital financially solvent, employ a variety of accounting maneuvers collectively known as "cost shifting" to cover the deficit areas with any excess revenues available (Table 1). To ensure the presence of a sufficient excess of revenues for this purpose, administrators may choose to raise the price for a cardiac catheterization procedure or an exercise radionuclide test substantially above the cost to the hospital of providing these services. These cost-shifting practices bring us to our second estimate of medical cost, which is the true dollar amount expended by the hospital or medical care provider to provide the given medical service (Table 1). This concept, termed "cost," should be clearly distinguished from the "charge" or price described previously.

The analogy we use to explain the charge versus cost distinction comes from the familiar domain of the automobile dealer. When a prospective buyer comes to a dealership to purchase a car, the salesman will often try to get him or her to pay

Table 1   Major Components of Hospital Charges For Medical Services

1.	True costs to hospital of resources consumed (e.g., supplies, personnel, capital equipment, utilities)
2.	Cost shifting accounting maneuvers Bad debts Free services (e.g., employees, indigent care) Disallowed costs by insurance companies
3.	Budgeting for expansion of services (e.g., more inpatient beds, more outpatient clinics)
4.	Acquisition of new technologies (e.g., PET scanner, digital angiographic equipment)
5.	Replacement of existing equipment (depreciation)

Item 1 = cost for given hospital service; items 1–5 = charge or price for given hospital service.

the sticker price for the vehicle. The dealer, however, has actually paid a lower price, the dealer's invoice price, to obtain the vehicle from the manufacturer. The difference between the two figures represents profit. In medicine, the charges that appear on the hospital bill are like a sticker price, whereas the hospital's actual costs for providing the given services are like the dealer's invoice price. The difference between charges and costs are accounted for largely by the hospital's need to shift the cost of the nonpaying segment of their patient population onto the paying segment. Thus, when we wish to determine how much a particular item of medical care costs (i.e., the dollar value of resources consumed), we must be wary of using the readily available charges on a hospital bill as surrogates for the true costs (13,14).

To facilitate the economic analysis of different clinical strategies, medical costs can be subdivided into variable and fixed components. Variable costs change with small changes in patient volume and include such things as disposable supplies and drugs. Fixed costs, on the other hand, do not change with patient volume. For example, the costs of building a cardiac care unit or an interventional catheterization laboratory are fixed and do not recur with each additional patient cared for. These concepts are particularly relevant when one begins to examine how many dollars can be saved by shifting patients from one treatment to another. For example, moving from a reperfusion strategy of thrombolytic therapy routinely followed by catheterization at 18–48 hr (i.e., the TIMI-2 intermediate strategy) to a strategy of thrombolytic therapy with catheterization reserved for patients with recurrent ischemia (i.e., the TIMI-2 conservative strategy) will save the variable costs of the extra catheterization procedures but not the fixed costs of having a catheterization suite with its specially trained personnel who must be paid whether one case or 10 are scheduled for the day.

Marginal cost analysis is a concept used by economists to examine the costs (or cost savings) of doing one additional (or one less) procedure or test (15,16). The marginal costs of doing one more procedure such as a coronary angioplasty cannot be simply determined from medical bills (hospital and physician). Rather, the resource consumption patterns associated with varying the volume of procedures must be examined to determine the cost components that are affected by small changes in patient volume (i.e., the variable costs). When larger patient volume changes occur, however, even costs previously regarded as fixed must be included in a marginal cost analysis. For example, shifting enough CAD patients from CABG to PTCA at a particular medical center will eventually result in the closing of an operating room with reassignment of the associated personnel (thereby reducing costs). When the PTCA volume gets large enough, a new PTCA laboratory will need to be built and new personnel will need to be hired (thus increasing costs).

The notion of one more or less procedure or test is useful in some types of economic analysis, but the more practical question usually relates to the costs of shifting a *group* of patients from one diagnostic or therapeutic strategy to another. In this setting the term "incremental" is often substituted for "marginal." (Some medical economics researchers do not distinguish between "marginal" and "incremental" (17) while others do (9), leading to potential confusion of the unwary.) Incremental cost analysis addresses the key question of how much will be saved (or added) by adopting one treatment strategy over another. The methodology for doing such an analysis, however, is relatively complex and has therefore been infrequently applied in practice. Most published medical cost analyses to date have only reported charge data. Measuring true incremental cost is time consuming and difficult. Therefore, many researchers in medical economics employ costs calculated from charges using Medicare ratios of costs to charges (RCCs) as a surrogate (18). Medicare RCCs are a product of the era when Medicare part A reimbursements to hospitals were "cost (charge) based" (i.e., prior to initiation of the current prospective payment system). Medicare sought to develop a means by which it could reimburse hospitals for the reasonable and necessary costs of providing care to covered patients (i.e., "dealer invoice price") rather than paying charges (i.e., "sticker price"). To meet this need, it derived an elaborate reporting system that required each hospital to file a Medicare Cost Report with the Health Care Financing Administration each year. This report details how hospital expenses for patient care, overhead, capital equipment, and so forth relate to billed charges and provides a set of ratios that can be used to convert charges to costs.

The advantage of the RCC cost methodology is that it can be applied to almost every hospital in the United States and thus is valuable for multicenter cost studies and for comparing costs measured in different hospitals. However, several limitations of the RCC approach should be noted. First, it provides estimates of average rather than marginal costs and thus may overestimate potential cost savings. Second, Medicare Cost Reports are like federal income tax forms in that the written rules for completing the Report and deriving the RCCs give different hospitals the discretion to interpret the instructions differently (just as different individuals may interpret IRS rules differently).

We recently compared charges for elective PTCA and CABG patients at Duke Hospital with RCC-derived costs and with marginal costs (19). RCC costs were equivalent to marginal costs that included departmental overhead but substantially overestimated the marginal costs of supplies and personnel. Thus, while RCC-based cost estimates do represent an improvement over charges, they have a number of important limitations which must be kept in mind.

Another major and often misunderstood concept in medical economics is cost-effectiveness (17). Clinicians have tended to use the term "cost-effective" in an intuitive sense, but it actually has a specific technical (and not particularly intuitive) meaning (20). Cost-effectiveness analysis *always* involves comparison with some explicit alternative investment of dollars, so it is incorrect to describe a treatment as cost-effective in isolation (as is often done in the medical literature) (9). Furthermore, cost-effectiveness analysis does not indicate whether a given health care expenditure is worthwhile, but merely how it stands in relation to other potential expenditures.

The measurements made in cost-effectiveness analysis are expressed in ratio form, with the numerator being the incremental costs, for example, of treatment A relative to treatment B and the denominator being the incremental health benefits of A relative to B (Table 2). These health benefits are most often measured in terms of changes in life expectancy, but may also be expressed in terms of changes in quality-adjusted life expectancy (which is also called cost-utility analysis) or in terms of the dollar value of changes in health status (which is also called cost-benefit analysis). The underlying tenet of all these forms of economic analysis is that the analyst wishes to *maximize the net health benefits for a particular population* under conditions of limited resources (i.e., where you cannot do everything for everyone). For example, if economic analysis showed that it was more cost-effective to give AZT to asymptomatic human immunodeficiency virus-positive patients than to give thrombolytic therapy to patients with an acute inferior MI, the resulting policy decision would be to buy more AZT and less t-PA (because this would buy more benefits per societal dollar spent on health care). Such analyses are, therefore, neutral to the specific patients and diseases under study, and the health benefits being maximized are abstractly conceptualized as belonging to a group or population.

The problem cost-effectiveness analysis poses for clinicians is that the goal of individual physicians is to *maximize the health of their own patients* with little or no regard for cost. This traditional patient advocate role is thus significantly at

Table 2   Calculation of Cost-Effectiveness: Example

Strategy	Treatment costs	Effectiveness (life expectancy)	Utility (QOL)	QOL adjusted life expectancy	Benefits
Rx A	$20,000	4.5 years	0.80	3.6 QALYs	$4000
Rx B	$10,000	3.5 years	0.90	3.15 QALYs	$2000

Incremental cost-effectiveness ratio $= \dfrac{\$20{,}000 - \$10{,}000}{4.5 \text{ years} - 3.5 \text{ years}}$

$= \$10{,}000$ per life-year saved

Incremental cost-utility ratio $= \dfrac{\$20{,}000 - \$10{,}000}{3.6 \text{ QALYs} - 3.15 \text{ QALYs}}$

$= \$22{,}222$ per QALY saved

Incremental cost-benefit ratio $= \dfrac{\$20{,}000 - \$10{,}000}{\$4{,}000 - \$2{,}000} = 5$

[a]Shows health benefits valued in dollars.
QALY = quality-adjusted life year; QOL = quality of life; Rx = treatment.
Source: From Detsky and Naglie (17).

odds with the societal objective of cost-effectiveness analysis to maximize the efficiency with which scarce health care resources are used (17). The ultimate problem, of course, is that as individual patients (and their physicians) we want all the health benefits that modern medical technology can supply; as the collection of all patients taken together (i.e., society), our resources are limited and we cannot afford to provide this for everyone (21,22). The more we provide for selected segments of the population (such as acute MI patients, acquired immunodeficiency syndrome patients, or renal failure patients), the higher the likelihood that other segments will ultimately be denied needed services. In the next section, we shall examine the costs and cost-effectiveness of treatment of acute MI, which has become a major focal point in the debate over medical costs in recent years.

COST STUDIES OF ACUTE MI THERAPIES

Despite the widespread attention currently focused on the cost of treatment of acute MI, very few cost analyses have been published in this area. The available studies can be classified into three major types: randomized trial comparisons of different treatment strategies, nonrandomized (i.e., observational) treatment comparisons, and cost-effectiveness models. In addition, the studies may be classified according to whether they *measured* costs directly on a group of patients or they assigned or imputed costs from starting assumptions, "standard charges," expert opinions, and so forth, without direct patient observation. In general, randomized trials and observational studies usually measure costs while cost-effectiveness analyses usually impute costs.

Costs (both measured and imputed) are influenced not only by what is wrong with the patient and what has been done for him or her, but also by such nonmedical factors as the cost of living in that particular region of the country, the type of institution in which the care is provided, and the specific care setting (e.g., rural or urban). In addition, measured costs of health care have only a loose relationship to underlying pathophysiological processes and associated treatment decisions. Thus, costs may be more variable from one institution or practice setting to the next than medical outcomes. To compensate for the relative "softness" of the data, cost and cost-effectiveness analyses often employ the technique of sensitivity analysis to determine the bottom-line impact of systematically varying one or more factors (e.g., the cost of a PTCA or CABG procedure) from their baseline value (9).

Cost of Thrombolytic Therapy

To date, the cost of thrombolytic therapy has been compared with conventional supportive care in six studies (Table 3). Three of these involved cost-effectiveness models in which estimates of costs and benefits were derived from the available medical literature, with expert medical opinion used to fill other necessary data (23-25). While all three models had access to the GISSI-1 results, none had the final ISIS-2 results or results from the other important megatrials, such as ASSET and AIMS. In evaluating these studies, it is therefore crucial to examine their starting assumptions carefully. Some of these basic assumptions were: (a) survival benefits from thrombolysis are a direct function of the time interval between symptom onset and duration of therapy, with little or no benefits evident after more than 4- 6 hr; (b) survival benefits of thrombolysis are a function of infarct size/prognosis, with the greatest benefits in the highest risk group; (c) survival benefits are a function of infarct vessel patency and reperfusion/reocclusion rates and are therefore greater with IV t-PA than IV SK, and (d) higher infarct vessel patency leads to more episodes of recurrent ischemia and ultimately to more revascularization procedures. The in-hospital mortality rates assigned to conventional therapy by Laffel and co-workers were 40% for a large/complicated infarct, 12% for a moderate infarct, and 3% for a small infarct (23). These authors further assumed that treatment with IV thrombolytic therapy within 1 hr of symptom onset would reduce the mortality rate of the large infarct group by ≥60% (somewhat more than subsequent empirical observations in ISIS-2). Steinberg and colleagues assumed an in-hospital mortality rate with conventional therapy of 11.3%, a 10%

Table 3 Cost Studies of Thrombolytic Therapy

Study	Pub. year	Type of analysis	Treatments compared	Sample size	Measure of costs
Laffel (23)	1987	Cost-effectiveness model	SK, t-PA, primary PTCA, conventional therapy	N/A	Estimated costs (RCC method) using Brigham and Women's Hospital data (1986 U.S. dollars)
Steinberg (24)	1988	Cost-effectiveness model	SK, t-PA, conventional therapy	N/A	DRG reimbursement rates for Baltimore (1988 U.S. dollars)
Liu (25)	1988	Cost-effectiveness model	SK, t-PA, conventional therapy	N/A	Estimated costs (1987 Canadian dollars)
Vermeer (31)	1988	Randomized trial	IC SK, conventional	533	Calculated from big ticket items (1984 Dutch guilders)
Herve (33)	1990	Observational treatment comparison	APSAC, conventional therapy	162	Medical bills, calculated (British pounds)
Naylor (26)	1990	Cost-effectiveness	SK, t-PA	N/A	Estimated costs (1988 Canadian dollars)
Jonsson (32)	1992	Randomized trial substudy	t-PA, conventional therapy	313	Calculated from big ticket items (Swedish crowns).
Machecourt (36)	1990	Randomized trial	t-PA, APSAC	180	Not specified
Mark (35)	1991	Randomized trial	t-PA, UK, t-PA/UK	575	Measured charges, costs from charges (RCC method)

rate with IV SK (a 12% reduction), and a 9.3% rate with IV t-PA (an 18% reduction) (24).

For the model by Laffel et al., costs were estimated from 1986 Brigham and Women's Hospital charges and physician fees converted (for the hospital charges) to costs using Medicare cost-to-charge ratios (23). These investigators assumed that IV SK would add $300 to conventional care costs, while IV t-PA would add $1500 (the analysis was published before t-PA was approved for use in the United States). Steinberg et al. did their analysis from the perspective of Medicare rather than society overall, and costs were assigned using the appropriate DRG reimbursement rates for metropolitan Baltimore hospitals in 1988 (24). Because Medicare had (and has) not adjusted DRG reimbursements to reflect the higher cost of t-PA, this analysis did not include the specific cost of thrombolytic therapy. Liu and colleagues used cost estimates (similar to the approach of Laffel et al.) based on 1987 Canadian dollars (25).

The major results of these three cost-effectiveness models are shown in Table 4, along with selected cost-effectiveness ratios from other areas of medicine for reference. Overall, the incremental cost per additional life-year saved with thrombolysis compared with conventional therapy was $50,000–75,000, although the amount of benefit (and consequently the cost-effectiveness ratio) was sensitive to the magnitude of mortality reduction assumed as well as the level of risk associated with conventional therapy. Smaller mortality reductions or treatment of lower-risk patients resulted in fewer lives saved over the study period and consequently a higher cost per each life-year saved. In general, the added cost per additional life-year saved of thrombolytic therapy over conventional treatment of acute MI appears comparable with that of other widely accepted forms of therapy, such as CABG for three-vessel disease with good left ventricular function and severe angina, and appears to substantially exceed the cost-effectiveness of other routine medical practices (such as the use of predischarge treadmill testing after acute MI or the use of nonionic contrast agents for angiography).

Two studies examined the cost-effectiveness of substituting t-PA for SK. In the model of Steinberg and co-workers, the cost of saving an additional year of life with t-PA over SK was $64,571 (24). In a sensitivity analysis, the authors concluded that this figure was primarily dependent on their assumption of a higher subsequent revascularization rate with t-PA. Goel and Naylor found the incremental cost for each additional survivor in 1988 Canadian dollars was $58,600 assuming that t-PA reduced short-term mortality from 8% (with SK) to 7% with no additional effect on long-term survival (26). With either a larger benefit on short-term survival or an additional improvement in long-term survival, the cost-effectiveness of substituting t-PA for SK ranged from $16,300 to $44,600 per year of life saved. The results of this analysis were principally dependent on the assumption of an added mortality reduction with t-PA relative to SK. If the survival equivalence of these two agents found in the recent International t-PA/SK and

Table 4   Cost-Effectiveness of Thrombolytic Therapy over Conventional Therapy

Treatment compared		Incremental cost per additional life saved ($)
a. IV SK versus conventional therapy		
Laffel (23)	Large MI, ≤4 hr	$27,000
	Moderate MI, ≤4hr	$171,000
	Small MI, ≤4hr	$682,000
Steinberg (24)		$52,796
Liu (25)		$78,676[a]
b. IV t-PA versus conventional therapy		
Laffel (23)	Large MI, ≤4hr	$30,000
	Moderate MI, ≤4hr	$158,000
	Small MI, ≤4hr	$631,000
Steinberg (24)		$56,900
Liu (25)		$61,000[a]
c. Other cost-effective figures (for illustration)		
Routine predischarge ETT post-MI versus no routine testing (48)		$255,726[a]
Nonionic contrast media for low-risk patients versus conventional contrast media (49)		$220,000
Bone marrow transplant for acute nonlymphocytic leukemia versus conventional chemotherapy (50)		$59,300
Treatment of severe diastolic hypertension versus no treatment (51)		$9,800
Drug therapy of cholesterol > 265 mg/dl in asymptomatic middle-aged men versus no treatment (52, 53)		$100,000–200,000
CABG for 3-vessel CAD with normal LV function and severe angina versus conservative therapy (54)		$65,000
PTCA for 1-vessel LAD disease with normal LV function and mild angina versus conservative therapy (54)		$75,000

[a]Costs measured in Canadian dollars.

GISSI-2 trials (27,28) is confirmed by the ongoing GUSTO trial, the issue will, of course, be moot. The work by Naylor and colleagues suggests, however, that even a very modest survival advantage for t-PA will translate into a competitive cost-effectiveness outcome. The other important point this study makes is that the cost-effectiveness of thrombolytic therapy may become more favorable when figured on the basis of long-term rather than hospital or 30-day survival.

Of course, the very long-term medical benefits of reperfusion therapy for acute MI (e.g., over 10–20 years) remain uncertain. It has been hypothesized that salvaging myocardium and keeping the infarct vessel patent during the initial MI will make any subsequent MIs more survivable with fewer cases of shock and fewer deaths (thus, improving the cost-effectiveness). Empirical validation of this hypothesis will require continued long-term follow-up of the megatrial cohorts (such as GISSI-1 and ISIS-2).

One controversial area in the comparison of SK and t-PA is the frequency of subsequent revascularization procedures. Steinberg and colleagues assumed in their analysis that substantially more PTCAs and CABGs would be performed in t-PA–treated patients than in their SK-treated counterparts (24). Naylor and Jaglal, in a recent meta-analysis of this issue, reported higher revascularization rates in patients receiving thrombolytic therapy relative to conservative therapy, with rates somewhat higher in the t-PA trials than the SK trials (29). However, cumulative 1-year revascularization rates (PTCA or CABG) in the TIMI-1 trial were 36% for the 143 t-PA patients and 39% for the 147 SK patients (30). Furthermore, in this study the 90-min patency status of the infarct vessel did not significantly affect the likelihood of subsequent revascularization. One of the goals of the ongoing GUSTO randomized trial is to collect empirical data on this issue in comparable patients randomly selected for t-PA, SK, or combination t-PA/SK therapy.

Three studies to date have compared costs of thrombolysis versus conventional care using direct patient observation (Table 3). All three were conducted in Europe, making extrapolation to equivalent United States results difficult due to markedly different health care systems. The largest was the Dutch Interuniversity Trial of Intracoronary Streptokinase (IC SK), which involved a total of 533 patients treated between 1981 and 1985 (31). The IC SK treatment arm, of course, necessitated acute angiography and 17% went on to acute PTCA. In addition, almost 80% of both groups had a subsequent elective catheterization, so the treatment strategies evaluated in this study are not strictly comparable with the cost-effectiveness models previously described. The rates of late PTCA and CABG were somewhat higher in the thrombolysis group (9% and 16% versus 5% and 12%, respectively). ICU days were also higher in the thrombolysis group, but general ward days did not differ between the two treatments. Overall, the costs out to 1 year were higher in the IC SKs group due particularly to the need for acute catheterization as well as the longer ICU stay. The investigators estimated that the gain in life expectancy with treatment of inferior MIs was 0.7 year, for anterior MIs was 2.4 years, and for large anterior MIs treated within 2 hr of symptom onset was 3.6 years. Subgroup analysis showed that IC SK was most cost-effective in patients with large anterior MI admitted within 2 hr of symptom onset (D fl 1,900 per extra year of life) and least cost-effective in patients with inferior MI (D fl 10,000 per extra year of life). (One Dutch guilder is equivalent to 50–60 cents in 1991 United States currency.) These data, thus, support the assumption of Laffel et al. (23) about sensitivity of the cost-effectiveness of thrombolysis to infarct size and time elapsed since pain onset.

Jonsson and colleagues examined the costs of t-PA versus placebo in 313 Swedish participants of the ASSET study (32). At the end of 1 year of follow-up, the t-PA group mean costs were 39,400 Swedish crowns and the placebo group costs were 29,530 (p = 0.03). (One Swedish crown is equivalent to 17 cents in 1991 United States currency.) Most of this difference was due to the cost of t-PA. Seven percent of the t-PA patients received coronary angiography, compared with 5% of the placebo patients. One percent in each group had a PTCA and 5% in each group had a CABG. The gain in life expectancy for the average patient treated with t-PA relative to placebo was estimated to be 1.25 years. The cost per additional year of life saved with t-PA relative to placebo in this study was thus less than $1400 (in United States currency). Herve and co-workers reported that the initial higher costs associated with APSAC therapy compared with conventional therapy were offset by fewer follow-up rehospitalization days (33).

Two studies have compared the costs associated with different thrombolytic regimens (Table 3). In the recently completed TAMI-5 study, patients were randomized to one of three thrombolytic regimens (t-PA monotherapy, UK monotherapy, or combination t-PA/UK) and to one of two angiography strategies (acute versus deferred) (34). Although analyses of the cost data for this study have not yet been completed, preliminary calculations have shown essentially identical hospital costs for the t-PA and UK monotherapy groups and a $1000 lower total cost for the combination therapy group, associated with lower rates of recurrent ischemia and emergency PTCA in the latter group (35). Preliminary data from a smaller French study failed to detect a difference in costs between t-PA and AP-SAC (36).

Cost of Direct Coronary Angioplasty

As yet, no published observational studies or randomized trials have measured the costs of treating acute MI with direct PTCA. The model of Laffel et al. estimated the costs per additional survivor with direct PTCA at $83,000 for large MIs, $268,000 for moderate MIs, and $988,000 for small MIs (23). Liu et al. reported a cost of $48,229 (Canadian $) per year of life saved with direct PTCA relative to supportive medical therapy (25). DeWood recently described preliminary results

Table 5   Randomized Trial of Direct PTCA Versus IV t-PA (Preliminary Results)

	t-PA (n = 27)	PTCA (n = 27)
Patency at 90 min	74%	67% (p = 0.50)
Sx onset to admission (hr)	2.6 ± 1.5	1.9 ± 0.09 (p = 0.04)
Admission to treatment (hr)	1.4 ± 0.5	2.2 ± 1.0 (p = 0.002)
Hospital charges[a]	$19,000 ± 10,800	$14,500 ± 5900 ($p$ = 0.06)
Cumulative 1-year charges[a]	$24,000 ± 12,400	$18,200 ± 7900 ($p$ = 0.03)

[a]18/20 (90%) t-PA-treated patients who were patent at 90 min underwent a revascularization procedure in the first year.
Sx = symptoms.
Source: From DeWood (37).

from a small randomized trial comparison of direct PTCA with IV t-PA (37). Ninety-minute patency in the direct PTCA arm was lower in this study than had been reported previously for this form of therapy (Table 5). In addition, initiation of thrombolytic therapy could clearly be accomplished more rapidly than direct PTCA in this experienced center. The hospital and cumulative 1-year charges for direct PTCA, on the other hand, were quite competitive with the t-PA arm (which included acute angiography for every patient) and with other studies of the cost of thrombolytic therapy in the United States (see Table 6). The multicenter Primary Angioplasty Revascularization (PAR) Study has measured the hospital and cumulative 6-month costs of 270 acute MI patients treated with direct PTCA; preliminary results presented at the 1991 American Heart Meetings showed that the mean baseline hospital costs were $14,022 with mean professional fees of $5,303 (37a). Thus, based on the limited data available, direct PTCA appears to have comparable cost-effectiveness to a treatment strategy starting with thrombolytic therapy.

Coronary Angioplasty Following Thrombolysis

While a number of randomized trials have examined the role of PTCA in patients who have received thrombolytic therapy, only TIMI-2 and TAMI-5 have included cost measurements. The TIMI-2 cost substudy (38) involved the 376 patients enrolled at the University of Alabama and at the Mayo Clinic. Follow-up cost data collection is still underway in this study, but preliminary results have been presented (Table 6). Two points are noteworthy about these data. First, the unfavorable medical outcomes reported for the 2-hr PTCA group in the overall trial (39,40) were associated with a trend toward a longer hospital stay in this substudy,

Table 6   TIMI-2 Cost Substudy (Preliminary Data)

	PTCA strategy		
	2 hr PTCA (n = 66)	18–48-PTCA (n = 160)	No PTCA (n = 150)
a. Initial hospitalization			
Hospital days	10	9	9
PTCA performed	67%	58%	21%
CABG performed	26%	16%	16%
Hospital costs[a]	$10,988	$10,496	$8,625
Hospital charges[a]	$14,552	$14,471	$13,372
Professional fees[a]	$4,548	$3,754	$2,698
Total charges[a]	$19,100	$18,226	$16,070
b. Follow-up resources use			
Cardiac catheterization	3.0%	13.6%	15.4%
PTCA	1.5%	7.2%	5.1%
CABG	6.6%	6.4%	6.8%
Cardiac rehospitalizations			
1	19.7%	20.0%	22.2%
>1	1.5%	7.2%	8.5%

[a]Figures shown are means.
Source: From Charles et al. (38).

thus eliminating one potential mechanism for recouping higher initial procedural costs. Second, two-thirds of the difference in charges between the three groups is due to a difference in professional fees. Furthermore, the $1200 difference in hospital charges between the 2-hr PTCA and no-PTCA groups is substantially less than would be expected from the significantly different rates of angiography and PTCA in these two groups. A similar dissociation between the use of expensive "big ticket" items (such as catheterization and PTCA) and the resulting hospital charges was reported in a case-control study from the University of Michigan (41). Despite a more than twofold difference in the rates of catheterization and PTCA in the acute-intervention patients (PTCA or thrombolytic therapy or both) compared with the nonintervention group in this latter study, the average hospital charges were only $1500 more.

Of the randomized trials involving acute angiography with the option for acute PTCA, only TAMI-5 has observed medical benefits in the acute intervention group (34), and none have been large enough to detect a survival benefit (in fact, most have observed a trend toward higher mortality in the acute group). Preliminary evaluation of the TAMI-5 cost data has shown higher costs in the acute angiography group, but these trends were influenced by the requirement for patients in both angiography groups to have a 7 to 10-day protocol angiogram, thus adding research-driven charges to many of the acute angiography patients.

Based on available data, it is likely that acute angiography with appropriate triage to PTCA or CABG will be most cost-effective if it can be targeted to patients with large or complicated MIs who have failed thrombolysis. Full analysis of the TAMI-5 and TIMI-2 cost data will provide a more complete database for estimating the costs and cost-effectiveness of acute angiography and PTCA strategies.

Adjunctive Medical Therapy Following Reperfusion

A number of medical interventions, including antiplatelet therapy with aspirin and antithrombin therapy with heparin, have become a standard part of current reperfusion therapy. In addition, intravenous nitrates and intravenous/oral beta-blockers are used routinely in many centers, while the role of calcium channel blockers in the acute MI patient continues to be debated (42). Of these, only long-term oral beta-blockers have been subjected to any cost or cost-effectiveness analysis. Goldman and colleagues constructed a cost-effectiveness model of oral propranolol therapy started before discharge and continued for 6–15 years (43). The average cost per patient for 240 mg/day of propranolol in 10 retail pharmacies in the Boston area in 1987 was $208/year. Assuming a 25% relative reduction in annual mortality with treatment, these investigators reported cost-effectiveness ratios of $23,400 per year of life saved in low-risk patients, $5900 in medium-risk patients, and $3600 in high-risk patients. Thus, compared with thrombolytic therapy, as well as other medical interventions such as treatment of severe hypertension or CABG for left main disease, long-term beta-blocker therapy appears quite cost effective. Because the costs of treatment are so low, even very small survival benefits result in a favorable cost-effectiveness ratio.

The survival benefits of IV and oral beta-blocker therapy in patients receiving thrombolysis or other forms of reperfusion therapy remain uncertain, partly because they have not been measured in an adequately sized randomized trial. If the benefits on ischemic endpoints observed in TIMI-2B (40) ultimately translate into a decreased mortality rate with an effect size similar to that of conservatively treated patients (e.g., ≥10–15% reduction in mortality for IV therapy, ≥20–25% additional reduction for long-term oral therapy), then the Goldman analysis suggests that this form of therapy will still be quite cost-effective.

Cost-Effectiveness Estimation: An Example

It is interesting to speculate about the economic effects that will result if some of our current adjunctive medical therapies are replaced over the next decade by more effective "high-tech" agents, such as hirudin for heparin or the glyco-protein IIb/IIIa receptor antibody for aspirin. We can expect all these newer agents to be priced substantially above the drugs they replace. Using some "back of the envelope" calculations, we can illustrate how new adjunctive therapies for acute MI might affect incremental costs and cost-effectiveness. In Table 7, we present several hypothetical scenarios involving a newly approved thrombolytic therapy (treatment B) and a cheaper "standard" thrombolytic therapy (treatment A). Table 7A demonstrates a crude method for calculating the denominator of the cost-effectiveness ratio, the number of lives saved in a given interval by treatment B relative to treatment A. If we calculate lives saved on the basis of *hospital* survival rates, a 2% absolute difference in the survival rates for two agents translates into two lives saved by B for every 100 patients treated. If we assumed that the survival rates out to 1 year are equal in the hospital survivors for the two groups (as has been frequently been observed in reperfusion trials), then at *1 year* treatment B still saves just two lives over treatment A for every 100 patients treated. If, however, by the end of *5 years*, group A hospital survivors have had an accelerated mortality rate compared with group B, then group B will be credited with saving additional lives (for a total of six lives saved over 5 years in our example, Table 7A.c). Thus, the incremental survival benefits of one treatment over another in a cost-effectiveness calculation may depend significantly on the length of follow-up being considered.

The calculation of incremental costs of treatment B over treatment A is illustrated in Table 7B. This figure will form the numerator of our cost-effectiveness ratio. For simplicity, our example starts with the assumption that the only difference in costs between the two groups is the $2000 difference in cost of the thrombolytic agents. Thus, we assume that rates of catheterization, revascularization (PTCA, CABG), and length of ICU and total hospital stay are equal in the two groups. In this highly simplified scenario, the incremental cost of substituting treatment B for treatment A would be $2000 per patient, or $200,000 per 100 patients treated. Dividing this figure by our previous estimate of two lives saved in hospital for every 100 patients treated yields a cost-effectiveness ratio of $100,000 per life saved for new treatment B relative to standard treatment A (Table 7C).

With this simplified starting scenario, we can now explore how departures from our initial assumptions would affect our cost-effectiveness calculations. First, it is clear that if treatment B had a smaller survival advantage over treatment A so that only one life was saved in hospital rather than two, the resulting cost-effectiveness ratio would double to $200,000 per life saved. Of course, if B were substantially more effective, so that it saved an additional four lives over A in-hospital, the cost-effectiveness ratio would decrease to $50,000 per life saved.

Second, if treatment B not only saved more lives than A in-hospital but also resulted in modest reductions in resource consumption, so that half the patients treated with B stayed in the CCU 1 day less and also stayed on the hospital ward 1 day less (i.e., total length of stay reduced by 2 days for half of treatment B pa-

Table 7   Simplified Cost-Effectiveness Worksheet

A. Calculation of survival benefits (denominator)

		Rx A	Rx B
a.	Based on hospital survival rates		
	Hospital survival rates	0.93	0.95
	Hospital deaths/100 patients	7	5
	Lives saved by Rx B in hospital/100 patients		2
b.	Based on 1-year survival rates		
	1-year survival rate	0.90	0.92
	1-year deaths/100 patients	10	8
	Lives saved by Rx B over 1 year/100 patients		2
c.	Based on 5-year survival rates		
	5-year survival rate	0.78	0.84
	5-year deaths/100 patients	22	16
	Lives saved by Rx B over 5 years/100 patients		6

B. Calculation of costs (numerator)

			Rx A	Rx B
a.	Based on initial hospitalization			
	i.	Unit costs of resources		
		Thrombolytic therapy	$200	$2200
		Adjunctive medical therapy	$250	$250
		Catheterization	$2000	$2000
		PTCA	$3000	$3000
		CABG	$8000	$8000
		CCU/ICU day	$300	$300
		Regular hospital room day	$100	$100
	ii.	Rates of resource consumption		
		Thrombolytic therapy dose	100%	100%
		Adjunctive therapy	100%	100%
		Cardiac catheterization	50%	50%
		PTCA	30%	30%
		CABG	15%	15%
		2 CCU days	100%	100%
		2 ICU days	20%	20%
		7 hospital ward days	100%	100%
	iii.	Costs per 100 patients		
		Thrombolytic therapy	$20,000	$220,000
		Adjunctive therapy	$25,000	$25,000
		Catheterization	$100,000	$100,000

Table 7   (continued)

PTCA	$100,000	$100,000
CABG	$160,000	$160,000
CCU days	$60,000	$60,000
ICU days	$12,000	$12,000
Hospital ward days	$70,000	$70,000
Total	$547,000	$747,000

C. Calculation of in-hospital cost-effectiveness ratio

   i. Incremental hospital costs of B over A for 100 pts = $200,000

   ii. Incremental hospital survival benefits of B over A for 100 patients = 2 lives saved

   iii. Cost-effectiveness ratio = $200,000/2 = $100,000 per life saved in-hospital by B over A

D. Calculation of 1-year cost-effectiveness ratio

   i. Total 1-year costs per 100 patients

Baseline hospital costs (see B1ii)	$547,000	$747,000
Follow-up hospitalization rates	30%	20%
Cost per follow-up hospitalization	$8,000	$8,000
Total follow-up hospitalizations costs	$240,000	$160,000
Total 1-year costs	$787,000	$907,000

   ii. Incremental 1-year costs of B over A for 100 patients = $120,000

   iii. Incremental 1-year survival benefits of B over A for 100 patients = 2 lives saved

   iv. Cost effectiveness ratio = $120,000/2 = $60,000 per year of life life saved by B over A

Rx = treatment.

tients), the total costs for treating 100 patients with B would be reduced by $20,000 from our hypothetical calculations in Table 7B. The new added hospital cost figure of B over A for 100 patients would thus be $180,000 and the cost-effectiveness ratio would be $90,000 per life saved.

From these first two examples, we can see that in the case of acute MI treatment, relatively small absolute changes in mortality rates will be associated with large changes in the cost-effectiveness ratios, while modest shifts in resource consumption will have a much smaller effect. Larger effects on the cost side of the ratio would be seen with shifts in the rates of catheterization and revascularization because of the higher unit prices of these items.

The final variation considered in our hypothetical scenario is the potential effect of taking a long-term rather than a short-term view to the calculation of costs and benefits (Table 7D). If the survival benefits of B relative to A are assumed to be constant over time (i.e., parallel survival curves), then only differential rates of follow-up health care use will affect the cost-effectiveness ratios. Assuming an average follow-up hospitalization cost per episode of $8000 for both treatments A and B, if the 1-year follow-up hospitalization rate for A is 30% and for B is 20%, then the cumulative 1-year costs (hospital and follow-up) for A will be $787,000 and for B will be $907,000. The resulting cost-effectiveness ratio of B relative to A is $120,000/two lives saved, or $60,000 per year of life saved. Thus, even though B saved no additional lives over the first year postdischarge, patients receiving treatment B were healthier and required fewer follow-up hospitalizations, thereby recouping some of the added costs of B relative to A. In long-term followup, therefore, a new, more expensive treatment can improve its cost-effectiveness ratio by either saving additional lives or having lower follow-up medical care costs (or both).

Caveats

The foregoing examples are extremely crude. They are meant only to provide a feel for how new adjunctive therapies for acute MI might fare in cost-effectiveness comparisons and not a guide for how to perform cost-effectiveness calculations. For therapies that have a large effect on survival (e.g., equal to or exceeding the benefits of thrombolysis relative to conventional care), an increment in hospital costs of the magnitude associated with t-PA or APSAC should still result in cost-effectiveness ratios $\leq$ $75,000 per year of life saved. New and improved reperfusion regimens, however, will have to be compared with current reperfusion regimens (which result in an average 5% hospital mortality rate) rather than with "conservative therapy" (10–12% average hospital mortality rates). Thus, it will be much harder for these improvements to have a large effect on survival, which is a more important determinant of the cost-effectiveness ratio than a several-thousand-dollar increase in the overall hospital costs.

Every clinician is aware that therapies can affect both the quantity of life remaining (i.e., survival or life expectancy) and the quality of life. Some cost-effectiveness analyses attempt to consider both these aspects by calculating so-called quality-adjusted life-years (QALYs) (Table 2). For example, if a year in full health is given a value of 1 QALY, a year with chronic stable angina would have some smaller value (e.g., 0.8 QALY). Such measures are appealing because they reduce the difficult problem of assessing and valuing different quality of life states to a single easily manipulated figure. There is, however, no consensus about how best to measure QALYs or how reliable or valid they are as indicators of patient or societal preference for different health states. In addition, use of QALYs raises serious ethical questions which may not be evident to the casual reader of cost-effectiveness research (44–46). Valuing health outcomes in dollars for cost-benefit analysis (Table 2) is, of course, even more problematic and has been generally avoided in the medical economics literature.

The fact that cost-effectiveness analysis provides a way to compare different clinical strategies for a given group of patients (e.g., thrombolysis versus direct angioplasty for acute MI patients) as well as diverse treatment programs for different groups of patients (e.g., thrombolysis for CAD patients versus dialysis for renal failure patients) is both its major advantage and its biggest potential liability. Cost-effectiveness studies often measure both cost and health outcomes in a variety of different ways and over varying follow-up periods (17). Yet the apparent similarity of the final measures created in these studies, dollars per additional year of life saved, tends to mask these differences in methodology and may lead clinicians and policy makers to assume incorrectly that the results of different cost-effectiveness studies can be compared directly (47). Such comparisons are no more valid than are comparisons of treatment mortality rates using raw survival figures and historical controls. The potential for bias and error in a cost-effectiveness analysis is, of course, just as great as in any other form of nonrandomized treatment comparison. Clinicians and clinical researchers must take the responsibility for ensuring that cost and cost-effectiveness studies are subjected to the same careful scrutiny and high standards expected of other types of clinical research.

CONCLUDING REMARKS

The economic analysis of medical care at a level relevant to the individual patient and practicing physician is a field still in its infancy. As government regulators, third-party payors, and hospitals exert increasing pressure for "cost containment," physicians are going to be increasingly called upon to exercise restraint in the use of new diagnostic and therapeutic technologies. The emphasis among many research and professional groups to develop practice guidelines may ultimately provide the blueprints, as some have feared, for practice restrictions and regimentation of care. We believe that it is now as important for clinicians to understand the economics of medical care and the benefits and limitations of cost-effectiveness analysis as it is for them to understand the pathophysiology of disease. Although it is still possible to practice medicine adequately without understanding either, both will be required for clinicians who wish to meet the challenges that lie ahead.

ACKNOWLEDGMENTS

This work was supported in part by Research Grants HS 05635 and HS 06503 from the Agency for Health Care Policy and Research, Rockville, MD; Research Grant HL 36587 from the National Heart Lung and Blood Institute, Bethesda, MD; and a grant from the Robert Wood Johnson Foundation, Princeton, NJ.

We are grateful to Dr. Ed Charles, Dr. David Naylor, and Dr. Bengt Jonsson for providing us with access to unpublished data and manuscripts. We are also grateful to Dr. Joe Lipscomb, Dr. Robert Califf, Dr. Chris Granger, Dr. David Frid, and Dr. Don Fortin for critical review of the chapter and to Ms. Alex Lubans for technical support.

REFERENCES

1. AP Wire Service. U.S. reports rise, to $604 billion, in health care spending in 1989. New York Times 1990; Dec 22:12.
2. Wennberg JE. Outcomes research, cost containment, and the fear of health care rationing. N Engl J Med 1990; 323:1202–4.
3. Wennberg JE, Freeman JL, Culp WJ. Are hospital services rationed in New Haven or over-utilised in Boston?. Lancet 1987; 1:1185–9.
4. Fuchs VR, Hahn JS. How does Canada do it? A comparison of expenditures for physicians' services in the United States and Canada. N Engl J Med 1990; 323:884–90.
5. Burda D. Cardiology leads hospital profitmaker list. Mod Healthcare 1988; September:4.
6. Harlan WR, Parsons, PE, Thomas JW, Murt HA, Lepkowski JM, Guire KE, Berki SE, Landis JR. Health care utilization and costs of adult cardiovascular conditions. Natl Med Care Util Expend Survey 1989; 7(Series C):1–69.
7. Rice DP, Hodgson TA, Kopstein AN. The economic cost of illness: A replication and update. Health Care Financ Rev 1985; 7:61–80.
8. Weinstein MC, Coxson PG, Williams LW, Pass TM, Stason WB, Goldman L. Forecasting coronary heart disease incidence, mortality, and cost: the coronary heart disease policy model. Am J Public Health 1987; 77: 1417–26.
9. Eisenberg JM. Allocating economics. A guide to the economic analysis of clinical practices. JAMA 1989; 262:2879–86.
10. Drummond MF. Clinical resources. Int J Tech Assess Health Care 1990; 6:77–92.
11. Robinson JC, Luft HS. Competition and the cost of hospital care, 1972 to 1982. JAMA 1987; 257:3241–5.
12. Newhouse JP, Manning WG, Morris CN, Orr LL, Duan N, Keeler EB, Leibowitz A, Marquis KH, Marquis MS, Phelps CE, Brook RH. Some interim results from a controlled trial cost sharing in health insurance. N Engl J Med 1981; 305:1501–7.
13. Finkler SA. The distinction between costs and charges. Ann Intern Med 1982; 96:102–9.
14. Conn RB, Aller RD, Lundberg GD. Identifying costs of medical care. An essential step in allocating resources. JAMA 1985; 253:1586–9.

15. Eisenberg JM. New drugs and clinical economics: analysis of cost effectiveness in the assessment of pharmaceutical innovations. Rev Infect Dis 1984; 6:S905–S908.
16. Luce BR, Elixhauser A. Estimating costs in the economic evaluation of medical technologies. Int J Tech Assess Health Care 1990; 6:57–75.
17. Detsky AS, Naglie IG. A clinician's guide to cost-effectiveness analysis. Ann Intern Med 1990; 113:147–54.
18. Newhouse JP, Cretin S, Witsberger CJ. Predicting hospital accounting costs. Health Care Financ Rev 1989; 11:25–33.
19. Hlatky MA, Lipscomb J, Nelson C, Califf RM, Pryor DB, Wallace AG, Mark DB. Resource use and cost of initial coronary revascularization. Coronary angioplasty versus coronary bypass surgery. Circulation 1990; 82(Suppl IV):IV-208–IV-213.
20. Doubilet P, Weinstein MC, McNeil BJ. Use and misuse of the term "cost effective" in medicine. N Engl J Med 1986; 314:253–6.
21. Ginzberg E. High-tech medicine and rising health care costs. JAMA 1990; 263:1820–2.
22. Eddy DM. Connecting value and costs. Whom do we ask, and what do we ask them?. JAMA 1990; 264:1737–9.
23. Laffel GL, Fineberg HV, Braunwald E. A cost-effectiveness model for coronary thrombolysis/reperfusion therapy. J Am Coll Cardiol 1987; 10: 79B–90B.
24. Steinberg EP, Topol EJ, Sakin JW, Kahane SN, Appel LJ, Powe NR, Anderson GF, Erickson JE, Guerci AD. Cost and procedure implications of thrombolytic therapy for acute myocardial infarction. J Am Coll Cardiol 1988; 12:58A–68A.
25. Liu P, Floras J, Haq A, Detsky A. Cost-effectiveness evaluation of thrombolytic therapy: comparison of current modalities and identification of critical cost factors—a Canadian perspective. J Am Coll Cardiol 1988; 11:186A (abstract).
26. Goel V, Naylor CD. Intravenous thrombolysis for acute myocardial infarction: importance of long-term results in cost-effectiveness analysis. Can J Cardiol 1991 (submitted).
27. International Study Group. In-hospital mortality and clinical course of 20,891 patients with suspected acute myocardial infarction randomised between alteplase and streptokinase with or without heparin. Lancet 1990; 336:71–5.
28. Gruppo Italiano per Lo Studio Della Sopravvivenza, Nell'Infarto Miocardico. GISSI-2: A factorial randomised trial of alteplase versus streptokinase and heparin versus no heparin among 12,490 patients with acute myocardial infarction. Lancet 1990; 336:65–71.

29. Naylor CD, Jaglal SB. Impact of intravenous thrombolysis on short-term coronary revascularization rates. A meta-analysis. JAMA 1990; 264: 697–702.

30. Dalen JE, Gore JM, Braunwald E, Borer J, Goldberg RJ, Passamani ER, Forman S, Knatterud G, TIMI Investigators. Six- and twelve-month follow-up of the Phase 1 Thrombolysis in Myocardial Infarction (TIMI) trial. Am J Cardiol 1988; 62:179–85.

31. Vermeer F, Simoons ML, de Zwaan C, van Es GA, Verheught FWA,van der Laarse A, van Hoogenhuyze DCA, Azar AJ, van Dalen FJ, Lubsen J, Hugenholtz PG. Cost benefit analysis of early thrombolytic treatment with intracoronary streptokinase: twelve month follow-up report of the randomised multicentre trial conducted by the Interuniversity Cardiology Institute of the Netherlands. Br Heart J 1988; 59:527–34.

32. Levin LA, Jönsson B. Cost-effectiveness of thrombolysis—a randomized study of intravenous rt-PA in suspected myocardial infarction. Eur Heart J 1992; 13:2–8.

33. Herve C, Castiel D, Gaillard M, Boisvert R, Leroux V. Cost-benefit analysis of thrombolytic therapy. Eur Heart J 1990; 11:1006–10.

34. Califf RM, Topol EJ, Stack RS, Ellis SG, George BS, Kereiakes DJ, Samaha JK, Worley SJ, Anderson JL, Woodlief LH, Wall TC, Phillips HR, Abbottsmith CW, Candela RJ, Flanagan WH, Sasahara A, Mantell SJ, Lee KL. Evaluation of combination thrombolytic therapy and timing of cardiac catheterization in acute myocardial infarction. Results of thrombolysis and angioplasty in myocardial infarction—phase 5 randomized trial. Circulation 1991; 83:1543–6.

35. Mark DB, Lam LC, Hlathy MA, Melton JR, Davidson-Ray L, Woodlief LH, Lipscomb J, Sasahara A, Califf RM. Effects of three thromboblytic regimens and two interventional strategies on acute MI costs: results from a prospective randomized trial. Circulation 1991; 84(Suppl IV):II-221 (abstract).

36. Machecourt J, Dumoulin J, Calop J, Foroni L, Terisse MP. Comparison of the cost and the efficacy of 2 thrombolytic agents (rTPA and APSAC) used at the acute stage of a myocardial infarction: results of a multicenter randomized trial. Eur Heart J 1990; 11:195 (abstract).

37. DeWood MA. Direct PTCA vs intravenous t-PA in acute myocardial infarction: results from a prospective randomized trial. Presented at 6th International Workshop on Thrombolysis and Interventional Therapy in Acute Myocardial Infarction, Dallas, TX 1990.

37a. Mark DB, Brodie B, Ivanhoe R, Knopf W, Taylor G, O'Keefe J, Davidson-Ray L, Knight D, O'Neill W. Effects of direct angioplasty on hospital costs in acute myocardial infarction: results from the multicenter PAR study. Circulation 1991(Suppl IV):II-257 (abstract).

38. Charles ED, Rogers WJ, Reeder GS, Chesebro JH, Papapietro SE, Maske L, Bartolucci AA. Economic advantages of a conservative strategy for AMI management: rt-PA without obligatory PTCA. J Am Coll Cardiol 1989; 13:152A (abstract).

39. Rogers WJ, Baim DS, Gore JM, Brown BG, Roberts R, Williams DO, Chesebro JH, Babb JD, Sheehan FL, Wackers FJTh, Zaret BL, Robertson TL, Passamani ER, Ross R, Knatterud GL, Braunwald E. Comparison of immediate invasive, delayed invasive, and conservative strategies after tissue-type plasminogen activator. Results of the Thrombolysis in Myocardial Infarction (TIMI) Phase II-A trial. Circulation 1990; 81:1457-76.

40. TIMI Study Group. Comparison of invasive and conservative strategies after treatment with intravenous tissue plasminogen activator in acute myocardial infarction. Results of the Thrombolysis in Myocardial Infarction (TIMI) Phase II Trial. N Engl J Med 1989; 320:618-27.

41. Chapekis AT, Burek K, Topol EJ. The cost:benefit ratio of acute intervention for myocardial infarction: results of a prospective, matched pair analysis. Am Heart J 1989; 118:878-92.

42. Yusuf S, Wittes J, Friedman L. Overview of results of randomized clinical trials in heart disease. I. Treatments following myocardial infarction. JAMA 1988; 260:2088-93.

43. Goldman L, Sia STB, Cook EF, Rutherfors JD, Weinstein MC. Costs and effectiveness of routine therapy with long-term beta-adrenergic antagonists after acute myocardial infarction. N Engl J Med 1988; 319:152-7.

44. Loomes G, McKenzie L. The use of QALYs in health care decision making. Soc Sci Med 1989; 28:299-308.

45. La Puma J, Lawlor EF. Quality-adjusted life-years. Ethical implications for physicians and policymakers. JAMA 1990; 263:2917-21.

46. Gafni A. The quality of QALYs (quality-adjusted-life-years): do QALYs measure what they at least intend to measure?. Health Policy 1989; 13:81-3.

47. Russell LB. Some of the tough decisions required by a national health plan. Science 1989; 246:892-6.

48. Laupacis A, LaBelle R, Goeree R, Cairns J. The cost-effectiveness of routine post myocardial infarction exercise stress testing. Can J Cardiol 1990; 6:157-63.

49. Goel V, Deber RB, Detsky AS. Nonionic contrast media: economic analysis and health policy development. Can Med Assoc J 1989; 140:389-95.

50. Welch HG, Larson EB. Cost effectiveness of bone marrow transplantation in acute nonlymphocytic leukemia. N Engl J Med 1989; 321:807-12.

51. Weinstein MC. Economics of prevention. The costs of prevention. J Gen Intern. Med 1990; 5(Suppl):S89–S92.
52. Oster G, Epstein AM. Cost-effectiveness of antihyperlipemic therapy in the prevention of coronary heart disease. JAMA 1987; 258:2381–7.
53. Toronto Working Group. Efficiency considerations: the cost-effectiveness of treating asymptomatic hypercholesterolemia. J Clin Epidemiol 1990; 43: 1093–1101.
54. Wong JB, Sonnenberg FA, Salem DN, Pauker SG. Myocardial revascularization for chronic angina. Analysis of the role of percutaneous transluminal coronary angioplasty based on data available in 1989. Ann Intern Med 1990; 113:852–71.

22

Treatment Recommendations for Acute Myocardial Infarction

Eric R. Bates
University of Michigan Medical Center, Ann Arbor, Michigan

THROMBOLYTIC THERAPY

Thrombolytic therapy has recently been shown to significantly reduce morbidity and mortality in patients with acute myocardial infarction (1). Unfortunately, carefully performed studies have established that approximately 2 hours elapse from the time a patient decides to seek medical assistance to the initiation of thrombolytic therapy (2,3). These delays persist despite public education measures directed toward encouraging early evaluation of chest pain syndromes and trials showing survival rates with thrombolytic therapy inversely proportional to symptom duration. Several studies are currently exploring the feasibility and cost-effectiveness of prehospital treatment with thrombolytic therapy administered by ambulance personnel to decrease this delay.

From the emergency room perspective, time to treatment could be reduced if patients presenting with chest pain could immediately have an electrocardiogram performed and interpreted. Patients with ST-segment elevation or left bundle branch block could undergo a quick 5- to 10-min evaluation with the goal of initiating thrombolytic therapy (Table 1) within 15 min of presentation in appropriate candidates (Table 2). Patients with nondiagnostic electrocardiograms could go through the regular evaluation process. Critically important to such a strategy would be to have both the electrocardiography machine and the thrombolytic agents available in the emergency room. Additionally, responsibility for interpret-

Table 1   Thrombolytic Therapy for Acute Myocardial Infarction

Agent	Dose
Alteplase (rt-PA)	6-mg bolus, 54 mg over 1 hr, 40 mg over 2 hr or 15-mg bolus, 50 mg over 30 min, 35 mg over 1 hr
Anistreplace (APSAC)	30 units over 5 min
Streptokinase	1.5 million units over 1 hr

APSAC = anisoylated plasminogen streptokinase activator complex; rt-PA = recombinant tissue plasminogen activator.

Table 2   Indications and Contraindications for Thrombolytic Therapy

Indications
1. Ischemic chest pain < 12 hr
2. ST-segment elevation in two contiguous leads or left bundle branch block
3. Low bleeding risk

Absolute contraindications
1. Active internal bleeding
2. Trauma or surgery less than 2 weeks previously
3. Suspected aortic dissection
4. Prolonged or traumatic cardiopulmonary resuscitation
5. Recent head trauma or known intracranial neoplasm
6. Diabetic hemorrhagic retinopathy or other hemorrhagic ophthalmic condition
7. Pregnancy
8. Previous allergic reaction to the thrombolytic agent (streptokinase or APSAC)
9. Recorded blood pressure higher than 200/120 mmHg
10. History of cerebrovascular accident known to be hemorrhagic

Relative contraindications
1. Recent trauma or surgery more than 2 weeks previously
2. History of chronic severe hypertension with or without drug therapy
3. Active peptic ulcer disease
4. History of cerebrovascular accident
5. Known bleeding diathesis or current use of anticoagulants
6. Severe liver dysfunction
7. Prior exposure to streptokinase or APSAC (especially in the initial 6- to 9-month period after streptokinase or APSAC administration)

ing emergency electrocardiograms would need to be clearly assigned and emergency room physicians would have to have the authority to initiate thrombolytic therapy without consulting a cardiologist.

Supplemental oxygen should be provided. Modest hypoxemia can be present even in patients with uncomplicated myocardial infarction, partly secondary to ventilation-perfusion mismatch. If sublingual nitroglycerin does not relieve ischemic chest pain, then intravenous doses of morphine sulfate, 2–5 mg every 5–30 min, can be given (4).

ADJUNCTIVE PHARMACOLOGICAL THERAPY

The critical role aspirin plays as an antiplatelet agent in the treatment of acute myocardial infarction has been obscured somewhat by the enthusiasm surrounding thrombolytic therapy. In fact, equal efficacy was demonstrated for both treatments in the ISIS-2 trial (5). Furthermore, meta-analyses of aspirin therapy (6) and thrombolytic therapy (1) confirm an equal benefit of the same magnitude with each intervention. Importantly, the benefit appears to be additive (5). Additionally, aspirin was associated with a 46% reduction in nonfatal reinfarction and a 40% reduction in nonfatal stroke in the ISIS-2 trial. Whereas thrombolytic therapy is associated with expense and bleeding risk, aspirin has no cost associated with it and is basically free of side effects if given as a buffered tablet. A dose of at least 160 mg should be given immediately and continued indefinitely because of the proven ability of aspirin to reduce subsequent reinfarction, stroke, and mortality rates. Although it has been noted several times that thrombolytic therapy has been given to only 20% of patients with acute myocardial infarction in the United States, compared with 60% of patients in Europe, it is shocking to find that only 30% of patients in the United States are receiving aspirin (Charles Hennekens, M.D., personal communication) when almost all are candidates for therapy independent of electrocardiographic findings.

There are many reasons to use heparin as a prophylactic anticoagulant agent in all patients with acute myocardial infarction, including decreasing risk for deep venous thrombosis, left ventricular mural thrombus formation, infarct artery reocclusion, and infarct extension (4). In the prethrombolytic era, a meta-analysis of 20 published studies found a 17% mortality reduction with heparin (7). There was also a 66% reduction in deep venous thrombosis, a 54% reduction in pulmonary embolism, a 22% reduction in reinfarction, and a 50% reduction in stroke. Survival benefit has also been shown in patients treated with heparin in the thrombolytic era, but the magnitude is less. Whereas aspirin and thrombolytic therapy each save approximately 25 lives per 1000 treated patients, delayed subcutaneous heparin saves approximately an additional five lives (8). In the United States, intravenous heparin is administered instead of subcutaneous heparin. A dose of 5000 units can be given acutely, followed by an intravenous infusion to maintain

Table 3   Adjunctive Pharmacological
Therapy for Acute Myocardial Infarction

Proven benefit
  Aspirin
  Heparin
  Beta-adrenergic blockers
Potential benefit
  Nitrates
  ACE inhibitors
  Magnesium
No Proven benefit
  Lidocaine
  Calcium channel blockers

---

the activated partial thromboplastin time from 60 to 85 sec. The potential benefit and risk of giving a monitored intravenous heparin infusion relative to subcutaneous heparin is being tested in the GUSTO trial in patients receiving streptokinase.

Beta-blockers decrease oxygen demand by lowering heart rate and blood pressure; they also have antiplatelet and antiarrhythmic effects. Intravenous beta-blocker therapy is recommended in patients with acute myocardial infarction (4), although there are no recent trials demonstrating survival benefit. In the prethrombolytic era, five lives per 1000 treated patients were saved (9), but high-risk patients were often excluded from therapy because of contraindications to beta-blocker use, such as bradycardia, hypotension, congestive heart failure, atrioventricular conduction delay, and bronchospastic lung disease. Given these exclusion criteria, half the patients with acute myocardial infarction are candidates for therapy which is given to decrease the risk of cardiac rupture, ventricular fibrillation, recurrent ischemia, and reinfarction. Therapy is particularly useful in patients with reflex tachycardia, systolic hypertension, continuous ischemic pain, or atrial fibrillation with fast ventricular response (4). Atenolol can be given in two 5-mg injections over 10 min, followed by a 50-mg tablet 10 min later. Alternatively, metoprolol can be given as three 5-mg injections over 10–15 min, and followed 10 min later with a 50-mg tablet. Oral therapy should be continued, if tolerated.

Nitrates decrease oxygen demand by reducing afterload and preload and increase blood supply by relieving coronary vascular tone and improving collateral flow. Approximately 3000 patients with acute myocardial infarction have been studied in small randomized trials of oral or intravenous nitrates (10). A 35% reduction in mortality found with intravenous nitrates was not statistically different from the 25% reduction with oral nitrates. Both GISSI-3 and ISIS-4 are studying the mortality results with oral nitrates given for several weeks.

Angiotension-converting enzyme inhibitors decrease oxygen demand and increase supply by decreasing systemic and coronary vascular tone. They also have a favorable effect on electrolytic balance and decrease catecholamine levels. Survival benefit has been shown in randomized trials in patients with congestive heart failure (11,12). GISSI-3, ISIS-4, and several other trials are now studying mortality results in patients with acute myocardial infarction.

Preliminary studies have suggested that magnesium infusions limit infarct size, decrease coronary and systemic vascular tone, and decrease ventricular arrhythmias. Small studies involving approximately 1300 patients have shown a reduction in mortality from 8% to 4% (13). ISIS-4 is studying the mortality results associated with a 24-hr magnesium infusion.

Prophylactic lidocaine has commonly been used to reduce the risk of ventricular fibrillation. A meta-analysis of 14 randomized trials with over 9000 patients found a 35% reduction in the odds of developing ventricular fibrillation (14). However, there was an increase in mortality, perhaps because of an increase in fatal asystole. Therefore, routine use of prophylactic therapy is not encouraged. Therapeutic use in patients with ventricular premature beats that are frequent (>6/min), closely coupled (R on T), multiform, or occurring in bursts of three or more is recommended (4).

Although calcium channel blockers reduce oxygen demand, increase blood supply, and prevent calcium overload of ischemic cells, routine use of these agents has not been shown to reduce morbidity or mortality in studies totaling over 18,000 patients (15). Probable explanations include the reflex tachycardia and diversion of blood flow from ischemic zones associated with nifedipine and the depression of myocardial contractility and sinoatrial and atrioventricular conduction associated with diltiazem and verapamil (1). Calcium channel blockers can be useful in the symptomatic treatment of postinfarction angina (4).

CARDIAC CATHETERIZATION, PTCA, AND OTHER TREATMENT OPTIONS

The routine use of diagnostic cardiac catheterization and percutaneous transluminal coronary angioplasty (PTCA) in patients with acute myocardial infarction has not been shown to be a valid clinical strategy (16-20). This topic has been reviewed by both Topol (21) and Ryan (22). However, these procedures are clinically important in selected patients, and guidelines exist to direct their appropriate use (4,23,24). A summary of these indications is presented in Tables 4 and 5. Guidelines have also been published for the use of intracardiac electrophysiological studies (25) and coronary bypass graft surgery (26).

Table 4   Indications for Cardiac Catheterization in Patients with Acute
Myocardial Infarction

1. Candidates for acute reperfusion utilizing PTCA or CABG who are not candidates for thrombolytic therapy
2. Severe pump failure or cardiogenic shock
3. Acute ventricular septal defect or acute mitral regurgitation causing heart failure or shock
4. Recurrent or persistent episodes of ischemic chest pain
5. Recurrent ventricular tachycardia or ventricular fibrillation despite antiarrhythmic therapy
6. Exercise-induced ischemia
7. Patients with unusually active and vigorous physical activities
8. Left ventricular ejection fraction < 40%

Table 5   Indications for PTCA in Patients with Acute Myocardial Infarction

Candidates for thrombolysis in whom thrombolytic therapy is contraindicated
Cardiogenic shock
Recurrent ventricular tachycardia or ventricular fibrillation related to ischemia
Recurrent postinfarction angina
Exercise-induced ischemia

Table 6   Pharmacological Therapy After
Hospital Discharge for Acute
Myocardial Infarction

Proven benefit
Aspirin
Beta-adrenergic blockers
ACE inhibitors
Lipid-lowering drugs
Potential benefit
Warfarin
No proven benefit
Class I antiarrhythmic agents
Dihydropyridine calcium channel blockers

A number of complications are associated with acute myocardial infarction. A thorough discussion of these is beyond the scope of this book, but treatment approaches are well summarized in two recent books (27,28). The important topic of risk stratification after myocardial infarction is also covered well in those books (27,28), and guidelines have been published for diagnostic testing (6,27–31).

Patients discharged from the hospital after acute myocardial infarction (Table 6) should be continued on aspirin (160–325 mg/day) for at least 2 years because of data showing a reduction in mortality and reinfarction rates of 15 and 31%, respectively (6). Likewise, beta-blockers decrease subsequent mortality by 21% and should be continued in all but low-risk patients who do not have a clear contraindication to use (9). Finally, angiotension-converting enzyme inhibitors decrease hospitalization and mortality rates in patients with systolic left ventricular dysfunction and heart failure (11,12).

The risk of recurrent cardiovascular events can be reduced by risk factor modification. Warfarin has been used effectively after myocardial infarction, but bleeding risk is higher than with aspirin and comparative trials showing superiority to aspirin have not been performed. The routine use of class I antiarrhythmic agents (32) and calcium channel blockers that raise heart rate (15) have been associated with increased mortality.

The preceding chapters have summarized the treatment options available for patients with acute myocardial infarction and suggested future possibilities. Although great progress has recently been made in reducing the morbidity and mortality associated with acute myocardial infarction, much work remains to be done. Patient triage, improved thrombolytic agents, noninvasive detection of infarct artery patency, reperfusion injury, prevention of reocclusion with better antiplatelet and antithrombin agents, and the role of invasive procedures are but a few of the important challenges currently being addressed by investigators.

REFERENCES

1. Yusuf S, Sleight P, Held P, MacMahon S. Routine medical management of acute myocardial infarction. Lessons from overviews of recent randomized controlled trials. Circulation 1990; 82(suppl II):II-117–II-134.

2. Weaver WD, Eisenberg MS, Martin JS, et al. Myocardial Infarction Triage and Intervention project—Phase I: Patient characteristics and feasibility of pre-hospital initiation of thrombolytic therapy. J Am Coll Cardiol 1990; 15:925–31.

3. Kereiakes DJ, Weaver WD, Anderson JL, et al. Time delays in the diagnosis and treatment of acute myocardial infarction: a tale of eight cities. Report of the Pre-hospital Study Group and the Cincinnati Heart Project. Am Heart J 1990; 120:773–80.

4. ACC/AHA Task Force Report. Guidelines for the early management of patients with acute myocardial infarction. J Am Coll Cardiol 1990; 16:249–92.

5. ISIS (Second International Study of Infarct Survival) Collaborative Group. Random-
    ized trial of intravenous streptokinase, oral aspirin, both or neither among 17,187
    cases of suspected acute myocardial infarction: ISIS-2. Lancet 1988; 2:349-60.
6. Hennekens CH, Buring JE, Sandercock P, Collins R, Peto R. Aspirin and other anti-
    platelet agents in the secondary and primary prevention of cardiovascular disease.
    Circulation 1989; 80:749-56.
7. MacMahon S, Collins R, Knight C, Yusuf S, Peto R. Reduction in major morbidity
    and mortality by heparin in acute myocardial infarction. Circulation 1988; 78(suppl
    II):II-98 (abstract).
8. Sleight P. ISIS-3 Trial: results of SK versus APSAC versus t-PA. Presented at the
    American College of Cardiology 40th Annual Scientific Session, Atlanta, GA, March
    5, 1991.
9. Yusuf S, Peto R, Lewis J, Collins R, Sleight P. Beta blockade during and after myocar-
    dial infarction: an overview of the randomized trials. Prog Cardiovasc Dis 1985;
    27:335-71.
10. Yusuf S, MacMahon S, Collins R, Peto R. Effect of intravenous nitrates on mortality
    in acute myocardial infarction: an overview of the randomized trials. Lancet 1988;
    1:1088-92.
11. The CONSENSUS Trial Study Group. Effects of enalapril on mortality in severe con-
    gestive heart failure. N Engl J Med 1987; 316:1429-35.
12. The SOLVD Investigators. Effect of enalapril on survival in patients with reduced left
    ventricular ejection fractions and congestive heart failure. N Engl J Med 1991; 325:
    293-302.
13. Teo K, Held P, Collins R, Yusuf S. Effect of intravenous magnesium on mortality in
    myocardial infarction. Circulation 1990; 82:III-393.
14. MacMahon S, Collins R, Peto R, Koster RW, Yusuf S. Effects of prophylactic
    lidocaine in suspected acute myocardial infarction: an overview of results from the
    randomized controlled trials. JAMA 1988; 260:1910-6.
15. Held P, Yusuf S, Furberg C. Effects of calcium antagonists on initial infarction,
    reinfarction and mortality in acute myocardial infarction and unstable angina. Br Med
    J 1989; 299:1187-92.
16. Topol EJ, Califf RM, George BS, et al. A randomized trial of immediate versus de-
    layed elective angioplasty after intravenous tissue plasminogen activator in acute
    myocardial infarction. N Engl J Med 1987; 317:581-8.
17. The TIMI Research Group. Immediate vs. delayed catheterization and angioplasty
    following thrombolytic therapy for acute myocardial infarction. TIMI IIA results.
    JAMA 1988; 260:2849-58.
18. Simoons ML, Betriu A, Col J, et al. Thrombolysis with tissue plasminogen activator
    in acute myocardial infarction: no additional benefit from immediate percutaneous
    coronary angioplasty. Lancet 1988; 2:197-202.
19. The TIMI Study Group. Comparison of invasive and conservative strategies after
    treatment with intravenous tissue plasminogen activator in acute myocardial infarct-
    ion. Results of the thrombolysis in myocardial infarction (TIMI) phase II trial. N Engl
    J Med 1989; 320:618-27.

20. SWIFT Trial Study Group. SWIFT trial of delayed elective intervention v conservative treatment after thrombolysis with anistreplase in acute myocardial infarction. Br Med J 1991; 302:555-60.

21. Topol EJ. Coronary angioplasty for acute myocardial infarction. Ann Intern Med 1988; 109:970-89.

22. Ryan TJ. Revascularization for acute myocardial infarction: strategies in need of revision. Circulation 1990; 82(suppl II):II-110-6.

23. ACC/AHA Task Force Report. Guidelines for coronary angioplasty. J Am Coll Cardiol 1987; 10:935-50.

24. ACC/AHA Task Force Report. Guidelines for percutaneous transluminal coronary angioplasty. J Am Coll Cardiol 1988; 12:529-45.

25. ACC/AHA Task Force Report. Guidelines for clinical intracardiac electrophysiologic studies. J Am Coll Cardiol 1989; 14:1827-42.

26. ACC/AHA Task Force Report. Guidelines and indications for coronary bypass graft surgery. J Am Coll Cardiol 1991; 17:543-89.

27. Califf RM, Mark DB, Wagner GS, eds. Acute coronary care in the thrombolytic era. Chicago: Year Book Medical Publishers, 1988.

28. Gersh BJ, Rahimtoola SH, eds. Acute myocardial infarction. New York: Elsevier, 1991.

29. ACC/AHA Task Force Report. Guidelines for ambulatory electrocardiography. J Am Coll Cardiol 1989; 13:249-58.

30. ACC/AHA Task Force Report. Guidelines for exercise testing. J Am Coll Cardiol 1986; 8:725-38.

31. ACC/AHA Task Force Report. Guidelines for clinical use of cardiac radionuclide imaging. J Am Coll Cardiol 1986; 8:1471-83.

32. The Cardiac Arrhythmia Suppression Trial (CAST) Investigators. Preliminary report: effect of encainide and flecainide on mortality in a randomized trial of arrhythmia suppression after myocardial infarction. N Engl J Med 1989; 321:406-12.

Index

About the Editor

ERIC R. BATES is Associate Professor of Internal Medicine, University of Michigan Medical School, Ann Arbor, and Staff Cardiologist, University Hospital, Ann Arbor, Michigan. A Fellow of the American College of Physicians, the American College of Cardiology, the American College of Angiology, the American College of Chest Physicians, and the Council on Clinical Cardiology and the Council on Circulation of the American Heart Association, he is the author or coauthor of over 70 book chapters and professional papers and more than 150 abstracts and presentations. Dr. Bates received the A.B. degree (1972) from Princeton University, New Jersey, and the M.D. degree (1976) from the University of Michigan Medical School, Ann Arbor. He is board certified in internal medicine and the subspecialty of cardiovascular diseases.